Archives of
TOXICOLOGY
Archiv für Toxikologie
Supplement 7

Disease, Metabolism and Reproduction in the Toxic Response to Drugs and Other Chemicals

Proceedings of the
European Society of Toxicology

Springer-Verlag Berlin Heidelberg New York Tokyo

Archives of Toxicology, Supplement 7

Disease, Metabolism and Reproduction in the Toxic Response to Drugs and Other Chemicals

Proceedings of the
European Society of Toxicology
Meeting Held in Rome, March 28 – 30, 1983

Edited by
P. L. Chambers, P. Preziosi and C. M. Chambers

With 117 Figures

Springer-Verlag
Berlin Heidelberg New York Tokyo 1984

Claire M. Chambers and Philip L. Chambers
University of Dublin, Department of Pharmacology, Trinity College, Dublin 2, Ireland

Paolo Preziosi
Department of Pharmacology, Catholic University of the Sacred Heart, Via della Pineta Sacchetti 644, 00168 Rome, Italy

ISBN 3-540-12452-7 Springer-Verlag Berlin Heidelberg New York Tokyo
ISBN 0-387-12452-7 Springer-Verlag Berlin Heidelberg New York Tokyo

Library of Congress Cataloging in Publication Data. European Society of Toxicology. Meeting (1983: Rome, Italy) Disease, metabolism and reproduction in the toxic response to drugs and other chemicals. (Archives of toxicology. Supplement 7) Includes bibliography and index. 1. Toxicology-Congresses. 2. Drugs-Toxicology-Congresses. 3. Drugs-Metabolism-Congresses. 4. Generative organs, Male-Effect of drugs on-Congresses. I. Chambers, P. L. (Philip L.), 1931. II. Preziosi, P. (Paolo) III. Chambers, C. M. (Claire M.) IV. Title. V. Series. [DNLM: 1. Drugs-adverse effects-congresses. 2. Drugs-metabolism-congresses. 3. Reproduction-drug effects-congresses. 4. Toxicology-congresses. W1 AR49GA v. 7/QV 38 E88d 1983] RA1190.E8 Suppl. vol. 7 615.9 s [615.9] 84-10638 [RA1191]

Printed in Germany.

Typesetting, printing, and bookbinding: v. Starck'sche Druckereigesellschaft m.b.H., 6200 Wiesbaden.
2127/3130-543210.

Contents

Metabolism and Toxicity

Toxicity of Non-steroidal Antirheumatic Drugs: Molecular Mechanisms and Clinical Assessment

Heavy Metal Toxicity

Indexed in Current Contents

Disease, Metabolism and Reproduction in the Toxic Response to Drugs and Other Chemicals
Arch. Toxicol., Suppl. 7, 1–15 (1984)

Plenary Lecture:

Drug-Induced Cardionecrosis

T. Godfraind

Laboratoire de Pharmacodynamie Générale et de Pharmacologie,
Université Catholique de Louvain, U.C.L. 7350,
Avenue Emmanuel Mounier, 73, 1200 Bruxelles, Belgium

Abstract. Cardiotoxicity may be defined as a drug action producing abnormalities in cardiac function, such as transitory disturbances or rhythm, conduction or contractility. Clearance of the drug is followed by recovery of the initial function. Cardionecrosis is the irreversible consequence of cardiotoxicity. Its appearance depends not only upon the toxicological potency of a given compound but may also depend upon the pathophysiological state of the heart. Therefore, two main categories may be recognized considering the influence of this state. Drugs may act on the processes controlling cellular structure such as protein biosynthesis in the case of antibiotics of the anthracycline group. Drugs may act at the level of metabolic regulation through a membranal or an intracellular action; in this case, the functional state of the heart plays a major role. This is mainly observed with sympathomimetics and with drugs interacting with the function of catecholamines. The cardiotoxicity observed in such conditions mimics the action of anoxia or of ischemia. The main determinant of the cardiac lesion is probably the disturbance of cellular calcium metabolism. This situation may be prevented (or treated) by the use of calcium entry blockers (calcium antagonists). A great part of this report will deal with the second group of drugs, because of their potential importance as a chemical hazard for the population and because of a possible preventive protection by calcium entry blockers (calcium antagonists).

Key words: Cardiotoxic drugs – Cardionecrotic drugs – Calcium antagonists – Calcium entry blockers

Most of the statistics on the cause of death in industrial countries show that cardiovascular diseases contribute a large proportion. In West Europe, 37–50% of deaths are due to those diseases and cardiac diseases participate in about 20–30% of the rest.

The aetiology of cardiac disease is complex and has been attributed to polyfactorial causes each contributing an unknown proportion.

This report will discuss the possibility that drugs could be part of these factors and that when the cardiac toxicity is due to an imbalance between O_2 supply and O_2 demand, it can be prevented by anti-ischemic drugs, most of which are related to calcium entry blockers (calcium antagonists).

Observations coming from both the clinical and the experimental side have described the change in sensitivity to cardiotoxic drugs of heart in ischemic or postischemic state. Although the exact role of drug toxicity in inducing or worsening cardiac disease is not quantitatively evaluated, the large utilisation of drugs with cardiotoxic potentialities justifies the analysis of their effects. This paper deals exclusively with drugs. However, similar problems of cardiotoxicity arise from contaminants within the environment, as reviewed by Rosenman (1979).

Evidence for the cardiotoxic action of a drug is more often obtained from observed disturbances in rhythm or conduction. It is more difficult to obtain information on contractility defects and even more on irreversible alterations of myocytes. Drugs and other exogenous compounds may affect the heart in various ways. A chronic biochemical disturbance may alter the lipid composition of the membrane (Stein et al. 1981). An exaggerated pharmacological action may cause directly or indirectly an anoxic or ischemic alteration of some of the cardiac structures. Although the mechanism of cardiotoxicity is still unclear for some agents, disturbance in calcium metabolism appears to be a major common event in drug toxicity. Therefore, the physiological calcium regulation will be examined, the disturbance of this metabolism, the pathological consequences for the heart and finally the cardioprotective drugs.

Cellular Calcium Metabolism in the Cardiovascular System

The regulation of calcium metabolism shows several similar features in different types of cells, with specific characteristics for a given type, mainly due to a better differentiation of one process of regulation.

In order to make this point clearer and because the reaction of the coronary arteries may be involved at least indirectly in cardionecrosis. The common mechanisms for heart and smooth muscle will be described and their differences will be shown.

In a resting muscle, the cytoplasmic free calcium concentration is not more than 10^{-7} M, so that the ratio of extracellular to intracellular Ca^{2+} exceeds 10^4. The calcium electrochemical gradient is oriented inward. This means that calcium tends to enter the cell. The low calcium concentration is due to a low permeability for calcium of the polarized membrane and to several buffering processes. The presence of intracellular structures able to bind, accumulate, and most probably release Ca^{2+} has long since been recognized in most cells. The cytoplasm itself, or some intracytoplasmic structures, possibly not organelles, might have calcium binding properties. This is mainly the case for cytoplasmic proteins such as parvalbumins. In most tissues, mitochondria are able to take up considerable amounts of Ca^{2+} and may serve as a Ca^{2+} sink. Calcium binding is in part energy independent. Half of the energy independent binding capacity is located in the outer membrane and is thus not considered as a transport mechanism. The energy-dependent uptake is coupled stoechiometrically either to substrate oxidation or to ATP hydrolysis: 1.7–2 Ca^{2+} are accumulated per pair of electrons flowing to each coupling site of the respiratory chain (see Ferrari et al. 1982). Mitochondria are also capable of releasing Ca^{2+} rapidly, but the efflux is very low when the energized state is maintained. These properties might allow mitochondria to play a role in the regulation of cellular metabolism and activity of calcium. The question that is not solved is whether they play in fast regulation or only act as long-term buffers (Godfraind-De Becker and Godfraind 1980). Sarcoplasmic reticulum (SR) of muscles is another intracellular structure able to accumulate and to release Ca^{2+}. An acidic protein that can bind up to 40 moles of Ca^{2+} per mole of protein, calsequestrin, has also been isolated from SR membranes. In cardiac muscle, it has been demonstrated by Katz and associates (1977) that Ca^{2+} transport in SR is a cAMP-dependent process. cAMP-dependent protein kinase mediates phosporylation of a specific site of SR: a 22,000-dalton protein, termed phospholamban, which when phosphorylated appears to enhance the Ca^{2+}-ATPase activity and Ca^{2+}-uptake by isolated cardiac SR. The constancy of the intracellular Ca^{2+} over long periods of time requires that Ca^{2+} efflux exactly balances Ca^{2+} influx. This may only be achieved by a Ca pump located in the plasma membrane. At least two types of mechanisms are feasible: a Ca pump that actively extrudes Ca^{2+} at the expense of ATP hydrolysis and a Ca exchange with Na moving down its electrochemical gradient (Na-Ca exchange). The former mechanism has been reported to be activated by calmodulin, the ubiquitous Ca binding protein, and a common feature of most types of cells. Na-Ca exchange probably occurs through a membrane carrier process. It is not sensitive to calmodulin and is of variable importance among different cells. In plasma membrane vesicles prepared from heart and from arteries, the relative efficacy of the Na-Ca exchange mechanism and of the Ca-ATP pump to transport calcium have been compared. It was observed that the Na-Ca exchange process is the most efficient in the heart, whereas Ca-ATP pump is of primary importance in smooth muscle (Morel and Godfraind 1982). Because of its stoechiometry (3 Na for 1 Ca), it is likely that this transport is electrogenic and that it also allows Ca entry when the cell is depolarized.

Excitation-contraction coupling is associated with important calcium fluxes from pools located inside or outside the cell.

As far as the cardiac cell is concerned, the present understanding of this process can be summarized as follows. During the course of a cardiac action potential, depolarization of the sarcolemma and T systems initiates calcium fluxes which are dependent upon an extracellular calcium source and which result in an increased concentration of ionized calcium within the cardiac cell. An increased permeability of the sarcolemma to calcium during the action potential plateau enables Ca^{2+} to move down its concentration gradient from outside to inside the cell via an electrogenic calcium mediated current. In addition to the ionized calcium of the extracellular phase, it is thought by some that superficially bound calcium of the sarcolemma is mobilized during depolarization and participates in the calcium influx associated with contraction.

The amount of calcium entering the cell during the plateau phase of the action potential is by itself not sufficient to produce a full contraction. To account for activation of myofilaments during the action potential, some amplification mechanism has been proposed. It is named Ca-Ca induced release, a terminology describing the mechanism by which the influx of calcium may mediate the release of intracellular stores of bound calcium from the sarcoplasmic reticulum and possibly, under certain circumstances, from the mitochondria. Heart relaxation occurs at the end of the activation process, primarily an enzymatic uptake mechanism of the sarcoplasmic reticulum that is activated by cyclic AMP. If the sarcoplasmic reticulum was the only mechanism responsible for relaxation, Ca entry during activation should produce an accumulation of cellular calcium. In the long term, mechanisms of Ca extrusion should compensate between Ca entry and Ca efflux. Calcium efflux from the cell occurs against a large concentration gradient which requires an active process and is also caused by the Na-Ca exchange mechanism already described (for ref. see Adams and Schwartz 1980).

As far as catecholamines are concerned, recent studies have demonstrated that at the postjunctional membrane α_1 and α_2 receptors are present. Contractions produced by α_1 receptor stimulation are dependent on the release of intracellular calcium whereas contractions produced by α_2 receptor stimulation depend on extracellular calcium, as are the contractions evoked by several other agonists such as histamine and by membrane depolarization with KCl solutions.

It is thought that stimuli, which evoke a contraction dependent on extracellular calcium, open membrane Ca channels thereby allowing Ca entry into the cell. An hypothesis based on several criteria, allows one to speculate on receptor operating channels (ROC) and potential operating channels (POC) in smooth muscle membrane (Godfraind 1982).

Drugs and Disturbances of Cardiac Metabolism and Structure

Cardiac cellular injury is characterized by alterations in electrical properties, alterations in contractility and cell death. The first two are easy to demonstrate and may be reversible. They are part of the symptoms of cardiotoxicity. The last is more difficult to demonstrate when it does not involve a large portion of the heart muscle; it is the irreversible consequence of the action of cardionecrotic drugs. There are three main mechanisms of cardionecrosis: ischemia (reduction of blood supply), anoxia (reduction of oxygen supply), direct toxic action on the heart. The rate at which cardionecrosis occurs and its extent are influenced by a number of factors including the dosage of the drug directly responsible for the severity of ischemia or hypoxia, age, sex, hormonal, nutritional and metabolic status of the tissue and the coexistence of other disease processes. A striking and important characteristic of ischemia and to a lesser extent of hypoxia, is its macroscopic and microscopic heterogeneity (Jennings 1969). Varying conditions of work load and tissue perfusion may create a transient or patchy ischemia. In the latter instance islands of severely ischemic tissue may be interspersed with, or lie adjacent to, areas of normal tissue. This is well illustrated by the multifocal distribution of the cardionecrotic areas resulting from the injection of large doses of catecholamines in rats (Godfraind and Sturbois 1979).

Immediately following the onset of ischemia, within a few seconds, there is a decline in contractile activity. This decline occurs at a time when excitability remains essentially normal (Kardesch et al. 1958). During these first few seconds in anoxic tissue or in severely ischemic tissue, the available oxygen dissolved in the cytoplasm will be utilized and anaerobic conditions will develop within the cell (Williamson et al. 1976). Associated with this will be a major reduction or even a complete abolition of oxidative metabolism, electron transport and mitochondrial ATP production and only the much less efficient anaerobic pathways of metabolism remain for the production of ATP.

Reduced mitochondrial metabolism will result in a rapid reduction in the flux through the beta oxidation pathway for fatty acids. Despite the reduction in utilization of fatty acids, uptake may not be diminished and as a result of these two factors, fatty acid acylCoA derivatives may accumulate during ischemia. This accumulation may be exacerbated by cyclic-AMP mediated lipolysis of endogenous triglyceride which itself may be triggered by the early, ischemia induced, release of catecholamines (Opie 1976). The stimulation of anaerobic glycolysis, the Pasteur effect, represents an attempt to maintain, through non-oxidative mechanisms of substrate-level phosphorylation, the declining myocardial ATP content. The stimulation of glycolysis in the face of reduced mitochondrial activity leads to the accumulation of glycolytic intermediate and reduced nicotinamide adenine dinucleotide phosphate (NADH). In an attempt to regenerate declining and limited reserved of NAD^+ for continued glycolytic activity, pyruvate is reduced to lactate, which accumulates and leaks from the cell (Opie et al. 1973).

An early feature of myocardial ischemia is the accumulation in the cytoplasm of protons and the progressive development of intracellular acidosis. In addition to their inhibitory effect upon glycolytic activity and their possible role in early contractile failure, protons may contribute to the development of the later stages of ischemic damage.

The progressive evolution of ischemia is associated with the loss of intracellular constituents to the extracellular space and ultimately to the circulating blood. This may be divided into three relative distinct phases: ions, metabolites and macromolecules.

The loss of ions, namely potassium reflects the deficit of the ion pumps and is associated with some electrical disturbances. The loss of metabolites, namely of adenine nucleotide precursors is of an extreme importance particularly for the interference with restoration of cell function when the aggression factor declines. The loss of macromolecules reflects the alteration of membrane integrity. Macromolecules such as creatine phosphokinase (CPK) may be detected in the blood as indicators for the lesion and its size. However, only large lesions can be recognized (Hearse and De Leiris 1979).

The alteration of the membrane is associated with the activation of phospholipases leading to a stimulation of the arachidonic acid cascade with the formation of potent vasoconstrictor products. It has been demonstrated that reperfusion or reoxygenation are associated with exagerated cell damage (oxygen paradox). This has been attributed to an accumulation of calcium into mitochondria. This results in a diminution of the capacity of these organelles to synthesize ATP (Poole-Wilson et al. 1982).

Inhalation Anaesthetics

Inhalation anaesthetics have been shown to present a major risk in patients with ischemic heart disease (Steen et al. 1978). This is due to the addition of several factors producing a mixed state of anoxia and ischemia, associated with direct actions on ionic metabolism.

Indeed, the cardiac risk is not identical for all the compounds utilized in anaesthesiology, the main points to be considered are their action on cardiac rate and rhythm, their effect on ventricular function and their interference with the balance between O_2 supply and O_2 demand. Because some may have vasodilating properties and because of the surgical shock, there may be some increase in the sympathetic tone. Catecholamine release may have a direct action on the heart and interact with the anaesthetics action.

During anaesthesia with cyclopropane, chloroform, trichlorethylene, halothane, the dose of β agonists necessary to produce ventricular arrhythmias is reduced, this is due to the classical sensitization of the myocardium (Zink et al. 1975). Anaesthetics also impair the ventricular performance by a depressive action on the SR function and by a direct action on the contractile machinery. The cardiac consequences are specific for each drug (Bristow et al. 1969; Filner et al. 1976). It has been demonstrated both in animal and in man that halothane and its parent compounds affect myocardial oxygenation and perfusion. It has indeed been shown in man that the potent negative inotropic effect of halothane is accompanied by a decrease in coronary blood flow. There is a decrease in oxygen extraction together with a slight increase in lactate extraction (Sonn et al. 1979).

Ethanol

Although ethanol is generally believed to alter hepatic function, there are many illustrations or its cardiotoxic effect, both in animal and man. Ethanol is acutely depressant to myocardium as shown by a depression of the force of heart muscle contraction for a midly intoxicating blood level of 75 mg/100 ml (Regan 1971). In contrast with alcoholics without clinical evidence of heart disease, the patient who has already had at least one episode of heart failure exhibits a much greater ventricular dysfunction than non cardiac subjects. This observation has also been made in subjects who are not alcoholic (Timmis et al. 1975). Potentiation of the acute cardiodepressive action of alcohol may occur in combination with other drugs, mainly the sympathoplegics which block the sympathetic reflex to cardiodepression. Ethanol impairs the cellular calcium metabolism. It also alters the transport of lipids in the myocardium. There is a reduction of free fatty acid uptake and an increase in triglyceride uptake resulting in accumulation of lipid in the myocardium. This implies a limit to the oxidative capacity of the myocardium when substantial uptake of triglyceride occurs (Retig et al. 1977; Ferrans et al. 1965).

The chronic consumption of ethanol may produce a cardiomyopathy characterized by cardiac dilatation including all chambers but particularly the ventricles, an increase in cardiac weight, a high incidence of mural thrombi and patent obstruction of the coronary arteries. Histologically, these hearts show some increase in the diameter of the muscle cells, variable degrees of interstitial fibrosis, small foci of myocytolysis and a variety of degenerative changes. Histochemistry demonstrates an increase in lipid droplets and a decrease in the activity of a number of enzymes of oxidative metabolism (Ferrans et al. 1965). Clinical studies show that cardiac arrhythmias occur during the preclinical states of alcoholic cardiomyopathy, they have mainly been attributed to an alteration of the Purkinje fibers (Ettinger et al. 1978). Of interest, in view of the traditional claim that ethanol has a coronary vasodilator effect, are observations on the influence of ethanol in nonalcoholic individuals suffering from classical stable angina pectoris and proven coronary artery disease. Ten minutes after consuming an alcohol-containing beverage or a non-caloric control, the patients underwent exercise stress testing. Ingestion of either 2 or 3 oz. of alcohol is associated with a decrease in the duration of exercise required to precipitate angina and a significant increase in ischemic ST segment depression (Orlando et al. 1976). The traditional claim seems to be based on the observation of facial arteries, but the evidence is that ethanol is a cardiac ischemia-inducing drug.

Antidepressants

Antidepressants are drugs used to treat mental depressive disorders. They are generally divided in three main groups: monoaminoxidase inhibitors (MAOI), tricyclic antidepressants and the new generation generally assumed to be less toxic than the former ones (Lechat 1978).

The most documented cardiotoxicity is reported for the tricyclic antidepressants. It is seen as an increase in heart rate, a fall in blood pressure, a decrease in myocardial contractility and output and a decrease in peripheral resistance. There are also arrhythmias and slowing in conduction velocity. These cardiac effects can be related to a mixture of anticholinergic atropine-like action, quinidine-like membrane action and to an enhanced catecholamine action resulting from inhibition of their reuptake. This last action tends to increase the risk factor in aged patients and in patients with coronary artery disease, with those drugs producing an enhanced sensitivity to the cold test. This test mimics the conditions in which an angina crisis can be produced in an ambulatory patient. With these drugs, there is a risk of cardiac ischemia (Moir 1973).

Antineoplasic Drugs

The cardiotoxicity of antineoplasic drugs is well documented for anthracycline antibiotics, cyclophosphamide and 5-fluorouracil, but the characteristics of toxicity differ between them.

Anthracycline Antibiotics

The anthracyclines, daunorubicin (daunomycin) and doxorubicin (adriamycin) are effective agents against acute lymphocytic and acute myelocytic leukemias. Doxorubicin appears to be especially effective in the therapy of solid tumors and is considered one of the most important drugs currently used in cancer chemotherapy (Blum and Carter 1974). Two distinct types of cardiac effects are produced by the administration of anthracyclines.

Acute cardiac changes which do not show dose-dependent relationship are characterized by non-specific electrocardiographic changes including sinus tachycardia, reduced QRS voltage, ST-segment depression, T wave alteration and ventricular premature beats (Von Hoff et al. 1977).

Chronic pathological alterations occurred in patients who received a dose of daunorubicin exceeding 550 mg/m^2. Cross pathological examination of patients who died from anthracycline-induced cardiomyopathy revealed the heart to be enlarged, pale and flaccid, with ventricular dilatation and hypertrophy. Mural thrombus associated with multiple pulmonary or systemic emboli and congestion of the lungs and visceral organs were also seen. Light microscopic examination showed that the number of myocardial cells was decreased and that the remaining cells had signs of degeneration (Ferrans 1978). The mechanism of cardiotoxicity has been attributed to decreased protein synthesis due to alterations in DNA, but there is evidence that adriamycin could stimulate Ca entry via stimulation of slow Ca channels. The resulting Ca overload could be toxic for the heart (see below) (Azuma et al. 1981).

Cyclophosphamide

The heart of patients studied at necropsy were generally dilated and exhibited transmural hemorrhages. There were myocyte lesions and fibrinous pericarditis. Fibrin deposition was also seen in the small intramural coronary vessels. It has been proposed that these alterations could lead to cardiac ischemic damage (Slavin et al. 1975).

5-Fluorouracil

The feature common to all clinical reports on fluorouracil has been chest pain. The pain varied in severity from mild angina to crushing chest pain similar to that experienced during myocardial infarction. Cardiac ischemia induced by fluorouracil may lead to cardiogenic shock (Soukop et al. 1978).

Antihypertensive Vasodilators

Antihypertensive vasodilators comprise hydralazine, diazoxide, sodium nitroprusside, minoxidil, converting enzyme inhibitors and the α blocking drug prazocin. Arrhythmia is the most common though often insigificant adverse reaction of antihypertensive drugs. Angina pectoris can be provoked with most antihypertensive drugs, particularly by diazoxide, hydralazine, prazocin and by withdrawal of propranolol (Brodgen et al. 1977). The main factors responsible for the appearance of angina is the ischemia caused by decrease of the perfusion pressure in the coronary vessels. Preexisting coronary heart disease renders patient more susceptible to these agents that aggravate angina pectoris. Reflex tachycardia by shortening the diastole will further diminish coronary circulation and at the same time increase cardiac work. Therefore, an antihypertensive like diazoxide without significant vasodilator effect is more likely to provoke angina than sodium nitroprusside which decreases venous return (Thirlwell and Zsoter 1972). Papillary and subendocardial necrosis with ischemic changes in the ECG has been produced when large doses of hydralazine, diazoxide or minoxidil were given to dogs (Balazs and Herman 1976).

Sympathomimetics

Sympathomimetics are widely used in therapy. The cardiotoxicity of catecholamines is well established (Raab et al. 1961). The cardiac lesions evoked by isoproterenol, the most commonly used for experimental study will be described below. Its human toxicity has been reported in asthmatic patients and β_2 receptor agonists have been introduced in therapy to reduce the toxicological risk. These drugs have also been recommended for the treatment of premature labour and cardiac insuffiency, because of their vasodilating action. Although their chronotropic effect is much lower than that of the non-specific β stimulants, the ratio between the smooth muscle relaxation and the cardiac action depends upon the drug. Most of the β_2 stimulants evoke a tachycardia and an increase in myocardial oxygen consumption (Canepa et al. 1982).

Because β stimulants are used to treat cardiac failure in patients with ischemic heart attack, inotropic agents with a weak chronotropic effect appear to be the most suitable. Dopamine and β_1 partial agonists (prenalterol and corwin) are proposed as being the most interesting. Indeed, it has been reported that the latter increase heart contractility but not myocardial oxygen consumption (Hjalmarson et al. 1982; Pouleur et al. 1982).

If the actual trends are confirmed, the new β stimulants could improve cardiac contractility without risk of enhanced ischemia. However, the large use of other sympathomimetics justifies the study of the cardionecrotic action of those drugs.

The most common model is the cardionecrotic action of isoprenaline in rats. This action can be studied with morphological techniques and with biochemical ones. Light microscopy shows observable changes 24 hours after isoprenaline injection. They are characterized by multifocal lesions disseminated in the ventricular wall with the highest incidence at the apex of the heart. Some cardiac cells are necrotic and are surrounded by interstitial oedema and cellular infiltration. The infiltration is constituted by histyocytic and fibroplastic cells. The lesions are surrounded by intact cardiac tissue. The cellular lesion occurs very early and is characterized by a generalised lipid vacuolization associated with alteration of mitochondria. The multifocal lesion is due to restoration of most of the cells. This tendency to restoration is faster in young rats than in old rats. Only with the latter, there is a residual fibroblastic lesion observable few days after isoprenaline injection (Godfraind and Sturbois 1979). Those morphological changes have been attributed to a dramatic decrease in the reserve of high energy phosphate leading to a disturbance of divalent cation metabolism: large increase in cell calcium and concommittent decrease in magnesium (Bloom and Davis 1972).

Preservation of the Myocardium

As shown in the preceding section, drug-induced cardionecrosis may be the result of a direct action on the myocytes or of an indirect one resulting from the decrease in coronary blood supply. The pathophysiological mechanisms involved in this toxicity are in essence similar to those activated by various disease processes leading to myocardial ischemia and infarction. It is noteworthy that patients suffering from angina pectoris or with an ancient infarction story are more susceptible to the cardiotoxic effect of the drugs reviewed above. In recent years, these cardiovascular disorders have been successfully treated by drugs interfering with calcium metabolism (calcium antagonists, calcium entry blockers).

The term Calcium entry blocker has been recently introduced in order to specify among the group of calcium antagonists those whose pharmacological actions result from the blockade of Ca entry through membrane channels opened during cell excitation (Godfraind 1981). The concept of calcium antagonism emerged from earlier studies with the antianginal drug lidoflazine and with cinnarizine which was introduced as an antihistaminic (Godfraind and Polster 1968). Calcium entry blockers have a broad spectrum of clinical uses (Table 1) mostly in the cardiovascular field, but it may be anticipated that their field of activity will be enlarged, especially to the central nervous system. Because the first "calcium antagonists", lidoflazine (Godfraind and Polster 1968) and verapamil (Fleckenstein 1971), were used to treat coronary insufficiency, a great deal of attention has been devoted to their action in ischemia and anoxia. Different experimental models have been utilized, the most documented are: in vivo: the cardionecrotic action of isoprenaline in rats, permanent or transitory coronary artery ligation in dogs, permanent coronary ligation in rats; in vitro: isolated heart from rat or rabbit perfused according to Langendorf or isolated working heart; such preparations are submitted to a period of anoxia followed by reoxygenation (oxygen paradox), to ischemia (suppression or reduction of the perfusion) followed by reperfusion or to Ca deprivation followed by a return to Ca (Ca paradox).

In the models where normal conditions were reestablished, most of the cardiac lesions occurred at this time (therefore, the term paradox was introduced). A good index to follow the time course of myocardial deterioration is the kinetic measure of ^{45}Ca accumulation. As recently shown by Poole-Wilson et al. (1972) for anoxia, Ca accumulation in the heart occurs at the time of

Table 1. Ca entry blockers with potential interest in therapy

A.	Specific Ca entry blockers
	Angina
	Lidoflazine, verapamil, diltiazem, nifedipine
	Hypertension
	Verapamil, nifedipine, diltiazem
	Arrhythmia
	Verapamil
	Peripheral vascular disorders
	Cinnarizine, flunarizine, nimodipine
	Under experimental study
	Nisoldipine, niludipine, nicardipine, tiapamil
B.	Ca entry blockers with a additional action
	1. On catecholamine receptors
	Chlorpromazine
	Rauwolscine and corynanthine
	Pimozide
	2. On fast Na channel
	Angina: Bepridil, perhexiline, prenylamine, fendiline, bencyclane
	3. On Ca calmodulin
	Felodipine
	4. On phosphodiesterase
	Papaverine
	Amrinone

reoxygenation. At this time, there is a sudden increase in high energy phosphate needs for the restablishment of the physiological regulation of the myocardium. During the deprivation phase, high energy phosphate stores have been utilized and the cell has generally lost its adenosine content (Berne 1982).

Because of adenosine lack, mitochondria cannot follow the ATP demand and cellular alteration occurs. It is characterized by calcium overload, phospholipases are activated leading to membrane disorganization and to the activation of the arachidonic acid cascade with the formation of vasoconstrictor products. Those products together with K ions released by cells in the ischemic state diffuse into the surrounding tissue area producing an action on adjacent cardiac cells and on the microcirculation. The latter is responsible for the so called no-reflow phenomenon and the former for the activation of abnormal cardiac pace-makers. This will result in the appearance of arrhythmias and in the extension of the initial lesion. The severity of this complex situation can be attenuated by calcium entry blockers, but also by a compound such as creatinol-O-phosphate which maintain the anaerobic metabolism in the anoxic heart (Godfraind and Sturbois 1979). The site of action of calcium entry blockers in this pathology is a matter of discussion.

Two anatomical structures may be involved as target sites: vessels and heart, because these drugs may act on both tissues.

In smooth muscle the simplest experimental procedure with which to assess the ability of a pharmacological compound to inhibit Ca^{2+} entry is to preincubate the muscle in Ca^{2+}-free physiological solution and then to depolarize it with a KCl rich solution and gradually increase the Ca^{2+} concentration in the bathing solution. This will result in an increase in tension dependent on Ca^{2+} concentration. When this procedure is repeated in the presence of a putative Ca entry blocker, the contractile responses are depressed in a concentration dependent manner (Godfraind and Kaba 1969). Recent experiments with ^{45}Ca have directly demonstrated that depression of the contraction due to these drugs is related to inhibition of calcium entry. Calcium entry blockers block not only Ca entry due to smooth muscle depolarization but also the entry dependent on tissue activation by various agonists. This is the basis for their antagonism to various vasoconstrictors, including catecholamines, serotonin, prostaglandins. They do not inhibit that component of the contraction dependent upon the release of intracellular calcium, so that part of the response to agonists is still present. Their action depends upon the anatomical origin of the vessel, an observation which explains why some are efficient in cerebral circulation and others are potent antihypertensive agents. In this respect they also show a selectivity for the slow Na-Ca channel in heart, where verapamil is the most potent drug. Hence, it is efficient in treating cardiac arrhythmias (Godfraind 1982; Fleckenstein 1971).

In the ischemic heart, calcium entry blockers may act on the slow Na-Ca channel to decrease Ca entry or on the coronary artery spasm. Another mechanism could be that of membrane stabilisation (Poole-Wilson et al. 1982). However, even if the exact nature of their mechanism of action is still under discussion, it is well established that some of them (verapamil, diltiazem, lidoflazine, nifedipine, cinnarizine and flunarizine) have potent cardioprotective actions against the various factors producing cardionecrosis.

Cigarette smoke evokes anoxia characterized by electrocardiographic changes (Tirlapu et al. 1982). It has been shown by van Nueten (1982) that anoxia evoked coronary constriction is blocked by calcium entry blockers. In obstetrics, it is now usual to use verapamil in association with β stimulants in order to decrease the β cardiac effects (see van Lierde et al. 1982).

Therefore, one is justified in treating patients at risk with one of these drugs, preferentially those which do not have any cardiodepressive action and in this respect, the calcium entry blockers cinnarizine and flunarizine could be utilized.

Concluding Remarks

From the data summarized above, it appears that some drugs may cause cardionecrosis. The pathophysiological mechanisms involved in this action resemble those involved in disease-induced cardiac ischemia or anoxia. By altering the balance between O_2 supply and demand or by a direct action on the heart muscle, these drugs induce a loss of high energy phosphate and of adenosine that is required for its resynthesis. This in turn is responsible for alterations of ionic gradients, arrhythmias and decrease in contractility. Furthermore, changes in membrane permeability and structure activate the arachidonic acid cascade, thereby inducing a vicious circle and the extension of the cardiac lesion. There is experimental and clinical evidence for the cardioprotective action of calcium entry blockers and of an antiischemic drug such as creatinol-O-phosphate. Their use as preventive agents in patients at risk appears to be justified.

References

Adams RJ, Schwartz A (1980) Comparative mechanisms for contraction of cardiac and skeletal muscle. Cest 78: 123–139

Azuma J, Sperelakis N, Hasegawa H, Tanimoto T, Vogel St, Ogura K, Awata N, Sawamura A, Harada H, Ishiyama T, Morita V, Yamamura Y (1981) Adriamycin cardiotoxicity: possible pathogenic mechanism. J Mol Cell Cardiol 13: 381–397

Balazs T, Herman EH (1976) Toxic cardiomyopathies. Ann Clin Lab Sci 6: 467–476

Berne RM, Belardinelli L, Winn HR, Rubio R (1982) The adenosine concept in ischemia of heart and brain. In: Wauquier A, Borgers M, Amery WK (eds) Protection of tissues against hypoxia. Elsevier Biomedical Press, Amsterdam New York Oxford, p 105

Bloom S, David DL (1972) Calcium as mediator of isoproterenol-induced myocardial necrosis. Am J Pathol 69: 459–470

Blum RS, Carter SK (1974) Adriamycin: a new anticancer drug with significant clinical activity. Ann Intern Med 80: 249–259

Bristow JD, Prys-Roberts C, Fisher A, Pickering TG, Sleight P (1969) Effects of anesthesia on baroreflex control of heart rate in man. Anesthesiology 31: 422–428

Brodgen RN, Heel RC, Speight TM, Avery GS (1977) Prazosin: a review of its pharmacological properties and therapeutic efficacy in hypertension. Drugs 14: 163–197

Canepa-Anson R, Dawson JR, Frankl WS, Kuan P, Sutton GC, Reuben S, Poole-Wilson PA (1982) β_2 adrenoceptors agonist pharmacology, metabolic effects and arrhythmias. Eur Heart J (Suppl D) 3: 129–134

Ettinger PO, Wu CF, De la Cruz C Jr, Weisse AB, Ahmed SS, Regan TJ (1978) Arrhythmias and the "holiday heart" alcohol-associated cardiac rhythm disorders. Am Heart J 95: 555–562

Ferrans VJ (1978) Overview of cardiac pathology in relation to anthracycline cardiotoxicity. Cancer Treat Rep 62: 955–961

Ferrans VJ, Hibbs RG, Weilbaecher DB, Black WC, Walsh J, Burch GE (1965) Alcoholic cardiomyopathy: a histochemical study. Am Heart J 69: 748–765

Ferrari R, Di Lisa F, Raddino R, Visioli O (1982) Effects of myocardial calcium overloading during ischaemia and reperfusion on ATP synthesis. In: Godfraind T, Albertini A, Paoletti R (eds) Calcium modulators. Elsevier Biomedical Press, Amsterdam New York Oxford, p 99

Filner BE, Karliner JS (1976) Alterations of normal left ventricular performance by general anesthesia. Anesthesiology 45: 610–621

Fleckenstein A (1982) Basic membrane actions of calcium antagonists with special reference to verapamil. In: Godfraind T, Albertini A, Paoletti R (eds) Calcium modulators. Elsevier Biomedical Press, Amsterdam New York Oxford, p 297

Godfraind T (1981) Mechanism of action of calcium entry blockers. Fed Proc 40: 2866–2871

Godfraind T (1982) Pharmacology of calcium entry blockers. In: Godfraind T, Albertini A, Paoletti R (eds) Calcium modulators. Elsevier Biomedical Press, Amsterdam New York Oxford, p 51

Godfraind T, Kaba A (1969) Blockade or reversal of contraction induced by calcium and adrenaline in depolarized arterial smooth muscle. Br J Pharmacol 36: 549–560

Godfraind T, Miller RC (1983) Specificity of action of Ca entry blockers, a comparison of their actions in rat arteries and human coronary arteries. Circ Res (in press)

Godfraind T, Polster P (1968) Etude comparative de médicaments inhibant la réponse contractile de vaisseaux isolés d'origine humaine ou animale. Thérapie 23: 1209–1220

Godfraind T, Sturbois (1979) An analysis of the reduction by creatinol-O-phosphate of the myocardial lesions evoked by isoprenaline in the rat. Arzneim Forsch Drug Res 29: 1457–1464

Godfraind-De Becker A, Godfraind T (1980) Calcium transport system: a comparative study in different cells. Int Rev Cytol 67: 141–170

Hearse DJ, De Leiris J (1979) Enzymes in cardiology. John Wiley & Sons, New York

Hjalmarson A, Avelardo N; Waagstein E (1982) Effects of prenalterol in congestive heart failure. Eur Heart J (Suppl D) 3: 115–121

Jennings RB (1969) Early phase of myocardial ischemic injury and infarction. Am J Cardiol 24: 753–765

Kardesch M, Hogancamp CE, Bing RJ (1958) The effect of complete ischemia on the intracellular electrical activity of the whole mammalian heart. Circ Res 6: 715–720

Katz AM, Repke DI, Dunmet J, Hasselbach W (1977) Relation of calcium permeability to the Ca^{2+} concentration gradient across the sarcoplasmic reticulum. In: Riecker G, Weber A, Goodwin J (eds) Myocardial Failure. Springer, Berlin Heidelberg New York, p 72

Lechat P (1978) Quelques données sur le chronotropisme, obtenues à l'aide de cellules cardiaques en culture. Bull Acad Natl Med 162: 401–406

Moir DC (1973) Tricyclic antidepressants and cardiac disease. Am Heart J 86: 841–842

Morel N, Godfraind T (1982) Na-Ca exchange in heart and smooth muscle microsomes. Arch Int Pharmacodyn Ther 258: 319–321

Opie LH (1976) Effects of regional ischemia on metabolism of glucose and fatty acids. Circ Res (Suppl 1) 38: 52–74

Opie LF, Owen P, Thomas M, Samson R (1973) Coronary sinus lactate measurements in assessment of myocardial ischemia. Am J Cardiol 32: 295–307

Orlando J, Aronew WS, Cassidy J, Prakash R (1976) Effect of ethanol on angina pectoris. Ann Intern Med 84: 652–655

Poole-Wilson PA, Harding D, Bourdillon P, Fleetwood G (1982) Mechanism of myocardial protection through Ca^{2+} blockade. In: Borgers M, Aremy WK (eds) Protection of tissue against hypoxia. Elsevier Biomedical Press, Amsterdam New York Oxford, p 351

Pouleur H, Rousseau MF, Mengeot P, Veriter C, Vincent MF, Brasseur LA (1982) Improvement of global and regional left ventricular function in patients with previous myocardial lesions. Am J Cardiol 8: 203–211

Regan T (1971) Ethyl alcohol and the heart. Circulation 44: 957–963

Retig JN, Kirchberger MA, Rubin E, Katz AM (1977) Effects of ethanol on calcium transport by microsomes phosphorylated by cyclic AMP-dependent protein kinase. Biochem Pharmacol 26: 393–396

Rosenman KD (1979) Cardiovascular disease and environmental exposure. Br J Industr Med 36: 85–97

Slavin RE, Millan JC, Mullins GM (1975) Pathology of high dose intermittent cyclophosphamide therapy. Hum Pathol 6: 693–709

Sonntag H, Merin RG, Donath U, Radke J, Schenk HD (1979) Myocardial metabolism and oxygenation in man awake and during halothane anesthesia. Anesthesiology 51: 204–210

Soukop M, McVie JG, Calman K (1978) Fluorouracil cardiotoxicity. Br Med J 1: 1422

Steen PA, Tinker JH, Tarhan S (1978) Myocardia reinfarction after anesthesia and surgery? JAMA 239: 2566–2570

Stein O, Hasin Y, Stein Y (1981) Membrane cholesterol and spontaneous depolarization in cultured cardia myocytes. In: Godfraind T, Meyer P (eds) Cell membrane in function and dysfunction of vascular tissue. Elsevier Biomedical Press, Amsterdam New York Oxford, p 266

Thirlwell MP, Zsoter TT (1972) The effect of diazoxide on the veins. Am Heart J 83: 512–517

Timmis CG, Ramos RC, Gordon S, Gangadharan V (1975) The basis for differences in ethanol-induced myocardial depression in normal subjects. Circulation 51: 1144–1148

Tirlapur VG, Charalambous BM, Evans PJ, Jones MK, Mir MA (1982) In: Wauquier A, Borgers M, Amery WK (eds) Protection of tissues against hypoxia. Elsevier Biomedical Press, Amsterdam New York Oxford, p 443

Van Lierde M, Jacquetin B, Boog G, Thomas K (1982) Aspects obstétricaux de la prématurité, vol 2. Excerpta Medica, p 655

van Nueten JM (1982) Selectivity of calcium entry blockers. In: Godfraind T, Albertini A, Paoletti (eds) Calcium modulators. Elsevier Biomedical Press, Amsterdam New York Oxford, p 199

Von Hoff DD, Rozencweig M, Layard M, Slavik M, Murria FM (1977) Daunomycin-induced cardiotoxicity in children and adults: review of 110 cases. Am J Med 62: 200–208
Williamson JR, Schaffer SW, Ford C, Safer B (1976) Contribution of tissue acidosis to ischemic injury in the perfused rat heart. Circulation (Suppl) 53: 3–14
Zink J, Sasyniuk BI, Dresel PE (1975) Halothane-epinephrine-induced cardiac arrhythmias and the role of heart rate. Anesthesiology 43: 548–555

Disease, Metabolism and Reproduction in the Toxic Response to Drugs and Other Chemicals
Arch. Toxicol., Suppl. 7, 16–29 (1984)

Young Scientists Award Lecture 1983:

Investigations into the Mechanism of Coumarin-Induced Hepatotoxicity in the Rat

B. G. Lake

Biochemistry Department, British Industrial Biological Research Association,
Woodmansterne Road, Carshalton, Surrey, SM5 4DS, England

Abstract. The administration of single doses of coumarin to the rat was found to produce hepatic centrilobular necrosis and also to depress a number of hepatic enzyme activities within 24 h. Coumarin-induced liver damage was diminished by pretreatment with cobaltous chloride but potentiated by the administration of diethyl maleate. Hepatic reduced non-protein sulphydryl levels were rapidly depleted following coumarin treatment whereas urinary mercapturic acid excretion was enhanced suggesting the formation of a coumarin metabolite or metabolites hitherto undetected in this species. In in vitro studies [3-^{14}C]coumarin was converted by rat hepatic microsomes to reactive intermediates which became bound covalently to microsomal proteins. Additional studies established that the formation of reactive metabolites was a cytochrome P-450 dependent process and that macromolecular binding could be inhibited by sulphydryl compounds (including reduced glutathione) and hepatic cytosol fractions. These results demonstrate that coumarin-induced hepatotoxicity in the rat is likely to be mediated via one or more reactive metabolites generated by cytochrome P-450 dependent enzymes and that reduced glutathione and other thiol agents constitute a detoxification pathway.

Key words: Coumarin – Hepatotoxicity – Cytochrome P-450 – Reduced glutathione

Introduction

Coumarin (1,2-benzopyrone; *cis-o*-coumarinic acid lactone) is a naturally occurring plant product which is used in various soaps, detergent and cosmetic preparations (Opdyke 1974). It is also present in certain tobaccos and alcoholic beverages (Cohen 1979). The use of coumarin as a food flavour was discontinued after it was found to be hepatotoxic in the rat and dog (Hazelton et al. 1956; Hagan et al. 1967).

Several aspects of the toxicology of coumarin merit attention. For example, coumarin appears to elicit interspecies differences in both metabolism and hepatotoxicity (Cohen 1979) and controversy exists as to the nature of the bile duct lesions observed after the prolonged administration of this compound to rats. Indeed these lesions have been diagnosed both as "bile duct carcinomas" (Bär and Griepentrog 1967; Griepentrog 1973) and as "cholangiofibrosis" (Hagan et al. 1967; Evans et al. 1982). As man and the rat metabolise coumarin differently, the significance of these lesions in predicting the hepatotoxic risk to man has been questioned (Cohen 1979).

In man and the baboon, coumarin is extensively metabolised to 7-hydroxycoumarin (Shilling et al. 1969; Gangolli et al. 1974) whereas in several other species examined, including the rat, hamster, dog and rabbit, 7-hydroxylation constitutes only a minor metabolic pathway (Cohen 1979). The major metabolic pathway in the rat appears to involve an initial 3-hydroxylation reaction with subsequent opening of the lactone ring and further metabolism to *o*-hydroxyphenylacetic acid (Kaighen and Williams 1961; Cohen 1979). A number of studies have suggested that 7-hydroxylation may constitute a detoxification pathway. For example, Endell and Seidel (1978) found that coumarin was less acutely toxic in DBA strain mice than in C3H/HeJ strain animals, which correlates with the known higher hepatic coumarin 7-hydroxylase activity determined both in vitro (Wood and Conney 1974; Wood and Taylor 1979) and in vivo (Lush and Andrews 1978) in DBA strain mice. However, coumarin hepatotoxicity cannot be explained simply in terms of hepatic coumarin 7-hydroxylase activities as the chronic administration of coumarin to the hamster did not result in significant hepatotoxic changes (Ueno and Hirono 1981). Like the rat this species is a poor 7-hydroxylator (Gangolli et al. 1974) and the dose level employed in the study (5,000 ppm in the diet for 2 years) is known to be sufficient to produce bile duct lesions and other hepatotoxic changes in the rat (Hagan ct al. 1967; Evans et al. 1982).

To date the mechanism of coumarin-induced hepatotoxicity has not been conclusively established (Cohen 1979). Whilst the studies of Endell and Seidel (1978) suggest that 7-hydroxylation may constitute a detoxification pathway, Gibbs et al. (1971) have suggested that hepatotoxicity is due to the parent compound per se. The aim of the present study was to assess the role of metabolism in the acute hepatotoxicity of coumarin in a sensitive species, namely the rat. A longer term aim would be to apply these findings with appropriate pharmacokinetic studies to other species which are apparently resistant to coumarin-induced hepatotoxicity.

Materials and Methods

Materials

Coumarin was purchased from the Aldrich Chemical Company, Gillingham, Dorset, England and [3-^{14}C] coumarin (specific activity 5.5 mCi/m mol) from Amersham International Ltd., Bucks, England. Enzymes, cofactors, sulphydryl compounds, buffers etc. were obtained from the Sigma Chemical Co., Poole, Dorset, England. Proadifen (SKF 525-A, 2-diethylaminoethyl-2,2-diphenylvalerate) and metyrapone (2-methyl-1,2-*bis*-(3-pyridyl)-1-propanone) were the generous gifts of Smith, Kline and French Laboratories, Welwyn Garden City, Herts, England and CIBA Laboratories, Horsham, Sussex, England, respectively.

Animals and Treatment

Male Sprague-Dawley rats (100–120 g) were purchased from Charles River U.K. Ltd., Margate, Kent, England. They were housed in accomodation maintained at 20 ± 2° C with a relative humidity of 30–70% and fed Spratt's (Barking, Essex, England) Laboratory Diet 1 and water. Coumarin was administered by either gastric intubation or intraperitoneal (i.p.) injection, control animals received corresponding quantities (5 ml/kg) of the corn oil vehicle. Animals were starved overnight and killed by cervical dislocation.

Biochemical Investigations

Whole liver homogenates (0.25 g fresh tissue/ml) were prepared in ice-cold 0.154 M KCl containing 50 mm Tris-HCl buffer pH 7.4 employing a Potter-type, Teflon-glass, motor-driven homogeniser (A. H. Thomas Co., Philadelphia, Pa., USA). A portion of the whole homogenate was mixed with an equal volume of 10% (w/v) trichloroacetic acid (TCA) containing 10 mM EDTA and the reduced non-protein sulphydryl content of the deproteinised supernatant was determined by the method of Ellman (1959), as modified by Sedlak and Lindsay (1968), using reduced glutathione as the standard. The homogenates were centrifuged at an average force of 10,000 *g*, for 20 min to obtain the postmitochondrial supernatants and subsequently at an average force of 158,000 *g* for 40 min to separate the microsomal fraction from the cytosol. The pellets were resuspended in fresh homogenising medium and again centrifuged at an average force of 158,000 *g* for 40 min. Washed microsomal fractions were assayed for the activities of ethylmorphine N-demethylase, 7-ethoxycoumarin O-deethylase and glucose-6-phosphatase and for the content of cytochrome P-450, cytochrome b_5 and haem as described previously (Lake et al. 1982). Protein was determined by the method of Lowry et al. (1951) employing bovine serum albumin as the standard. The spectral interaction of coumarin with microsomal cytochrome P-450 was studied by the method of Schenkman et al. (1967).

In the studies on the covalent binding of coumarin metabolites to microsomal proteins incubation mixtures contained 1.5 mM nicotinamide adenosine diphosphate ($NADP^+$), 7.5 mM DL-isocitric acid, 0.5 U/ml isocitrate dehydrogenase, 2.5 mg/ml microsomal protein, either 0.05 or 0.5 mM [3-^{14}C] coumarin (300,000 dpm/tube) and 0.1 M phosphate buffer pH 7.6 in a final volume of 2 ml. Blank tubes were incubated with [3-^{14}C] coumarin but in the absence of the NADPH-generating system. After incubating for 15 min at 37° C in a shaking water bath the incubations were terminated with 2 ml of 10% (w/v) TCA and the macromolecular bound [3-^{14}C] coumarin metabolites determined by exhaustive solvent extraction of the pellets as described previously (Lake et al. 1981).

In the urinary mercapturic acid excretion studies 24 h urine samples were collected from rats caged singly in "Metabowls" (Jencons Scientific, Hemel Hempstead, Herts, England). Urinary thioethers and creatinine were estimated by the methods of Summer et al. (1979) and Bonsnes and Taussky (1945), respectively.

Serum activities of glutamic-oxaloacetic transaminase (GOT) and glutamic-pyruvic transaminase (GPT) were determined by standard methods (Bechtler 1974).

Morphological Investigations

Liver slices were fixed in neutral buffered formalin. Paraffin sections of about 5 μm thickness were cut and stained with haematoxylin and eosin. Five sections of liver from each animal were examined by light microscopy and the extent of necrosis scored on an arbitrary scale as described in the legend to Table 2.

Results

Coumarin-Induced Hepatotoxicity

The administration of single oral 125–500 mg/kg doses of coumarin to rats were hepatotoxic within 24 h. Morphological investigations revealed necrosis of the centrilobular cells of the liver lobule (Fig. 1), the severity of which was dose dependent. There was a dose dependent increase in relative liver weight and a depression of microsomal glucose-6-phosphatase, ethylmorphine N-demethylase, 7-ethoxycoumarin O-deethylase and cytochrome P-450 content (Fig. 2). The depression of cytochrome P-450 content was accompanied by losses of cytochrome b_5 and haem (Table 1). In microsomes from both control and coumarin treated rats the combined amounts of cytochromes P-450 and b_5 largely accounted for the total haem content, indicating the absence of cytochrome P-420 from these preparations. Coumarin administration also produced a small decrease in microsomal protein content (Table 1).

Studies on the Mechanism of Coumarin-Induced Hepatotoxicity

Coumarin was found to elicit the formation of a Type I binding spectrum (Schenkman et al., 1967) with rat hepatic microsomal cytochrome P-450. The value of the apparent spectral dissociation constant (K_s) was calculated to be 1.7 ± 0.2 mM (mean ± SEM of 3 microsomal preparations). Previous studies have shown that both the 3- and 7-hydroxylation of coumarin by rodent microsomes are cytochrome P-450 dependent processes (Feuer 1970; Wood 1979). In order to investigate the possibility that coumarin is bioactivated to toxic products by cytochrome P-450 dependent mixed function oxidase (m.f.o.)

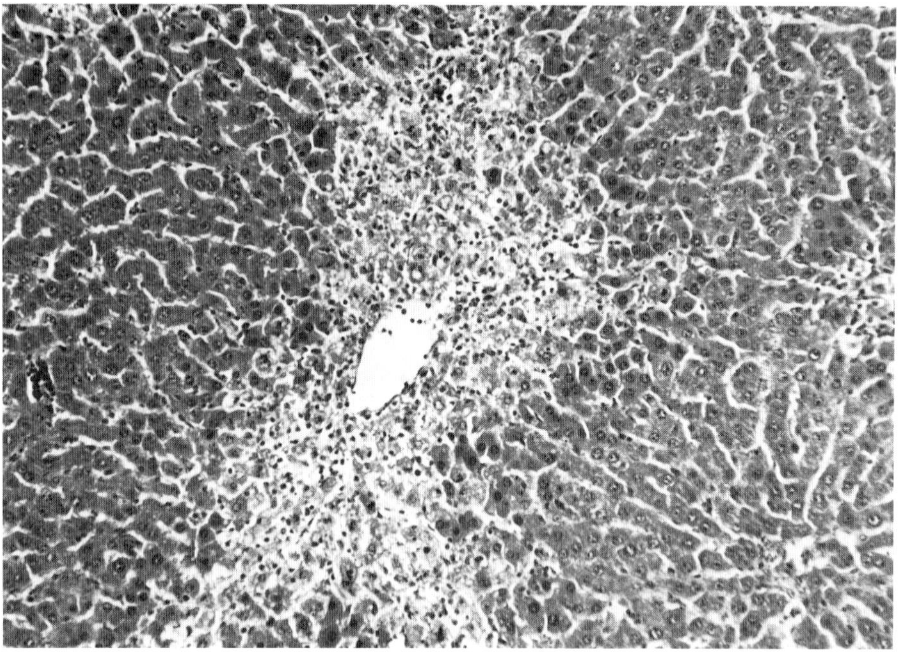

Fig. 1. Liver section from a rat given a single oral 500 mg/kg dose of coumarin and killed 24 h later. There is extensive necrosis of the centrilobular area of the liver lobule. Haematoxylin and eosin. × 250

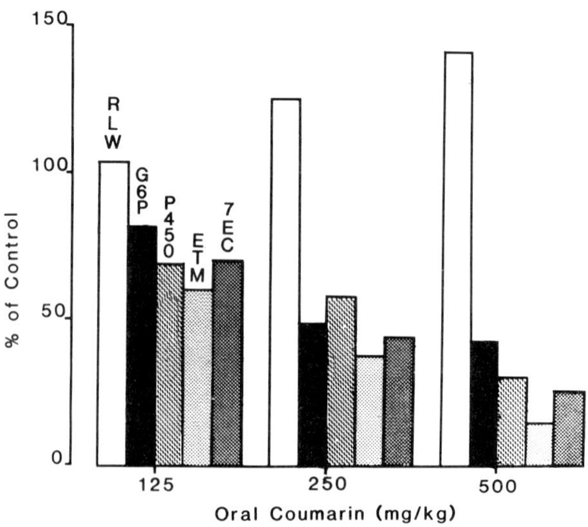

Fig. 2. The effect of single oral 125–500 mg/kg doses of coumarin on some hepatic parameters in the rat. Animals were killed 24 h after coumarin treatment and the relative liver weight (g liver/100 g body wt, RLW) and hepatic microsomal glucose-6-phosphatase (G6P), cytochrome P-450 content (P450), ethylmorphine N-demethylase (ETM) and 7-ethoxycoumarin O-deethylase (7 EC) activities were determined. Results are presented as percentage of control (corn oil treated) activities for groups of either six control or five coumarin treated animals

Table 1. The effect of a single oral dose of coumarin on some hepatic microsomal parameters in the rat

Parameter	Treatment[a]	
	Control (corn oil)	Coumarin (375 mg/kg)
Cytochrome P-450[b]	0.92 ± 0.03	0.50 ± 0.07[c]
Cytochrome b_5[b]	0.49 ± 0.01	0.34 ± 0.02[c]
Haem[b]	1.45 ± 0.01	0.92 ± 0.03[c]
Protein (mg/g liver)	31.0 ± 0.9	26.7 ± 1.3[d]

[a] Rats were killed 24 h after treatment. Results are presented as mean ± SEM of four animals
[b] In units of nmol/mg microsomal protein
[c] Significantly different (Student's *t*-test) from control: $p < 0.01$
[d] Significantly different (Student's *t*-test) from control: $p < 0.05$

enzymes, the effect of cobaltous chloride pretreatment on coumarin-induced hepatotoxicity was determined. Cobaltous chloride is known to deplete hepatic cytochrome P-450 levels by affecting haem biosynthesis and catabolism (Tephly et al. 1978). The oral administration of 250 and 500 mg/kg coumarin to control (saline pretreated) rats produced a dose dependent increase in relative liver weight, in the extent of hepatic necrosis and in the elevation of serum GOT and GPT activities (Table 2). In contrast, the hepatotoxicity of coumarin assessed by any of these criteria was markedly reduced in animals pretreated with cobaltous chloride.

Preliminary experiments established that coumarin administration depletes hepatic reduced non-protein sulphydryl (NPS) concentrations within 2 h. Indeed the treatment of rats with 125–500 mg/kg coumarin produced a dose dependent depletion of hepatic NPS levels, the depletion being more marked after i.p. administration than after oral administration (Fig. 3). As previous studies (Moron et al. 1979) have shown that hepatic NPS levels measured by the method of Ellman (1959) largely represent reduced glutathione, it is likely that this sulphydryl compound is involved in the hepatotoxicity of coumarin. This hypothesis was investigated by treating rats with diethyl maleate, a compound known to markedly reduce hepatic reduced glutathione concentrations (Boyland and Chasseaud 1970). Rats were treated with 0.2 ml/kg doses of diethyl maleate i.p. 0.5 h before and 4 h after i.p. doses of either corn oil (control) or 50 mg/kg coumarin. The diethyl maleate treatment regime was chosen to minimise the known inhibitory effects of this compound on cytochrome P-450 dependent m.f.o. enzyme activities (Anders 1978; Suarez et al. 1981). At this dose level coumarin produced no effect on relative liver weight, microsomal cytochrome P-450 content or glucose-6-phosphatase activity (Table 3). In contrast, significant changes in these parameters were observed in rats treated with both coumarin and diethyl maleate. Whilst coumarin treatment alone reduced microsomal ethylmorphine N-demethylase activity, a greater effect was observed after the co-administration of coumarin and diethyl maleate. The

Table 2. The effect of cobaltous chloride pretreatment on coumarin-induced hepatotoxicity in the rat

Pretreatment[a]	Coumarin (mg/kg)	Relative liver wt (g liver/100 g body wt)[b]	Extent of hepatic necrosis[c]				Serum enzyme (μmol/min/l)[b]	
			0	+	++	+++	GOT	GPT
Control (saline)	0	3.6 ± 0.2	5	–	–	–	120 ± 16	30 ± 4
	250	4.6 ± 0.3[d]	–	2	2	1	880 ± 490	300 ± 115[d]
	500	5.2 ± 0.1[e]	–	–	1	4	4,100 ± 770[e]	800 ± 190[e]
Cobaltous chloride	0	3.9 ± 0.1	5	–	–	–	210 ± 46	38 ± 9
	250	4.3 ± 0.2	1	4	–	–	129 ± 33	57 ± 5
	500	4.8 ± 0.2[f]	2	3	–	–	157 ± 27	135 ± 54

[a] Rats were pretreated with either 0.9% (w/v) saline or cobaltous chloride (40 mg/kg/day) by s.c. injections for 2 days. Animals were then treated with coumarin orally at the dose levels indicated and killed 24 h later

[b] Results are presented as mean ± SEM of five animals

[c] Hepatic necrosis was assessed in five sections from each liver averaged to provide an overall value. Figures refer to the number of rats from each group ($n = 5$) showing liver lesions classified as: 0, no necrosis; +, subcapsular or occasional single cell necrosis; ++, necrosis of 5–20% of hepatocytes; +++, necrosis of > 20% of hepatocytes

[d] Significantly different (Student's t-test) from control (saline pretreated) group: $p < 0.05$

[e] Significantly different (Student's t-test) from control (saline pretreated) group: $p < 0.01$

[f] Significantly different (Student's t-test) from control (cobaltous chloride pretreated) group: $p < 0.01$

Table 3. The effect of diethyl maleate treatment on coumarin-induced hepatotoxicity in the rat

Treatment[a]	Coumarin (mg/kg)	Relative liver wt (g liver/100 g body wt)	Cytochrome P-450 (nmol/mg protein)	Ethylmorphine N-demethylase (nmol/h/mg protein)	Glucose-6-phosphatase (nmol/min/mg protein)
Control (corn oil)	0	3.5 ± 0.1	0.99 ± 0.05	1,080 ± 47	761 ± 54
	50	3.6 ± 0.1	0.86 ± 0.06	784 ± 67[b]	730 ± 19
Diethyl maleate	0	3.5 ± 0.1	0.89 ± 0.03	1,130 ± 150	712 ± 27
	50	3.9 ± 0.1[c]	0.64 ± 0.07[d]	532 ± 58[d]	562 ± 42[c]

[a] Rats were treated with either corn oil or diethyl maleate (0.2 ml/kg) by i.p. injections 0.5 h before and 4 h after i.p. treatment with either corn oil or coumarin (50 mg/kg) and subsequently killed 24 h later. Results are presented as mean ± SEM of five animals

[b] Significantly different (Student's t-test) from control (corn oil treated) group: $p < 0.01$

[c] Significantly different (Student's t-test) from control (diethyl maleate treated) group: $p < 0.05$

[d] [illegible]

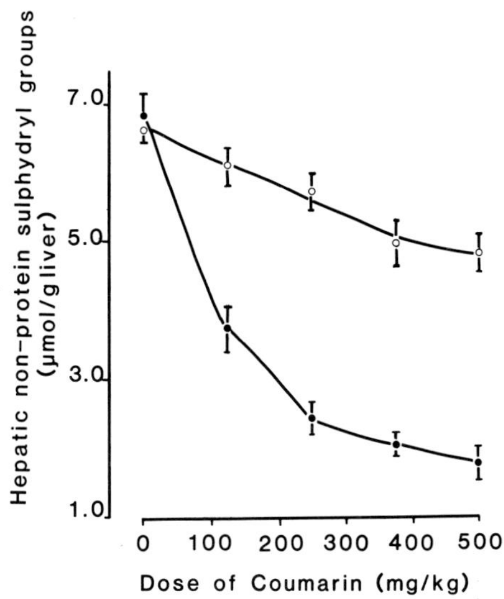

Fig. 3. The depletion of hepatic non-protein sulphydryl levels by coumarin. Rats were treated with 0–500 mg/kg coumarin by either oral intubation (○) or i.p. injection (●) and killed 2 h later. Each point representes the mean ± SEM of six to eight animals

potentiation of coumarin-induced hepatotoxicity by diethyl maleate was confirmed by additional morphological investigations (data not shown).

Coumarin did not appear to react non-enzymatically with reduced glutathione since no depletion of sulphydryl groups was observed when 1–5 mM coumarin was incubated with either 0.5 or 2 mM reduced glutathione in pH 7.4 buffer at 37° C for 60 min. Under these conditions significant nonenzymic conjugation of 1 mM diethyl maleate with reduced glutathione was observed in agreement with the findings of Boyland and Chasseaud (1967).

A number of compounds whose metabolism includes the formation of glutathione conjugates are known to increase urinary mercapturic acid excretion in the rat. To determine if coumarin treatment increased urinary mercapturic acid excretion, rats were treated orally with 50–500 mg/kg doses of coumarin, 24 h urine samples were collected and analysed for thioether and creatinine content. A group of rats were also treated orally with a 250 mg/kg dose of naphthalene as a positive control (Summer et al. 1979). Compared with the control animals, naphthalene treatment significantly increased urinary thioether excretion (Table 4). In addition, coumarin administration produced a dose related increase in urinary thioether excretion.

In Vitro Covalent Binding Studies

When [3-^{14}C] coumarin was incubated with washed rat hepatic microsomes and an NADPH-generating system [3-^{14}C] coumarin metabolites became irreversibly bound to the microsomal proteins. Macromolecular binding was linear with respect to the incubation time (up to 20 min) and the microsomal protein concentration (up to 3 mg/ml in the incubation mixture). A double reciprocal plot of coumarin covalent binding over a substrate concentration range of

0.011–3.0 mM yielded two kinetic lines (Fig. 4). Apparent K_m values were calculated to be 0.056 ± 0.006 and 0.78 ± 0.13 mM (mean ± SEM of 4 microsomal preparations) with corresponding maximal velocities of 4.7 ± 1.0 and 20.2 ± 0.8 nmol metabolites bound/h/mg microsomal protein respectively. In order to investigate the nature of the enzyme or enzymes responsible for the coumarin metabolite covalent binding, further studies were conducted at [3-^{14}C] coumarin substrate concentrations of 0.05 and 0.5 mM, i.e., at concentrations representative of both kinetic lines. Macromolecular binding at both substrate concentrations was found to be enzyme mediated and NADPH-dependent, since no binding was obtained with boiled microsomes and NADH could not substitute for NADPH as the electron donor (Table 5). Covalent binding was markedly diminished under anaerobic conditions (nitrogen atmosphere) and by the cytochrome P-450 inhibitors carbon monoxide, proadifen (SKF 525-A) and metyrapone (Table 5). In contrast, the addition of either 0.08 or 0.8 mM 3,3,3,-trichloropropylene oxide, an inhibitor (Oesch 1974) of epoxide hydratase (EC 3.3.2.3), had little effect (data not shown). A number of sulphydryl compounds including reduced glutathione, cysteamine, L-cysteine and homocysteine inhibited covalent binding whereas L-methionine had no significant effect, indicating a requirement for a free thiol group (Table 5). Hepatic cytosol fractions also inhibited macromolecular binding, the extent of inhibition being less when boiled cytosol fractions were employed, indicating a requirement for both heat stable and heat labile components. The inhibition of covalent binding of coumarin metabolites by cytosol was still significant even when the results

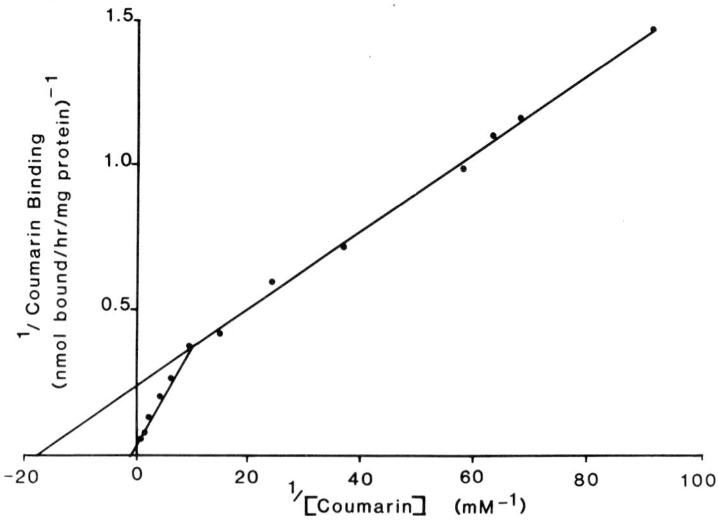

Fig. 4. Kinetics of the NADPH-dependent covalent binding of [3-^{14}C] coumarin metabolites to rat hepatic microsomes. Macromolecular binding was determined as described in the Materials and Methods section over a [3-^{14}C] coumarin substrate concentration range of 0.011–3.0 mM. Apparent K_m values were calculated to be 0.056 ± 0.006 and 0.78 ± 0.13 mM (mean ± SEM of four microsomal preparations) with corresponding maximal velocities of 4.7 ± 1.0 and 20.2 ± 0.8 nmol metabolites bound/h/mg protein respectively

Table 4. The effect of administration of coumarin and naphthalene on urinary mercapturic acid excretion in the rat

Treatment[a]	Urinary thioethers[b] (μmol/mg creatinine)
Control (corn oil)	1.16 ± 0.09 (100)
Coumarin (50 mg/kg)	1.76 ± 0.21[c] (152)
Coumarin (250 mg/kg)	3.90 ± 0.56[d] (336)
Coumarin (500 mg/kg)	8.08 ± 1.05[d] (697)
Naphthalene (250 mg/kg)	2.00 ± 0.19[d] (172)

[a] Compounds were administered orally at the dose levels indicated and 24 h urine samples collected and analysed for thioethers and creatinine
[b] Results are presented as mean ± SEM of either six control or five treated animals with percentage of control values being shown in parentheses
[c] Significantly different (Student's *t*-test) from control: $p < 0.05$
[d] Significantly different (Student's *t*-test) from control: $p < 0.01$

Table 5. The inhibition of the covalent binding of [3-^{14}C]coumarin metabolites to rat hepatic microsomes in vitro

Addition[a]	Covalent binding (% of control)[b]	
	0.05 mM substrate	0.5 mM substrate
+ Boiled microsomes	0.2 ± 0.1[c]	0.4 ± 0.3[c]
+ 1 mM NADH	77 ± 5[c]	100 ± 10
– NADPH + 1 mM NADH	4 ± 0.3[c]	5 ± 2[c]
– O_2 (100% N_2 atmosphere)	8 ± 0.5[c]	6 ± 1[c]
+ CO (80% CO, 20% O_2 atmosphere)	5 ± 2[c]	13 ± 4[c]
+ 0.1 mM SKF 525-A	50 ± 1[c]	48 ± 5[c]
+ 1 mM Metyrapone	38 ± 3[c]	30 ± 5[c]
+ 0.5 mM Reduced glutathione	41 ± 1[c]	36 ± 3[c]
+ 0.5 mM Cysteamine	22 ± 2[c]	33 ± 2[c]
+ 0.5 mM L-Cysteine	56 ± 1[c]	49 ± 5[c]
+ 0.5 mM Homocysteine	65 ± 4[c]	59 ± 6[c]
+ 0.5 mM L-Methionine	92 ± 5	85 ± 6
+ 2.5 mg Cytosol (158,000 *g* av. supt.) protein	24 ± 3[c]	28 ± 6[c]
+ 2.5 mg Boiled cytosol protein	52 ± 7[c]	55 ± 7[c]
+ 10 mM Sodium benzoate	104 ± 8	112 ± 4[c]
+ 20 mM Sodium benzoate	122 ± 3[c]	105 ± 6
+ 20 mM Ethylenediamine	59 ± 4[c]	67 ± 1[c]
+ 50 mM Ethylenediamine	30 ± 2[c]	35 ± 7[c]
+ 1 Mm L-Ascorbic acid	68 ± 4[c]	60 ± 5[c]
+ 10 mM L-Ascorbic acid	48 ± 2[c]	45 ± 8[c]

[a] The macromolecular binding of [3-^{14}C]coumarin metabolites was determined with either 0.05 or 0.5 mM substrate, an NADPH-generating system and rat hepatic microsomes at 37° C under air as described in the Materials and Methods section
[b] Results are presented as percentage of control activities as mean ± SEM of four microsomal preparations. Typical control (100%) rates of 0.05 and 0.5 mM [3-^{14}C]coumarin metabolite binding were 2.7 ± 0.3 and 7.4 ± 0.3 nmol metabolites bound/h/mg protein respectively
[c] Significantly different (paired Student's *t*-test) from control: $p < 0.01$

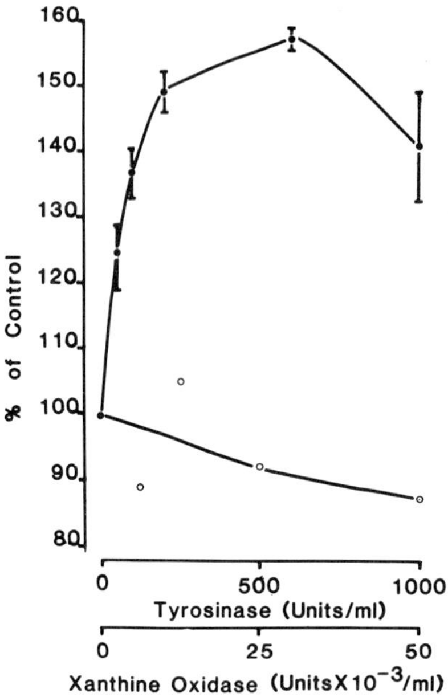

Fig. 5. The effect of mushroom tyrosinase (●) and 0.25 mM xanthine/xanthine oxidase (○) on the NADPH-dependent covalent binding of [3-^{14}C]coumarin metabolites to rat hepatic microsomes. Macromolecular binding was determined as described in the Materials and Methods section at a [3-^{14}C] coumarin substrate concentration of 0.05 mM. Results are presented as the mean ± SEM of three microsomal preparations for mushroom tyrosinase and as the mean of two microsomal preparations for 0.25 mM xanthine/xanthine oxidase

were calculated per incubation vessel to allow for the increased total (microsomal and cytosol) protein content (data not shown).

Whilst the addition of sodium benzoate had no inhibitory effect on covalent binding, both ethylenediamine and L-ascorbic acid inhibited macromolecular binding in a concentration dependent manner (Table 5). Even though high (20 and 50 mM) concentrations of ethylenediamine were employed these had no effect on rat microsomal m.f.o. enzyme activities as indicated by the lack of inhibition of 7-ethoxycoumarin O-deethylase activity (data not shown). Whilst the addition of 0.25 mM xanthine/xanthine oxidase (EC 1.2.3.2) had little effect, mushroom tyrosinase (EC 1.14.18.1) enhanced the NADPH-dependent rate of [3-^{14}C] coumarin metabolite covalent binding (Fig. 5). No macromolecular binding was observed when hepatic microsomes were incubated with either 0.25 mM xanthine/xanthine oxidase or mushroom tyrosinase in the absence of an NADPH generating system. Finally, the addition of either catalase (EC 1.11.1.6., 360 U/ml) or superoxide dismutase (EC 1.15.1.1., 3−145 U/ml) had little effect on the NADPH-dependent covalent binding of coumarin metabolites (data not shown).

Discussion

Single doses of coumarin produced hepatotoxic changes in the rat within 24 h. These changes consisted of centrilobular hepatic necrosis, the elevation of serum GOT and GPT activities and the depression of several hepatic enzyme activities. The reduction in coumarin-induced hepatotoxicity observed after cobaltous chloride pretreatment suggests the involvement of a cytochrome P-450 generated metabolite or metabolites in this process. However, it should be noted that cobaltous chloride is not a specific inhibitor of cytochrome P-450 dependent biotransformations and also enhances hepatic reduced glutathione levels (Sasame and Boyd 1978). Indeed the results also demonstrate a role for reduced glutathione with or without other NPS compounds in protecting against liver damage, since coumarin administration rapidly depletes hepatic NPS levels and coumarin-induced hepatotoxicity was potentiated by diethyl maleate. The elevation of urinary thioether excretion by coumarin treatment may be taken as evidence of the excretion of a coumarin metabolite or metabolites conjugated with mercapturic acid, although the nature of such a metabolite or metabolites requires identification. No mercapturic acid conjugates have been reported in previous studies on the metabolism of coumarin in the rat and other species (Cohen 1979).

In vitro studies reactive [3-^{14}C] coumarin metabolite or metabolites, generated by cytochrome P-450 dependent m.f.o. enzymes, were found to bind covalently to microsomal proteins. As would be expected from the in vivo studies reduced glutathione and other NPS compounds inhibited the macromolecular binding of these metabolites. The inhibition obtained with hepatic cytosol fractions may have been due to both the presence of reduced NPS compounds and to the action of glutathione S-transferase enzymes. Investigations into the kinetics of macromolecular binding revealed a biphasic plot which may indicate either the participation of multiple cytochrome P-450 forms in the bioactivation process or the formation of two or more distinct reactive intermediates. However, in the inhibition studies essentially similar effects were observed on both kinetic processes.

Assuming the in vitro covalent binding of coumarin metabolites is associated with coumarin-induced hepatotoxicity in vivo, then these studies may suggest a possible mechanism of coumarin bioactivation. The lack of effect of sodium benzoate, superoxide dismutase, catalase and xanthine/xanthine oxidase would tend to discount the involvement of either hydroxyl radicals, superoxide anions or hydrogen peroxide in the formation of reactive [3-^{14}C] coumarin metabolites. However, inhibition was observed with L-ascorbic acid which can reduce superoxide anions, semiquinones and quinones (Deamer et al. 1971; Nishikimi 1975) and with ethylenediamine which is a known *o*-quinone trapping agent (Jellinck and Irwin 1963). The possible involvement of quinone or semiquinone intermediates in macromolecular binding was also indicated by the enhancement of the NADPH-dependent rate of [3-^{14}C] coumarin metabolite binding by mushroom tyrosinase, an enzyme which possesses a variety of oxidase activities (Zeffren and Hall 1973). The lack of effect of this enzyme in the absence of an NADPH-generating system indicates that it is activating a metabolite of coumarin rather than the parent compound, although it remains to be demonstrated that mushroom tyrosinase leads to the formation of the same reactive metabolite or metabolites as are produced by an NADPH-generating system alone. No evidence was obtained for the formation of a reactive coumarin 3,4 – or other – epoxides since 3,3,3-trichloropropylene oxide failed to enhance the rate of covalent binding. However, the 3,4-double bond appears to be required for coumarin-induced hepatotoxicity as dihydrocoumarin (1,2-benzohydropyrone) possesses little or no hepatotoxicity in the rat after either acute (B. G. Lake, unpublished observations) or chronic (Hagan et al. 1967) administration. Since the major pathway of coumarin metabolism in the rat comprises an initial cytochrome P-450 dependent 3-hydroxylation (Feuer 1970), the reactive metabolite or metabolites may be formed by further oxidation of 3-hydroxycoumarin. Whether this would involve the formation of quinone or semiquinone derivatives merits further investigation.

In conclusion, the results of these studies demonstrate that coumarin-induced hepatotoxicity in the rat is unlikely to be due to the parent compound, as suggested by Gibbs et al. (1971), but rather to one or more cytochrome P-450 generated metabolites which may be detoxified by reduced NPS compounds. Further studies are required to confirm and extend these findings. Additional studies into species differences in metabolism, pharmacokinetics and hepatotoxicity of this compound may permit the better assessment of the hazard of coumarin to man.

References

Anders MW (1978) Inhibition and enhancement of microsomal drug metabolism by diethyl maleate. Biochem Pharmacol 27: 1098–1101

Bär F, Griepentrog F (1967) Die Situation in der gesundheitlichen Beurteilung der Aromatisierungsmittel für Lebensmittel. Medizin Ernähr 8: 244–251

Bechtler G (1974) UV-Assay, automated method (for glutamate-oxalacetate and glutamate-pyruvate transaminases). In: Bergmeyer HU (ed) Methods of enzymatic analysis, vol 2. Academic Press, New York, pp 733–735, 758–760

Bonsnes RW, Taussky HH (1945) On the colorimetric determination of creatinine by the Jaffe reaction. J Biol Chem 158: 581–591

Boyland E, Chasseaud LF (1967) Enzyme-catalysed conjugations of glutathione with unsaturated compounds. Biochem J 104: 95–102

Boyland E, Chasseaud LF (1970) The effect of some carbonyl compounds on rat liver glutathione levels. Biochem Pharmacol 19: 1526–1528

Cohen AJ (1979) Critical review of the toxicology of coumarin with special reference to interspecies differences in metabolism and hepatotoxic response and their significance to man. Food Cosmet Toxicol 17: 277–289

Deamer DW, Heikkila RE, Panganamala RV, Cohen G, Cornwell DG (1971) The alloxan-dialuric acid cycle and the generation of hydrogen peroxide. Physiol Chem Phys 3: 426–430

Ellman GL (1959) Tissue sulfhydryl groups. Arch Biochem Biophys 82: 70–77

Endell W, Seidel G (1978) Coumarin toxicity in different strains of mice. Agents Action 8: 299–302

Evans JG, Lake BG, Conning DM (1982) The pathogenesis of coumarin induced cholangiofibrosis in the rat. Toxicologist 2: 100

Feuer G (1970) 3-Hydroxylation of coumarin or 4-methylcoumarin by rat-liver microsomes and its induction by 4-methylcoumarin given orally. Chem Biol Interact 2: 203–216

Gangolli SD, Shilling WH, Grasso P, Gaunt IF (1974) Studies on the metabolism and hepatotoxicity of coumarin in the baboon. Biochem Soc Trans 2: 310–312

Gibbs PA, Janakidevi K, Feuer G (1971) Metabolism of coumarin and 4-methylcoumarin by rat-liver microsomes. Can J Biochem 49: 177–184

Griepentrog F (1973) Pathologisch-anatomische Befunde zur karzinogenen Wirkung von Cumarin im Tierversuch. Toxicology 1: 93–102

Hagan EC, Hansen WH, Fitzhugh OG, Jenner PM, Jones WI, Taylor JM, Long EL, Nelson AA, Brouwer JB (1967) Food flavourings and compounds of related structure. II. Subacute and chronic toxicity. Food Cosmet Toxicol 5 : 141–157

Hazelton LW, Tusing TW, Zeitlin BR, Thiessen R Jr, Murer HK (1956) Toxicity of coumarin. J Pharmacol Exp Ther 118 : 348–358

Jellinck PH, Irwin L (1963) The interaction of oestrogen quinones with ethylene diamine. Biochim Biophys Acta 78 : 778–780

Kaighen M, Williams RT (1961) The metabolism of [3-^{14}C] coumarin. J Med Chem 3 : 25–43

Lake BG, Harris RA, Phillips JC, Gangolli SD (1981) Studies on the effects of L-ascorbic acid on acetaminophen-induced hepatotoxicity. 1. Inhibition of the covalent binding of acetaminophen metabolites to hepatic microsomes in vitro. Toxicol Appl Pharmacol 60 : 229–240

Lake BG, Foster JR, Collins MA, Stubberfield CR, Gangolli SD, Srivastava SP (1982) Studies on the effect of orally administered dicyclohexyl phthalate in the rat. Acta Pharmacol Toxicol 51 : 217–226

Lowry OH, Rosebrough NJ, Farr AL, Randall RJ (1951) Protein measurement with the Folin phenol reagent. J Biol Chem 193 : 265–275

Lush IE, Andrews KM (1978) Genetic variation between mice in their metabolism of coumarin and its derivatives. Genet Res 31 : 177–186

Moron MS, DePierre JW, Mannervik B (1979) Levels of glutathione, glutathione reductase and glutathione S-transferase activities in rat lung and liver. Biochim Biophys Acta 582 : 67–78

Nishikimi M (1975) Oxidation of ascorbic acid with superoxide anion generated by the xanthine-xanthine oxidase system. Biochem Biophys Res Commun 63 : 463–468

Oesch F (1974) Purification and specificity of a human microsomal epoxide hydratase. Biochem J 139 : 77–88

Opdyke DLJ (1974) Monographs on fragrance raw materials: coumarin. Food Cosmet Toxicol 12 : 385–405

Sasame HA, Boyd MR (1978) Paradoxical effects of cobaltous chloride and salts of other divalent metals on tissue levels of reduced glutathione and microsomal mixed-function oxidase components. J Pharmacol Exp Ther 205 : 718–724

Schenkman JB, Remmer H, Estabrook RW (1967) Spectral studies of drug interaction with hepatic microsomal cytochrome. Mol Pharmacol 3 : 113–123

Sedlak J, Lindsay RH (1968) Estimation of total, protein-bound, and nonprotein sulfhydryl groups in tissue with Ellman's reagent. Anal Biochem 25 : 192–205

Shilling WH, Crampton RF, Longland RC (1969) Metabolism of coumarin in man. Nature 221 : 664–665

Suarez KA, Griffin K, Kopplin RP, Bhonsle P (1981) Protective effect of diethylmaleate pretreatment on carbon tetrachloride hepatotoxicity. Toxicol Appl Pharmacol 57 : 318–324

Summer KH, Rozman K, Coulston F, Greim H (1979) Urinary excretion of mercapturic acids in chimpanzees and rats. Toxicol Appl Pharmacol 50 : 207–212

Tephly TR, Wagner G, Sedman R, Piper W (1978) Effects of metals on heme biosynthesis and metabolism. Fed Proc 37 : 35–39

Ueno I, Hirono I (1981) Non-carcinogenic response to coumarin in Syrian golden hamsters. Food Cosmet Toxicol 19 : 353–355

Wood AW (1979) Genetic regulation of coumarin hydroxylase activity in mice. Biochemical characterization of the enzyme from two inbred strains and their F_1 hybrid. J Biol Chem 254 : 5641–5646

Wood AW, Conney AH (1974) Genetic variation in coumarin hydroxylase activity in the mouse (*Mus musculus*). Science 185 : 612–614

Wood AW, Taylor BA (1979) Genetic regulation of coumarin hydroxylase activity in mice. Evidence for single locus control on chromosome 7. J Biol Chem 254 : 5647–5651

Zeffren E, Hall PL (1973) In: The study of enzyme mechanisms. Wiley-Interscience, New York, pp 224–236

Alteration of Drug Toxicity in Disease States

Disease, Metabolism and Reproduction in the Toxic Response to Drugs and Other Chemicals
Arch. Toxicol., Suppl. 7, 33–38 (1984)

Influence of Disease on Drug Toxicity

P. Turner

Department of Clinical Pharmacology, St. Bartholomews' Hospital,
London, EC1A 7BE, Great Britain

Abstract. Disease can influence the actions of a drug, both therapeutic and undesired, in many ways. These include changes in the rate and extent of its absorption from the gastrointestinal tract and other sites, its disposition throughout body compartments, its hepatic uptake and metabolism, and its clearance from the body by one of more routes of elimination. In addition to these pharmacokinetic changes, disease may modify the pharmacological action of a drug, for example by influencing receptor number and responsiveness. However, the mechanisms underlying some adverse drug effects related to certain inherited and acquired diseases remain unexplained.

Key words: Disease toxicity – Pharmacokinetics

The actions of a drug, both therapeutic, non-therapeutic and adverse may be influenced by factors that alter its pharmacokinetics or its mechanism of action at a cellular molecular level. Although in most instances it is impossible to resolve observed changes into either pharmacokinetic or pharmacodynamic elements, it may be possible to identify the major factors responsible for them. This certainly applies to several disease states in which enhanced drug toxicity can be explained predominently in terms of kinetic or dynamic changes induced by disease.

Disease and Pharmacokinetics

Some of the disease states that are known to produce clinically significant changes in pharmacokinetics which in turn can result in enhanced drug effects are shown in Table 1.

Gastrointestinal disease can modify drug absorption by producing changes in regional pH, absorptive surface, motility and in pancreatic secretion.

Table 1. Disease states which may influence pharmacokinetics

Gastrointestinal disease	Liver disease	Cancer
Cardiac infarction and failure	Thyroid disease	Surgery
Pulmonary disease	Anaemia	Malnutrition
Renal disease	Inflammatory disease	

Cardiac failure and infarction influence pharmacokinetics in several different ways. Drug absorption tends to be reduced by mucosal oedema, splanchnic vasoconstruction and reduced epithelial perfusion.

The volumes of distribution of several drugs are markedly reduced, probably by changes in protein and tissue binding. Marked changes in alpha-1 acid glycoprotein levels have been found in patients following myocardial infarction (Johnston et al. 1983), associated with increases in the binding of disopyramide and flecainide, leading to reduced free drug concentrations. In the case of disopyramide the increased binding at day 5 after an infarction was equivalent to a decrease of about 50% in free disopyramide levels which may have clinical significance.

Hepatic elimination may be impaired because of reduced perfusion and metabolism, and renal elimination because of decreased glomerular filtration and increased tubular reabsorption.

Observed changes in drug kinetics will depend on the relative magnitude of these various factors in individual patients with heart disease. The nature of the heart disease is an important factor, changes in protein binding probably being of major importance after an infarction or inflammatory cardiac condition, and in tissue and organ perfusion in the presence of failure.

Pulmonary disease might be predicted to influence drug kinetics through acute or chronic hypoxic effects on the organs of absorption and excretion. Few controlled studies have been carried out, however, and the changes described in clearance of several drugs are difficult to resolve into a clear picture of consistent effects (Wilson and Bromberg 1981). This may be due in part ot the presence of other factors, for example, cardiac impairment, fever, and acute inflammatory responses, which may be essential components of pulmonary disease and influence drug kinetics in the various ways discussed here.

Renal disease not only influences pharmacokinetics through changes in glomerular filtration and tubular reabsorption, but also by altering protein binding and metabolism. Changes in plasma albumin content and structure lead to reduced binding of acidic drugs, for example of phenytoin and azapropazone (Reidenberg 1976; Jahnchen et al. 1981), with a consequent risk of drug toxicity. Extrarenal metabolism of drugs may be increased in uraemic patients, although the mechanisms involved are poorly understood.

Liver disease may influence pharmacokinetics through reduced first pass uptake, leading to increased bioavailability of drugs normally taken up avidly by that mechanism, for example chlormethiazole (Pentikainen et al. 1978). This may result from impaired hepatocellular function, as in hepatic necrosis, or by portosystemic shunting as may occur in hepatic cirrhosis; reduced protein binding may occur because of decreased hepatic synthesis and decreased elimination.

These factors are interdependent and all tend to increase the total and free systemic levels of many drugs. Drugs may conveniently be classified into those whose liver metabolism is determined primarily by hepatic blood flow, and whose clearance is therefore markedly sensitive to factors which influence it, such as lignocaine, propranolol and morphine, and those whose metabolism is primarily dependent on the capacity of the liver enzymes to metabolise them, such as phenytoin, warfarin and theophylline (Shand 1978).

Thyroid disease is known to influence the kinetics and action of several drugs, probably in part by effects on protein binding, hepatic metabolism and renal function. Hypothyroid patients tend to be very sensitive to the effects of digitalis, and hyperthyroid patients, on the other hand, require larger doses than normal to control atrial fibrillation (Rogers et al. 1981), but the mechanisms involved are not clear. Changes in antipyrine and steroid clearance are thought to be due to increased hepatic metabolism. Increased propranolol clearance appears to involve both increased hepatic metabolism and decreased plasma protein binding (Feely et al. 1981).

The influence of anaemia on drug kinetics appears to have received little attention, although it might reasonably be expected to produce effects through changes in cardiac function and tissue nutrition. Recent studies in patients with severe anaemia secondary to hookworm infestation have shown a reduced half-life and increased clearance of antipyrine which were reversed by correction of their anaemia (Desai et al. 1982). The importance of these observations on the therapeutic and toxic effects of other drugs, and an explanation of their mechanisms, await elucidation.

Inflammatory disease, both acute and chronic, may produce marked changes in pharmacokinetics. Acute febrile illness in children is associated with a significant reduction in antipyrine clearance (Forsyth et al. 1982), and experimentally induced fever in adults increases plasma levels of quinine (Trenholme et al. 1976). Chronic inflammatory disorders such as Crohn's disease (Schneider et al. 1976) and rheumatoid arthritis (Schneider et al. 1979) have been shown to be associated with increases in plasma levels of propranolol. In rheumatoid arthritis, the increases were shown to be related to the erythrocyte sedimentation rate, and are probably due to changes in plasma proteins associated with the acute phase inflammatory response. The implications of these findings in terms of drug efficacy and toxicity are not yet clear.

Cancer can be associated with increased plasma concentrations of alpha-1 acid glycoprotein and reduced levels of albumin, and it is not surprising, therefore, that changes in plasma binding of some drugs have been described in patients with malignant disease. Lignocaine, a basic drug, binds predominantly to alpha-1 acid glycoprotein, and its free fraction has been found to be significantly lower in plasma from cancer patients compared with controls. In contrast, the free fraction of tolbutamide, an acidic drug which binds mainly to albumin, was significantly higher in cancer patients than in control plasma (Jackson et al. 1982). The therapeutic and toxicological significance of these observations is being investigated.

Table 2. Some examples of enhanced drug toxicity associated with inherited diseases (after Rawlins and Thompson 1981)

Inherited disease	Drug	Effect
Hereditary methaemoglobinaemia	Oxidising drugs	Methaemoglobinaemia, cyanosis
Porphyria	Barbiturates, oestrogens, etc.	Porphyric crisis
Haemophilia and von Willeband's	Salicylates	Prolongs bleeding time
Malignant hyperpyrexia	Halothane, caffeine, succinylcholine, KCl	Hyperpyrexic syndrome
Osteogenesis imperfecta	Halothane, succinylcholine	Pyrexia
Periodic paralysis	KCl, insulin, adrenaline, ethanol, licorice derivatives	Paralysis
Familial dysautonomia	Cholinergic and adrenergic agonists	Denervation supersensitivity

Surgery and anaesthesia significantly alter antipyrine clearance (Pessayne et al. 1978) and profound bradycardia after partial thyroidectomy has been described in a thyrotoxic patient receiving a constant dose of digoxin and propranolol. Marked increases were found in serum digoxin and plasma propranolol steady state levels compared with preoperative levels (Feely 1982).

Malnutrition may not be considered as a disease process, but several studies have shown that drug absorption may be impaired, plasma steady state levels reduced, and pharmacokinetics changed in undernourished subjects (Raghuram and Krishnaswamy 1982).

Disease and Pharmacodynamics

Disease processes are known to have a significant influence on the effects of many drugs, but in only relatively few are the mechanisms understood.

An example already referred to is the enhanced sensitivity to digitalis found in hypothyroid patients.

Enhanced drug toxicity associated with inherited diseases, some examples of which are given in Table 2. The enzymatic basis of some of these disorders is understood, but that of others awaits elucidation.

Changes in receptor density and function have been reviewed elsewhere (Turner 1980), and may explain the enhanced bronchoconstrictor effects of beta-adrenoceptor antagonists in asthamtic patients, and the sensitivity of patients with myasthenia gravis to the neuromuscular blocking effects of streptomycin, neomycin or kanamycin (Rawlins and Thompson 1981).

Pseudo-allergic reactions happen in which histamine release occurs from mast cells without the mediation of immunological processes. An example of

Table 3. Some examples of enhanced drug toxicity associated with disease states, the nature of which is not yet understood (after Prescott 1978)

Disease	Drug	Toxicological result
Hypothyroidism	CNS depressants	Enhanced CNS depression
Respiratory failure	CNS depressants	and respiratory failure
Burns	Succinylcholine	Release of potassium
Renal failure	Succinylcholine	producing cardiac arrhythmias
Peripheral neuropathy	Succinylcholine	
Rheumatoid arthritis and other collagen diseases	Salicylates	Hepatotoxicity
Cystic fibrosis	Isoprenaline	Bronchospasm
Cystic fibrosis	Theophylline	Bronchospasm
Renal failure	Clofibrate	Severe myopathy
Renal failure	Benzodiazepines	Fatal dialysis
Renal failure	Monoamine reuptake inhibiting antidepressives	Dementia

such a reaction is that seen in a patient with urticaria pigmentosa with generalised mastocytosis in which acetylsalicylic acid produced an anaphylactic-like reaction (Waldenstrom 1980).

Other examples of enhanced drug toxicity associated with disease, but at present not understood in pharmacological or kinetic terms, are shown in Table 3.

In conclusion, it is evident that many mechanisms are already understood by which disease may interfere with the therapeutic effects of drugs and enhance their toxicity, but their importance in clinical practice still awaits careful prospective investigation.

References

Desai NK, Karbhari K, Paul T, Kshirsagar NA, Sheth UK (1982) Prolongation of antipyrine half-life after correction of severe anaemia due to hook-worm infection. Br J Clin Pharmacol 13 : 745–746

Feely J (1982) Increased drug effect induced by surgery. Hum Toxicol 1 : 447–449

Feely J, Crooks J, Stevenson IH (1981) The influence of age, smoking and hyperthyroidism on plasma propranolol steady state concentration. Br J Clin Pharmacol 12 : 73–78

Forsyth JS, Moreland TA, Rylance GW (1982) The effect of fever on antipyrine metabolism in children. Br J Clin Pharmacol 13 : 811–815

Jackson PR, Tucker GT, Woods HF (1982) Plasma binding of drugs in patients with cancer. Br J Clin Pharmacol 13 : 263P–264P

Jähnchen E, Blanck KJ, Breuing KH, Gilfrich HJ, Meinertz T, Trenk D (1981) Plasma protein binding of azapropazone in patients with kidney and liver disease. Br J Clin Pharmacol 11 : 361–367

Johnston A, Caplin JL, Hamer J, Camm AJ (1983) The serum protein binding of disopyramide and flecainide following acute myocardial infarction. Br J Clin Pharmacol 15 : 601P

Pentikainen P, Neuvonen PJ, Tarpila S, Syvalahti E (1978) Effect of cirrhosis of the liver on the pharmacokinetics of chlormethiazole. Br Med J 2 : 861–863

Pessayre D, Allemand H, Benoist C, Afifi F, Francoise M, Benhamou JP (1978) Effect of surgery under general anaethesia on antipyrine clearance. Br J Clin Pharmacol 6: 505–513

Prescott LF (1978) Drug toxicity. In: Turner P, Shand DG (eds) Recent advances in clinical pharmacology, vol 1. Churchill Livingstone, Edinburgh, pp 189–204

Raghuram TC, Krishnaswamy K (1982) Pharmacokinetics and plasma steady state levels of doxycycline in undernutrition. Br J Clin Pharmacol 14: 785–789

Rawlins MD, Thompson JW (1981) Pathogenesis of adverse drug reactions. In: Davies DM (ed) Textbook of adverse drug reactions, 2nd ed. Oxford University Press, Oxford, pp 11–34

Reidenberg MM (1976) The binding of drugs to plasma proteins from patients with poor renal function. Clin Pharmacokin 1: 121–125

Rogers HJ, Spector RG, Trounce JR (1981) A textbook of clinical pharmacology. Hodder & Stoughton, London, pp 141–142

Schneider RE, Babb J, Bishop H, Mitchard M, Hoare AM, Hawkins CF (1976) Plasma levels of propranolol in treated patients with coeliac disease and patients with Crohn's disease. Br Med J 2: 794–795

Schneider RE, Bishop H, Hawkins CF (1979) Plasma propranolol concentrations and the erythrocyte sedimentation rate. Br J Clin Pharmacol 8: 43–47

Shand DG (1978) Recent advances in pharmacokinetics. In: Turner P, Shand DG (eds) Recent advances in clinical pharmacology, vol 1. Churchill Livingstone, Edinburgh, pp 1–11

Trenholme GM, Williams RL, Rieckmann KH, Frischer H, Casson PE (1976) Quinine disposition during malaria and during induced fever. Clin Pharmacol Ther 19: 459–467

Turner P (1980) Some clinical implications of the receptor concept. Circ Res 46: 10–14

Waldenstrom JG (1980) Urticaria pigmentosa and acetylsalicyline acid intolerance. In: Pseudo-allergic reactions. Involvement of drugs and chemicals, vol 1. Karger, Basel, pp 204–218

Wilson K, Bromberg T (1981) The influence of some disease states on drug disposition. Methods Find Exp Clin Pharmacol 3: 189–200

Disease, Metabolism and Reproduction in the Toxic Response to Drugs and Other Chemicals
Arch. Toxicol., Suppl. 7, 39–47 (1984)

Drug Toxicity and Hormonal Dysfunction

M. Eichelbaum

Medizinische Klinik, Universität Bonn,
Sigmund-Freud-Strasse 25, 5300 Bonn-Venusberg, Federal Republic of Germany

Abstract. Abnormal levels of hormones can exert profound changes in drug disposition and the number and affinity of receptors. In endocrine diseases a variety of organ functions change. These disease related changes in the function of organs involved with the distribution, metabolism and excretion of drugs can profoundly alter drug disposition. If not taken into account when devising dosage regimens drug toxicity can result.

Key words: Hormonal dysfunction – Drug toxicity – Drug disposition

Introduction

Alterations in drug action and drug toxicity have been observed in a variety of disease processes due to disease related changes in organ function. Since abnormal levels of some hormones are associated with changes in cardiac, hepatic and renal function, it can be envisioned that alterations in the function of organs involved with the metabolism and excretion of drugs will interfere with drug disposition. In addition to altered drug disposition changes in the number and affinity of receptors or both might occur in endocrine disease. If these disease related changes in drug disposition and receptor number and sensitivity are not taken into account when devising dosage regimens drug toxicity can result. It should also be kept in mind that disease is a dynamic process and therefore time dependent changes in organ function will occur as the condition of the patient deteriorates or improves. Thus, the situation may arise that a given dose of a drug which was appropriate for the patient a fortnight previously might no longer be appropriate. For instance, in hypothyroidism, cardiac output, liver blood flow, hepatic drug metabolism, glomerular filtration rate and renal plasma flow are decreased and return to normal as the patient becomes euthyroid with thyroxine treatment, thus necessitating dose adjustment in relation to changing organ function. While in animals numerous studies on the influence of abnormal levels of hormones on drug metabolism, drug response, and drug toxicity have been carried out (Carrier and Buday 1961; Prange and Lipton 1962; Ellingwood and Prange 1964; Prange et al. 1964, 1966; Gillette 1965; Kato and Gillette 1965; Kato 1977) little definitive information is available about altered drug disposition and drug toxicity in man in endocrine disorders (Eichelbaum 1976, 1981; Marble et al. 1980; Shenfield 1981; Feely 1983). Most of the studies have focused on altered drug disposition. There is a paucity of information whether or not these disease related changes in drug disposition may result in drug toxicity. This is mainly due to the fact that for most endocrine diseases with the exceptions of diabetes mellitus, hyperthyroidism, and myxoedema, the incidence is too low to allow detailed studies to be carried out in a sufficient number of patients.

To overcome these difficulties, studies in animals could be carried out. These animal models, however, might be of limited value in tackling the problem since the spontaneously occurring disease in man might elicit differing effects when compared with the animal disease model. In addition, the dose of exogenously administered hormones might far exceed the hormone levels occurring in the disease in man. Thus, Rumbaugh and others (1978) have observed a dose dependency of thyroxine on hepatic ethylmorphine demethylase, benzo(a)pyrene hydroxylase and aniline hydroxylase activity. While small doses of thyroxine (2.5–5 μg/100 g body weight) increased activity of these reactions, larger amounts of thyroxine (12.5–50 μg) reversed the stimulatory effects of the smaller doses.

This review will focus primarily on data obtained in man and an attempt will be made to evaluate whether or not disease related changes in drug disposition and drug sensitivity can be held responsible for drug toxicity in endocrine disorders.

Thyroid Disease

Thyroid disease is associated with pronounced changes in the function of several organs. It has been demonstrated that cardiac output, hepatic blood flow, hepatic drug metabolizing enzyme activity, glomerular filtration rate and renal plasma flow are increased in hyperthyroidism and decreased in hypothyroidism. Therefore, it can be anticipated that disease related changes in the function of the organs responsible for drug distribution, metabolism and elimination will affect drug disposition. Although the data available do not always allow an accurate prediction as to what extent thyroid disorders will affect drug disposition, studies both in animals and man have shown alterations in drug disposition in relation to thyroid function (Eichelbaum 1976, 1982; Shenfield 1981; Feely 1983). Hepatic drug metabolism has been shown to be altered in thyroid disease. Antipyrine clearance was greatly increased in hyperthyroidism and reduced in hypothyroidism. Antipyrine clearance returned to normal after treatment of thyroid dysfunction. The alterations in the disposition of this drug seen during thyroid dysfunction could be ascribed to changes in the rate of its metabolism which was controlled by the levels of circulating thyroxine (Crooks et al. 1973; Eichelbaum et al. 1974). The fact, however, that hepatic metabolism of one drug is influenced by thyroid dysfunction does not necessarily imply that the metabolism of other drugs being also metabolized by the hepatic monooxygenases might also be altered. Thus, while the rate of elimination of tolbutamide and methimazole is increased bishydroxycoumarin, warfarin, phenytoin, and diazepam clearance are not altered by changes in thyroid function (Eichelbaum 1976, 1982; Shenfield 1981; Feely 1983). Since cardiac glycosides and β-adrenoreceptor blocking agents are among the most commonly used drugs in thyroid disease, changes in their disposition and its relation to drug toxicity will be discussed in more detail.

Interest in the pharmacokinetics of cardiac glycosides has been stimulated by the reports that unusually high doses of cardiac glycosides are required to control ventricular rate in hyperthyroid patients with atrial fibrillation (Wenckebach 1927; Boas 1931; Frye and Braunwald 1961; Morrow et al. 1963). Hypothyroid patients, however, are much more sensitive to glycosides and smaller doses than usual are required to treat congestive heart failure. The altered sensitivity to digitalis in patients with thyroid disease has been attributed to a change in intrinsic myocardial function (Buccino et al. 1967; Peacock and Morran 1963; Morrow et al. 1963). In addition, alterations in glycoside pharmacokinetics which were demonstrated by several investigators could be another possible explanation for the altered glycoside sensitivity in thyroid disease. In patients with thyrotoxicosis lower digoxin plasma levels have been observed, and in patients with myxoedema these levels are higher. Changes in renal and non-renal clearance and volume of distribution have been implicated for these changes in the pharmacokinetics of cardiac glycosides (for review see: Eichelbaum 1976, 1982; Shenfield 1981). Patients with thyrotoxicosis have, on average, shorter digoxin half-lives and an increased total plasma clearance. This increase in total clearance is due to both an increase in renal and metabolic clearance of digoxin. In addition, increased volumes of distribution were reported during thyrotoxicosis. But these changes in the volume of distribution seem to be due to some shortcomings in the pharmacokinetic analysis of the data. When the volume of distribution was calculated using a model independent method, no significant differences in volume of distribution could be observed in hyperthyroidism.

In hypothyroidism, digoxin half-lives are increased and total plasma clearance is decreased. These changes in the pharmacokinetics of digoxin in myxoedema can be attributed to both a decrease in renal and nonrenal clearance of digoxin. These findings may be the kinetic correlate for the clinical observation that larger than the usual dose of digitalis is required in thyrotoxic patients and lower in hypothyroid patients (Table 1).

In hypothyroidism, the likelihood of digitalis toxicity is increased due to the lower renal and metabolic clearance. In addition, there is evidence to suggest that in hypothyroidism the heart is more sensitive to cardiac glycosides. If these changes in drug disposition and sensitivity are not taken into account and the dose is reduced accordingly, toxicity will result.

Some of the clinical symptoms of thyrotoxicosis such as tachycardia, arrhythmias, sweating, nervousness, tremor and diarrhoea resemble signs of overactivity of the sympathetic nervous system and β-adrenoreceptor blocking

Table 1. Digoxin pharmacokinetic parameters in thyroid disease

Thyroid function	$t_{1/2}$ (h)	Cl_p (ml/min)	Cl_{ren} (ml/min)	Cl_{met} (ml/min)	V_{dss} (l)
eu[a]	33.3	–	90.3	–	–
hy[a]	35.7	–	158.0	–	–
ho[a]	42.2	–	83.0	–	–
hy[b]	30.0	–	–	–	–
ho[b]	43.3	–	–	–	–
hy[c]	24.9*	–	–	–	–
eu[c]	40.0*	–	–	–	–
hy[d]	24.2	270.3	119.6	150.7	387
eu[d]	38.7	137.9	69.7	68.2	253
hy[e]	28.9**	142.9	92.0	50.9	–
ho[e]	38.5**	103.5	48.5	55.0	–

eu: euthyroid, hy: hyperthyroid, ho: hypothyroid; Cl_p: total plasma clearance; Cl_{ren}: renal clearance; Cl_{met}: nonrenal clearance; V_{dss}: volume of distribution at steady-state. * Based on urinary excretion rates; ** Calculated assuming a V_{dss} of 350 l; –, no data available

[a] Doherty and Perkins (1966)
[b] Croxson and Ibbertson (1975)
[c] Gilfrich (1976)
[d] Bonelli et al. (1978); Koup (1980)
[e] Lawrence et al. (1977)

agents have been successfully used to relieve these symptoms although they do not appear to affect the underlying thyrotoxicosis itself. The effects of propranolol in thyrotoxicosis have been firmly established in a number of studies (for review: McDevitt 1976).

Although studies in animals with experimental thyrotoxicosis have demonstrated an increased number of β-adrenoceptors in the myocardium (Williams et al. 1977) the evidence for an increased number of β-adrenoceptors in thyrotoxic patients is still controversial. No changes in receptor numbers on peripheral leucocytes in thyrotoxicosis were reported by Williams et al. (1979) whereas Ginsberg et al. (1981) observed an increase in receptor numbers in subjects with triiodothyronine (T_3) induced thyrotoxicosis. Sensitivity to physiological concentrations of exogenous catecholamines in patients with hypothyroidism and hyperthyroidism seems to be unaltered (McDevitt et al. 1978).

Due to the widespread use of β-adrenoreceptor antagonists a great deal of studies has focused on the alterations of the pharmacokinetics of this group of drugs in thyroid disease (for review: Feely 1983). As in euthyroid patients, propranolol levels have been shown to be highly variable in hyperthyroid patients (Rubenfeld et al. 1979; Feely et al. 1980). Thus, the therapeutic failure of propranolol in controlling thyrotoxic symptoms in some hyperthyroid patients at propranolol dosages which achieves β-adrenoreceptor blockade, in most euthyroid patients could be due to an altered propranolol disposition in thyrotoxicosis. The question whether or not thyrotoxicosis can cause a change in propranolol disposition has been a matter of controversy. Bell et al. (1977),

Ishizaki et al. (1980), and Tawara et al. (1981) could not observe any significant alterations in propranolol half-life and oral clearance in hyperthyroid patients. Recent studies by Feely et al. (for review: Feely 1983) have clearly demonstrated that the systemic clearance of propranolol in hyperthyroidism is increased by approximately 50%, which seems to be due to an increase in liver blood flow. Since clearance of propranolol given orally was also increased in thyrotoxicosis resulting in a lower bioavailability, these findings indicate an increase in hepatic drug metabolism.

With regard to the effect of hypothyroidism on the disposition of β-blockers little information is available. Although single dose studies could not demonstrate significant changes in the pharmacokinetics of propranolol, data by Feely, Crooks and Stevenson (1981) suggest an influence of myxoedema on propranolol steady-state concentrations (C_{ss}). In hypothyroid patients treated with an oral dose of 160 mg propranolol daily, propranolol C_{ss} were on average higher (116.8 ± 20.4 ng/ml) as compared to hyperthyroid patients (38.3 ± 6.2 ng/ml). Following thyroxine treatment, C_{ss} declined to 69 ± 16.3 ng/ml.

Myxoedema is often associated with coronary artery disease. Aggravation of angina pectoris or precipitation of acute myocardial infarction has been described after attempting thyroid replacement therapy (Levine 1980). Therefore, treatment with a β-adrenoceptor antagonist is indicated. When initiating such a therapy it should be kept in mind that hypothyroid patients often have compromised cardiac function and therefore administration of a β-adrenoceptor antagonist might precipitate congestive heart failure. In addition, clearance after oral dosing with propranolol is decreased in hypothyroidism as compared to clearance after normalization of thyroid function in the same patient, thus requiring a lower dose of β-blockers in myxoedema. On the other hand, correction of hypothyroidism reduces steady-state concentrations of propranolol and therefore requires dose adjustment.

Mice and rat have been observed to have an enhanced toxicity and mortality with imipramine, desipramine, monoamine oxidase inhibitors and barbiturates following administration of thyroxine (Carrier and Buday 1961; Prange and Lipton 1962; Prange et al. 1964; Ellingwood and Prange 1964; Coville and Telford 1969). In agreement with these animal studies, potentiated extrapyramidal reactions to fluphenazine and neurotoxic effects of haloperidol in thyrotoxic patients have been reported. Sudden death has been observed following administration of haloperidol or phenothiazines to hyperthyroid patients due to aspiration asphyxia as a consequence of laryngeal-pharyngeal dystonia (Lake and Fann 1973; Hamadah and Teggin 1974; Weiner 1979; Witschy and Redmond 1981).

The prolonged prothrombin time in patients treated with coumarin-type anticoagulants concurrently suffering from hyperthyroidism seems to be the result of a increased catabolism of the vitamin K-dependent clotting factors, rather than inhibition of drug metabolism of the anticoagulants. In hypothyroid patients their hypothrombinaemic action is decreased due to an unusually slow rate of decay of the vitamin K-dependent clotting factors (Self et al. 1975).

Diabetes

Although diabetes mellitus is a very common disease, the incidence being 3–4% in the population, there is a paucity of information about this endocrine disorder on drug disposition and drug toxicity. Diabetes mellitus and insulin treatment have been shown to alter drug metabolism in man. Thus, the rate of O-dealkylation of phenacetin to paracetamol and its subsequent conjugation are impaired in untreated diabetic patients. If the impaired rate of O-dealkylation of phenacetin leads to an increased rate of formation of 2-hydroxy phenetidin, thus resulting in an increased methemoglobinaemia has not been evaluated. Treatment with insulin reverted phenacetin metabolism to normal (Dajani et al. 1974). In accordance with this observation are the findings of Daintith et al. (1976) who observed an increased rate of elimination of antipyrine in insulin treated patients, but not by chlorpropamide or tolbutamide treatment. It remains to be proven, however, if these changes in drug metabolism are a common phenomenon and if they are of relevance to drug toxicity in diabetic patients.

Hypoparathyroidism

There is a lack of data concerning the influence of this endocrine disorder on drug toxicity. Precipitation of congestive heart failure has been reported in a 6-year-old girl suffering from idiopathic hypoparathyroidism treated with anticonvulsant drugs. Although calcium ions play an essential role in the excitation-contraction process of the myocardium, heart failure due to hypocalcemia is rare. It seems that additional factors which further lower serum calcium concentration are required for the precipitation of heart failure in hypoparathyroidism. Thus, treatment with anticonvulsant drugs could lower serum calcium by its effect on vitamin D metabolism. Since, due to the concomitant anticonvulsant drug treatment, susceptibility to the convulsive manifestation of hypocalcemia is masked, severe hypocalcemia can develop and may cause heart failure (Benderly et al. 1980).

Acute dystonic reactions to prochlorperazine at small doses have been observed by Schaaf and Payne (1966) in hypoparathyroid patients, thus indicating a striking phenothiazine toxicity in this disease. Some patients experienced dangerous laryngospasm and asphyxia. This phenothiazine sensitivity may persist after treatment of hypoparathyroidism. An acute dystonic reaction to phenothiazines should suggest the possibility of this rare disease. If this increased toxicity is due to altered drug disposition or sensitivity is not clear since no studies have been carried out.

Hyperparathyroidism

Hypercalcemia has been demonstrated to increase the toxicity of cardiac glycosides, and therefore when treatment with these glycosides is necessary smaller doses should be administered and the patient carefully evaluated for signs of toxicity.

Pheochromocytoma

Pheochromocytome is often associated with persistent tachycardia, arrhythmias and angina pectoris and therefore treatment with a β-adrenoreceptor antagonist is indicated. It should be kept in mind, however, that β-blockade should never be induced without initially inducing α-blockade. If β-adrenoceptor blockers are administered in the absence of α-blockade a life-threatening hypertensive crisis can be elicited which is due to a vasoconstriction caused by the stimulation of α-receptors by the excessive high levels of catecholamines (Grago et al. 1967; Manger and Gifford 1977).

Heart failure may be precipitated by the administration of β-adrenoceptor antagonists in patients with catecholamine-induced cardiomyopathy due to pheochromocytoma.

Increased digitalis toxicity has also been observed in this condition due to the augmented myocardial irritability by excessive circulating catecholamines (Manger and Gifford 1977).

Conclusions

Endocrine disorders can influence cardiac, hepatic and renal function, thus leading to changes in drug disposition which in turn can lead to altered drug response and toxicity. The data available so far do not allow general prediction of how dosage modifications in endocrine disease are required in order to avoid drug toxicity.

References

Bell JM, Russell CJ, Nelson JK, Kelly JE, McDevitt DG (1977) Studies on the effect of thyroid dysfunction on the elimination of β-adrenoceptor blocking drugs. Br J Clin Pharmacol 4: 79–82

Benderly A, Etzioni A, Levy J (1980) Idiopathic hypoparathyroidism and anticonvulsive treatment as a possible cause for cardiac failure. Helv Paediatr Acta 35: 501–504

Boas EP (1931) Digitalis dosage in auricular fibrillation. Am Heart J 6: 788–803

Bonelli J, Haydl H, Hruby K, Kaik G (1978) The pharmacokinetics of digoxin in patients with manifest hyperthyroidism and after normalization of thyroid function. Int J Clin Pharmacol 16: 302–306

Buccino RA, Spann JR, Pool PE, Sonnenblick EH, Braunwald E (1967) Influence of the thyroid state on the intrinsic contractile properties and energy stores of the myocardium. J Clin Invest 46: 1669–1682

Carrier RN, Buday PV (1961) Augmentation of toxicity of monoamine oxidase inhibitor by thyroid feeding. Nature 191: 1107

Coville PF, Telford JM (1969) Changes in drug sensitivity in hyperthyroidism. Br J Pharmacol 36: 189P

Crooks J, Hedley SJ, Macnee C, Stevenson IH (1973) Changes in drug metabolising ability in thyroid disease. Br J Clin Pharmacol 49: 156P–157P

Croxson MS, Ibbertson HK (1975) Serum digoxin in patients with thyroid disease. Br Med J 3: 566–568

Daintith H, Stevenson IH, O'Malley K (1976) Influence of diabetes mellitus on drug metabolism in man. Int J Clin Pharmacol 13: 55–58

Dajani RM, Kayyali S, Saheb SE, Birbari (1974) A study of the physiological disposition of acetophenitidin by the diabetic man. Comp Gen Pharmacol 5: 1

Doherty JE, Perkins WH (1966) Digoxin metabolism in hypo- and hyperthyroidism – Studies with tritiated digoxin in thyroid disease. Ann Intern Med 64: 3

Eichelbaum M (1976) Drug metabolism in thyroid disease. Clin Pharmacokin 1: 339–350

Eichelbaum M (1982) Dosage modification in patients with hormonal dysfunction. In: Yoshida H, Hagihara Y, Ebashi S (eds) Advances in pharmacology and therapeutics II, vol 6. Pergamon Press, Oxford New York, pp 187–196

Eichelbaum M, Bodem G, Gugler R, Schneider-Deters Ch, Dengler HJ (1974) Influence of thyroid status on plasma half-life of antipyrine in man. N Engl J Med 290: 1040–1042

Ellinwood EH, Prange AJ (1964) Effect of epinephrine pretreatment on pentobarbital sleeping time of mice with altered thyroid status. Nature 201: 305–306

Feely J, Stevenson IH, Crooks J (1980) Propranolol dynamics in thyrotoxicosis. Clin Pharmacol Ther 28: 40–44

Feely J, Crooks J, Stevenson IH (1981) Plasma propranolol steady-state concentrations in thyroid disorders. Eur J Clin Pharmacol 19: 329–333

Feely J (1983) Clinical pharmacokinetics of β-adrenoceptor blocking drugs in thyroid disease. Clin Pharmacokin 8: 1–16

Frye RL, Braunwald E (1961) Studies on digitalis III – The influence of tri-iodothyronine on digitalis requirements. Circulation 23: 376

Gilfrich HJ (1976) Untersuchungen zur Pharmakokinetik von Digoxin bei hyperthyreoten Patienten. Verh Dtsch Ges. Inn Med 82: 1726–1728

Gillette JR (1965) Drug toxicity as a result of interference with physiological control mechanisms. Ann NY Acad Sci 123: 42–54

Ginsberg AM, Clutter WE, Shah SD, Cryer PE (1981) Triiodothyronine-induced thyrotoxicosis increases mononuclear leukocyte β-adrenergic receptor density in man. J Clin Invest 67: 1785–1791

Grago RM, Eckholt JW, Wiswell JG (1967) Pheochromocytoma – treatment with – and β-adrenergic blocking drugs. JAMA 202: 104–108

Hamadah K, Teggin AF (1974) Haloperidol, thyrotoxicosis, and neurotoxicity. Lancet 2: 1019–1020

Ishizaki T, Masuno M, Tawara K (1980) No enhanced elimination of propranolol in patients with hypothyroidism. Res Commun Chem Pathol Pharmacol 29: 473–485

Kato R (1977) Drug metabolism under pathological and abnormal physiological states in animals and man. Xenobiotica 7: 25–92

Kato R, Gillette JR (1965) Sex differences in the effects of abnormal physiological states on the metabolism of drugs by rat liver microsomes. J Pharmacol Exp Ther 150: 285–291

Koup JR (1980) Distribution of digoxin in hyperthyroid patients. Int J Clin Pharmacol Biopharm 18: 236

Lake CR, Fann WE (1973) Possible potentiation of haloperidol neurotoxicity in acute hyperthyroidism. Br J Psychiatry 123: 523–525

Lawrence JR, Sumner DJ, Kalk WJ, Ratcliffe WA, Whiting B, Gray K, Lindsay M (1977) Digoxin kinetics in patients with thyroid dysfunction. Clin Pharmacol Ther 22: 7–13

Levine HD (1980) Compromise therapy in the patient with angina pectoris and hypothyroidism. A clinical assessment. Am J Med 69: 411–418

Manger WM, Gifford RW (1977) Pheochromocytoma. In: Manger WM, Gifford RW (eds) Pheochromocytoma. Springer, New York Heidelberg Berlin, pp 306–315

Marble A, Selenkow HA, Rose LI, Dluhy RG, Williams GH (1980) In: Avery GS (ed) Drug treatment. Churchill Livingstone, Edinburgh London, pp 496–498

McDevitt DG (1976) Propranolol in the treatment of thyrotoxicosis: a review. Postgrad Med J (Suppl 4) 52: 157–161

McDevitt DG, Riddell SG, Hadden DR, Montgomery DAD (1978) Catecholamine sensitivity in hyperthyroidism and hypothyroidism. Br J Clin Pharmacol 6: 297–301
Morrow DH, Gaffney TE, Braunwald E (1963) Influence of hyper- and hypothyroidism on the myocardial response of ouabain. J Pharmacol Exp Ther 140: 324–328
Peacock WF, Moran NC (1963) Influence of thyroid state on positive inotropic effect of ouabain on isolated ventricle strips. Proc Soc Exp Biol Med 113: 526–530
Prange AJ, Lipton MA (1962) Enhancement of imipramine mortality in hyperthyroid mice. Nature 196: 588–589
Prange AJ, Lipton MA, Love GN (1964) Effect of altered thyroid status on desmethylimipramine mortality in mice. Nature 204: 1205–1206
Prange AJ, Lipton MA, Shearin RB, Love GN (1966) The influence of thyroid status on the effects and metabolism of pentobarbital and thiopental. Biochem Pharmacol 15: 237–248
Rumbaugh RC, Kramer PE, Colby HD (1978) Dose-dependent actions of thyroxine on hepatic drug metabolism in male and female rats. Biochem Pharmacol 27: 2027–2031
Schaaf M, Payne CA (1966) Dystonic reactions to prochlorpenazine in hypoparathyroidism. N Engl J Med 275: 991–995
Self T, Weissburst M, Wooten E, Straughn A, Oliver J (1975) Warfarin-induced hypoprothrombinaemia: potentiation by hyperthyroidism. JAMA 231: 1165
Shenfield GM, Thompson J, Horn DB (1977) Plasma and urinary digoxin in thyroid dysfunction. Eur J Clin Pharmacol 12: 437–443
Shenfield GM (1981) Influence of thyroid dysfunction on drug pharmacokinetics. Clin Pharmacokin 6: 275–297
Tawara K, Kawashima K, Ishikawa H, Yamamoto K, Saito K, Ebihara A, Yoshida S (1981) Pharmacokinetics and pharmacodynamics of propranolol stereoisomers and hyperthyroid patients. Eur J Clin Pharmacol 19: 197–203
Weiner ME (1979) Haloperidol, hyperthyroidism, and sudden death. Am J Psychiatry 136: 717–718
Wenckebach KF, Winterberg H (1927) Die unregelmäßige Herztätigkeit. Wilhelm Engelmann, Leipzig, S 493
Williams LT, Lefkowitz RJ, Watanabe AM, Hathaway DR, Besch HR Jr (1977) Thyroid hormone regulation of β-adrenergic receptor number. J Biol Chem 252: 2787–2789
Williams RS, Guthrow CE, Lefkowitz RJ (1979) β-adrenergic receptors of human lymphocytes are unaltered by hyperthyroidism. J Clin Endocrinol Metab 48: 503–505
Witschy JK, Redmond FC (1981) Extrapyramidal reaction to fluphenazine potentiated by thyrotoxicosis. Am J Psychiatry 138: 246–247

Disease, Metabolism and Reproduction in the Toxic Response to Drugs and Other Chemicals
Arch. Toxicol., Suppl. 7, 48–57 (1984)

Alterations of Drug Toxicity in Neuropsychiatric Disease States

E. Perucca[1] and A. Richens[2]

[1] Institute of Medical Pharmacology, University of Pavia, Piazza Botta, 10, 27100 Pavia, Italy
[2] Department of Pharmacology and Therapeutics, Welsh National School of Medicine, Heath Park, Cardiff CF4 4XN, Great Britain

Abstract. Potentially adverse alterations in drug response in patients with neuropsychiatric disease can be divided into two categories: those arising from the pathological state itself (e.g., enhanced responsiveness to phenylephrine in patients with chronic autonomic failure) and those arising from interactions with the pharmacological treatment used for such disease (e.g., reversal of the antihypertensive action of guanethidine by imipramine). Sound knowledge of the pharmacological profile of individual compounds and of the pathophysiology of the disease is essential if drug therapy is to be used safely and effectively in these patients.

Key words: Neuropsychiatry – Interactions – Neurological disorders

Introduction

The importance of disease states as a factor predisposing to drug toxicity is widely recognized. The greatest emphasis, however, is usually placed on the implications of altered drug kinetics in conditions such as renal failure, hepatic dysfunction and cardiovascular disorders. Relatively little attention, on the other hand, is paid to the role of neurological and psychiatric disease.

Potentially adverse alterations in drug response are not uncommon in neuropsychiatric patients. Since the function of virtually every physiological system is under nervous control, it is not surprising that these alterations are seen at various sites and with a wide variety of drugs.

Adverse reactions related to altered drug response in patients with neuropsychiatric disorders can be classified into two categories: those arising from the pathological state itself and those resulting from an interaction with the pharmacological treatment used in such disorders.

Alterations in Drug Response Caused by the Pathological State

Almost invariably, adverse reactions caused by this mechanism represent an exaggeration of an otherwise normal pharmacological effect. In most cases, these exaggerated responses can be easily explained and predicted on the basis of the drug's pharmacology and of the known functional disturbances caused by the disease. Examples include the precipitation of severe muscle weakness by aminoglycoside antibiotics in patients with myasthenia gravis, or the occurrence of marked supine hypertension following conventional doses of directly acting sympathomimetic agents in patients with chronic autonomic failure.

Examples of altered drug responses in selected neuropsychiatric disease states will be discussed below.

Parkinson's Disease

Levo-dopa Induced Dyskinesias. It has been reported that L-dopa induced dyskinesias are far more common in patients with Parkinson's disease than in those with apparently intact nigrostriatal pathways (Chase et al. 1973; Parke 1981). These dyskinesias, that are characterized by abnormal involuntary movements of the limbs, hands, trunk and lingual-facial-buccal musculature, are generally considered to result from an excessive dopaminergic stimulation in the basal ganglia. There is evidence that, as nigro-striatal neurones degenerate, the receptors in the post-synaptic membrane innervated by the degenerating fibres become supersensitive to dopamine (Anden 1970). The increased susceptibility of Parkinsonian patients to this disabling adverse effect of L-dopa therapy can therefore be explained as a consequence of denervation supersensitivity in the striatum (Weiner and Bergen 1977).

Several lines of evidence support this hypothesis. In animal models, apparently similar dyskinesias can be induced by experimental procedures resulting in striatal dopamine supersensitivity (Ungerstedt et al. 1975). In Parkinsonian patients the prevalence and the severity of the dyskinesias appear to be related to the duration of the disease (Weiner and Bergen 1977). Presumably, the patients with the longest duration of the disease are also those with the greatest degree of nigro-striatal degeneration and, hence, the greatest degree of dopamine supersensitivity. This interpretation is also supported by the observation that the dyskinesias usually start on the side first affected by the disease (Weiner and Bergen 1977).

Administration of non-selective dopamine receptor blockers such as the phenothiazines effectively controls the dyskinesias, but this form of treatment is not recommended because of the concurrent worsening of the Parkinsonian symptoms. More promising results have been obtained with selective dopamine$_2$-receptor antagonists such as oxperomide and tiapride (Parkes 1981).

Exaggerated Response to Pressor Drugs. Many patients with Parkinson's disease show degenerative changes in the autonomic system. The altered drug responses seen in this condition are discussed below under the heading Chronic Autonomic Failure.

Aggravation of Parkinsonian Symptoms by Antipsychotic Agents. Most antipsychotic agents and many anti-emetic drugs are potent dopamine-receptor blockers. Therefore, it is not surprising that the administration of even small doses of these agents can markedly aggravate the primary biochemical defect of Parkinson's disease, with worsening of the clinical picture.

Huntington's Chorea

Induction or Worsening of Chorea by L-Dopa. L-Dopa aggravates the abnormal movements of Huntington's chorea and can be used to identify individuals at risk with a family history of the disease. Individuals at risk of developing Huntington's chorea appear to be much more sensitive to induction of abnormal movements by L-dopa than those not at risk (Kutt and McDowell 1980).

Dementia and Degenerative CNS Disease

Drug-Induced Toxic Delirium. Patients with dementia or degenerative CNS disease appear to be more susceptible to develop toxic delirium. This condition is a drug-induced syndrome characterized by disorientation, confusion, anxiety, delusions and hallucinations. The drugs more commonly implicated include sedatives, antidepressants, tranquilizers, reserpine, methyldopa, anticholinergics, alcohol, digitalis and cimetidine (Kutt and McDowell 1980).

Multiple Sclerosis

Hypersensitivity to Opiates. Patients with multiple sclerosis are reported to show an increased susceptibility to the depressant effects of morphine (Jaffe and Martin 1980).

Hyperkalaemic Reactions to Succinylcholine. Patients with multiple sclerosis may show an exaggerated hyperkalaemic response to succinylcholine (Cooperman 1970). The mechanisms responsible for this reaction will be discussed below (see Miscellaneous Neurological Disorders).

CNS Infections

Altered Permeability of the Blood-Brain Barrier. Meningeal inflammation is associated with an increased permeability of the blood brain barrier. This results in increased CNS penetration of a number of drugs. This phenomenon may have positive therapeutic implications (e.g., better availability of antimicrobials at the sites of infection) but may also predispose to adverse CNS reactions.

Epilepsy

Precipitation of Seizures. Several drugs, including nalidixic acid, isoniazid, tricyclic antidepressants, phenothiazines and baclofen have been reported to precipitate seizures. At therapeutic dosages, this effect appears to be relatively rare, at least with some of these agents.

Migraine

Aggravation of Migraine. Oral contraceptives may aggravate or precipitate attacks of migraine (Ryan 1978).

Cerebrovascular Disease

Precipitation of Ischemic Attacks. Ergotamine is contraindicated in patients with cerebrovascular disease because it may precipitate ischemic episodes. Antihypertensive drugs and other drugs causing a fall in blood pressure (e.g., phenothiazines) should also be used cautiously in these patients.

Increased Sensitivity to CNS Depressants. Patients with cerebrovascular disease are considered to be especially sensitive to the effects of sedatives.

Endocranial Hypertension

Aggravation by Respiratory Depressants. Respiratory depressants (e.g., morphine) may further increase the raised intracranial pressure due to cerebral tumours or trauma. This effect is due to cerebral vasodilation secondary to CO_2 retention.

Chronic Autonomic Failure

Hypersensitivity to Pressor Amines and Angiotensin. Chronic autonomic failure may occur as an isolated entity (idiopathic postural hypotension) and in association with Parkinson's disease or other neurological abnormalities (multiple system atrophy or the Shy-Drager syndrome). In all these conditions, postural hypotension may be the major presenting symptom.

Several studies have demonstrated that patients with chronic autonomic failure show a markedly exaggerated pressor response to noradrenaline, ephedrine, phenylephrine and other sympathomimetic agents (Bannister et al. 1979; Davies et al. 1979). This abnormality may result from a number of factors, namely: a decreased neuronal uptake (with termination of effect) of the amine due to degeneration of the sympathetic nerve terminals, the denervation supersensitivity of vascular smooth muscle (and myocardium) and an impaired baroreceptor control (Wilcox and Aminoff 1976; Bannister et al. 1979). Because of the latter defect, the pressor response to sympathetic amines may be accompanied in these patients by paradoxical tachycardia (Davies et al. 1978).

There is evidence that the pressor response to angiotensin II is also increased in patients with autonomic failure (Scroop and Whelan 1968; Bannister et al. 1969; Davies et al. 1979). Since angiotensin II can increase noradrenaline release and interact with the sympathetic nervous system in other ways, the enhanced responsiveness to this peptide may be explained, at least in part, by the development of denervation supersensitivity to catecholamines. This explanation is supported by the finding that the blood pressure rise caused by angiotensin can be antagonized in part by phentolamine. Other lines of evidence, on the other hand, seem to indicate the occurrence of a direct supersensitivity of angiotensin vascular receptors in patients with chronic autonomic failure (Davies et al. 1979).

Interestingly, fludrocortisone, a mineralocorticoid frequently used for the treatment of the postural hypotension, can increase further the pressor response to noradrenaline, but not to angiotensin II, in these patients (Davies et al. 1979).

Paradoxical Pressor Response to Saralasin. The presence of an altered sensitivity to drugs affecting vascular resistance in patients with chronic autonomic failure is underlined by the observation that these patients show a consistent dose-dependent pressor response to the angiotensin receptor blocker saralasin. This paradoxical response, that may also be seen in hypertensive patients, is probably mediated by a drug-induced adrenergic discharge. The possible additional role of a partial agonist action of saralasin on supersensitive angiotensin receptors has also been discussed (Davies et al. 1979).

Fludrocortisone treatment has been shown to potentiate the pressor response to saralasin in these patients (Davies et al. 1979).

Miscellaneous Neurological Disorders

Exaggerated Hyperkalaemic Reactions to Succinylcholine in Neurological Patients. Administration of succinylcholine may cause a transient hyperkalaemia, which is due to release of intracellular potassium into the general circulation. In some patients this response may be exaggerated to the point of resulting in life-treatening hyperkalaemic reactions. Patients particularly susceptible appear to be those with burns, uraemia, severe abdominal infections, trauma, denervation injuries, spinal cord injuries, central nervous system disease (including multiple sclerosis), neuromuscular disease and head injury (for review: see Brass and Thompson 1982).

The primary source of the potassium released by succinylcholine is muscle. The suggestion has been made that the exaggerated hyperkalaemic response in the injury states listed above is due to enhanced cellular efflux of potassium from the neuromuscular end-plates during generalized depolarization (Gronert and Theye 1975). This theory is supported by the evidence that several types of nerve injuries result in an increased number of neuromuscular end-plates (Axelsson and Thesleff 1959). The observation that there may be a delay of several days in the development of the "vulnerability" to succinylcholine after the injury is also consistent with the time period required for end-plate proliferation (Gronert and Theye 1975). Alternatively, it may simply be postulated that the exaggerated hyperkalaemic response after injury is related to enhanced potassium release from the damaged muscle following stimulation (Cooperman 1970).

Psychiatric Disorders

Aggravation of Psychiatric Disease. A wide variety of drugs may cause or aggravate psychotic symptoms. Examples include L-dopa, bromocriptine, antidepressants, anticholinergics, pentazocine and corticosteroids.

A latent depressive disease can be precipitated by a number of therapeutic agents, including clonidine, methyldopa, reserpine, L-dopa, propranolol and oral contraceptives.

Patients with a previous history of psychiatric disease appear to be much more susceptible to these adverse effects.

Myasthenia Gravis

Aggravation or Unmasking of a Myasthenic Syndrome. In view of the pathophysiology of myasthenia gravis, it is not surprising that patients with this disease, even in subclinical or latent form, show an increased sensitivity to drugs depressing the neuromuscular transmission, e.g., curariform agents and general anaesthetics. This may result in failure of respiration to become adequate in the postoperative period.

The increased sensitivity of myasthenic patients to curariform agents can be exploited diagnostically in the provocative test with d-tubocurarine. Worsening of the muscle weakness after intravenous d-tubocurarine chloride (0.1–0.5 mg) in patients with minimal symptoms is strongly suggestive of myasthenia; since this test is potentially hazardous, it is important that the symptoms be reversed immediately by intravenous neostigmine. Moreover, an anesthesiologist with adequate resuscitatory facilities should be available at the bedside.

Several antibiotics, including streptomycin, neomycin, tobramycin, kanamycin, gentamycin, colistin, polimyxin B, bacitracin, clindomycin, lincomycin and tetracyclines have a weak neuromuscular blocking effect and may precipitate severe muscle weakness in myasthenic patients (Argov and Mastaglia 1979). Beta-blockers also have been shown to interfere with neuromuscular transmission (Larsen 1978) and occasionally to induce or unmask a myasthenic syndrome (Herishanu and Rosenberg 1975). Other drugs that can cause or exacerbate a pre-existing myasthenic syndrome include penicillamine, quinine, quinidine, chloroquine, lithium, chlorpromazine, phenytoin, thyroid hormones and magnesium containing carthartics (Mastaglia 1982).

Enhanced Susceptibility to CNS Depressants. There is some evidence that patients with myasthenia gravis are particularly sensitive to CNS depressants such as morphine, barbiturates and tranquilizers (Flacke 1973).

Miscellaneous Muscular Disorders

Aggravation or Unmasking of a Myotonic Syndrome. A number of drugs have been shown to exacerbate or to unmask a myotonic syndrome. These include depolarizing muscle relaxants (e.g., succinylcholine), beta-blockers, and the β_2-adrenergic agonist fenoterol. Diuretics are also likely to cause a similar effect (Mastaglia 1982).

The precipitation of myotonic symptoms by depolarizing muscle relaxants appears to be particularly hazardous, because it may lead to problems with tracheal intubation and ventilation (Mitchell et al. 1978). Therefore patients with myotonia congenita, myotonic dystrophy and other myotonic disorders should preferentially be given, in the event of a surgical operation, a non-depolarizing neuromuscular blocking drug.

Susceptibility to Malignant Hyperthermia in Muscular Disease. Malignant hyperthermia is a potentially lethal adverse drug reaction that can be precipitated by various anaesthetic agents, succinylcholine and other muscle relaxants. Predisposition to this reaction is genetically determined. Susceptible individuals may have a clinical or more often subclinical myopathy associated with elevated serum creatin phosphokinase levels and abnormal findings at electromyography or biopsy. Attacks of malignant hyperpyrexia have also been described in patients with progressive congenital myopathy, central core disease, myotonia congenita, myotonic dystrophy, Duchenne muscular dystrophy, Schwartz-Jampel syndrome and osteogenesis imperfecta (for review: see Mastaglia 1982).

Alterations in Response Caused by Drug Interactions

Many neurological and psychiatric diseases require long-term pharmacological treatment. Therefore, these patients are particularly liable to receive multiple drug therapy.

Alterations in response caused by interactions with drugs used in neuropsychiatric disorders are a common source of drug toxicity. A number of illustrative examples are listed in Table 1. It is important that the clinician

Table 1. Examples of important adverse drug interactions in neuropsychiatric patients

Interacting drugs	Mechanism and/or effect of interaction
Antianxiety agents and hypnotics	
CNS depressants (including alcohol)	Impairment of psychomotor skills and increased CNS depression
Anticonvulsants	
Sulthiame Valproic acid Chloramphenicol Disulfiram Isoniazid Phenylbutazone Propoxyphene	These drugs inhibit the metabolism of various anticonvulsants, with consequent potentiation of effect
Oral anticoagulants	Some anticonvulsants may induce the metabolism of dicoumarol and other anticoagulants, leading to decreased response
Vitamin D	Anticonvulsants stimulate vitamin D metabolism and cause osteomalacia
Glucocorticoids Metyrapone Oral contraceptives	Anticonvulsants may stimulate the metabolism of these agents resulting in failure of diagnostic tests and loss of prophylactic or therapeutic efficacy
Griseofulvin Frusemide	Some anticonvulsants decrease the gastrointestinal absorption of these drugs
Antimigraine agents	
Antihypertensive agents	Some patients are more sensitive to vasoconstrictors. Pizotifen may antagonise the effect of guanethidine and other adrenergic neurone blocking drugs

Table 1 (continued)

Interacting drugs	Mechanism and/or effect of interaction
CNS depressants	Potentiation of CNS depression induced by clonidine
Hypoglycaemic agents	Hypoglycaemia potentiated by propranolol
Phenothiazines	Chlorpromazine inhibits propranolol metabolism
Antiparkinsonian agents	
Antipsychotics	Precipitation of parkinsonian symptoms Aggravation of anticholinergic side effects
Decarboxylase inhibitors (peripheral)	Potentiation of the central effect of L-dopa (interaction usually beneficial since it allows reduction of L-dopa dose and peripheral side effects)
Monoamine oxidase inhibitors	Exaggeration of L-dopa effects (hypertensive crisis and hyperpyrexia may occur). Aggravation of anticholinergic side effects
Pyridoxine	Reversal of the effects of L-dopa (interaction does not occur if L-dopa is associated with a decarboxylase inhibitor)
Antipsychotic agents (apart from lithium)	
Antihypertensive agents	Chlorpromazine and some other antipsychotics can antagonize the effects of guanethidine. Antipsychotic drugs with α-receptor blocking properties can enhance the fall in blood pressure caused by some antihypertensives. Methyldopa potentiates the toxicity of haloperidol
Lithium	See below
Antiparkinsonian agents	See above
Propranolol	Chlorpromazine inhibits propranolol metabolism
Lithium	
Diuretics	By causing loss of sodium, diuretics can cause retention of lithium and intoxication
Methyldopa	Toxicity at relatively low lithium levels may occur
Pancuronium	Enhanced neuromuscular blockade
Antipsychotic drugs	Lithium may decrease the bioavailability of chlorpromazine and potentiate the toxicity of haloperidol
Sodium chloride	Intake of large amounts of sodium enhances the elimination of lithium
Monoamine oxidase inhibitors (MAOI)	
Alcoholic drinks and certain foods	Tyramine content results in increased noradrenaline levels (severe hypertension, etc.)
Amphetamines, indirectly acting sympathomimetic agents, guanethidine (initial doses), methyldopa, etc.	Increased noradrenaline levels. Severe hypertension. headaches, etc.
L-dopa and anticholinergics	See above
CNS depressants	Potentiation of CNS depression
Oral hypoglycaemic agents	Potentiation of hypoglycaemia
Pethidine	Severe reaction (excitation, sweating, hyper- or hypotension, etc.)

Table 1 (continued)

Interacting drugs	Mechanism and/or effect of interaction
Tricyclic antidepressants	Increased noradrenaline levels (severe hypertension, etc.), hyperpyrexia, coma
Non-MAOI antidepressants	
Anticholinergic agents (including some anti-parkinsonian drugs, antipsychotic, antihistamines)	Potentiation of anticholinergic effects
Antihypertensive agents	Tricyclic antidepressants and some of the newer antidepressants antagonize the effects of guanethidine, debrisoquine, bethanidine, clonidine and sometimes methyldopa (severe overshoot in blood pressure may occur). Antidepressants with α-adrenergic blocking properties may enhance the fall in blood pressure caused by some antihypertensive agents
CNS-depressants (including alcohol)	Impairment of psychomotor skills
Monoamine oxidase inhibitors	See above
Sympathomimetic amines	Potentiation of pressor response

familiarizes himself with the most important among these interactions, some of which can have even lethal clinical consequences.

Avoidance of the more hazardous combinations, reduction of unnecessary polypharmacy and careful clinical observation represent the mainstay for a safer use of drug therapy in these patients.

References

Anden NE (1970) Pharmacological and anatomical implications of induced abnormal movements with L-dopa. In: Barbeau A, McDowell F (eds) L-dopa and parkinsonism. FA Davis, Philadelphia, pp 132–143

Argov Z, Mastaglia FL (1979) Drug-induced disorders of neuromuscular transmission. Adverse Drug Reaction Bull 74: 264–267

Axelsson J, Thesleff S (1959) A study of supersensitivity in denervated mammalian skeletal muscle. J Physiol 147: 178–193

Bannister R, Ardill L, Fentem P (1969) An assessment of various methods of treatment of idiopathic orthostatic hypotension. Q J Med 38: 377–395

Bannister R, Davies B, Holly E, Rosenthal T, Sever P (1979) Defective cardiovascular reflexes and supersensitivity to sympathomimetic drugs in autonomic failure. Brain 102: 163–176

Brass EP, Thompson WL (1982) Drug-induced electrolyte abnormalities. Drugs 24: 207–228

Chase TN, Holden EM, Brody JA (1973) Levodopa-induced dyskinesias. Arch Neurol 29: 328–330

Cooperman LH (1970) Succinylcholine-induced hyperkalaemia in neuromuscular disease. JAMA 213: 1767–1871

Davies B, Bannister R, Sever P (1978) Pressor amines and monoamine oxidase inhibitors for treatment of postural hypotension in autonomic failure. Lancet 1: 172–175

Davies B, Bannister R, Sever P, Wilcox C (1979) The pressor actions of noradrenaline, angiotensin II and saralasin in chronic autonomic failure treated with fludrocortisone. Br J Clin Pharmacol 8: 253–260

Flacke W (1973) Treatment of myasthenia gravis. N Engl J Med 288: 27–29
Gronert GA, Theye RA (1975) Pathophysiology of hyperkalaemia induced by succinylcholine. Anesthesiology 43: 89–99
Herishanu Y, Rosenberg P (1975) Beta-blockers and myasthenia gravis. Ann Intern Med 83: 834–835
Jaffe JH, Martin WR (1980) Opioid analgesics and antagonists. In: Goodman Gilman A, Goodman LS, Gilman A (eds) The pharmacological basis of therapeutics. MacMillan, New York, pp 494–534
Kutt H, McDowell FH (1980) Neurological disease. In: Avery G (ed) Drug treatment. Adis Press, Sydney New York, pp 1010–1056
Larsen A (1978) On the neuromuscular effects of pindolol and sotalol in the rat. Acta Physiol Scand 102: 35–40
Mastaglia FL (1982) Adverse effects of drugs on muscle. Drugs 24: 304–321
Mitchell MM, Ali HH, Savarese JJ (1978) Myotonia and neuromuscular blocking agents. Anesthesiology 49: 44–48
Parke JD (1981) Adverse effects of antiparkinsonian drugs. Drugs 21: 341–353
Ryan RF (1978) A controlled study of the effect of oral contraceptives on migraine. Headache 17: 250
Scroop GG, Whelan RF (1968) The effects of alpha-adrenergic receptor blockade and sympathetic denervation on the pressor action of angiotensin in man. Aust J Exp Biol Med Sci 46: 563–572
Ungerstedt U, Ljunberg T, Hoffer B, Siggins S (1975) Dopaminergic supersensitivity in the striatum. In: Calne DB, Chase TN, Barbeau A (eds) Advances in neurology. Dopaminergic mechanisms, vol 9. Raven Press, New York, pp 57–65
Weiner WJ, Bergen D (1977) Prevention and management of the side effects of levodopa. In: Klawans HL (ed) Clinical neuropharmacology, vol 2. Raven Press, New York, pp 1–23
Wilcox CS, Aminoff MJ (1976) Blood pressure responses to noradrenaline and dopamine infusions in Parkinson's disease and the Shy-Drager syndrome. Br J Clin Pharmacol 3: 207–214

Disease, Metabolism and Reproduction in the Toxic Response to Drugs and Other Chemicals
Arch. Toxicol., Suppl. 7, 58–65 (1984)

Alterations of Drug Toxicity in Cardiovascular Disease

F. Ledda

Department of Pharmacology and Clinical Toxicology, University of Florence,
Viale G.B. Morgagni, 65, 50134 Florence, Italy

Abstract. The past ten years have seen a rapid expansion in the field of cardiovascular pharmacology. New indications for old agents have appeared and new powerful drugs have been introduced, including entirely new classes of compounds. The availability of so many agents has considerably expanded the risk of life-threatening adverse reactions due to overdosage or to inappropriate drug associations. The liability to encounter severe side effects is often enhanced in patients with underlying cardiovascular diseases, which may change the usual drug action either by inducing modifications of the drug pharmacokinetic or by altering the receptor sensitivity. In most cases these kind of reactions are predictable on the ground of the knowledge of both the drug mechanism of action and the functional alterations induced by the disease. However entirely unexpected adverse reactions may also occur in cases in which unrecognized alterations exist, whose pathophysiology has not been fully elucidated. Recent demonstrations that some physiopathological influences, as well as prolonged drug treatment, can modulate the number of adrenergic receptors in the cardiovascular system has offered a clue to a better understanding of at least some episodes of altered responsiveness to cardiovascular drugs, previously considered of unknown origin. The possibility of obtaining some indications of the adrenoceptor status in man, by the assessment of the receptor density in circulating blood cells, seems to represent a promising diagnostic approach to the problem of disease induced adrenergic regulation and its possible consequences in terms of altered drug responsiveness.

Key words: Digitalis – Calcium-entry blockers – Antiarrhythmic agents – Beta-adrenoceptor antagonists – Adverse effects

The problem of adverse drug reactions in cardiovascular disease states has been widely recognised since the introduction of digitalis glycosides and quinidine in cardiac therapy.

The chance of encountering severe untoward reactions has been considerably increased in subsequent years, mainly as a consequence of the introduction of entirely new classes of powerful compounds, which often have narrow therapeutic indices. The list of drugs able to lead to cardiovascular complications has become quite impressive (for two recent reviews see Deglin et al. 1977; Opie 1980); at present it includes old and new cardiovascular drugs (such as digitalis glycosides, antiarrhythmic agents, calcium-entry blockers and beta-adrenoceptor antagonists) as well as drugs used to treat non-cardiac problems (tricyclic antidepressants, phenothiazine antipsychotics, anthracycline antibiotics and so on). Moreover, many reports have alerted the cardiology medical community to the possibility that some specific cardiovascular diseases may be predisposed to adverse reactions to the above-mentioned classes of drugs. However, the ability to prevent such events obviously depends not simply on the delineation of the circumstances under which adverse reactions may occur, but chiefly on the knowledge of the mechanisms which are possibly involved in any given kind of reaction.

Although the designation of these mechanisms is not always easy, some remarkable advances have been made recently in this field. For instance, it has been recently recognized that cardiac diseases may directly influence drug pharmacokinetics (Benowitz et al. 1976) by producing marked alterations in renal and hepatic blood flow. Since the blood flow to an organ of elimination is an important determinant of the disposition of compounds which are highly extracted by that organ, a reduction in cardiac output in patients with heart failure may result in a decrease in systemic clearance and in an increase in the drug concentration at the steady state (Williams et al. 1980). Lidocaine (Stenson et al. 1971), prazosin (Baughman et al. 1979) and furosemide (Andreasen et al. 1977) are only a few examples of drugs whose disposition may be affected by cardiac disease. The distribution of drugs which are not significantly extracted by the liver may also be changed; for instance it has been found that the volume of distribution of quinidine is decreased in subjects with heart failure, with the consequence of a plasma concentration higher than in normal subjects (Ueda et al. 1978). However, adverse reactions due to alterations of pharmacokinetic processes can be easily detected and even prevented by careful attention to the blood levels of the drug in the subjects at risk.

On the contrary, real problems arise in cases in which severe adverse reactions are suddenly induced by usual drug doses able to produce therapeutic or even subtherapeutic, blood levels. Lack of adequate knowledge of the mechanism of drug action and of the existence of anatomical or functional predisposing factors, are the commonest causes of these events. In this connection, it is necessary to point out that instances of adverse drug reactions attributable to the existence of anatomical abnormalities of the cardiovascular system are indeed uncommon; the presence in some subjects of anomalous pathways which bypass the atrioventricular node (Durrer et al. 1970) is one of these rare instances. In fact, it is well known that in this kind of abnormality (Wolfe Parkinson Whyte syndrome) the rapid conduction of impulses through the anomalous pathway can induce a high ventricular rate in response to atrial flutter or fibrillation. Since digitalis is able to slow the conduction through the bundle of His, but is ineffective on the accessory pathway, the usual slowing of ventricular rate by digitalis glycosides is absent in patients with W.P.W. syndrome. On the contrary, the refractory period of the accessory pathway may be decreased by digitalis, the result being a "paradox effect" consisting of an increased ventricular rate (Sellers et al. 1977).

However, as previously stated, most cases of adverse reactions to drugs in cardiovascular disease states may simply result from the same mechanism of action which is responsible for the pharmacological effects.

For instance, the pharmacological effects of organic calcium-entry blockers are due to an inhibition of the slow inward calcium current, which contributes to the depolarization phase of sino-atrial and upper atrio-ventricular nodal cells, and is responsible for the excitation-contraction coupling in myocardial working cells (Fleckenstein 1977). Because of this "selective" mechanism of action serious complications have been induced by intravenous verapamil in patients with a pre-existing impaired function of the sinus node or of atrio-ventricular conduction (Hagemaeijer 1978). Although the depression of myocardial contractility in patients with a well preserved heart function is usually compensated for by a sympathetic reflex stimulation of the myocardium in response to the peripheral vasodilating effect (Singh et al. 1977), a marked cardiodepression has been induced in patients with an impaired ventricular function (Chew et al. 1981). It may be of some interest to recall that the ability to block calcium channels in myocardial fibers is shared by some cations, such as manganese, nickel and cobalt (Kohlhardt et al. 1973). Cobalt cardiomyopathy in heavy beer drinkers, a syndrome characterized by sudden heart failure, first observed in Canada, is still an interesting example of how the adverse effects of a noxious agent can be facilitated by underlying biochemical and functional alterations. In fact, experimental studies have suggested that the clinical manifestations of cobalt cardiotoxicity were mainly due to the potentiating effects of thiamine deficiency and myocardial damage induced by a chronic ethanol abuse (Alexander 1972).

In a review on drug cardiotoxicity it is almost obligatory to mention digitalis glycosides, since it is widely known that this class of drugs has a narrow therapeutic index. The many reported instances of digitalis toxicity due to pharmacokinetic interactions with quinidine (Doherty 1982) represent a further confirmation of the risk associated with the therapeutic use of cardioactive glycosides. The heart's sensitivity to the toxic effects of digitalis may be altered by a number of predisposing pathological conditions; among them electrolyte disorders (such as hypokalemia and hypocalcemia), hypoxemia and ischemia have been shown to reduce the heart's tolerance to cardioactive glycosides (Akera et al. 1981). An increased sensitivity to digitalis has been detected in patients with chronic pulmonary diseases and hypoxemia (Baum et al. 1959; Morrison et al. 1971); the use of cardiac glycosides in "cor pulmonale" may lead to a high incidence of arrhythmias (Green et al. 1977). Recent in vitro electrophysiological studies have shown (Ferrier et al. 1973) that the main mechanism by which digitalis enhances ventricular automaticity consists in the appearance of oscillatory after-potentials in ventricular cells and in the specialized conducting system. According to recent views (Kass et al. 1978) this kind of abnormal automaticity results from the simple extension of the therapeutic mechanism of action. In fact, the oscillatory after-potentials are due to the induction of transient inward currents associated with a cellular calcium overload which, in turn, depends on the inhibition of Na^+-K^+-ATPase. It is quite obvious that the long chain of events, linking the drug interaction with the receptor to the ultimate electrophysiological phenomena, offers many points of attack for a variety of possible potentiating factors. For instance, hypoxemia and ischemia may act, at least in part, by further reducing the number of functioning sodium pump units (Balasubramanian et al. 1973; Beller et al. 1976). Moreover, the increase in sympathetic discharge possibly present in an ischemic or hypoxic heart, as well as hypocalcemia, may increase the amplitude of the oscillatory potentials by increasing the intracellular calcium overload (Kass et al. 1978).

The electrophysiological derangements underlying digitalis toxicity are probably quite simple, if compared with the complicated functional and structural abnormalities underlying dysrhythmias associated with cardiac diseases. Although considerable information about the electrophysiological derangements of automaticity and conduction in diseased hearts has been recently obtained (Singer et al. 1981), the mechanisms underlying chronic complex arrhythmias in patients with ischemic and diseased hearts are still only poorly understood (Singer and Ten Eick 1981). Experimental models, which are largely obtained from normal heart tissues, are obviously inadequate in reproducing the complicated and highly integrated electrophysiological, biochemical and structural alterations responsible for arrhythmias in chronic heart diseases.

The unpredictability of the response of these kinds of arrhythmias to drug therapy is often the consequence of this situation: for instance, recent careful studies have documented an aggravation of chronic ventricular arrhythmias in 11% of patients tested with nine currently used anti-arrhythmic drugs at doses producing blood levels in the therapeutic range (Velebit et al. 1982). Drugs interfering with cardiac conduction and refractoriness (such as quinidine, procainamide, amiodarone, phenothiazine derivatives and tricyclic antidepressants) are also able to induce, in some patients, a characteristic syndrome consisting of a prolongation of the Q-T interval of the electrocardiogram (long Q-T syndrome) which is associated with an extremely high incidence of ventricular fibrillation and sudden death (Schwartz et al. 1975; Reynolds and Vander Ark 1976). The drug induced long Q-T syndrome is not different from that which may be found in ischemic heart diseases, electrolyte disorders, neurological diseases and in a congenital form associated with deafness, syncope and sudden death (Abidskow 1979). It is now quite clear that Q-T prolongation is due to a delayed repolarization phase of ventricular cells, sometimes associated with a sympathetic imbalance, which may lead to an increased degree of temporal dispersion of cardiac refractoriness, and thus to a prolongation of the vulnerable ventricular period (Schwartz and Stone 1978). However, the reasons for the susceptibility of some patients to Q-T prolongation by drugs is completely unclear, although the presence of some anatomical or functional predisposing factors must obviously be admitted; a difference in action potential duration due to a differential drug response of normal and diseased cardiac tissues might be a possible explanation.

In consequence of the lack of clues for identifying which patients are susceptible to this kind of highly individual complication, reports of drug induced long Q-T syndrome continue to increase, even with previously unsuspected drugs; for instance, at the Division of Cardiology of this hospital, typical cases of Q-T prolongation-syncope and ventricular fibrillation have been observed in patients treated with prenylamine (Fazzini et al. 1973) and with lidoflazine. Beta blockers are another class of drugs which have been frequently implicated in serious cardiovascular complications. A severe syndrome characterized by arrhythmias, worsening of anginal symptoms, myocardial infarction and sudden death, has been described in patients with angina treated with beta-blockers following the withdrawal of the therapy (Shand and Wood 1978). A number of suggestions have been made to explain the pathogenesis of this beta antagonist withdrawal phenomenon; however, recent reports indicate that an increase in the cardiac sensitivity to catecholamines due to an "up-grading" of beta-adrenoceptors, might be an important factor (Boudoulas et al. 1977). In support of this suggestion, it has been demonstrated that several days of treatment of human subjects with propranolol is able to induce a 40% increase in the number of peripheral beta-adrenoceptors (Aarons et al. 1980). Life-threatening reactions consisting of cardiac failure and shock have also been documented in 1–2% of patients receiving propranolol (Greenblatt and Kock-Weser 1973; Stephen 1966). Most of these adverse effects did not correlate with high doses, and occurred suddenly after the first drug administration. In view of the widespread use of beta-blockers in patients with cardiovascular diseases, even such a small percentage of adverse reactions becomes quantitatively relevant. However it is quite clear that such an incidence might be significantly reduced by an appropriate selection of patients, since subjects at risk are chiefly identifiable as those who are dependent on an increased sympathetic tone to maintain an adequate or suboptimal cardiac output (Jackson and Harrison 1980). Patients with a latent heart failure can be obviously included in this group, since the cardiac function in heart failure is highly dependent on beta-adrenoceptor stimulation (Gaffney and Braumwald 1963). In fact, an increased level of circulating catecholamines has been consistently detected in these kinds of patients (Thomas and Marks 1978). The vulnerability to beta blockade of patients with impaired ventricular function may even be increased by the existence of a "down-grading" phenomenon resulting in a decrease in the number of peripheral beta-adrenoceptors (Bristow et al. 1982). Such a reduction may represent a crucial point in the regulation of the cardiac sensitivity to catecholamines since the human heart probably does not have "spare" beta-adrenoceptors. The possibility that modifications of cardiovascular function homeostasis similar to those depicted above may be present in other clinical conditions, different from organic heart disease, thus predisposing them to deleterious effect of beta blockade, must be kept in mind. For instance, it has been repeatedly demonstrated that in hypothyroidism a cardiac subsensitivity to catecholamines exists, despite an increased level of circulating catecholamines (Christensen 1972). Recent studies in isolated heart preparations have raised the possibility that the altered catecholamine sensitivity of the heart in hypothyroidism might be secondary to a decrease in the density of cardiac beta-adrenoceptors (Stiles and Lefkowitz 1981).

However, the awareness that a latent altered heart function may be present in hypothyroid state is still not fully recognized, although severe complications induced by beta-blockers in patients with hypothyroidism have been recently observed (Murakami et al. 1982). At the Clinical Toxicology Unit of this Hospital, two cases of severe cardiogenic shock precipitated by a single oral dose of a beta-blocker in hypothyroid subjects have been observed. Both patients were females, 56 and 64 years old, respectively, without any previous history of cardiac dysfunction, for whom a beta-blocker was prescribed for therapeutic purposes ("palpitations" in the former, hypertension in the latter); in both, thyroid function tests indicated a low free thyroxine index (1.10 and 1.32 respectively) and an increased level of thyroid stimulating hormone (higher than 68 μU/ml). It is noteworthy that in both patients a slow heart rate was observed, in spite of the presence of a profound hypertensive state.

Following these two observations it was decided to evaluate the peripheral beta adrenergic status in hypothyroid subjects. With this aim the density and the affinity of beta-adrenoceptors in intact lymphocytes of hypothyroid patients have been determined by the (^{3}H) dihydroalprenolol binding technique (Williams et al. 1976); beta receptor assays have been performed immediately after the diagnosis of hypothyroidism, and after the patients were rendered euthyroid. Preliminary results obtained in five patients studied sequentially, have shown that the improvement in both the hormonal and the clinical conditions, during a three-month period of therapy, was associated, in four out of the five subjects, with an evident decrease in the levels of circulating noradrenaline and to a mean increase in beta receptor density of about 100%, without any significant change in the affinity. Therefore, these findings seem to confirm that an alteration in peripheral beta-adrenoceptors may be detectable also in human subjects with hypothyroidism, thus offering a clue to a better understanding of episodes of abnormal responsiveness to beta-blockers in this pathological condition.

Acknowledgements. Cases of previously undescribed drug induced long Q-T syndrome are due to the courtesy of Prof. P. F. Fazzini and Prof. F. Marchi, to whom I am very grateful. Preliminary findings regarding the beta adrenoceptor density in lymphocytes of hypothyroid subjects have been obtained from a study which is now in progress and on which the following colleagues collaborated: Prof. R. Fantozzi and Dr. S. Brunelleschi (Department of Pharmacology and Toxicology, University of Florence); Prof. M. Serio, Dr. S. Cuomo, Dr. L. Defeo, Dr. M. Maggi, and Dr. M. Mannelli (Institute of Endocrinology, University of Florence).

References

Aarons RD, Nies AS, Gal J, Hegstrand LR, Molinoff PB (1980) Elevation of beta adrenergic receptor density in human lymphocytes after propranolol administration. J Clin Invest 65: 949–957

Akera T, Brown BS (1982) Cardiovascular toxicology of cardiotonic drugs and chemicals. In: Van Stee EW (ed) Cardiovascular toxicology. Raven Press, New York, p 109

Alexander CS (1972) Cobalt beer cardiomyopathy – A clinical and pathologic study on twenty-eight cases. Am J Med 53: 395–417

Andreasen F, Mikkelsen E (1977) Distribution, elimination and effect of furosemide in normal subjects and in patients with heart failure. Eur J Clin Pharmacol 12: 15–22

Balasubramanian V, McNamara DB, Singh JN, Dhalla NS (1973) Biochemical basis of heart function. Reduction in the Na^+-K^+-stimulated ATPase activity in failing rat heart to hypoxia. Can J Physiol Pharmacol 51: 504–510

Baughman RA, Lin ET, Williams RL, Benet LZ (1979) Prazosin disposition in patients with congestive heart failure and in healthy controls. Clin Pharmacol Ther 25: 213

Baum GL, Dick MM, Blum A, Kaupe A, Carballo J (1959) Factors involved in digitalis sensitivity in chronic pulmonary insufficiency. Am Heart J 57: 460–462

Beller GA, Conroy J, Smith TW (1976) Ischemia induced alterations in myocardial (Na^+-K^+)-ATPase and cardiac glycoside binding. J Clin Invest 57: 341–350

Benowitz NL, Meister W (1976) Pharmacokinetics in patients with cardiac failure. Clin Pharmacokinet 1: 389–405

Boudoulas M, Lewis RP, Kates RE, Dalamangas G (1977) Hypersensitivity to adrenergic stimulation after propranolol withdrawal in normal subjects. Ann Intern Med 87: 433–436

Bristow MR, Ginsburg R, Minobe W, Cubicciotti RS, Sageman WS, Lurie K, Billingham ME, Harrison DC, Stinson EB (1982) Decreased catecholamine sensitivity and beta adrenergic-receptor density in failing human hearts. N Engl J Med 307: 205–211

Chew CYC, Hecht HS, Collett JT, McAllister RG, Singh BN (1981) Influence of severity of ventricular function on hemodynamic responses to intravenously administered verapamil in ischemic heart disease. Am J Cardiol 47: 917–922

Christensen NJ (1972) Increased levels of plasma noradrenaline in hypothyroidism. J Clin Endocrinol Metab 35: 359–363

Cluff LE (1966) Adverse reactions to drugs: methods of study. In: Lasagna L (ed) International encyclopedia of pharmacology and therapeutics, sect 6, vol II. Pergamon Press, Oxford London, p 655

Deglin SM, Deglin JM, Chung EK (1977) Drug induced cardiovascular diseases. Drugs 14: 29–40

Doherty JE (1982) The digoxin-quinidine interaction. Annu Rev Med 33: 163–170

Durrer D, Schuillenburg RM, Wellens HJJ (1970) Preexcitation revisited. Am J Cardiol 25: 690–697

Fazzini PF, Marchi F, Pucci P (1973) Q-T lungo, sincope e prenilamina. Giorn It Cardiol 3: 233–239

Ferrier GR, Saunders JM, Mendez C (1973) A cellular mechanism for the generation of ventricular arrhythmias by acetylstrophantidin. Circ Res 33: 508–515

Fleckenstein A (1977) Specific pharmacology of calcium in myocardium, cardiac pacemakers and vascular smooth muscle. Ann Rev Pharmacol Toxicol 17: 149–166

Gaffney TE, Braunwald E (1963) Importance of the adrenergic nervous system in the support of circulatory function in patients with congestive heart failure. Am J Med 34: 320–324

Green LH, Smith TW (1977) The use of digitalis in patients with pulmonary disease. Ann Intern Med 87: 459–465

Greenblatt DJ, Koch-Weser J (1974) Adverse reactions to beta adrenergic blocking drugs: A report from the Boston Collaborative Drug Surveillance Program. Drugs 7: 118–129

Hagemeijer F (1978) Verapamil in the management of supraventricular tachyarrhythmias occurring after a recent myocardial infarction. Circulation 57: 751–755

Jackson G, Harrison DC (1980) Adverse effects of beta-adrenergic blocking drugs. In: Bristow MR (ed) Drug-induced heart disease. Elsevier-North Holland, Amsterdam New York Oxford, p 323

Kass RS, Lederer WJ, Tsien RW, Weingart R (1978) Role of calcium ions in transient inward currents and aftercontractions induced by strophantidin in cardiac Purkinje fibers. J Physiol 281: 187–208

Kohlhardt M, Bauer B, Krause H, Fleckenstein A (1973) Selective inhibition of the transmembrane Ca conductivity of mammalian myocardial fibers by Ni, Co and Mn ions. Pflügers Arch 338: 115–123

Morrison J, Killip T (1971) Hypoxemia and digitalis toxicity in patients with chronic lung disease. Circulation 43/44: II 44

Murakami K, Kasama T, Hayashi R, Tsushima M, Nishiomeda Y, Koh H, Nambu S, Ikeda M (1982) Myxoedema coma induced by beta-adrenoceptor-blocking agent. Br Med J 285: 543–544

Opie LH (1980) Metabolic and drug-induced injury to the myocardium. In: Bristow MR (ed) Drug-induced heart disease. Elsevier-North Holland Biomedical Press, Amsterdam New York Oxford, p 81

Reynolds EW, Vander Ark CR (1976) Quinidine syncope and the delayed repolarization syndromes. Mod Concepts Cardiovasc Dis 45: 117–122

Schwartz PJ, Stone HL (1978) Unilateral stellectomy and sudden death. In: Schwartz PJ, Brown AM, Malliani A, Zanchetti A (eds) Neural mechanisms in cardiac arrhythmias. Raven Press, New York, p 107

Schwartz PJ, Periti M, Malliani A (1975) The long Q-T syndrome. Am Heart J 89: 378–390

Sellers DT Jr, Basmore TM, Gallagher JJ (1977) Digitalis in the pre-excitation syndrome. Analysis during atrial fibrillation. Circulation 56: 260–267

Shand DG, Wood AJJ (1978) Editorial: propranolol withdrawal syndrome: why? Circulation 58: 202–203

Singer DH, Ten Eick RE (1981) Chronic dysrhythmias: A new look at old questions. Prog Cardiovasc Dis 24: 91–96

Singer DH, Baumgarten CM, Ten Eick RE (1981) Cellular electrophysiology of ventricular and other dysrhythmias: Studies on diseased and ischemic heart. Prog Cardiovasc Dis 24: 97–156

Singh BN, Roche AHG (1977) Effects of intravenous verapamil on hemodynamics in patients with heart disease. Am Heart J 94: 79–85

Stenson RE, Constantino RT, Harrison DC (1971) Interrelationships of hepatic blood flow, cardiac output and blood levels of lidocaine in man. Circulation 43: 205–211

Stephen SA (1966) Unwanted effects of propranolol. Am J Cardiol 18: 463–468

Stiles GL, Lefkowitz RJ (1981) Thyroid hormone modulation of agonist-beta adrenergic receptor interaction in the rat heart. Life Sci 28: 2529–2536

Thomas JA, Marks BH (1978) Plasma norepinephrine in congestive heart failure. Am J Cardiol 41: 233–243

Ueda CT, Dzindzio BS (1978) Quinidine kinetics in congestive heart failure. Clin Pharmacol Ther 23: 158–164

Velebit V, Podrid P, Lown B, Cohen BM, Graboys TB (1982) Aggravation and provocation of ventricular arrhythmias by antiarrhythmic drugs. Circulation 65: 886–894

Williams RL, Benet LZ (1980) Drug pharmacokinetics in cardiac and hepatic disease. Ann Rev. Pharmacol Toxicol 20: 389–413

Williams LT, Snyderman R, Lefkowitz RJ (1976) Identification of beta adrenergic receptors in human lymphocytes by (^{3}H) alprenolol binding. J Clin Invest 57: 149–155

Disease, Metabolism and Reproduction in the Toxic Response to Drugs and Other Chemicals
Arch. Toxicol., Suppl. 7, 66–87 (1984)

The Diseased Lung and Drugs

Ph. Camus and L. Jeannin

Department of Respiratory Diseases, University Hospital, 21000 Dijon, France

Abstract. Among the numerous ways by which drug-lung relationships can be discussed we chose to examine three questions:

1) Is the lung capable of directly modulating drug pharmacokinetics?

Knowing that the pulmonary circulation can exert very selective and efficient clearance and catabolism of biogenic molecules such as serotonin (5-HT), norepinephrine (N.E.), prostaglandins PGE_2 and $PGF_{2}\alpha$, and bradykinin, as well as activation of angiotensin (A)I to AII, a similar behavior has been sought for drugs. *Uptake* of circulating drugs occurs in a very efficient manner in the lung; basic amines, especially if amphiphilic, are significantly retained and build up tissue levels 1 to 3 orders of magnitude higher than blood levels, depending on the compound and duration of administration. Pharmacokinetic studies have shown a rapidly-exchanging pool, presumably representing binding to cell membranes, and a pool with low influx and efflux rate suggesting binding to subcellular fractions. Inhibitor studies suggest that no carrier is involved in the uptake process, the opposite to what occurs for biogenic amines. We review the influence of lung disease on these properties, emphasizing the potential role of these molecules as indicators of endothelial cell surface and/or function. Potential pharmacokinetic consequences of drug uptake include smoothing out of the systemic arterial peak drug concentration, particularly during intravenous administration, and drug-drug displacement during sequential injection of structurally related compounds. Therapeutic effect may be reinforced by accumulation in the lung, as has been demonstrated for ibuterol, doxorubicin and certain antibiotics. Harmful consequences consist of (i) the transient impairment of the clearance of biogenic amines, the significance of which remains to be fully evaluated, and (ii) iatrogenic phospholipidosis localization of which in the lung might result from the elevated drug concentration in the tissue.

Lung cells contain enzymes, among them mixed function oxidases (MFO), which enables them to *metabolize* xenobiotics even in the intact organ. Although blood supply to the lung is higher than that to the liver, the comparatively low MFO content of the former organ predicts only a marginal pulmonary metabolic contribution in vivo. On the other hand, enzymatic activity upon drugs can generate instable reactive metabolites which, even in minute amounts, are toxic and can damage cells; furthermore, it is hypothesized that the relatively high bronchiolar Clara cell MFO content explains the striking susceptibility of the lung to xenobiotics.

2) Do lung diseases indirectly influence drug pharmacokinetics?

Hindrance to blood flow is common in respiratory failure (R.F.), from both reduced area and hypoxic vasoconstriction, resulting in altered flow distribution to the liver and kidney. Altered drug elimination may ensue. Due to the extraordinarily numerous factors involved, the results from clinical studies still remain difficult to interpret, but sufficient data exist to recommend careful use of drugs such as theophylline and digitalis, since R.F. additionally alters protein binding, volume of distribution and possibly receptor sensitivity and thus increases the risk of unwanted effects.

3) How do drugs damage the lung?

In the final question, we offer a current review of common drug-induced respiratory diseases. We use a clinical classification and provide mechanistic explanations whenever possible some of them being related to the properties described in the first chapter.

Key words: Drugs – Drug-induced lung disease – Endothelial cell – Lung metabolism – Pharmacokinetics – Pulmonary circulation

There are many reasons for dealing with the topic of drugs and the lung. Even this apparently limited field in pulmonary medicine is extremely vast. It is clearly beyond the scope of the present paper to fully review how drugs and lungs interact; three main points will be dealt with, summarized into the three following questions:

Is the lung itself a significant determinant of drug pharmacokinetics?

The well studied metabolic functions of the pulmonary circulation concern both endogenous molecules and drugs for which significant storage has been demonstrated. Whether or not this pharmacokinetic property of the lung endothelium modulates the fate of drugs in healthy and diseased lungs will be developed in the first part.

Do lung diseases have distant consequences relevant to drug disposition?

Diseased lungs may oppose an elevated resistance to blood flow and, as a consequence reduce the flow devoted to upstream organs such as the liver. Additionally, hypoxemia may alter the distribution of blood flow within distant organs, and impair the function of enzymatic systems which require oxygen. An attempt to answer this question will be in the second part.

How do some drugs attack the lung?

The respiratory system, and particularly the lung is not an unusual target for the deleterious effects of drugs. The drugs involved, the patients exposed and the mechanistic pathways will be dealt with in the third part.

The Metabolic Functions of the Pulmonary Circulation in Health and in Disease

The first recognized function of the lung was the exchange of gases and later, evidence was found of metabolic activities within the pulmonary circulation. In the past decade, a great amount of work has accumulated on this topic. The lung and particularly the pulmonary circulation have been shown to be capable of processing a wide number of endogenous molecules (Bakhle and Vane 1974) such as vasoactive amines, as well as drugs and foreign compounds (Brandenburger-Brown 1974; Philpot et al. 1977). These metabolic and pharmacokinetic functions of the pulmonary circulation are favored by the large endothelial surface which is in excess of 70 m^2 and by the amount of blood flowing through the lung which equals cardiac output. These metabolic functions are mostly performed by the endothelial cell (E. Cell) (Mellins 1982), the best studied among the 42 different types present in the lung.

Although the present paper is mostly devoted to drugs, some data relative to the metabolic properties of the pulmonary circulation on both endogenous and foreign molecules are presented. For several reasons the processing of endogenous amines and that of drugs cannot be dissociated; their respective uptakes, although accounted for by different mechanisms, probably occur at the same anatomic level. Furthermore each of these uptake processes may be selectively altered in different experimental lung diseases, and their study in such situations undoubtedly enhances the knowledge and comprehension of the behavior of the pulmonary circulation in disease. Similarly, several clinical conditions in humans are characterized by an attack to the pulmonary E. Cell. These diseases are usually severe and the study of the derangements of the metabolic functions of the pulmonary circulation they induce may help to recognize them at an earlier stage than is currently possible.

It must be stressed that the present paper cannot provide a full review of each of the points which will be discussed. Each of them has already deserved previous reviews many of them exhaustive to which the interested reader will be referred whenever possible. Attention should also be drawn to the fact that care must prevail when analyzing animal data, for extrapolations to humans are not yet justified (Junod 1981), except when stated otherwise.

The Pharmacokinetic Functions of the Normal Lung

Although suspected by Starling in the early 20's, metabolic functions were convincingly demonstrated 30 years ago when Gaddum and his associates (Gaddum et al. 1953) discovered 5 hydroxytryptamine (5-HT) removal within the lung. During the time elapsed, formidable advances have occurred in the comprehension of the metabolic capacities of the lung which are now far better understood. Blood 5-HT and norepinephrine (NE) are substantially removed during their passage through the lung in most if not all mammalian species including man (Bakhle and Vane 1974). They are transported by a distinct rate-limiting, Na^+-dependent carrier into the endothelial cell where subsequent metabolism occurs by the action of monoamine oxidase (MAO) and cathechol-O-methyl transferase (COMT). 5-HT transport can be blocked by Na^+ depletion, cold, anoxia and several drugs (imipramine, chlorpromazine) (Junod 1981) whereas that of NE can be blocked by desipramine and also by cocaine.

Numerous other endogenous compounds are subjected to metabolism within the pulmonary circulation (Junod 1982; Mellins 1982). Angiotensin I (AI) is converted into AII by the virtue of angiotensin converting enzyme (ACE), the activity of which is more prominent within the lung vessels than in any other vascular bed (Block and Stalcup 1982); ACE also processes the potent inflammatory mediator bradykinin into inactive metabolites (Block and Stalcup 1982). Prostaglandins (PG) E2 and PG F2α, steroids and cyclic nucleotides are also inactivated (Junod 1974, 1982). In contrast, epinephrine, histamine and AII leave the lung unaltered (Mellins 1982).

The physiological importance of these metabolic functions of the pulmonary circulation are difficult to interpret. It has been suggested that in baseline conditions they play only a small role (Junod 1982): if, for example, ACE activity is blocked by a synthetic inhibitor in man or in animals, there is very little change in resting blood pressure. On the other hand, resting norepinephrine blood levels only moderately differ between the pulmonary artery and vein (Sole et al. 1979) which does not argue for a significant removal of this cathecholamine in the normal state. However these metabolic functions may be involved in particular conditions: exercise, during which ACE activity and AII production may participate in the control of blood pressure and flow distribution to the muscles, respiratory distress syndrome during which the relative inability of the pulmonary circulation to degrade bradykinin may enhance its inflammatory properties and favor pulmonary edema (Mellins 1982), and therapeutic i.v. administration of NE the pressor effects of which are markedly higher in subjects receiving imipramine than is the case in controls.

Uptake, storage, and even metabolism have also been demonstrated for drugs (Bakhle and Vane 1974). Several reviews are available for the interested reader (Brandenburger-Brown 1974). They discuss uptake (Junod 1981) metabolism (Hook and Bend 1976) and release (Junod 1981) of drugs from the lung vascular network. Basic amines, and among them imipramine, are significantly retained by the lung (Orton et al. 1973) and may concentrate up to 100 times or more. In experiments designed to assess the precise mechanism of 5-HT uptake, Junod observed that imipramine inhibited 5-HT uptake competitively (Junod 1981). Hence the question arose of whether the transport of the drug and that of the amine were dependent on the same carrier. In a series of experiments he was able to demonstrate that in contrast to 5-HT, Na^+ concentration had no significant effect on imipramine uptake, and gave strong evidence for different uptake processes for the two compounds. It is presently thought that the mechanism of imipramine, and more generally basic amines, concentration within the lung mostly occurs by binding to endothelial cell membranes and also by diffusion and binding outside the vascular lumen. However, the kinetic and magnitude of the uptake mechanisms probably differs between drugs since their respective time-concentration curves exhibit different slopes. As has been said before, other basic amines especially when amphiphilic (methadone, chlorphentermine, amphetamine) are also subjected to strong uptake whereas neutral amines (aniline, imidazole, propazone) are not (Orton et al. 1973). An interesting feature of the pulmonary circulation is its striking ability to concentrate propranolol which is also a basic amine (Dollery and Junod 1976; Pang et al. 1982b). During in vivo experiments conducted in dogs as well as in humans, Pang et al. (1982b) and Geddes et al. (1979) were able to demonstrate a 75% first-pass removal of this drug by the lung without any significant metabolism.

The uptake properties extend, at least in animals, to numerous other drugs such as adrenergic compounds, antihistamines, antimalarial, antipsychotics, synthetic analgesics and also to some anorectics, tricyclic antidepressants, barbiturates, local anesthetics and antiarrythmic drugs (Brandenburger-Brown 1974).

Interestingly the uptake of drugs can be altered by other compounds. A decreased propranolol uptake may result from concurrent administration of chlorpromazine, imipramine, nortryptyline or desmethylimipramine whereas lidocaine increases propranolol uptake in vitro (Junod 1981).

These interesting studies, mainly performed on animal preparations, still require further advances for a full understanding of how and to what extent each drug is captured by the pulmonary circulation. Although it may be reasonably proposed that their uptake does not primarily depend on a carrier (Junod 1981), possibly important factors such as lipid solubility, partition coefficient and pKa of each drug, as determinants of the kinetics of their removal and concentration within the lung, have to be carefully studied (Junod 1981).

The actual impact of drug accumulation in clinical practice is difficult to establish firmly due to the scarcity of human studies. However the remarkable experimental accumulation observed for several drugs justifies addressing this question. As recently stressed by Junod (1981), the substantial uptake of some drugs may help to dampen any abrupt variation in their plasma level particularly when they are given by the i.v. route. On a long term administration however, lung storage is unlikely to critically affect drug disposition which is mainly modulated by the liver and kidney. Drug-drug interactions may occur in situations where a drug bound to endothelial surface can be displaced either by another drug, or by one of its own metabolites. This is theoretically possible for imipramine with propranolol and imipramine with chlorcyclizine (Junod 1981) and has been demonstrated in man, lidocaine displacing previously bound mepivacaine (Jorfeldt et al. 1983).

In addition to their accumulation, drugs can be metabolized within lung cells (Hook and Bend 1976). Mixed function oxidases (MFO's) were first described in liver cells but are also present within some lung cells (Hook and Bend 1976) e.g., the Clara MFO's present in lung cell microsomes appear qualitatively similar to liver MFO's but are contained in a much lesser extent on a weight basis (Hook and Bend 1976). Accordingly, lung MFO's overall activity is lower than liver MFO's for most compounds except for benzphetamine whose N-demethylation occurs at a much higher rate than expected from the lung MFO's content (Hook and Bend 1976). The general qualitative properties of MFO'S (wide spectrum of drug oxidation capacities, induction and inhibition) apply to lung MFO's (Hook and Bend 1976), and it is generally thought that lung and liver MFO's are closely comparable except perhaps with regard to Δ-9 tetrahydrocannabinol, the metabolism of which could be specific for lung MFO's (Junod 1981). Numerous other enzymatic systems have been described in lung cells (Hook and Bend 1976). Amine oxidases, epoxide-metabolizing systems, glucuronyl-transferases and N-acetyl transferases are some of them. Experiments conducted on the whole organ have confirmed some of the metabolic activities observed on lung microsomal preparations (Hook and Bend 1976) these activities are directed toward several drugs which may or may not be concomitantly concentrated within the lung. Methadone and pentobarbital are metabolized by the isolated perfused lung (IPL) whereas this is not the case for imipramine or chlorcyclizine (Junod 1981). However, the two latter compounds are subjected to metabolism by lung MFO's on microsomal preparations which further emphasizes that caution must be exerted when comparing different experimental settings (Junod 1981) and may indicate that these drugs fail to reach the endoplasmic reticulum in the IPL.

Based on differences in MFO's content of the liver and that of the lung, the latter organ should not be regarded as a major site for drug metabolism in man, at least for drugs administered enterally or parenterally (Junod 1981); in contrast a few inhaled substances are degraded by lung enzymatic systems as has been demonstrated for some bronchodilators of the β adrenergic stimulating class (Junod 1981). Future work will perhaps invalidate the aforementioned statement and provide further insight on the extent of drug metabolism within the lung as well as information regarding the exact location and cell type(s) responsible for these processes.

The Pharmacokinetic Functions of the Lung in Disease

Several models of lung diseases or injury have been developed in animals. Their marked effect on the processes referred to in the preceding paragraph for endogenous molecules led some investigators to study drug uptake in these models (Pang et al. 1982b) and also in a few patients with lung diseases (Pang et al. 1982a). This chapter is considered important because animal models and human disease share some anatomical and/or metabolic abnormalities and data obtained in animals can provide suggestions and stimulate new areas of research in man.

Although many classifications of lung disease exist, none appears entirely satisfactory for the purpose of this present discussion, hence the list in Table 1 in which the prominent feature of the disease and examples are given together with possible consequences. Given the major role of the E. cell in numerous uptake and metabolic processes, attention has been paid to the metabolic behavior of the damaged or injured pulmonary endothelium as well as during reduction in vascular area or derangements of blood gases compared with normal.

Damaged Endothelium

The widely recognized toxicity of breathing high concentrations of oxygen upon E. Cell, has frequently led investigators to use O_2 as the damaging agent (Dobuler et al. 1982). In addition, investigators have used such toxicants as paraquat, alphanaphtylthiourea (see Pang et al. 1982), bleomycin or monocrotalin. After exposure, impairment of 5-HT and NE uptake is a usual feature in such experiments. In rabbits inhaling pure oxygen, Dobuler (1982) demonstrated a striking reduction in 5-HT clearance and ACE activity in vivo. These results were in keeping with those reported earlier in an IPL (Block and Fisher 1977) preparation as well as on cultured E. cells (Block and Stalcup 1981), in the same environmental conditions. Similar effects on 5-HT uptake have been reported after endothelial damage with chemicals (Block and Schoen 1981). Since the altered amine uptake seems to occur before any visible histological or electron microscopic abnormality takes place, 5-HT and NE uptake are regarded as sensitive indices of endothelial function (Block and Stalcup 1982), and some authors believe it could be an early in vivo indicator of E. cell dysfunction (Block and Stalcup 1982, Dobuler et al. 1982). If this proves true, endothelial attack, which is part of several diseases in man (see Table 1) could be detected earlier

Table 1

Prominent feature	Example	Concequences relevant to the metabolic functions of the lung
Damage to endothelial cells	R.D.S.* Oxygen toxicity Some drug induced lung diseases	Decreased metabolic functions of the pulmonary circulation
Reduced vascular surface	R.D.S.* Emphysema (panacinar)	Loss of pulmonary endothelial cells ? Decreased metabolic functions of the pulmonary circulation
Respiratory failure[a]		
Acute	R.D.S.* Severe pneumonia	Decrease in the functional vascular area by hypoxic pulmonary vasoconstriction
Chronic	Advanced chronic airflow obstruction (CAO) Advanced lung fibrosis	Loss of pulmonary endothelial cells Alteration of enzymatic function of lung enzymes (Robin and Theodore 1982)
Elevated pulmonary arterial pressure	Advanced CAO Primary pulmonary hypertension Pulmonary embolism Left sided valvular disease	Loss of vascular surface Altered morphometry of pulmonary vessels ? Decreased metabolic functions of the pulmonary circulation

* R.D.S. = respiratory distress syndrome

[a] Defined by a reduced arterial oxygen partial pressure (paO_2) with or without carbon dioxide retention and respiratory acidosis

than is currently the case with conventional means such as chest X-ray and blood gases which, when abnormal, express gross, ominous and frequently irreversible lung damage. Current investigation will probably attempt to evaluate the role of an impaired amine uptake as a predictive tool in the management of patients prone to develop adult respiratory disease syndrome (ARDS) as are those with sepsis, shock and trauma (A. F. Junod, personal communication).

Propranolol uptake has also been studied in animals with presumed endothelial damage (Pang et al. 1982b). They reported on dogs with lung shock in which they were able to show a substantial decrease in propranolol uptake. However these experiments were not designed to specifically induce E. cell damage and thus the results cannot readily be extrapolated to what actually occurs in that situation and, a fortiori in man. Given the imperfect knowledge of the kinetics of accumulation mechanisms of other drugs, even on normal lungs, the net result for any of them in this condition cannot be presently anticipated.

Reduced Vascular Surface

The lung's metabolic properties have also been studied in experimentally induced reduction of vascular area, a widely recognized hallmark of human pulmonary emphysema of panacinar type (Weibel 1973). Emphysematous models are easy to induce in animals and have been used, as well as pulmonary vascular occlusions. On an IPL preparation of emphysematous hamsters, Ryerson et al. (1981) were unable to show any significant impairment of 5-HT uptake, whereas Stalcup et al. (1981) demonstrated a slight but significant decrease in ACE activity in in vivo measurements performed in emphysematous dogs. Flink and associates performed a pulmonary artery ligation but failed to observe any change in 5-HT or NE extraction until only one lobe remained perfused (Flink et al. 1982) suggesting that the reserve of the pulmonary circulation is enormous. In parallel experiments these investigators embolized the pulmonary bed with glass beads, and this maneuver selectively reduced 5-HT uptake leading these authors to postulate that a reduced vascular surface per se does not significantly affect the uptake of amines in contrast with a vascular damage which does. In much the same way, as for endogenous amines, propranolol uptake has been studied in animals and in man with reduced vascular area. A 20% decrease in propranolol uptake has been reported in patients with emphysema (Pang et al. 1982a) and a reversible decrease of comparable magnitude has been recorded in dogs during pulmonary arterial occlusion (Pang et al. 1982b).

From these pooled results it may be hypothesized that the specific carrier dependent uptake of 5-HT and NE critically depends upon an intact endothelial cell function whereas the binding and diffusional processes which probably govern amine extraction may preferentially depend upon vascular surface (A. F. Junod, personal communication).

Hypoxemia

Hypoxemia is a frequent finding in patients with lung disease and has a significant effect on some metabolic pathways. It has been shown that a low pO_2 consistently decreases ACE activity in cultured endothelial cells (Stalcup et al. 1979), in dogs in vivo breathing hypoxic gas mixtures (Leuenberger et al. 1978), and in hypoxemic emphysematous dogs (Stalcup et al. 1981). That ACE activity returned to normal when hypoxemia was reversed in all the dogs (Leuenberger et al. 1978; Stalcup et al. 1981) strongly suggests that hypoxemia and not emphysema is responsible for the decreased ACE activity, by altering either E. cell shape or the configuration of caveolae which harbor the enzyme.

Pulmonary Arterial Pressure

Finally an increased pulmonary arterial pressure (PAP) may play a role (see Table 1). Gillis et al. (1974) found an increased amine uptake in patients with secondary pulmonary hypertension, which returned to normal after correction of the causative valvular disease. Postoperative derecruitment of pulmonary vessels was an explanation but does not agree with the previously mentioned limited role of vascular surface as compared with integrity in amine uptake.

Jose et al. (1976) have described one patient with primary pulmonary hypertension in whom prostaglandin metabolism was nil. Sole and associates (1979) have reported on patients with either primary or secondary pulmonary hypertension who removed little or no NE from their blood. It is, to date, only possible to suspect altered metabolic properties of the pulmonary circulation in patients with elevated PAP; drug uptake is not known in this condition but may also be altered given the decreased propranolol uptake described in one such patient in Pang's series (Pang et al. 1982a).

In summary, although the lung has remarkable properties concerning the accumulation and even metabolism of drugs and despite significant evidence that some of these properties are impaired in disease, it should not be regarded in itself as a significant modulating factor in drug disposition until the contrary is demonstrated. However, this very interesting feature of drug accumulation might prove useful in the future in the evaluation of the vascular surface of the lung and together with amine uptake provide a sensitive index of endothelial function.

Consequences of Lung Diseases on Distant Drug Metabolizing Organs and Systems

From this standpoint two main abnormalities associated with lung disease may potentially influence drug disposition. The first of them is hydrodynamic in nature: the reduction in vascular area due to loss of alveolar capillary units and hypoxic pulmonary vasoconstriction are responsible for an increased resistance in the pulmonary vascular bed and hence an increase in pressure upstream of the pulmonary capillary. When this hindrance to flow is marked, upstream organs may suffer from increased back-pressure and have their own blood flow reduced (Wilkinson 1976). This is particularly important for the liver and to a lesser extent for the kidney. These situations will be discussed by Dr. Ledda in a separate paper. Here the second consequence, which is hypoxemia, will be concentrated upon.

Consequences of Hypoxemia Relevant to Drug Disposition

The consequences of hypoxemia are very numerous and remain to a great extent imperfectly known in conscious humans. Hypoxemia has been shown to profoundly alter the flow within the splanchnic bed and the liver, and to reduce liver blood flow (Roth and Rubin 1976). However it has been shown that although hypoxemia reduces hepatic arterial blood flow it increases portal flow in such a way that total liver blood flow (LBF) remains practically unchanged (Richardson and Withrington 1981). It is presently thought that a hydrodynamic balance exists between the portal circulation on the one hand and the arterial circulation on the other which ensures the maintenance of LBF under different circumstances (Richardson and Withrington 1981). It is thus not proved that a reduced LBF actually takes place during chronic hypoxemia in conscious humans; the data is lacking (P. C. Withrington, personal communication). However, since hypoxemia and increased venous pressure frequently go hand in hand, the effects of a reduced LBF on drug elimination may be examined. Wilkinson and Shand (1975) and Wilkinson (1976) stated that drugs having a high hepatic extraction ratio (E.R.) (i.e., in the 0.8–0.9 range) were critically dependent upon blood flow whereas those having a low E.R. were virtually independent of LBF. Drugs with a high E.R. include propoxyphen, propranolol, alprenolol and lidocaine while antipyrine, tolbutamide and warfarin have a low E.R. But additional parameters influence LBF dependence of drugs. According to Gilette, only those drugs with a low ratio half-life ($t_{1/2}$ in minutes) to volume of distribution (vd in liters) are significantly affected by LBF, Figures of less than 4.3 being necessary in his analysis (Gilette 1971). Such low values for this ratio seldom occur for drugs used in practice (Gilette 1971).

To conclude on this point, if hypoxemia actually modulates blood flow to the liver in chronically hypoxemic conscious humans, which remains to be demonstrated, its effect would mostly affect drugs with a high extraction ratio and low $t_{1/2}$/vd ratio.

Hypoxemia has adverse effects on some enzymatic systems. As pointed out by Jösbis (1974), brain 5-hydroxy-tryptophane synthesis decreases linearly with venous PO_2, within the 50 to 20 mm Hg range. MAO activity is also sensitive to minor decreases in PO_2, and alterations in brain cytochrome a and a3 properties have been recorded in experimental lung diseases in animals (Jösbis and Lamanna 1978). Cytochrome P-450 function has also been shown to be dependent upon a normal O_2 supply. Since cytochrome P-450 is the most powerful drug-metabolizing system in animals and man (Burke 1981), one can wonder whether hypoxemia actually impairs the metabolism of drugs on the basis of enzymatic dysfunction. Undoubtedly acute oxygen lack can impede enzymatic systems but, in contrast, chronic hypoxemia can induce changes in enzymatic and metabolic functions (Sjostrom and Crapo 1983) and may promote induction of some enzymatic complexes (Merrit and Medina 1968; Sotaniemi et al. 1971). Thus hypoxemia may elicit opposite effects on the basis of its duration.

The analysis in patients is further complicated by other factors. During chronic hypoxemia compensatory mechanisms develop, the purpose of which is to enhance oxygen supply despite the lowered PaO_2. They include increased cardiac output which improves oxygen transport, increased blood hemoglobin content and red blood cell mass which ameliorate arterial oxygen content, and decreased hemoglobin affinity for O_2 which promotes O_2 tissue delivery. Ideally such factors should be taken into account when interpreting the data in patients.

In addition, patients may require and receive drugs for the treatment of their lung disease such as steroids which are powerful inducers (Conney 1967). Further difficulties of interpretation arise when patients do not give up smoking, because tobacco smoke exposure has inductive effects (Junod 1981) and also raises blood carbon monoxide which is a well known cytochrome P-450 inhibitor (Burke 1981).

It can be well appreciated from the arguments presented above that the net effects of hypoxemia on drug-metabolizing enzymes in any individual will be difficult to predict. Are their multiplicity an explanation for the wide interindividual differences and discrepancies between studies?

Additional Factors

Plasma albumin concentration has been reported to be decreased in patients with chronic bronchitis possibly because of bronchial protein loss (Jusko 1976). This may be responsible for a reduction in the amount of protein-bound drug. This in turn increases tissue binding and volume of distribution (Jusko 1976), while decreasing plasma drug level. The increased tissue binding might explain in part the reported enhanced activity or toxicity observed in patients with respiratory failure, particularly with theophylline (Clozel and du Souich 1982) and cardiac glycosides (du Souich et al. 1978). In addition protein binding of drugs may be affected by the α-1-glycoprotein level (du Souich et al. 1978) which is reported to be increased in some patients with diseased lungs (du Souich et al. 1978). Additionally the respiratory acidosis demonstrated by some patients with respiratory failure, can actually change the ratio of ionized to non-ionized forms of some drugs (Wallner et al. 1979), as a function of their pKa (Roth and Wiersma 1979), and thus alter their diffusional properties.

Clinical Data

It has been shown that during respiratory failure (RF) absorption of procainamide may be decreased (du Souich et al. 1978). Several studies have provided values of drug plasma half-life during R.F. For some drugs (aminopyrine, amikacin, amoxicillin), the half-life was increased whereas that of tolbutamide was decreased (du Souich et al. 1978; Sotaniemi et al. 1971). That tolbutamide's (a drug with a low hepatic extraction ratio), half-life decreased in R.F. cannot be explained by changes in liver perfusion as has been discussed before. This decreased half-life may have resulted in part from enzymatic induction from hypoxemia (Sotaniemi et al. 1971).

Theophylline deserves particular comment for several reasons. This very useful drug is widely used in the treatment of asthma and more generally of diseases characterized by airflow limitation in order to relieve an element of bronchospasm. The therapeutic index of this drug is low which in turn indicates that toxic effects are not a remote possibility. Since toxic effects are frequently hazardous and related to plasma drug level (Zwillich et al. 1975; Hendeles and Weinberger 1980) careful administration and pharmacokinetic monitoring seem advisable.

A huge number of reports on the pharmacokinetics of theophylline has accumulated in the past few years. Right heart failure seems a significant factor of reduced clearance, and commands lower dosages (du Souich et al. 1978). Severe airway obstruction has also been shown to decrease theophylline clearance (Powell et al. 1978) whereas the effect of hypoxemia alone is not precisely known. The presence of respiratory acidosis does not seem to directly influence the pharmacokinetics of theophyline in dogs or in humans (Clozel et al. 1981; Rizzo et al. 1982) a finding in opposition to that of Rezar et al. (Rezar et al. 1979) who showed that acidotic patients had a larger Vd and required more theophylline to achieve the same plasma drug level than patients with elevated pH. In contrast, smoking and phenobarbital increase theophylline clearance probably because of enzymatic induction (Powell et al. 1977; Hendeles and Weinberger 1980).

Some experimental data have been published on the bronchodilator effects of theophylline at different pH. The bronchodilator response of acidotic cats to a beta agonist or theophylline was reduced (Baisset et al. 1971) suggesting possible differences in receptor behavior.

Though imperfect, knowledge of theophylline pharmacokinetics in respiratory disease has however some immediate applications for the treatment of patients with airway obstruction. Adverse effects will be significantly reduced by the careful observance of published administration rules (Piafsky and Ogilvie 1975; Powell et al. 1977, 1978; Svedmyr and Simonsson 1981). Maintenance doses have to be reduced by 20% in patients with chronic airflow obstruction, by at least 30% in those with congestive heart failure and more than halved in patients with liver insufficiency (Svedmyr and Simonsson 1981).

A study concerning the pharmacokinetics of the acidic drug sulphamethazine in patients with respiratory failure has very recently appeared in the literature (du Souich et al. 1983). In this study, no demonstrable changes in drug absorption were recorded as compared with normal volunteers. Bioavailability was decreased and V_D increased in the patients, probably because of a higher free fraction which apparently correlated with arterial PCO_2. These observations have important conceptual implications since if V_D and tissue binding increase in patients with respiratory failure, the efficacy and the toxicity, when the therapeutic index is narrow, may increase without change in the plasma level of the drug. One may thus not entirely rely on drug levels in such disease states since the changes in protein binding alter the pharmacokinetics and the pharmacodynamic properties of drugs. The observations presented by du Souich and his associates may well apply to other acidic drugs, particularly those which are highly bound to proteins and which render patients with respiratory failure particularly prone to toxic effects. To such a compound class theophylline belongs.

In conclusion, though the lung is not a significant metabolic organ, derangements within its structure have marked consequences. Due to the location of the pulmonary vascular network which is connected in series within the circulation, every marked elevation in pulmonary vascular resistance will tend to affect cardiac output and consequently blood flow within distant organs. Furthermore, hypoxemia, which frequently develops in patients with lung diseases, has significant consequences on distant drug metabolizing systems and organs. This may in part explain the still confusing field of drug pharmacokinetics in lung disease. In such disease, caution should be exerted when prescribing widely used drugs such as cardiac glycosides and theophylline.

How Do Some Drugs Attack the Lung?

The topic of drug-induced respiratory disease has received, in the last few years, an impressive number of reviews which should be included with benefit in the bibliography of everyone interested in iatrogenic disease. An attempt is made here to describe the present status of drug-induced respiratory manifestations, a quite rapidly developing field of pathology.

The Past and Present of Drug-associated Respiratory Disease

The rapid development of this field in pulmonary medicine is best seen by comparing reviews written in the early 70's and now. Advances have been made in the recognition of the iatrogenic nature of some lung diseases as well as in the identification of previously unsuspected agents. Strong epidemiological evidence led for example to the withdrawal of aminorex, a drug implicated in the development of pulmonary hypertension (Gurtner 1979). The severe burden of adverse effects attributed to chemotherapeutic agents used in the treatment of cancer is a growing problem and few of these drugs remain innocent. Other recently recognized toxicants such as D-penicillamine (Geddes et al. 1977) or amiodarone (Marchlinski et al. 1982) become a matter of concern.

Classification of Drug-induced Respiratory Diseases (DIRD)

DIRD are particularly difficult to classify because the determinant of the classification may be the drug (Rosenow 1972, 1977; Whitcomb 1973; Sostman et al. 1977; Lipman 1977; Weiss and Muggia 1980; Collis 1980; Batist and Andrews 1981), the mechanism of its noxious effect (Brettner et al. 1970; Touraine 1977; Cole 1977), the clinical picture of the DIRD (Brettner et al. 1970; Saltiel and Chretien 1972; Akoun et al. 1976; Camus et al. 1981) or the X-ray symptomatology (Sostman et al. 1981). Each of these classifications is useful for the recognition of DIRD as a function of each determinant observed in patients. For example if the drug-induced nature of a bronchospasm or diffuse parenchymal disease is discussed one should refer to clinical classifications. On the other hand if one wishes to examine the pulmonary adverse effect of any particular drug, reference should be made to classification of the drug. Here a classification will be developed taking into account the patient himself (Camus et al. 1981): it must be emphasized that all the elements of the respiratory system (lung, airways, pleura, vessels, neuro-muscular apparatus) may be the prime target for adverse reactions to drugs.

The Drug-induced Respiratory Diseases in Clinical Practice

Cancer Patients

A growing number of such patients receive combination chemotherapy; and other non-neoplastic diseases such as severe collagen vascular disease or transplantation may also require similar potent myelosuppressive immunosuppressive drugs.

In fact the huge majority of antineoplastic drugs has been reported to produce pulmonary complications.

The most frequent disease induced by these drugs is pneumonitis. Clinical signs are nonspecific and include cough, fever and dyspnea.

At radiography the picture is variable between a subnormal chest X-ray and a diffuse interstitial or alveolar pattern. Several eminent radiologists have focused their attention upon the chest X-ray during chemotherapy of lung disease (Brettner et al. 1970; Sostman et al. 1981), but no specific pattern can be attributed to any particular drug. Methotrexate pneumonitis is sometimes associated with mediastinal lymph node enlargement and pleural effusion (Sostman et al. 1976); bibasilar linear shadows have been reported in bleomycin and cyclophosphamide pneumonitis (Sostman et al. 1981; Balikian et al. 1982) whereas misleading pseudotumors have been reported as a complication of bleomycin therapy (Glazier and Siegel 1981). Chest X-ray are among the first detectable signs concurrent with clinical symptoms but they usually express gross lung damage.

Biological data are few. Interestingly, a significant peripheral eosinophilia has been reported in a little less than 50% of cases with methotrexate pneumonitis (Camus et al. 1982). Arterial blood gases evaluate the gas exchanging function of the lung and usually show hypoxemia with frequent hypocapnia.

The differential diagnosis is difficult because of the lack of clinical or radiological specificity of DI lung disease. Similar symptoms could be accounted for by (i) opportunistic pneumonia (Bode et al. 1974), for which a systematic search for pathogens should be undertaken, (ii) pulmonary extension of the primary neoplastic disease, (iii) even diffuse pulmonary hemorrhage. A systematic search for an iatrogenic cause when such patients develop diffuse lung opacities should be undertaken with a review of all drug schedules, and previous chest X-rays. The reviews mentioned earlier in this text sometimes allow a definite diagnosis of chemotherapy lung disease, especially when patients are placed on single agent chemotherapy. Solving the differential diagnosis sometimes requires an open lung biopsy procedure which gives a reasonable 65–75% specific diagnosis at the expense of a low mortality rate.

The histologic picture of DI pneumonitis varies as a function of the drug and the stage at which the sample is obtained (Batist and Andrews 1981). Endothelial cell damage, interstitial or alveolar edema, interstitial cell infiltration and fibrosis are among the most frequently reported with dysplasia of type II alveolar pneumocytes which desquamate into the alveolar lumen. These features are thought to reflect a toxic effect of the drugs first directed toward the endothelial cell. Some drugs (bleomycin, nitrosourea) may show a dose dependent toxicity but for most other drugs there is no clear relationship of this type and susceptibility varies greatly from one individual to another. For a few drugs (methotrexate [MTX], procarbazine), granuloma and eosinophils are observed within the lung tissue (Sostman et al. 1976) which supports the concept of an allergic reaction to these agents. However reintroduction of MTX in patients with previous MTX pneumonitis does not lead to relapse (Sostman et al. 1976) which is against a purely allergic reaction.

Prognosis is related to the underlying disease, and to the extent of pulmonary damage from the drug which may lead to severe respiratory insufficiency or diffuse irreversible lung fibrosis.

Cardiac Patients

Different questions arise with cardiac patients. When they develop diffuse opacities the possibility of a drug-induced manifestation should be raised. These opacities may be related to a DI pulmonary edema during the use of β blocking agents or antiarrhythmic drugs which all demonstrate more or less depressive action on the myocardium. Withdrawal of the suspected agent with appropriate evaluation of myocardial function should allow confirmation of the diagnosis. Diffuse opacities are also part of a possible pulmonary localization of a DI lupus erythematosus (LE). Procainamide is a frequently cited agent in inducing LE among numerous drugs sharing this property (Cole et al. 1977); the diagnosis is supported by positive antinuclear antibodies in the serum or in the associated pleurisy. The symptoms and pulmonary infiltration usually disappear on the withdrawal of the drug.

Amiodarone pneumonitis is an interesting emerging pathology observed in patients receiving rather elevated dosages of this drug (Marchlinsky et al. 1982). Recent evidence has been given of a disturbance in lipid storage and turnover or both within lung cells (pneumocytes, endothelial cells, and fibroblasts) possibly induced by the drug. If this holds true, amiodarone could be included in the group of phospholipidosis-inducing agents (Marchlinsky et al. 1982).

A rare but threatening complication is pulmonary hemorrhage which may result from uncontrolled anticoagulation therapy, drug interactions or drug induced thrombocytemia.

Bronchospasm is another threat for these patients when exposed to nonselective β blocking agents, especially in former or current asthmatics. This risk can be reasonably expected to decrease in following the ever increasing use of β 1 selective drugs which allow their use without untoward effects even in asthmatics, provided they receive adequate β 2 airway stimulation (Svedmyr and Simonsson 1981).

Rheumatology

In this category, patients with adverse effects are less numerous but the pattern of DIRD in this field has changed in the past few years.

Diffuse pulmonary infiltrates have been observed with several antiinflammatory or antirheumatic drugs. Gold salts are sometimes associated with acutely developing lung shadows which fortunately usually disappear when the drug is discontinued. Several mechanisms have been put forward including DI-LE, immediate or late hypersensitivity. Pulmonary opacities have also been described in a small number of patients receiving D-penicillamine and histological abnormalities seem comparable with those found during chemotherapy lung disease (Camus et al. 1982), but pathogenesis remains poorly understood.

Numerous recently reviewed respiratory problems (Camus 1982) have been ascribed to D-penicillamine, a drug mainly used in the treatment of rheumatoid arthritis. The most worrying manifestation is undoubtedly bronchiolitis obliterans, a rapidly progressive diffuse and severe airway narrowing resulting from inflammation and scarring within the small-airway walls. Afflicted patients develop respiratory insufficiency and impairment in a matter of months but the respective responsibility of the underlying rheumatoid arthritis and of the drug are not yet entirely clear.

Non-steroidal anti-inflammatory drugs as well as aspirin are capable of inducing severe asthmatic reactions in particularly susceptible patients; interference of these compounds with prostaglandin metabolism is one possible mechanism.

Pneumonology

During the evaluation of nearly every respiratory problem, the systematic search for a possible DI etiology sometimes proves fruitful. In addition to the patients referred to in the previous paragraphs DI opacities are seen with a wide spectrum of different drugs which exert their unwanted effect by various mechanistic pathways, many of them remaining poorly understood. These other DI pneumonitides include:

Pulmonary eosinophilia, characterized by diffuse fluffy lung shadows with a frequently elevated eosinophil blood count. Drugs are one of the many possible causes for this phenomenon and several compounds have been identified (Leitch 1979). Although the attraction of eosinophils by the release of chemotactic factors from degranulating drug-sensitized mast cells is a coherent explanation, the reason for their striking accumulation within the lung is not clear.

DI-LE has been previously mentioned but it must be stressed that patients who receive a drug and have lung opacities and ANA do not inevitably have DI-LE since the presence of ANA can sometimes be accounted for by the underlying disease such as rheumatoid arthritis (Camus et al. 1982).

Cardiogenic pulmonary edema from drugs has been discussed above in cardiac patients. A particular form of such edema can be observed during or more likely after chemotherapy with high doses of doxorubicin (adriamycin) owing to the peculiar cardiac toxicity of this drug (Young et al. 1981). Non-cardiogenic pulmonary edema has been ascribed to several unrelated compounds such as aspirin, hydrochorothiazide, cytosine-arabinoside, haloperidol, and methotrexate.

Disturbances in the respiratory neuromuscular system also deserve further comments. Ventilatory depression is a frequent occurrence during analgesia and general anesthesia (Tech et al. 1980). This does not seem to be due to an altered output from the respiratory centers but rather to marked changes in the elastic properties of the lung and chest wall (Schmidt and Rehder 1981) following anesthesia. The deleterious effects on PCO_2 and pH during high flow oxygen therapy in patients with respiratory failure were for long ascribed to O_2 itself, due to a respiratory center depression. However, O_2 only induces a moderate and transient decrease in minute ventilation and the responsibility of the rise in PCO_2 seems to be shared in common with increased ventilation-perfusion mismatch and Haldane effect (Aubier et al. 1980).

Aminoside antibiotics, particularly when inappropriately used in association with or during renal failure, can markedly depress the conduction through the neuromuscular plaque and promote alveolar hypoventilation; the same result is observed with drugs inducing myasthenia.

Pulmonary embolism has been suspected during prolonged oestrogen use and pulmonary vascular obstruction is increasingly observed in drug addicts practicing IV injection of crushed tablets containing talc (Tomashefski and Hirsch 1980).

Finally isolated pleurisy or pleuritis is an unusual manifestation except during DI-LE. Otherwise pleural thickening or effusions have been described with dantrolene and methysergide therapy (Camus et al. 1981).

The Future of Drug-Induced Respiratory Disease

Significant advances are anticipated the comprehension of the involved mechanisms. The respective influence of each type of allergy, or of their association, the exact determinant of the adverse reaction (drug, metabolite, drug-modified autologous tissue, haptenic molecule), the pathogenic role of recently implicated free radicals (Housset and Junod 1983), the time course of toxic versus allergic events, the factors governing the susceptibility of the host as well as the magnitude of the reaction, all require further clarification. Epidemiological data as well as experimental studies will hopefully provide information with regard to associations believed or suspected to be harmful such as bleomycin plus oxygen (Tryka et al. 1982) and radiotherapy plus adriamycin.

Reports of individual cases seems necessary to help future epidemiological studies, provided each case record is critically documented and substantiated in order to avoid false-alarms.

DI manifestations are difficult to recognize and a fortiori to predict. Pulmonary function tests have proved to date either ineffective or even misleading (Lewis and Izbicki 1980).

Early recognition could theoretically be based on changes in the metabolic functions of the pulmonary circulation, since, as has been said before, several chemotherapeutic agents exert their toxic effect upon the endothelial cell; strong evidence has been given in this way by a bleomycin lung model in rabbits, where a decreased amine uptake was recorded before any evidence of irreversible lung fibrosis was apparent (Gillis and Catravas 1982).

To begin with, three apparently unrelated questions were posed concerning drugs and the lung. All aspects of this wide topic have not been detailed here. Important subjects such as the behavior of drug receptors in disease which are an important field of current research have not been included.

However, the present data from the literature indicate that, if the metabolic functions of the pulmonary circulation do not seem to influence the pharmacokinetics of drugs taken on a long term schedule, they may be valuable in the study of diseases states. The endothelial attack which is part of some severe diseases in man will perhaps be based on these metabolic activities, some of which are markedly impaired during such conditions. Metabolic derangements seem to occur much earlier than microscopic alterations and could help to detect endothelial damage in vivo long before chest X-ray abnormalities or blood gas disturbances develop. A somewhat theoretical view rests on the removal of altered endogenous amines by the lungs of animals given bleomycin which could hopefully become a means for evaluating the pulmonary toxicity of other chemotherapeutic agents in man if some difficulties and drawbacks in the method are overcome. If this occurs in the future, a very significant advance in the early detection of chemotherapy lung will be available, but the relatively limited number of patients with DI lung disease would require a great many patients to be tested which does not seem a reasonable goal for the foreseeable future. Finally, pulmonary drug uptake, if not a major determinant of drug pharmacokinetics, will probably become one method of study of the behavior of the pulmonary circulation in experimental animals, in health and in disease. Whether or not drug uptake will help to evaluate pulmonary vascular surface in man during disease states is not predictable; however, it is presently doubtful that it will dethrone the study of carbon monoxide diffusion as a non-invasive and reasonably accurate estimate of the functional vascular area.

Finally when prescribing a drug to any patient some questions should be raised regarding the potential storage of the drug used in the lung of the patient, the potential role of concomitant lung disease on the fate of the drug administered, and the possible deleterious consequences of this drug on the respiratory system.

Acknowledgements: The invaluable and refined advice, carefully provided by Drs. Y. S. Bakhle, D. M. Geddes, A. F. Junod, G. Mack, H. M. McRendale and P. C. Withrington is gratefully acknowledged.

References

Akoun G, Huchon G, Herson S (1976) La pathologie respiratoire iatrogène. Ann Med Interne (Paris) 127: 644–655

Aubier M, Murciano D, Milic-Emili J, Touaty E, Daghfous J, Pariente R, Derenne JPh (1980) Effects of the administration of O_2 on ventilation and blood gases in patients with chronic obstructive pulmonary disease during acute respiratory failure. Am Rev Respir Dis 122: 747–754

Baisset A, Montastruc P, Tran MA (1971) Etude expérimentale de l'influence des variations de pH sanguin sur les effets bronchiques de divers médicaments. Pathol Biol (Paris) 19: 1061–1067

Bakhle YS, Vane JR (1974) Pharmacokinetic function of the pulmonary circulation. Physiol Rev 54: 1007–1045

Balikian JP, Jochelson MS, Bauer KA, Skarkin AT, Garnick MB, Canellos GP, Smith EH (1982) Pulmonary complications of chemotherapy regimens containing bleomycin. Am J Roentgenol 139: 455–461

Batist G, Andrews JL Jr (1981) Pulmonary toxicity of antineoplastic drugs. JAMA 246: 1449–1453

Block ER, Fisher AB (1977) Depression of serotonin clearance by rat lungs during oxygen exposure. J Appl Physiol Respira Environ Exercise Physiol 42: 33–38

Block ER, Schoen FJ (1981) Effect of alphanaphtylthiourea on uptake of 5 hydroxytryptamine from the pulmonary circulation. Am Rev Respir Dis 123: 69–73

Block ER, Stalcup SA (1981) Depression of serotonin uptake by cultured endothelial cells exposed to high oxygen tension. J Appl Physiol Respir Environ Exercise Physiol 50: 1212–129

Block ER, Stalcup SA (1982) Metabolic functions of the lung: Of what clinical relevance. Chest 81: 215–223

Bode FR, Pare JAP, Fraser RG (1974) Pulmonary diseases in the compromised host. Medicine (Baltimore) 53: 255–293

Brandenburger-Brown EA (1974) The localization, metabolism and effects of drugs and toxicants in lung. Drug Metab Rev 3: 33–87

Brettner A, Heitzman ER, Woodin WG (1970) Pulmonary complications of drug therapy. Radiology 96: 31–38

Burke MD (1981) Cytochrome P-450 a pharmacological necessity or a biochemical curiosity? Biochem Pharmacol 30: 181–187

Camus Ph (1982) Manifestations respiratoires associées aux traitements par la D-Penicillamine. Rev Fr Mal Respir 10: 7–20

Camus Ph, Reybet Degat O, Vanoli A, Jeannin L (1981) L'appareil respiratoire face au médicament. Med Hygiène 39: 4338–4346

Camus Ph, Reybet Degat O, Justrabo E, Jeannin L (1982) D-Penicillamine induced severe pneumonitis. Chest 81: 376–378

Clozel JP, du Souich P (1982) Insuffisance respiratoire et pharmacologie de la Théophylline. Bull Eur Physiopathol Respir 18: 807–810

Clozel JP, Saunier C, Royer-Morot MJ, Royer RJ, Sadoul P (1981) Respiratory acidemia and theophylline pharmacokinetics in the awake dog. Chest 80: 631–633

Cole P (1977) Drug induced lung disease. Drugs 13: 422–444

Collis CH (1980) Lung damage from cytotoxic drugs. Cancer Chemother Pharmacol 4: 17–27

Conney AH (1967) Pharmacological implications of microsomal enzyme induction. Pharmacol Rev 19: 317–357
Dobuler KJ, Catravas JD, Gillis CN (1982) Early detection of oxygen induced lung injury in conscious rabbits. Am Rev Respir Dis 126: 534–539
Dollery CT, Junod AF (1976) Concentration of (±) Propranolol in isolated perfused lungs of rat. Br J Pharmacol 57: 67–71
du Souich P, McLean AJ, Lalka D, Erill S, Gibaldi M (1978) Pulmonary disease and drug kinetics. Clin Pharmacokinet 3: 257–266
du Souich P, Amyot R, Julien M, Desjardins R, Latour J, Leblanc P (1983) Influence of chronic obstructive lung disease on the disposition of an acidic drug (Sulfamethazine). Arch Intern Med 143: 233–236
Flink JR, Pitt BR, Hammond GL, Gillis CN (1982) Selective effect of microembolization on pulmonary removal of biogenic amines. J Appl Physiol Respir Environ Exercise Physiol 52: 421–427
Gaddum JH, Hebb CO, Silver A, Swan AAB (1953) 5 hydroxytryptamine: pharmacological action and destruction in perfused lungs. J Exp Physiol 38: 255–262
Geddes DM, Corrin B, Brewerton DA, Davies RJ, Turner-Warwick M (1977) Progressive airway obliteration in adults and its association with rheumatoid disease. Q J Med (NS) 46: 427–444
Geddes DM, Nesbitt K, Trail T, Blackburn JP (1979) First pass uptake of 14 C-propranolol by the lung. Thorax 34: 810–813
Gilette JR (1971) Factors affecting drug metabolism. Ann NY Acad Sci 179: 43–66
Gillis CN, Catravas JD (1982) Altered removal of vasoactive substances in the injured lung: detection of lung microvascular injury. Ann NY Acad Sci 384: 458–474
Gillis CN, Cronau LH, Greene NM, Hammond GL (1974) Removal of 5 Hydroxytryptamine and Norepinephrine from the pulmonary vascular space of man: influence of cardiopulmonary by pass and pulmonary arterial pressure on these processes. Surgery 76: 608–616
Glazier CM, Siegel MJ (1981) Multiple pulmonary nodules: unusual manifestation of bleomycin toxicity. Am J Roentgenol 137: 155–156
Gurtner HP (1979) Pulmonary hypertension; "Plexogenic pulmonary arteriopathy" and the appetite depressant drug aminorex: post or propter? Bull Eur Physiolpathol Respir 15: 897–923
Hendeles L, Weinberger H (1980) Avoidance of adverse effects during chronic therapy with Theophylline. Drug Intell Clin Pharm 14: 522–530
Hook GER, Bend JR (1976) Pulmonary metabolism of xenobiotics. Life Sci 18: 279–290
Housset B, Junod A (1983) Toxicité pulmonaire des radicaux libres de l'oxygène. Rev Fr Mal Respir 11: 3–17
Jorfeldt L, Lewis DH, Löfström JB, Post C (1983) Lung uptake of lidocaine in man as influenced by anesthesia mepivacaine infusion on lung insufficiency Acta Anesthesiol. Scand. 27: 5–9
Josbis FF (1974) Intracellular metabolism of oxygen. Am Rev Respir Dis 110: 58–63
Josbis FF, Lamanna JC (1978) Kinetic aspects of intracellular redox reactions. In: Robin ED (ed) Extrapulmonary manifestations of respiratory disease, vol VIII. Dekker, New York Basel, p 63
Jose P, Niederhauser U, Piper P, Robinson C, Smith AP (1976) Degradation of prostaglandin F2 α in the human pulmonary circulation. Thorax 31: 713–719
Junod AF (1974) Metabolism, production, and release of hormones and mediators in the lung. In: Murray JF (ed) Lung disease: State of the art 1974–1975. American Lung Association, New York, p 305
Junod AF (1981) Uptake, release and metabolism of drugs in the lung. In: Widdicombe JG (ed) Respiratory pharmacology. Pergamon Press, Oxford New York Toronto Sydney Paris Frankfurt, IEPT Section 104, p 733
Junod AF (1982) Metabolism of the intact pulmonary circulation. Ann NY Acad Sci 384: 66–71
Jusko WJ (1976) Pharmacokinetics in disease states changing protein binding. In: Benet LZ (ed) The effects of disease states on drug pharmacokinetics. American Pharmaceutical Association, Academy of Pharmaceutical Sciences, Washington, p 99
Leitch AG (1979) Pulmonary eosinophilia. ATS News 22–26

Leuenberger PhJ, Stalcup SA, Mellins RB, Greenbaum LM, Turino GM (1978) Decrease in angiotensin I conversion by acute hypoxemia in dogs. Proc Soc Exp Biol Med 158: 586–589
Lewis BM, Izbicki R (1980) Routine pulmonary function tests during bleomycin therapy. JAMA 243: 347–351
Lippmann M (1977) Pulmonary reactions to drugs. Med Clin North Am 61: 1353–1367
Marchlinski FE, Gansler TS, Waxman HL, Josephson ME (1982) Amiodarone pulmonary toxicity. Ann Intern Med 97: 839–845
Mellins RB (1982) Metabolic functions of the lung and their clinical relevance. Am J Roentgenol 138: 999–1009
Merritt JH, Medina MA (1968) Altitude-induced alterations in drug action and metabolism. Life Sci 7: 1163–1169
Orton TC, Anderson MW, Pickett RD, Eling TE, Fouts JR (1973) Xenobiotic accumulation and metabolism by isolated perfused rabbit lungs. J Pharm Exp Ther 186: 482–497
Pang JA, Butland RJA, Brooks N, Cattell M, Geddes DM (1982a) Impaired lung uptake of propranolol in human pulmonary emphysema. Am Rev Respir Dis 125: 194–198
Pang JA, Blackburn JP, Butland RJA, Corrin B, Williams TR, Geddes DM (1982b) Propranolol uptake by dog lung: Effect of pulmonary artery occlusion and shock lung. J Appl Physiol Respir Environ Exercise Physiol 52: 393–402
Philpot RM, Anderson MW, Eling TE (1977) Uptake, accumulation, and metabolism of chemicals by the lung. In: Y. S. Bakhle and J. R. Vane (ed) Metabolic functions of the lung, vol IV. Dekker, New York Basel, p 123
Piafsky KM, Ogilvie RI (1975) Dosage of Theophylline in bronchial asthma. N Engl J Med 292: 1218–1221
Powell JR, Thiercelin JF, Vozeh S, Sansom L, Riegelman S (1977) The influence of cigarette smoking and sex on theophylline disposition. Am Rev Respir Dis 116: 17–22
Powell JR, Vozeh S, Hopewell P, Costello J, Sheiner LB, Riegelman S (1978) Theophylline disposition in acutely ill hospitalized patients. Am Rev Respir Dis 118: 229–603
Resar RK, Walson PD, Fritz WL, Perry DF, Barbee RA (1979) Kinetics of Theophylline. Variability and effect of arterial pH in chronic obstructive lung disease. Chest 76: 11–16
Richardson PDI, Withrington PC (1981) Liver blood flow I-Intrinsic and nervous control of liver blood flow. Gastroenterology 81: 159–173
Rizzo A, Mirabella A, Ferrara G, Pipitone P, Bellia V, Bonsignore G (1982) Theophylline pharmacokinetics in patients with mild or severe airway obstruction. Bull Eur Physiopathol Respir 18: 811–818
Robin ED, Theodore J (1982) Are there ischemic lung diseases? Arch Intern Med 142: 1791–1793
Rosenow ED III (1972) The spectrum of drug-induced pulmonary disease. Ann Intern Med 77: 977–991
Rosenow ED III (1977) Drug-induced pulmonary disease. Clin Notes Respir Dis 16: 3–11
Roth RA, Rubin RJ (1976) Role of blood flow in carbon monoxide and hypoxic hypoxia induced alterations in hexobarbital metabolism in rats. Drug Metab Dispos 4: 460–467
Roth RA, Wiersma DA (1979) Role of the lung in total body clearance of circulating drugs. Clin Pharmacokinet 4: 355–367
Rierson G, Block ER, Harris JO, Cannon JK (1981) 5-Hydroxytryptamine uptake by lungs of hamsters with pulmonary emphysema. Exp Lung Res 2: 241–248
Saltiel JC, Chretien J (1972) Pathogénie pulmonaire médicamenteuse. Med Hygiène 30: 1864–1866
Schmid ER, Rehder K (1981) Anesthesia and the chest wall. Anesthesiology 55: 668–675
Sjostrom K, Crapo JD (1983) Structural and biochemical adaptative changes in rat lungs after exposure to hypoxia. Lab Invest 48: 68–79
Sole MJ, Drobac M, Schwartz L, Hussain MN, Vaughan-Neil EF (1979) The extraction of circulating catecholamines by the lungs in normal man and in patients with pulmonary hypertension. Circulation 60: 160–163
Sostman HD, Matthay RA, Putman CE (1976) Methotrexate pneumonitis. Medicine (Baltimore) 55: 371–388
Sostman HD, Matthay RA, Putman CE (1977) Cytotoxic drug-induced lung disease. Am J Med 62: 608–615
Sostman HD, Putman CE, Gamsu G (1981) Diagnosis of chemotherapy lung. Am J Roentgenol 136: 33–40

Sotaniemi E, Arvela P, Huhti E, Koivisto O (1971) Half-life of tolbutamide in patients with chronic respiratory failure. Eur J Clin Pharmacol 4: 29–31

Stalcup SA, Lipset JS, Woan JM, Leuenberger PhJ, Mellins RB (1979) Inhibition of angiotensin converting enzyme activity in cultured endothelial cells by hypoxia. J Clin Invest 63: 966–976

Stalcup SA, Leuenberger PhJ, Lipset JS, Osman MM, Cerreta JM, Mellins RB, Turino GM (1981) Impaired angiotensin conversion and bradykinin clearance in experimental canine emphysema. J Clin Invest 67: 201–209

Svedmyr N, Simonsson NS (1981) Drugs in the treatment of asthma. In: Widdicombe JG (ed) Respiratory pharmacology. Pergamon Press, Oxford New York Toronto Sydney Paris Frankfurt, IEPT, Section 104, p 657

Tech CJ, Lehane JR, Jones JG (1980) Respiratory depression following diazepam. Anesthesiology 53: 293–298

Tomashefski JF Jr, Hirsch CS (1980) The pulmonary vascular lesions of intravenous drug abuse. Hum Pathol 11: 133–145

Touraine R (1977) Les accidents respiratoires d'origine médicamenteuse. Lyon Med 238: 451–455

Tryka AF, Skornik WA, Godleski JJ, Brain JD (1982) Potentiation of Bleomycin-induced lung injury by exposure to 70% oxygen: Morphologic assessment. Am Rev Respir Dis 126: 1074–1079

Weibel ER (1973) Morphological basis of alveolar-capillary gas exchange. Physiol Rev 53: 419–495

Weiss RB, Muggia FM (1980) Cytotoxic drug induced pulmonary disease: Update 1980. Am J Med 68: 259–266

Whitcomb ME (1973) Drug-induced lung disease. Chest 63: 418–422

Wilkinson GR (1976) Pharmacokinetics in disease states modifying body perfusion. In: Benet LZ (ed) The effect of disease states on drug pharmacokinetics. American Pharmaceutical Association, Academy of Pharmaceutical Sciences, Washington D.C., p 13

Wilkinson GR, Shand DG (1975) A physiological approach to hepatic drug clearance. Clin Pharmacol Ther 18: 377–390

Young RC, Ozols RF, Myers CE (1981) The anthracycline antineoplastic drugs. N Engl J Med 305: 139–153

Zwillich CW, Sutton FD Jr, Neff TA, Cohn WM, Matthay RA, Weinberger MM (1975) Theophylline-induced seizures in adults. Ann Intern Med 82: 784–787

Note added in proof. In this brief note we mention how the pharmacokinetic function of the pulmonary circulation (P.C.) can place the lung at risk of toxicity from xenobiotic molecules. The phospholipidosis induced by the amphiphilic drugs may prominantly involve the lung just because they are subjected to strong pulmonary accumulation, their lung tissue concentration usually leading that found in most other organs. On the other hand, as exemplified by Mehendale's group (1983), once accumulated, some drugs markedly depress the normal clearance function of the P.C. toward vasoactive andogenous amines 5-HT and NE; since these amines influence pulmonary vascular tone, the pulmonary hypertension observed following long-term use of highly accumulated anorectics (e.g.; Chlorphentermine) could conceivably result from long-standing impaired amine clearance. The potential toxicity of metabolic activation has been recently masterly reviewed (Minchin and Boyd 1983); oxidation of xenobiotics particularly aromatic hydrocarbons by e.g. monoxygenases can form instable electrophiles apt to bind covalently to cell constituents thereby inducing damage; on the other hand, during reduction, electron-redundant metabolites form, which are likely to generate highly reactive oxygen species from O_2, their toxicity relying upon lipid peroxidation. Very interestingly, the cell-specific toxicity of some compounds according to whether they are activated by oxidation or reduction is likely to stem from the unequal lung-cell content in the responsible enzymes. Teleologically speaking, the lung may have been given a pharmacokinetic function to specifically process autologous molecules, which occurs without any harmful consequences; the involvement of the same function during the handling of xenobiotics however, can form one basis for lung toxicity.

Minchin RF, Boyd MR (1983) Localization of metabolic activation and deactivation systems in the lung, significance to the pulmonary toxicity of xenobiotics, Annu Rev Pharmacol Toxicol 23: 217–238

Morita T, Mehendale HM (1983) Drug-specificity in the perturbation of pulmonary disposition of serotonin in Rabbit in vivo, Pharmacology 27: 289–297

Disease, Metabolism and Reproduction in the Toxic Response to Drugs and Other Chemicals
Arch. Toxicol., Suppl. 7, 88–89 (1984)

Lead in Cerebrospinal Fluid in Cerebrovascular Disease: Its Possible Diagnostic, Prognostic and Toxic Significance

K. G. Kjellin†

Department of Neurology, Karolinska Hospital, 104 01 Stockholm, Sweden

Abstract. The reports on cerebrospinal fluid (CSF) lead are rather few and the results mostly divergent. Unfortunately, the collection procedure is often inadequately described. Using a low-contaminating device for lumbar puncture, the author had previously found "normal" CSF lead to be < 1 μg/dl. The potential value of CSF-lead analysis in cerebrovascular disease (CVD), combined with "quantitative CSF spectrophotometry" (CSF-SPE) elaborated by the author and shown to be very effective for clinical use, was studied. Anρdic stripping voltammetry (ASV), a fast, simple and sensitive method, requiring rather inexpensive equipment, was used for CSF and serum analyses of lead and cadmium. Increased lead levels in CSFs withdrawn by the above mentioned device were found in CVD. Considering the possible introduction of CSF-lead analysis for routine clinical use, the CSF was also withdrawn by conventional stainless-steel needles. Three intervals of CSF-lead levels were observed in non-vascular cases, ischaemic infarction, and haemorrhagic infarction, respectively. The results indicate that determination of CSF lead may be valuable in CVD in addition to CSF-SPE. An extended study could confirm the trend found with a correlation between the increase of CSF lead and the extent of brain damage. CSF-lead analysis may then turn out to be of prognostic importance. The conceivable pathophysiological effects of CSF trace-element increases, have been discussed previously. Moreover, recent reports on the interactions of lead with different cell components are to be considered. Increased CSF lead, probably combined with increased levels in the extracellular fluid, may be a risk factor for partly damaged and non-damaged brain tissue.

Key words: Cerebrospinal fluid – CSF Lead – CSF Cadmium – Cerebrovascular disease – Anodic stripping voltammetry – Trace element CSF-analyses

Acknowledgements. The investigation was supported by grants from the Karolinska Institute.

References

Kjellin KG (1981) Trace elements in the cerebrospinal fluid in neurological diseases. Clin Toxicol 18: 1237–1245

Kjellin KG (1983) Xanthochromic compounds in cerebrospinal fluid: Quantitative spectrophotometry and electromigration. In: Wood JH (ed) Neurobiology of cerebrospinal fluid 2, chapt 33. Plenum Press, New York, pp 559–570

Kjellin KG, Sidén Å (1983) Cerebrospinal fluid proteins in infectious neurological diseases and Guillain-Barré syndrome. In: Wood JH (ed) Neurobiology of cerebrospinal fluid 2, chapt 20. Plenum Press, New York, pp 369–386

Disease, Metabolism and Reproduction in the Toxic Response to Drugs and Other Chemicals
Arch. Toxicol., Suppl. 7, 90–93 (1984)

A Comparative Study of Acute Toxicity of Drugs Used During Anticancer Therapy in Healthy and Tumor-Bearing Mice

P. Scorza Barcellona, A. Campana, V. Rossi, C. Corradino, and B. Silvestrini

F. Angelini Research Institute, Viale Amelia 70, 00181 Rome, Italy

Abstract. A comparative study was performed, in healthy and Ehrlich ascites bearing mice, to ascertain if the acute toxicity of drugs can change in disease conditions. Adriamycin, cis-platinum, cyclophosphamide, 5-fluorouracil, vinblastine, morphine and cefoxitin were administered intravenously; prochlorperazine and acetylsalicylic acid were given orally, and dexamethasone and lonidamine were given by both routes. With the exception of morphine, the LD_{50}'s significantly decreased in tumor bearing animals. The highest potency ratios (about 4–6) were observed with prochlorperazine and cyclophosphamide and the lowest (1.3–1.4) with lonidamine given intravenously, adriamycin and acetylsalicylic acid. These results confirm that the toxic response may be strongly influenced by pathological states.

Key words: Acute toxicity – Antineoplastic agents – Ehrlich ascites tumor-bearing mice – Acetylsalicylic acid – Adriamycin – Cefoxitin – cis-Platinum – Cyclophosphamide – 5-Fluorouracil – Dexamethasone – Lonidamine – Morphine – Prochlorperazine – Vinblastine

Introduction

The toxicity of drugs is currently evaluated on the basis of tests carried out in healthy animals, whereas medicines are intended for subjects with various disease conditions. Since these deviations from the normal state of health are likely to influence the toxic response in the exposed individual (Doull 1980), it was decided to perform a comparative acute toxicity study in healthy and sick animals. For this purpose, highly toxic compounds, such as antitumor drugs, were tested in healthy and tumor bearing mice. Moreover, some other commonly used drugs, which may also be administered during anticancer therapy, were also studied.

Materials and Methods

Swiss CD-1 mice (Charles River, Calco, Italy) of both sexes, weighing 26–33 g, were used. The tumor bearing mice were prepared by injecting intraperitoneally 0.25 ml of sterile saline containing 6×10^6 Ehrlich ascites carcinoma (EAC) cells. Seven days later the animals in which an evident abdominal swelling developed were considered affected by tumor.

Groups consisting of 10 males and 10 females, both healthy and 7-day EAC bearing mice, were treated once with a range of 5–8 dose levels of the following drugs: lonidamine (LON) (ACRAF, Rome) suspended in 0.5% methylcellulose solution (MTC) for the oral route, or dissolved in H_2O as arginine salt for the intravenous route; cis-platinum diammine dichloride (CPDD) (Platinex, Bristol, Sermoneta), adriamycin (ADR) (Adriablastina, Farmitalia, Milan), vinblastine (VBL) (Velbe, Lilly, Sesto Fiorentino), cyclophosphamide (CYC) (Endoxan-Asta, Schering, Milan), 5-fluorouracil (5-FU) (Fluoro-Uracile, Roche, Milan), cefoxitin (CEF) (Mefoxin, Merck Sharp & Dohme, Rome), morphine HCl (MOR) (ACRAF, Rome), all dissolved in H_2O and administered intravenously; prochlorperazine maleate (PCP) (Agrar, Rome) and acetylsalicylic acid (ASA) (Agrar, Rome) both suspended in MTC and administered orally; dexamethasone disodic phosphate (DEX) (Agrar, Rome) dissolved in H_2O for the intravenous and oral route. All drugs were administered in a constant volume of 10 ml/kg, which when given by the intravenous route was injected over a constant time of 15 s.

After dosing, the animals were checked for 7 days to assess mortality. Both, the mice which died during the observation period and the survivors on day 7, were submitted to postmortem. To ascertain the contribution of the diseased state to the mortality trend, 32 or 42 EAC bearing mice of both sexes were treated with 10 ml/kg of MTC by the oral route and 10 ml/kg of H_2O by the intravenous route, respectively, and observed until all died.

LD_{50}'s and all related values were calculated according to Litchfield and Wilcoxon (1949).

Results

The LD_{50}'s were calculated on the cumulative mortality at day 7, as after this time the lethality in untreated EAC bearing mice increased dramatically to 50% as opposed to 10% on day 7. Significantly different LD_{50} values (Table 1) between the two sexes were observed for LON by the oral route in healthy mice, with a greater sensitivity in females. However, in the EAC bearing mice, the males receiving DEX intravenously, VLB and CYC were more sensitive. The acute toxicity of the majority of the compounds studied was generally increased in the EAC bearing mice. The greatest increase was detected for PCP, with a potency ratio of 5.9; the other drugs increased the toxicity by 1.3 times in the case of LON given intravenously, and 2.8 times for CPDD. With the compounds which showed a different toxicity in the two sexes, the greater increase was detected in males, the potency ratio being between 2.0 for DEX intravenously

Table 1. Comparative acute toxicity of representative anticancer agents and some other drugs in healthy and tumor bearing mice

Drug	Route	Healthy mice LD_{50} in mg/kg (confidence limits)			EAC bearing mice LD_{50} in mg/kg (confidence limits)			Potency ratio[a] (healthy mice/ EAC bearing mice)
		M	F	M + F	M	F	M + F	
ADR	i.v.	13.5 (11.8–15.5)	12.8 (10.9–15.0)	13.0 (11.7–14.4)	7.4 (5.8–9.3)	9.6 (7.7–11.9)	9.1 (7.4–11.2)	1.4
CPDD	i.v.	12.2 (10.6–14.0)	11.3 (9.1–12.9)	11.0 (10.0–12.0)	4.1 (3.0–5.6)	3.4 (2.8–4.2)	3.9 (3.3–4.6)	2.8
CYC	i.v.	425 (390–462)	550 (363–833)	460 (385–548)	80* (72–89)	148* (115–190)	–	M 5.3 F 3.7
5-FU	i.v.	229 (186–281)	229 (181–290)	229 (193–272)	156 (101–240)	132 (99–176)	141 (108–183)	1.6
VBL	i.v.	17.5 (16.8–22.1)	16.5 (13.2–20.6)	17.0 (14.6–19.8)	5.6* (4.3–7.2)	10.8* (7.8–14.6)	–	M 3.1 F 1.5
LON	p.o.	2,050* (1,690–2,487)	1,490* (1,175–1,889)	–	570 (394–824)	790 (644–968)	730 (586–909)	M 3.6 F 1.9
	i.v.	150 (130–172)	145 (131–161)	142 (132–153)	113 (94–136)	118 (103–135)	110 (99–122)	1.3
DEX	p.o.	1,800 (1,400–2,314)	2,000 (1,637–2,443)	1,900 (1,659–2,176)	710 (531–949)	1,210 (785–1,866)	900 (701–1,155)	2.1
	i.v.	550 (443–682)	660 (563–773)	620 (542–709)	280* (213–360)	475* (367–615)	–	M 2.0 F 1.4
ASA	p.o.	1,700 (1,335–2,164)	1,670 (1,308–2,140)	1,750 (1,474–2,078)	1,350 (1,044–1,746)	1,050 (873–1,263)	1,250 (1,074–1,455)	1.4
CEF	i.v.	> 3,920	> 3,920	> 3,920	> 3,920	> 3,920	> 3,920	–
MOR	i.v.	180 (155–209)	185 (167–205)	183 (167–201)	218 (148–321)	164 (134–200)	180 (148–219)	1.0
PCP	p.o.	1,250 (960–1,628)	1,200 (968–1,488)	1,210 (1,437–1,019)	210 (164–267)	226 (176–289)	205 (169–248)	5.9

* Significant difference between males and females at $p < 0.05$
[a] All potency ratios greater than 1 are statistically significant

and 5.3 for CYC. No increase in toxicity was observed for MOR and CEF. For the latter, it was impossible to calculate the LD_{50}'s due to the drug's poor solubility above the dose of 3,920 mg/kg which produced lethal effects below 50%.

No differences in both the incidence and severity of the structural pathological changes were observed between healthy and EAC bearing mice.

Discussion

These experiments show that the acute toxicity of some drugs in tumor bearing animals is consistently higher than in healthy mice. Among antitumor drugs, CYC has the highest toxicity ratio (around 4.5), ADR the lowest one (1.4). With the other drugs, PCP has the highest (5.9) ratio, MOR the lowest (1.0). These results suggest that the drug toxicity in humans may vary in relation to the intended medical use. Since chronic toxicity studies in animals with specific pathological conditions are unrealistic, it is suggested that, whenever possible, acute toxicity studies should be performed in animal models mimicking the pathological conditions in which drugs are to be used.

References

Doull J (1980) Factors influencing toxicology. In: Doull J, Klaassen CD, Amdur MO (eds) Casarett and Doull's toxicology: The basic science of poisons. Macmillan Publishing Co., New York, p 70

Litchfield JT, Wilcoxon FA (1949) A simplified method for evaluating dose-effect experiments. J Pharmacol Exp Ther 96: 99–113

Disease, Metabolism and Reproduction in the Toxic Response to Drugs and Other Chemicals
Arch. Toxicol., Suppl. 7, 94–97 (1984)

Antitumour Drug Toxicity in Pituitary or Adrenal-Ablated Rats

M. Vacca, P. L. Navarra, and P. Preziosi

Department of Pharmacology, Medical Faculty of the Catholic University of the Sacred Heart
Largo F. Vito 1, 00168 Rome, Italy

Abstract. Hypophysectomy or adrenalectomy increase the toxicity of the antitumour drug hydroxyurea (HYD) given by the oral route at daily doses/kg over 5 days, 10 times higher (10 Htd) than that employed in daily schedules for humans (100% and 85% lethality against 0% in intact controls). No differences were found between intact or hypophysectomized rats in their ability to tolerate a 5-day treatment with 1 Htd HYD given orally, 1–10 Htd of procarbazine (i.v.) and cisplatinum (i.v.) at a dose per kg/day equivalent to that recommended for protocols providing daily drug schedules in humans. L-asparaginase (10 Htd) induce 45% lethality in adrenalectomized animals. All the above drugs in intact rats induce significant ($p < 0.01$) adrenocortical activation after single, and in the case of hydroxyurea after 5-days, treatment at the above dosages. Replacement therapy with corticosterone may reduce HYD toxicity in adrenalectomized (20% lethality) but less so (90% lethality) in hypophysectomized rats.

Key words: L-Asparaginase – Cisplatinum – Hydroxyurea – Procarbazine – Corticosterone – Hypophyseal-adrenal axis – Adrenalectomy – Hypophysectomy – Cancer chemotherapy – Oestrogen receptor positive advanced breast cancer – Proliferative lymphoid diseases – Immunosuppression

Introduction

Hypophysectomy and adrenalectomy are two major endocrine ablations sometimes performed as ultimate therapeutic procedures for selected neoplasias (Robin and Dalton 1977). Anticancer drugs may interfere with the adrenocortical function both at suprahypophyseal, hypophyseal and adrenocortical level (Preziosi et al. 1978). An investigation was carried out to see whether or not hypophysectomy or adrenalectomy could modify the previously settled ability of intact male adults rats to tolerate a 5-day treatment with four antitumour drugs [L-asparaginase (Asp), cisplatinum (*c*P), hydroxyurea (HYD) and procarbazine (PRC)]. These drugs had previously been found capable of eliciting a significant adrenocortical activation, 2 and 4 h after a single dose 10 times higher than those employed per kg in humans (10 × Human therapeutic dose, Htd) (Salmon 1980). This activation may be considered a possibly detrimental "alarm" or stress reaction with consequent immunosuppressive effects (Craddock 1978) and release by the adrenals of sex hormone precursors (e.g., androstenedione) undesirable in post-menopausal women with oestrogen-receptor positive advanced breast cancer for which hypophysectomy or adrenalectomy is suggested (Henderson Craig 1981; Robin and Dalton 1977). On the other hand it may be a useful physiological mechanism to increase blood glucocorticoid in neoplastic involvement of lymphoid tissue against which some glucocorticoids are valuable therapeutic agents (Calabresi and Parks 1980).

Materials and Methods

Animals (♂ Wistar rats, 200–250 g), housing, blood analysis (plasma corticosterone) have been previously described (Preziosi and Vacca 1982). The rats were hypophysectomized by the transauricular approach and adrenalectomized by the dorsal approach. The rats were employed not less than 5 days after hypophysectomy or 2 days after adrenalectomy. Food (commercial rat chow) and water were available ad libitum. The rats drank 0.9% saline with 5% glucose added. Lethality, behaviour, weight, food and water consumption were recorded throughout the experiments (5-days).

Experiment A. The following drugs were given (in mg if not otherwise specified), according to the recommended route in human therapy, to intact hypophysectomized or adrenalectomized rats:

	Dose/kg/day	Htd
Asp (i.v.) (Crasnitin, 10,000 U vials)	514–5,140	1–10
*c*P (i.v.) (Platinex, 10 mg/10 ml ampoules)	0.5–5	1–10
HYD (os) (Oncocarbide, 500 mg/capsule)	80–800	1–10
PRC (os) (Natulan, 50 mg/capsule)	2.8–28	1–10

Because of the toxicity on repeated treatment with 10 Htd single doses (18 mg/kg) *c*P was given at a dose of 0.5 mg/kg/day equivalent, like the dosages of the other above antitumour drugs, to that recommended for protocols providing a daily *c*P schedule in humans and at a dose 10 times higher (5 mg/kg/day).

Experiment B. Replacement therapy with corticosterone (Sigma) 1–2 mg/kg once or twice daily i.m. × 5 days was given to HYD (10 Htd) treated hypophysectomized or adrenalectomized rats. The corticosterone was dissolved in olive oil for injection (1 mg/ml).

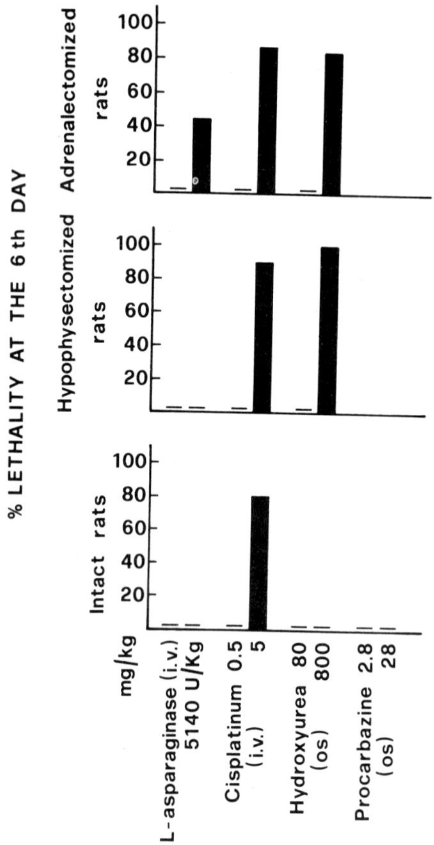

Fig. 1. Lethality in intact, hypophysectomized and adrenalectomized rats after a 5-day-treatment with antitumour drugs capable of eliciting in intact rats an adrenocortical activation following single and repeated (only 10 Htd HYD) treatments. Dark columns refer to a dose 10 times higher than human therapeutic dose. No lethality was observed for the human therapeutic dose of the above antitumour drugs

Results and Discussion

Neither hypophysectomy nor adrenalectomy produced a lethality or appreciably changed the weight, behaviour and food and water consumption over the 5-day period. None of the antitumour drugs produced a lethality or changed the behaviour of the hypophysectomised or the adrenalectomised rats at a dose per kg corresponding to the Htd. Weight changes were within ± 10% for all the antitumour drugs employed. Only HYD (10 Htd) displayed a unique marked toxicity in both the hypophysectomized and adrenalectomized animals (Fig. 1). Asp (10 Htd) induced 45% lethality in adrenalectomized animals on the 6th day. *c*P (10 Htd) induced high lethality both in intact and in endocrine-ablated animals (Fig. 1).

In intact rats HYD (10 Htd) retained the ability to elicit adrenocortial activation 2 and 4 h after the last of 5 daily administrations. The plasma corticosterone levels were +103 and +84%, respectively, compared with the vehicle-treated controls (in press). This might represent a useful mechanism to counteract a peculiar drug toxicity. In the absence of the pituitary or the adrenals this mechanism could be lacking, thus increasing HYD toxicity. Replacement

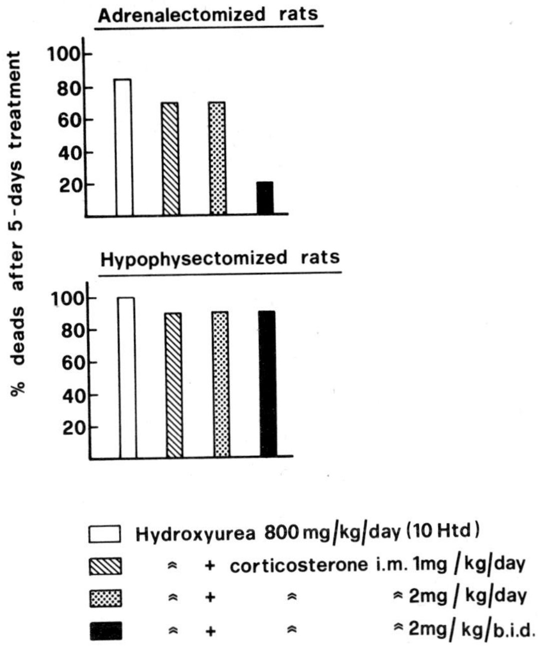

Fig. 2. Lethality in hydroxyurea (10 Htd × 5 days) treated hypophysectomized or adrenalectomized rats with or without the replacement therapy of corticosterone in oil by intramuscular route

therapy with the main adrenocortical rat hormone, corticosterone (2 mg/kg × 2 daily × 5 days), seems able to reduce the effects of adrenalectomy (Fig. 2) but not or much less so, the effects of hypophysectomy (Fig. 2) on HYD toxicity.

Acknowledgements. Supported by CNR contract n. 81.001443.96 Progetto Finalizzato "Controllo Crescita Neoplastica" c/o UCSC. M. Vacca and P. Preziosi members of the above project.

References

Calabresi P, Parks RE JR (1980) Chemotherapy of neoplastic disease. In: Gilman AG, Goodman LS, Gilman A (eds) The pharmacological basis of therapeutics, 6th ed. Saunders, New York, p 1301

Craddock CG (1978) Corticosteroid-induced lymphopenia, immunosuppression and body defense. Ann Intern Med 88: 564–566

Henderson Craig I (1981) Selection of therapy for metastatic breast cancer. In: Santen RJ, Henderson Craig I (eds) A comprehensive guide to the therapeutic use of aminoglutethimide. Karger, Basel, pp 58–63

Preziosi P, Vacca M (1982) Etomidate and corticotrophic axis. Arch Inter Pharmacodyn Ther 256: 308–310

Preziosi P, Scapagnini U, Di Renzo GF, Schettini G, Annunziato L (1978) Effetti neuroendocrini di chemiantibiotici antiblastici. Giorn Ital Chemioter 25: 127–133

Robin PE, Dalton GA (1977) The role of major endocrine ablation. In: Stoll BA (ed) Breast cancer managements: Early and late. Year Book Med Publ, Chicago, pp 147–153

Salmon SE (1980) Cancer chemotherapy. In: Meyers FH, Jawetz E, Goldfien A (eds) Medical pharmacology. Lange Med Publ, Los Altos, California, pp 477–513

Disease, Metabolism and Reproduction in the Toxic Response to Drugs and Other Chemicals
Arch. Toxicol., Suppl. 7, 98–102 (1984)

Tolerance to Pituitary-Adrenal Axis Activation by Anticancer Drugs in Normal and Tumour-Bearing Rats

M. Vacca and P. Preziosi

Department of Pharmacology, Medical Faculty of the Catholic University of the Sacred Heart, Largo F. Vito 1, 00168 Rome, Italy

Abstract. Cisplatinum given intravenously (i.v.), hydroxyurea given orally (os), procarbazine (os) and L-asparaginase (i.v.), on a decreasing scale, produce significant ($p < 0.01$) adrenocortical activation over 4-h period at a single dose per kg 10 times higher than those employed in human therapy. Only hydroxyurea retained this activity after a 5-day treatment both in normal and Walker carcinosarcoma-bearing rats. Adrenocortical activation depends on the presence of pituitary ACTH both after single or repeated treatments.

Key words: L-Asparaginase – Cisplatinum – Hydroxyurea – Procarbazine – ACTH – Hypothalamus-hypophyseal-adrenal axis – Adrenal cortex – Cancer chemotherapy – Drug effects – Tolerance – Walter carcinosarcoma

Introduction

The possible induction of tolerance of the adrenocortical activation seen after a single injection of antitumour drugs (Vacca et al. 1982), the target endocrine structure involved in such an activation and drugs displaying no tolerance as regards adrenocortical activation have been investigated. The possible persistence of this in tumour-bearing rats as well as the possible appearance of such an activation for drugs unable to retain this activation following repeated treatment has also been studied.

Materials and Methods

Animals (♂ Wistar rats, 200–250 g), housing, blood analysis (plasma corticosterone, plasma B) as previously (Preziosi and Vacca 1982). The rats were hypophysectomized by transauricular approach and employed not less than five days after the intervention. Walker carcinosarcomas were grafted according to Preziosi and Marmo (1960) and the animals employed after 25 days bearing a non-ulcered neoplastic mass of approximately the same size. The rats were sacrificed by decapitation 2–4 h after administration of the drugs. To prevent stress in the remaining rats sampling was performed in an area adjacent to the rat holding room.

Drugs. The drugs were given by the intravenous (i.v.) or oral (os) route according to the recommended route in human therapy (Salmon 1980). The volume used was 1–5 ml/kg body weight. The following drugs, found able, after a single administration at doses per kg 10 times higher than those employed in the human (10 × human therapeutic dose, Htd) (Salmon 1980), to elicit a significant ($p < 0.01$) adrenocortical activation over a period of 4 h (Vacca et al. 1982) were given daily for 5 days (doses in mg if not otherwise indicated):

	Dose/kg × 5 days
L-asparaginase (Asp) (i.v.) (Crasnitin, 10,000 U/10 ml ampoul)	5,140 U
Hydroxyurea (HYD) (os) (Oncocarbide, 500 mg/capsule)	800
Procarbazine (PRC) (os) (Natulan, 50 mg/capsule)	28

Because of the toxicity on repeated treatment with 10 Htd (18 mg/kg), cis-platinum (*c*P) was given at a dose of 0.5 mg/k/day equivalent to that recommended for protocols providing daily instead of single-dose schedule in humans (Salmon 1980). Drugs able to elicit an adrenocortical activation after a single administration were also given for 5-day treatment to hypophysectomized rats. $ACTH_{1-24}$ [Synachten, 0.25 mg (25 UI)/ampoul] was given to the hypophysectomized rats by the intramuscular route at a dose of 700 mU/kg either as a single dose or repeated doses over 5 days.

All the results are expressed as group arithmetic means and standard error of the means (SE). Analysis of variance and Student-Newmann-Keul's test for multiple comparison among groups were used to analyze the data. Differences between group means were considered significant if $p < 0.05$.

Results and Discussion

After repeated treatment, adrenocortical activation continued only with HYD (Table 1). A weak, not statistically significant adrenal activation was observed for *c*P given because of its high toxicity at a dose of 0.5 mg per kg/day; this corresponds to the dose employed in the repeated treatment schedule in cancer chemotherapy; it is lower than that (18 mg/kg) capable of eliciting a strong adrenocortical activation after a single i.v. injection (Vacca et al. 1982).

The adrenocortical activation seen 2 and 4 h after the 5th daily HYD administration is more evident in Walker carcinosarcoma-bearing rats (Fig. 1). PRC is unable to elicit a significant adrenocortical activation after a 5-day treatment either in intact or tumour-bearing rats.

The adrenocortical response to Asp, *c*P and PRC seems to depend on the presence of pituitary ACTH since it does not occur after single and repeated

Table 1. Percentage variations of plasma corticosterone against the respective vehicle-treated controls after single and repeated treatments with anticancer drugs capable of inducing statistically significant adrenocortical activation after single treatment

Drugs	mg/kg	Route	Single treatment		5-day treatment	
			2 h	4 h	2 h	4 h
L-asparaginase	5140 (U)	i.v.	+ 37[a]	+ 35[a]	+ 3.3	− 24
Cisplatinum	18−0.5*	i.v.	+ 61[a]	+ 37[b]	+ 43	+ 9
Hydroxyurea	800	os	+ 40[a]	+ 104[a]	+ 84[a]	+ 66[a]
Procarbazine	28	os	+ 103[a]	+ 92[a]	+ 15	− 31

[a] Significant for $p < 0.01$ against the respective controls
[b] Significant for $p < 0.05$ against the respective controls
* Dosage employed in daily treatment schedule

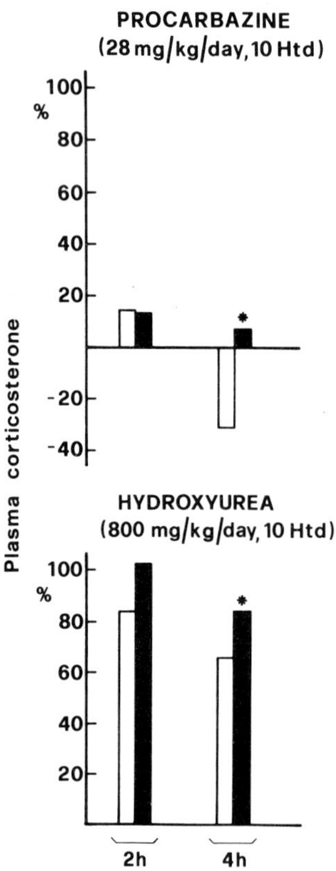

Fig. 1. Effect on plasma corticosterone of 5-day oral treatment with two antitumour drugs capable of eliciting a remarkable adrenocortical activation after single dose 2 and 4 h following the last administration in intact and Walker carcinosarcoma-bearing rats. Vertical bars represent the % change of plasma corticosterone against the relevant vehicle-treated controls for each group: □, intact rats; ■, Walker carcinosarcoma-bearing rats. * Significant for $p < 0.01$ against the intact rats

treatments if the rats are hypophysectomized prior to the administration of the drugs, in the presence of retained adrenocortical activation to exogenous ACTH (Fig. 2). Unexpected drug toxicity after pituitary ablation prevented repeated treatment with the only drug (HYD 10 Htd) capable of retaining adrenocortical activation after the 5-day-treatment.

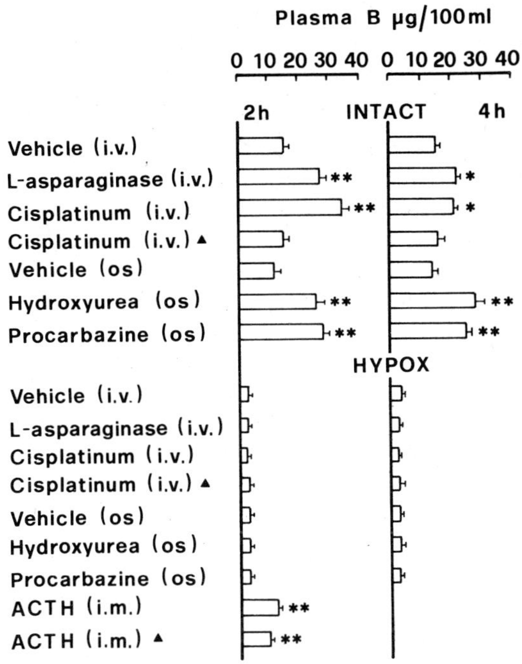

Fig. 2. Effect on plasma corticosterone (plasma B) of a single or repeated treatment with anticancer drugs in intact or hypophysectomized male rats. Each group consisted of at least eight animals. Vertical bars represent the standard error of the mean. The doses per kg employed [L-asparaginase 5140 U/kg; cisplatinum 18 mg/kg; hydroxyurea 800 mg/kg; procarbazine 28 mg/kg] are 10 times higher than those employed in human therapy. Cisplatinum was also given at doses of 0.5 mg/kg/day for 5 days (▲) the rats being killed 2 and 4 h after the 5th drug administration. 700 mU/kg ACTH was given as single or repeated (▲) treatments and the animals were killed 60 min thereafter (ACTH effect diminishes afterward). Significant for $p < 0.01$ (**) or $p < 0.05$ (*) against the relevant vehicle given rats. ACTH values are significant ($p < 0.01$) against vehicle and antitumour drugs-treated hypophysectomized rats

Hypophyseal activation may also be a unique feature of some anticancer drugs which may be explained as a stress reaction fitting into the systemic disturbance ensuing from administration of antitumour drugs. If this response is also present in man, tolerance to hypophyseal adrenal activation by antiproliferative agents may minimize a drug-induced detrimental change [in post-menopausal oestrogen receptor positive breast cancers, in patients exhibiting a proteocatabolic state and for possible immunosuppression (Craddox 1978) due to an advanced neoplasia], but it may nullify a possibly useful long-lasting increase in glucocorticoid release in acute leukaemia in children and in lymphoma disease (Calabresi and Park 1980).

Acknowledgements. Supported by CNR contract n. 81.01443.96 Progetto Finalizzato "Controllo Crescita Neoplastica" c/o UCSC. M. Vacca and P. Preziosi were members of the above project.

References

Calabresi P, Parks RE Jr (1980) Chemotherapy of neoplastic disease. In: Gilman AG, Goodman LS, Gilman A (eds) The pharmacological basis of therapeutics, 6th edn. Saunders, New York, p 1301

Craddock CG (1978) Corticosteroid-induced lymphopenia, immunosuppression and body defense. Ann Intern Med 28: 564–566

Preziosi P, Marmo E (1960) Effets de la dexaméthasone et de l'association dexaméthasone-tétracycline sur certaines tumeurs expérimentales. Chemotherapia 2: 89–112

Preziosi P, Vacca M (1982) Etomidate and corticotrophic axis. Arch Int Pharmacodyn Ther 256: 308–310

Salmon SE (1980) Cancer chemotherapy. In: Meyers FH, Jawetz E, Goldfien A (eds) Medical pharmacology. Lange Med Publ, Los Altos, California, pp 477–513

Vacca M, Cerrito F, Balzamo S, Preziosi P (1982) Pituitary adrenal axis and plasma prolactin following administration of clinically-useful anticancer drugs. Presented at the XXI Ital Cong of Pharmacology, June 2–5, 1982, Naples, Italy. Abs Book, p 191 (abstr. 51)

Disease, Metabolism and Reproduction in the Toxic Response to Drugs and Other Chemicals
Arch. Toxicol., Suppl. 7, 103–105 (1984)

Toxins in Hepatic Encephalopathy: The Role of the Synergistic Effect of Ammonia, Mercaptans and Short Chain Fatty Acids

M. Baraldi[1], G. Pinelli[2], P. Ricci[2], and M. L. Zeneroli[2]

[1] Istituto di Farmacologia, Università di Modena, Via Campi 287, 41100 Modena, Italy
[2] Clinica Medica III, Università di Modena, Via del Pozzo, 41100 Modena, Italy

Abstract. Evidence has been recently produced that neurological changes which characterize hepatic encephalopathy due to fulminant hepatic failure in rats are linked with a pathology of GABA receptors. In the search for the peripheral toxins responsible for the CNS impairment present in hepatic encephalopathy it has been shown that the administration of ammonia and mercaptans and octanoic acid in normal rats reproduced behavioural and electrophysiological changes similar to those seen in galactosamine induced encephalopathy. The present report shows that a subacute administration of the above toxins induced a marked alteration of the GABA receptor complex which may account for the CNS derangement of hepatic encephalopathy.

Key words: Ammonium chloride – Dimethyldisulfide – GABA receptors – Hepatic encephalopathy – Octanoic acid

Hepatic encephalopathy (HE) due to fulminant hepatic failure (FHF) is a very complex syndrome characterized by agitation followed by lethargy, somnolence, stupor and finally coma (Conn and Lieberthal 1979; Zieve 1981). The symptoms are paralleled by the appearance of hyperplastic astrocytes, degeneration of nerve cells and demyelinating processes (Diemer, 1978). The syndrome occurs when overall liver function is grossly subnormal and, as a consequence, many metabolic changes occur and several toxins accumulate in the blood but the primary factor or factors causing HE is still unknown.

In this context, researches carried out in order to define the neuronal mechanism of HE, demonstrated, in the brain of rabbits and rats with HE due to galactosamine injection, a pathology of GABA receptors (Schafer and Jones 1982; Baraldi and Zeneroli 1982). Rats with mild HE showed an increase in low and high affinity GABA receptors that may be interpreted as a denervation

Correspondence address: Dr. M. Baraldi at the above address.

supersensitivity phenomenon, while in the severe stage of HE there is a loss of low affinity GABA receptors with a selection of only high affinity GABA receptors (Baraldi and Zeneroli 1982; Zeneroli et al. 1982a). Other studies carried out to evaluate the electrophysiological changes occurring both in HE due to FHF and in coma-like states produced in normal animals by the injection of toxins presumably involved in the pathogenesis of HE, demonstrated that the subacute injection of substances, that accumulate during HE, ammonia, mercaptans and octanoic acid, can mimic the visual evoked potential pattern of HE when injected in combination (Zeneroli et al. 1982b).

The aim of the present study was to verify whether the above mentioned toxins, injected alone or in combination in normal rats could reproduce GABA receptor changes similar to those described in rats with HE and, as a consequence, to ascertain their primary role in the pathogenesis of HE.

Fifty rats, divided into five groups, were treated with saline or with a solution containing NH_4Cl (2.3 mmoles/kg) or octanoic acid (OA) (0.5 mmoles/kg) or dimethyldisulfide (DMDS) (230 μmoles/kg) or NH_4Cl + OA + DMDS (2.3 mmoles/kg + 0.5 mmoles/kg + 230 μmoles/kg) every 6 h × 4 times. This pretreatment was carried out in order to mimic somewhat better the prolonged exposure of the brain structures to toxins occurring in liver failure. It was followed 6 h later by a fifth injection of a solution containing the same toxins alone or in combination at three times higher concentrations. Fifteen minutes after this last injection 50% of the rats were sacrificed by decapitation; the brain was immediately removed and frozen. ^{3}H-GABA binding studies were performed on whole brain crude synaptic membrane preparation that had been three times frozen, thawed, treated with Triton X 100 and washed several times with Tris citrate buffer pH 7.1, as previously described (Baraldi et al. 1979; Baraldi and Zeneroli 1982).

The administration of the first doses did not produce gross behavioural alterations in any of the treated rats, whilst, after the last injection, different changes were observed depending on the injected toxin or the combination. In particular, as reported in Table 1, NH_4Cl and OA induced a sedative effect while DMDS elicited an hyperkinetic state. The three toxins injected in combination produced a nonconvulsive comatose state and death within 15–20 min.

The kinetic characteristics of ^{3}H-GABA binding, derived from the saturation curves performed on the brain membranes of each group of rats and the relative Scatchard plots, indicate, as shown in Table 1, that all the three toxins affected the number of GABA binding sites without changing the affinity constants. In comparison with the controls, NH_4Cl and OA increased significantly ($p < 0.01$) the high affinity GABA receptors, while DMDS abolished the low affinity binding sites. The combined injection of the three toxins resulted in a complete loss of low affinity GABA receptors which parallelled the presence of an increased number of high affinity GABA recognition sites. These data closely resemble the changes in GABA receptors seen in the severe stage of galactosamine-induced HE.

Ammonia, mercaptans and short chain fatty acids are neurotoxic agents capable of inducing a coma-like state when given alone at concentrations which induce brain levels higher than those reached in human and in experimental HE

Table 1. Effects of subacute administration of ammonia, octanoic acid (OA) and dimethyldisulfide (DMDS) alone and in combination on behavioral and on GABA receptor characteristics in rat

Toxins	Behaviour (5th injection)	^{3}H-GABA Kinetic components			
		Low affinity		High affinity	
		K_{D1} (nM)	B_{max1} (pmol/mg protein)	K_{D2} (nM)	B_{max2} (pmol/mg protein)
Saline	None	171 ± 25	5.5 ± 1.2	16 ± 4.0	1.2 ± 0.2
NH_4Cl	Sedation	188 ± 12	5.4 ± 0.8	19 ± 0.5	1.9 ± 0.1**
OA	Sedation	186 ± 30	6.9 ± 0.5	18 ± 1.2	2.0 ± 0.3**
DMDS	Hyperkinesia	–	–	15 ± 3.0	0.9 ± 0.3
NH_4Cl + OA + DMDS	Coma and death	–	–	25 ± 4.0	1.8 ± 0.2*

Reported values are mean ± SD. Student's *t*-test: * $p < 0.05$, ** $p < 0.01$ vs saline

(Zieve et al. 1974). Moreover two of them, NH_4Cl and DMDS, induce per se a convulsive coma. When given alone at low doses, by inducing brain concentrations very close to those found in HE (Zeneroli et al. 1982b), these three toxins alone do not induce a full coma in normal animals. However, when given in combination they produce a coma state which is characterized by GABA receptor alterations similar to those found in HE, thus suggesting their synergistic action and their primary role in the development of the neurological dysfunction of hepatic coma.

References

Baraldi M, Zeneroli ML (1982) Experimental hepatic encephalopathy: changes in γ-aminobutyric acid. Science 216: 427–429

Baraldi M, Guidotti A, Schwartz JP, Costa E (1979) GABA receptors in clonal cell lines: A model for study of benzodiazepine action at molecular level. Science 205: 821–823

Conn H, Lieberthal MM (1979) Management of fulminant hepatic failure. In: Conn H, Lieberthal MM (eds) The hepatic coma syndromes and Lactulose. Williams & Wilkins, Baltimore, pp 241–247

Schafer DF, Jones EA (1982) Hepatic encephalopathy and the γ-aminobutyric acid neurotransmitter system. Lancet 1: 18–20

Zeneroli ML, Iuliano E, Racagni G, Baraldi M (1982a) Metabolism and brain uptake of γ-aminobutyric acid in galactosamine-induced hepatic encephalopathy. J Neurochem 38: 1219–1222

Zeneroli ML, Ventura E, Baraldi M, Penne A, Messori E, Zieve L (1982b) Visual evoked potentials in encephalopathy induced by galactosamine, ammonia, dimethyldisulfide, and octanoic acid. Hepatology 2: 532–538

Zieve L (1981) The mechanism of hepatic coma. Hepatology 1: 360–365

Zieve L, Doizaki WM, Zieve FJ (1974) Synergism between mercaptans and ammonia or fatty acids in in the production of coma: a possible role for mercaptans in the pathogenesis of hepatic coma. J Lab Clin Med 83: 16–28

Toxic Effects on the Male Reproductive System

Disease, Metabolism and Reproduction in the Toxic Response to Drugs and Other Chemicals
Arch. Toxicol., Suppl. 7, 109–117 (1984)

Effects of Drugs and Chemicals on Spermatogenesis

F. Neumann

Research Laboratories of Schering AG, Department of Endocrine Pharmacology,
Müllerstrasse 170–178, 1000 Berlin 65, Federal Republic of Germany

Abstract. Many drugs and chemicals have been found which interfere with the process of spermatogenesis.

Among these substances are, for example, sex-hormones (androgens, antiandrogens, estrogens, progestogens, anabolics), chemotherapeutics, antibiotics, antifungal drugs, anticancer drugs, nonsteroidal antiinflammatory drugs, antihypertensives, neuroleptics, dopaminantagonists, indols, tranquilizers, tricyclic antidepressives, heavy metals (Co, Cd), MAO-inhibitors, antimetabolites, barbiturates, immunosuppressives (glucocorticoids), aldosteronantagonists, anticonvulsives, and perhaps alcohol and nicotine.

Concerning the mechanism by which spermatogenesis is effected several points of interference have to be considered: inhibition of gonadotrophin secretion, inhibition of enzymes involved in androgen biosynthesis, direct effects on the germinal epithelium or on Sertoli cell function, competitive inhibition of hormone action, damage of the blood-testes barrier and other mechanisms.

Some of these mechanisms will be discussed.

Key words: Drugs – Spermatogenesis

The germinal epithelium is one of the most proliferating tissues in the body capable of producing millions of spermatozoa every hour. It is also a very sensitive tissue and the regulation of testes function and spermatogenesis is very complex. For this reason, many drugs and chemicals have been described which interfere with this process and which might even induce sterility. Some of these substances are listed in Table 1.

The list is far from complete but should serve to give an impression about the variety of drugs and substances which can affect testes function. It includes, for example sex hormones, androgens, antiandrogens, estrogens, progestogens, anabolics, chemotherapeutics, antibiotics, antifungal drugs, anticancer drugs,

Table 1. Drugs and chemicals which effect or might effect spermatogenesis and fertility

Steroids Androgens Antiandrogens Estrogens Progestogens Anabolics **Chemotherapeutic agents and antibiotics** Thiophene Dinitrofuran Furadantin Furacin Actinomycin Chlorambucil Neomycin Gentamycin Trimethoprim **Inhibition of mitosis, alkylating agents** Cholchicine Vinblastine Busulphane Cyclophosphamide N-lost-derivatives Methan sulfonic acid ester	**Nonsteroidal antiphlogistic drugs** Aspirin? Indomethacin **Antihypertensives** Reserpine **Neuroleptics, dopamin-antagonists** Sulpiride **Indoles** Serotonin Melatonin **Tranquilizer** Chlorpromacine **Tricyclic antidepressives** **Heavy metals** Zn Cd Co	**MAO-inhibitors** **Antimetabolites** 5-Thio-glucose Folic acid antagonists Purine derivatives **PG $F_{2\alpha}$** **Barbiturates** **Immunosuppressives** Glucocorticoids **Aldosterone antagonists** Spironolactone **Anticonvulsives** Aminoglutethimide Alcohol? Nicotine?

non-steroidal antiphlogistic drugs, antihypertensives, neuroleptics, dopamine antagonists, indoles, tranquilizers, tricyclic antidepressives, heavy metals, monoaminooxydase inhibitors, antimetabolites, barbiturates, immunosuppressives, glucocorticoids, aldosterone antagonists, anticonvulsives, and also perhaps alcohol and nicotine.

For the toxicologist, it is very important to know the mechanism by which these substances interfere with testicular function because the severity and reversability of the disturbance depends on the process being disrupted. The toxicologist is involved in calculating the benefit-risk ratio. For this reason, one must know whether the effect on the male reproductive system in general and specificially the function of the testis is reversible or not reversible.

Briefly the various aspects of drug control or disruption of spermatogenesis will be discussed. The substances or substance classes affecting spermatogenesis act either directly or indirectly and the mechanism of action vary quite markedly.

It is well-known, that the function of the testis is mainly androgen dependent and because biosynthesis of androgens is regulated by the pituitary luteinizing hormone, any drug or compound which inhibits gonadotrophin secretion induces indirectly an androgen deficiency.

It should also be noted that the need for androgens within the testes is at least eight to 10 times higher when compared with other androgen target organs, for example, the prostate gland.

Table 2. Concentration of testosterone in serum and in testes cytosol of rats

nmol Testosterone/ml	
Serum 11 ± 2	Tests cytosol 83 ± 14

n = 12; I = standard error of the means

Table 2 shows the androgen concentrations in normal male rats in the serum and in testis cytosol. The testosterone concentration in testis cytosol is eight times higher compared with the serum concentration. Therefore, it becomes quite clear, that testosterone deficiency has a deleterious effect on spermatogenesis.

The inhibiton of spermatogenesis resulting from treatment with androgens, estrogens or synthetic progestogens is based on the long-known principle of negative feedback action (Gaarenstroom 1939; Greene and Burrill 1940; Greep and Chester-Jones 1950; Ludwig 1950; Rössle and Zahler 1938; Rubinstein and Kurland 1941; Yasuda and Johnson 1965; Zahler 1947a, b).

Various antihypertensive drugs (reserpine) and probably a number of antianxiety drugs (diazepam) or antipsychotic drugs (chlorpromazine), barbiturates and neuroleptics may interfere with gonadotrophin secretion (Tuchmann-Duplessis 1956).

The effect of some of these drugs seems to be mediated by a dopamine antagonism by stimulation of prolactin secretion. For example, neuroleptics or reserpine stimulate prolactin secretion by interfering with the dopaminergic system. High prolactin levels have an inhibitory effect on gonadotrophins as is known from animal experiments as well as from infertile patients. The effect of all these drugs acting by inhibition of gonadotrophin secretion seems to be fully reversible.

Other substances are capable of inhibiting enzymes involved in androgen biosynthesis. Spironolactone and aminoglutethimide belong in this category (Cash et al. 1967; Sitteri et al. 1974).

Figure 1 gives one example; it shows the inhibitory effect of spironolactone on testosterone biosynthesis in an in vitro system using testicular homogenates. Leydig cell function was stimulated by human chorionic gonadotrophin (HCG). The dose dependent decrease of testosterone biosynthesis by spironolactone is quite impressive.

Simultaneously, precursor molecules such as progesterone, androstendione and hydroxyprogesterone are found to accumulate. These hormones were measured in the medium. Again, the effect of these inhibitors is fully reversible.

Heavy metals, for example, cadmium, lead to a destruction of the blood-testis-barrier. The germinal epithelium undergoes total necrosis and does not recover (Favino et al. 1966; Gunn et al. 1961, 1963, 1965; Parizek 1957, 1960; Reddy et al. 1973). The Leydig cells seem to be less sensitive to heavy metals. There is some restoration of Leydig cell function as measured by the increase of testosterone synthesis several weeks after the administration of cadmium.

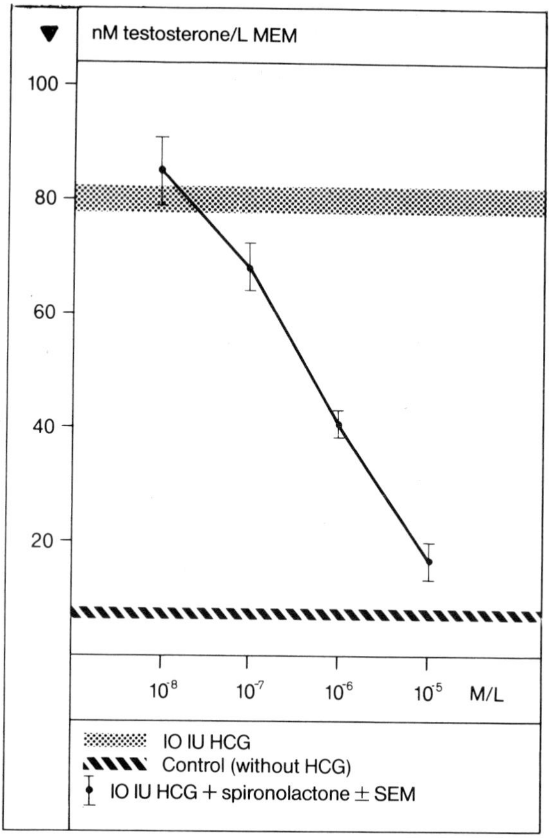

Fig. 1. Effect of spironolactone on testicular testosterone biosynthesis. $n = 12$ (from Nauert 1982)

Antimetabolites interfere with testicular function by causing nutritional disturbances (Chen and Whistler 1975; Neumann and Schenk 1976, 1977; Zysk et al. 1975). In studies with thioglucose and as is shown in Fig. 2, there is an extremely severe damaging effect on germ cells. It is not known whether this effect is fully reversible or not.

The effect of antimitotic and anticancer drugs including alkylating agents will be discussed in detail by other participants. Antimitotic and anticancer drugs are found to act directly on the germ cells (Buchanan et al. 1975; Hinkes and Plotkin 1973; Kumar 1972; Miller 1972; Qureshi et al. 1972; Weissbach et al. 1974; Rytter 1970).

Nitrofurane derivatives and some antibiotics and chemotherapeutics (for example gentamycin, oxytetracycline, trimethoprim) act in the same way (Dokov and Timmermanns 1970; Timmermanns 1974).

Several antiandrogens have an inhibitory effect on spermatogenesis. The extent of the inhibition of spermatogenesis is dose dependent and naturally varies from species to species. A consistent finding, however, is that only spermatid maturation (spermiogenesis) is affected initially by administration of medium doses. Meiosis fails to take place at higher doses and secondary

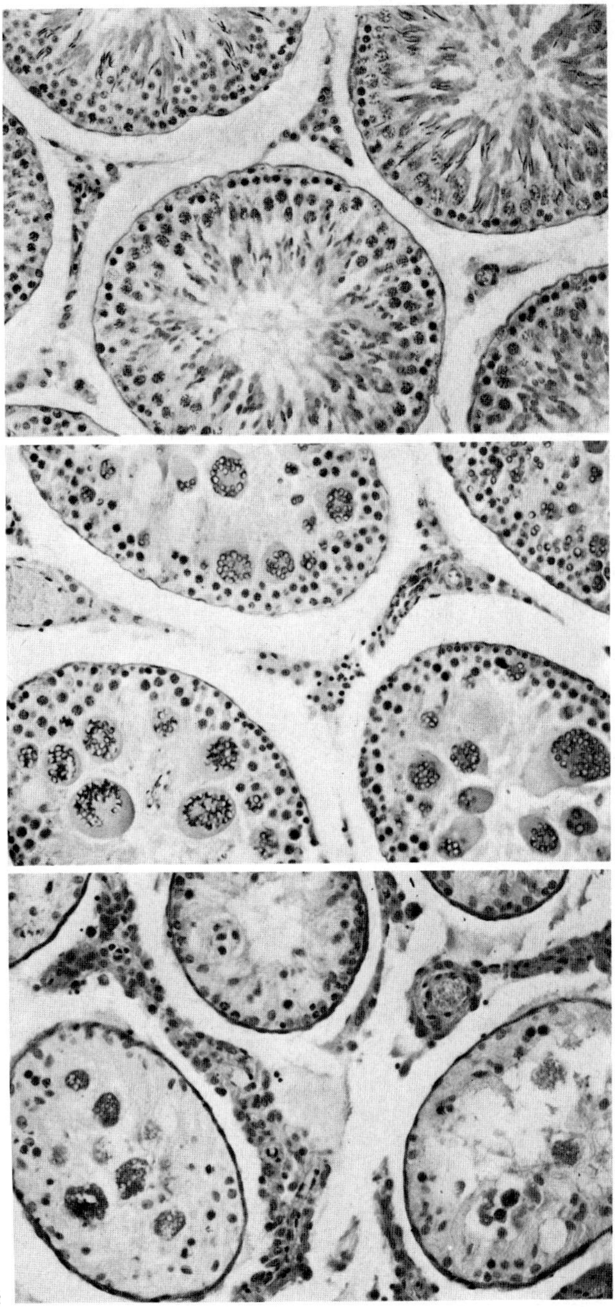

a b c

Fig. 2a–c. Rat testes. **a** Control; **b** 4 weeks after 5-thioglucose treatment (twice daily 40 mg/kg body weight s.c.). Note the formation of so-called giant cells; **c** 8 weeks after 5-thioglucose treatment (dose as described under **b**). Optically empty spaces delineate the previous presence of giant cells. Staining: **a,** Hematoxylin/Eosin; **b** and **c,** PAS-Lichtgrün. × 560

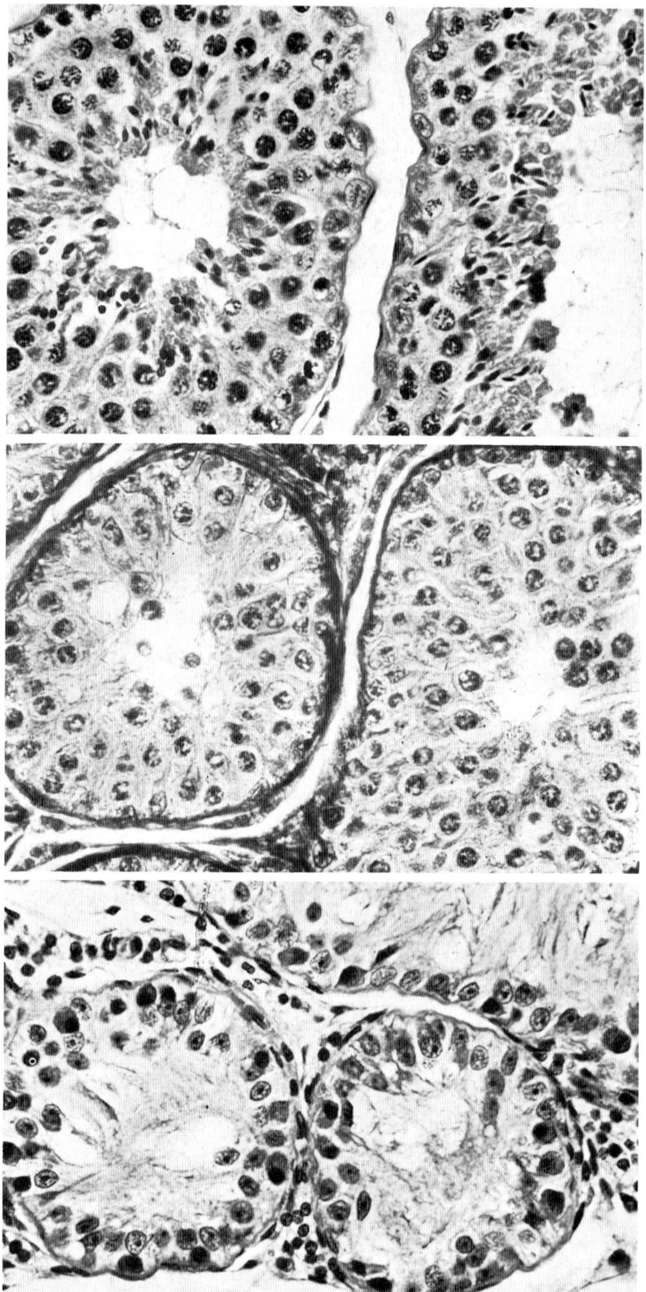

Fig. 3a–c. Testicular changes in the dog. **a** Control; **b** after 30 days intramuscular administration of 10 mg/day/kg body weight of cyproterone acetate, spermatogenesis is inhibited; **c** after approximately 12 months oral administration of 100 mg/day/kg body weight of cyproterone acetate, meiosis is also inhibited. Note the tubular atrophy and depopulation of the germinal epithelium. Staining: Hematoxylin/Eosin. × 304

spermatocytes are the most advanced stages of spermatogenesis which are found under these conditions. At extremely high doses, the convoluted tubules are completely depopulated and apart from Leydig cells, only spermatogonia and early spermatocyte forms are recognizable (Fig. 3a–c).

There is evidence that the point of attack of antiandrogens like cyproterone acetate is primarily at the androgen dependent Sertoli cells (Schenck and Neumann 1978).

It is well-known, that a specific secretory product of the Sertoli cells, the androgen binding protein (ABP) is important for the intratesticular transport of androgens and for the transport of androgens through the blood-testis barrier. It was assumed that antiandrogens also compete with androgens for binding sites on ABP. This is virtually not the case (Schenck and Neumann 1978). But ABP production is inhibited in a dose dependent manner by antiandrogens of the cyproterone acetate type and this effect is accompanied by decrease in testis weight as is shown in Fig. 4. According to this concept, the disturbance of spermatogenesis by antiandrogens would be a secondary effect attributable to limited secretory activity of the Sertoli cells. This assumption is supported by the observation that the follicle stimulating hormone (FSH) binding capacity of the Sertoli cells also decreases after treatment with cyproterone acetate (Neumann et al. 1976). The electron microscopic findings in the rat testes – namely, increased amounts of droplets and lyosome-like organelles in Sertoli cells – confirm this assumption (Hovatta and Koskimies 1978).

The effect of antiandrogens on spermatogenesis is fully reversible as has been shown experimentally and in men. So-called pure antiandrogens behave differently, but this will not be discussed here (for review: see Neumann and Schenck 1980).

The last effect to be mentioned is the influence of alcohol and nicotine on testicular function. Nicotine will not be commented upon. However, several years ago the effect of alcohol on spermatogenesis and fertility in rats was tested. The rats were allowed to drink only water containing 15% alcohol (a higher concentration of alcohol was not tolerated) for 6 months, and during this time fertility tests were performed by placing the "treated" males with fertile females. The outcome of this experiment was unexpected. Although the rats were always inebriated and slept almost all the time, fertility and spermatogenesis were never

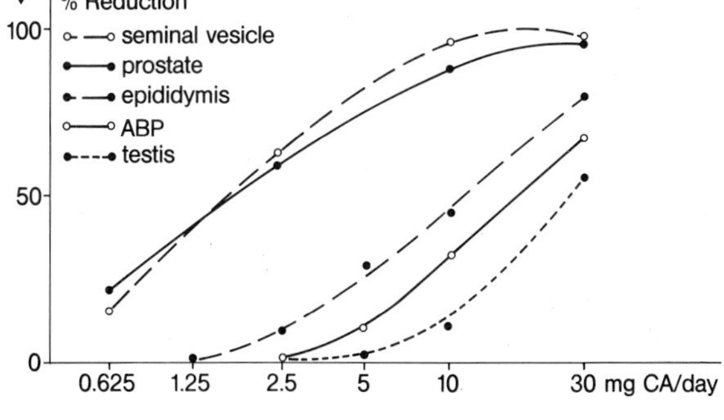

Fig. 4. Percent reduction of organ weights and ABP content in capita epididymides of intact rats treated for 6 weeks with cyproterone acetate (CA) related to hypophysectomized rats. (100% = reduction 6 weeks after hypophysectomy)

impaired. Other studies in which a deleterious effect of alcohol on spermatogenesis has been described were not confirmed.

Finally, it should be mentioned that all drugs and chemicals which inhibit testosterone synthesis directly or indirectly or which inhibit the effect of testosterone in the target organs, affect also the process of sperm maturation within the epididymis and the secretory activity of the accessory sexual glands, prostate and seminal vesicles.

References

Buchanan JE, Fairley KF, Barrie JU (1975) Return of spermatogenesis after stopping cyclophosphamide therapy. Lancet 7926: 156–157

Cash R, Brough AJ, Cohen MNP, Satoh PS (1967) Aminogluthetimide (elipten-Ciba) as an inhibitor of adrenal steroidogenesis: Mechanism of action and therapeutic trial. J Clin Endocrinol 27: 1239–1248

Chen M, Whistler RL (1975) Action of 5-thio-D-glucose and its 1-phosphate with hexokinase and phosphoglucomutase. Arch Biochem Biophys 169: 392–396

Dokov VK, Timmermanns L (1970) Arrêt de la spermatogénèse par certains antibiotiques recherches expérimentalis préliminaires. Acta Urol Belg 38: 277

Favino A, Baillie AH, Griffiths K (1966) Androgen synthesis by the testes and adrenal gland of rats poison with cadmium chloride. J Endocrinol 35: 185–192

Gaarenstroom JH (1939) Inhibition of the "antimasculine effect" of oestrone by testosterone propionate. Acta Brev Neerl Physiol 9: 134–135

Greene RR, Burrill WM (1940) The recovery of testes after androgen-induced inhibition. Endocrinology 26: 516–518

Greep RO, Chester Jones I (1950) Steroid control of pituitary function. Recent Prog Horm Res 5: 197

Gunn SA, Gould TC, Anderson WAD (1961) Zinc protection against cadmium injury to rat testis. Arch Pathol 71: 274–281

Gunn SA, Gould TC, Anderson WAD (1963) Cadmium induced interstitial cell tumors in rats and their prevention by zinc. J Natl Cancer Inst 31: 745–759

Gunn SA, Gould TC, Anderson WAD (1965) Comparative study of interstitial cell tumors of rat testis induced by cadmium intoxication and by vascular ligation. J Natl Cancer Inst 35: 329–337

Hinkes E, Plotkin D (1973) Reversible drug-induced sterility in a patient with acute leukaemia. JAMA 223: 1490–1491

Hovatta O, Koskimies AI (1978) Functional and structural aspects of the rat seminiferous tubules after treatment with exogenous cyproterone acetate, testosterone, progesterone and oestradiol. Int J Androl 1: 61

Kumar R, Biggart JD, McEvoy J, McGeown MG (1972) Cyclophosphamide and reproductive function. Lancet 7762: 1212–1214

Ludwig DJ (1950) The effect of androgen on spermatogenesis. Endocrinology 46: 453

Miller DG (1971/1972) Alkylating agents and human spermatogenesis. JAMA 217: 1662–1665; Fortschr Med 90: 316

Nauert Ch, Nishino Y (1982) Influence of steroidal aldosterone antagonists on testosterone biosynthesis in the testis of immature rats, in vitro. (Abstract No. 110) Acta Endocrinol [Suppl] (Kbh) 246: 98

Neumann F, Schenck B (1976) Pharmakologische Beeinflussung der Spermatogenese. 2. Cansteiner Colloquium. Arbeitstagung „Physiologie und Pathophysiologie der Hodenfunktion", Canstein/Sauerland

Neumann F, Schenck B (1980) Antiandrogens: Basic concepts and clinical trials. In: Cunningham GR, Schill WB, Hafez ESE (eds) Regulation of male fertility. Martinus Nijhoff Publishers, The Hague, Boston, London, p 93

Neumann F, Diallo FA, Hasan SH, Schenck B, Traore I (1976) The influence of pharmaceutical compunds on male fertility. Andrologia 8 : 203
Parizek J (1957) The destructive effect of cadmium ions on testicular tissue and its prevention by zinc. J Endocrinol 15 : 56–63
Parizek J (1960) Sterilization of the male by cadmium salts. J Reprod Fertil 1 : 294
Qureshi MSA, Pennington JH, Goldsmith HJ, Cox PE (1972) Cyclophosphamide therapy and sterility. Lancet 7790 : 1290
Reddy J, Svoboda D, Azarnoff D, Dawar R (1973) Cadmium induced Leydig cell tumors of rat testis – Morphologic and histochemical study. J Natl Cancer Inst 51 : 891–903
Rössle R, Zahler H (1938) Experimentelle Untersuchungen über Hoden- und Prostataveränderungen durch Zufuhr von Hodenwirkstoffen. Virchows Arch [Pathol Anat] 302 : 251
Rubinstein HS, Kurland AA (1941) The effect of small doses of testosterone propionate on the testis and accessory sex organs. J Urol 45 : 780–784
Rytter M (1970) Ejakulatveränderungen unter der Behandlung mit dem Folsäureantagonisten Methotrexat. Dermatol Monatsschr 56 : 898–906
Schenck B, Neumann F (1978) Influence of antiandrogens on Sertoli cell function and intratesticular androgen transport. Int J Androl 1 : 459–470
Sitteri PK, Brenner P, MacDonald PC (1974) Mechanism of spironolactone induced gynecomastia. 56th Annual Meeting of the Endocrine Society, Abstract No. 187
Timmermanns L (1974) Influence of antibiotics on spermatogenesis. J Urol 112 : 348–349
Tuchmann-Duplessis H (1956) Action de la réserpine sur le testicule et le tractus genital du rat. C R Acad Sci (Paris) 242 : 1651
Weissbach L, Lange CE, Meyhöfer W (1974) Hodenhistologie, Ejakulat und Nukleoproteidgehalt der Spermatozoen behandelter Hodentumorpatienten. Andrologica 6 : 135
Yasuda M, Johnson DC (1965) Effects of exogenous androgen and gonadotrophins on the testes and hypophyseal follicle-stimulating hormone content of the immature male rat. Endocrinology 76 : 1033–1040
Zahler H (1947a) Über die Wirkung verschiedener Gaben von Testosteronpropionat auf infantile Rattenhoden. Virchows Arch [Pathol Anat] 314 : 23
Zahler H (1947b) Über das Verhalten der Hoden und Hypophysen A-vitaminotischer Ratten und ihre Beeinflußbarkeit durch androgenen Wirkstoff. Virchows Arch [Pathol Anat] 314 : 45
Zysk JR, Bushway AA, Whistler RL, Carlton WW (1975) Temporary sterility produced in male mice by 5-thio-D-glucose. J Reprod Fertil 45 : 69

Disease, Metabolism and Reproduction in the Toxic Response to Drugs and Other Chemicals
Arch. Toxicol., Suppl. 7, 118–127 (1984)

Assessment of Chemicals Affecting the Male Reproductive System

R. L. Dixon

Laboratory of Reproductive and Developmental Toxicology,
National Institute of Environmental Health Sciences,
P.O. Box 12233, Research Triangle Park, North Carolina 27709, USA

Abstract. The reproductive toxicologist must be more concerned with the ability of laboratory models to predict human reproductive hazards and to estimate human health risks. Although more than a hundred chemicals have been reported to affect the reproductive capacity of male laboratory animals, fewer than 15 environmental chemicals have been shown conlusively to affect man and many of these are known mutagens, carcinogens or otherwise generally toxic agents. Pharmacokinetic and adaptive factors must be considered. More attention also needs to be directed towards processes other than spermatogenesis and towards mechanisms of toxicity other than cytotoxicity. The male component necessary for successful reproduction depends on a large variety of biological processes working in concert. The ability to assess chemically-induced reproductive effects needs to be refined and modern molecular and cellular approaches should be developed and validated. This paper summarizes aspects of the pharmacokinetic and adaptive factors involved in testicular toxicity, some current laboratory assessment techniques, and newer test procedures such as monoclonal antibodies for sperm surface proteins and the interspecies (human/hamster) sperm penetration assay.

Key words: Male – Reproductive toxicity – Pharmacokinetics – Laboratory models – Environmental chemicals

Although a vast number of drugs and other environmental chemicals have been linked to reproductive effects through laboratory reports, clinical studies, and epidemiological investigations, only a few, perhaps less than a dozen, environmental chemicals have been demonstrated conclusively to be the cause of reproductive dysfunction.

Two recent reports are especially helpful when considering this area: the Council of Environmental Quality's Chemicals Affecting Human Reproduction (CEQ, 1981) and Health Effects of Environmental Chemicals on the Adult

Human Reproductive System prepared in cooperation with the National Library of Medicine for the Information Response to Chemical Crises Project by the Federation of American Societies for Experimental Biology (Pruett and Winslow 1982). The text, Reproductive Hazards of Industrial Chemicals (Barlow and Sullivan 1982) is likewise a quality effort to describe this area of concern. The Laboratory of Reproductive and Developmental Toxicology also maintains a reproductive toxicity information file at the NIEHS in Research Triangle Park, N.C. This general area has also been discussed in recently published textbooks (Dixon 1980; Dixon and Hall 1982).

Table 1 lists categories of therapeutic agents reported to affect male reproductive capacity and includes both laboratory and clinical reports. The variety of therapeutic agents presented suggest many different mechanisms of action. Centrally-acting drugs are likely to disrupt the hypothalamo-pituitary-gonadal axis. Antineoplastic agents and other cytotoxic drugs generally affect spermatogenesis. Other agents or drugs might affect sperm maturation and motility or both. By altering the autonomic nervous system the erectile and ejaculatory processes can be disrupted.

Table 2 lists categories of environmental agents reported to affect the reproductive capacity of male laboratory animals. Those occupational chemicals which are thought to affect the ability of the human male to reproduce is much shorter. Less than a dozen chemicals are listed in Table 3.

Establishing cause and effect relationships for reproductive toxicants is inherently difficult. In the clinic, humans are sporadically exposed to a combination of agents in relatively low concentrations. The situation with environmental and occupational exposure is even more difficult than that experienced with therapeutic agents. Although the endpoints that can be monitored are multiple, most of these vary widely under "normal" circum-

Table 1. Categories of therapeutic agents reported to affect male reproduction. (Laboratory studies and clinical reports)

Adrenergic blocking agents (guanethidine)
Treatment of alcoholism (antabuse)
Analgesics/antipyretics (phenacetin)
Anticonvulsants (phenytoin)
Anti-infective agents (amphotericin B, nitrofurans, hycanthone, niridazole)
Antineoplastic agents (cyclophosphamide, procarbazine)
Antispermatogenic drugs-investigational (chlorosugars, thioglucose, gossypol)
Diuretics (aldactone, thiazides)
Gout suppressants (colchicine)
Hormones used in threatened abortion (DES)
Oral hypoglycemic agents (chlorpropamide)
Psychopharmacological agents (monoamine oxidase inhibitors, phenothiazines, reserpine)
Volatile anesthetics (halothane, methoxyflurane)
Xanthines (caffeine, theobromine)

Table 2. Categories of environmental chemicals reported to affect male reproduction. (Laboratory studies)

Food additives and contaminants (DES, nitrofurans, aflatoxins)
Fungicides, fumigants, and sterilants (DBCP, ethylene dibromide)
Fire retardants (TRIS, PBBs)
Herbicides (2,4-D, 2,4,5-T)
Heat transfer agents (PCBs)
Insecticides (DDT, lindane, dieldrin)
Metals and trace elemets (cadmium, methylmercury)
Plasticizers (phthalate esters)
Rodenticides (fluoroacetate)

Table 3. Occupational chemical exposures associated with male reproductive dysfunction. (Clinical reports)

Anesthetic gases	Lead (and other smelter emissions)
Boric acid	Pesticides (unspecified)
Carbon disulfide	Polybrominated biphenyls (PBBs)
Dibromochloropropane (DBCP)	Solvents (benzene and toluene)
Ethylene dibromide	Vinyl chloride
Kepone	

stances. Small sample sizes further weaken the confidence associated with any conclusion about human effects.

Therefore, in the laboratory, the reproductive toxicologist must be increasingly concerned with the ability of laboratory models to accurately predict human reproductive hazards and to reliably estimate human health risks. It is time to focus more attention on processes other than spermatogenesis and on mechanisms of toxicity other than cytotoxicity. The male component necessary for successful reproduction depends on a variety of biological processes working in concert. These include the hypothalamo-pituitary-gonadal axis, testicular Leydig and Sertoli cell function and spermatogenesis, epididymal sperm maturation and storage, and the fluid milieu and smooth muscle function of the male accessory sex organs. Each of these processes involves genetic, molecular, and cellular targets which, when perturbed by chemicals, result in reproductive dysfunction. Too much study seems to be directed toward chemicals which are already known to be mutagenic, carcinogenic, or otherwise generally toxic. It would appear that answers to important questions are being looked for only in the area where the light is the brightest. In developing the area of reproductive toxicology, a number of additional avenues of study deserve mention. These include pharmacokinetic and adaptive factors affecting testicular toxicity, laboratory procedures for identifying hazardous chemicals, and newer test procedures currently being developed and validated.

Pharmacokinetic and Adaptive Factors

Pharmacokinetic and adaptive factors are important modifiers of testicular toxicity and risk estimation. The objective of the toxicological study of a target organ is to discover the qualitative and quantitative toxic effects of a chemical on that organ. The ultimate objective is to assess the toxic effects of a chemical in laboratory animals and to extrapolate the experimental data pertinent to man. To accomplish these objectives, one must consider the main factors which may influence and modulate the toxic effects of chemicals in the organs. In gonads, such modifying factors are the pharmacokinetic parameters governing chemical absorption, distribution, activation, and detoxication, covalent bindings to macromolecules, and DNA damage as well as DNA repair of damaged germ cells. Phenomena such as biological barriers, biotransformation mechanisms which can decrease or increase the toxicity of a chemical, and the capacity of the germ cells to repair DNA damage, are each important pharmacokinetic and adaptive aspects to be examined. Both male and female gonads have been considered, although more data are available concerning the testis than the ovary (Dixon and Lee 1980).

An attempt has been made to model the pharmacokinetic and adaptive factors which affect testicular toxicity. The model is presented in Fig. 1. Efforts are under way to quantify the roles of the blood-testis barrier, biotransformation, and DNA repair in the male gonad to facilitate the extrapolation of laboratory animal data to man. It should be possible in the future to mathematically predict, with a reasonable degree of certainty, what toxic effects, if any, are associated with a known chemical exposure.

Biological Barriers. The blood-testis barrier (BTB) regulates the penetration of exogenous chemicals to male germ cells in the seminiferous tubules. Permeability of nonelectrolytes across the BTB is dependent upon molecular size, suggesting bulk flow through waterfilled pores. On the other hand, permeability of ionic drugs with varying pK_a values correlates best with the lipid solubility (partition coefficients) of their nonionized form. The transfer rate constants of chemicals from blood to seminiferous tubules closely resembles their transport rate from blood to cerebrospinal fluid. It appears that the BTB is a complex multicellular system composed of membranes surrounding the seminiferous tubules and the several layers of Sertoli and spermatogenic cells organized within the tubules which restrict the penetrability of many foreign compounds to the male germ cells (Okumura et al. 1975; Dixon and Lee 1981).

Biotransformation. Exogenous chemicals can be chemically transformed by the organism. Biotransformation is accomplished by enzymes in many organs and results in either the alteration of the foreign molecule or the formation of conjugated products. The new product is usually more polar, water soluble, and may be more or less toxic than the parent compound. The toxic effects of certain polycyclic aromatic hydrocarbons, in tissues other than germ cells, have been demonstrated to be due to reactive metabolites which interact with DNA, RNA, and other macromolecules. A steady state level of reactive metabolites within

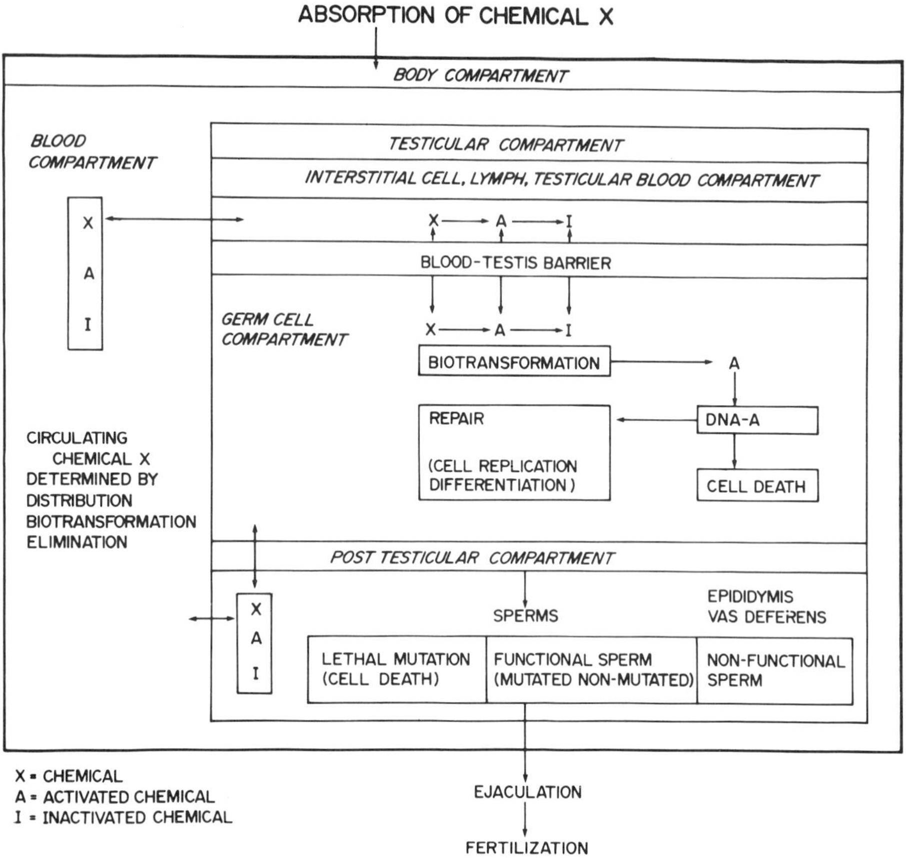

Fig. 1. Diagrammatic presentation of the pharmacokinetic and adaptive factors involved in testicular toxicity

the cells of a target organ is obviously a function of the competing rates of synthesis and degradation.

The relative specific activities of aryl hydrocarbon hydroxylase (AHH), epoxide hydrase (EH), glutathione transferase (GSH-ST), and cytochrome P-450 in the adult rat testis and liver have been studied by Mukhtar and coworkers (Mukhtar et al. 1978a, b). Appreciable activities of both mixed-function oxidases and epoxide degrading enzymes, as well as cytochrome P-450, have been found in testicular tissue. Glutathione transferase activity is especially high. The distribution of these enzymes and cytochrome P-450 in the interstitial and germ cell compartments indicates that AHH activity and cytochrome P-450 content of microsomes from the interstitial cells are nearly twice that in the tubules. In contrast, the specific activity of the detoxication enzymes EH and GSH-ST in tubules is twice that in the interstitial cells. Although AHH activity in interstitial cell microsomes has been found to be only 5% that of hepatic microsomes, its close proximity to the germ cells may increase its importance with regard to enzyme-activated toxic chemicals. Factors affecting induction of AHH and cytochrome P-450 may also play a significant role in germ cell toxicity. Data analyses also suggest that the isolated perfused testis may be a more reliable predictor of whole animal metabolism than are in vitro studies which utilize testicular tissue homogenates and microsomes (Dixon and Lee 1981).

DNA Repair. There are many indications that the mammalian cell recognizes and removes DNA damaged from exposure to a variety of chemical agents. Moreover, there appear to be distinct mechanisms by which this repair of mammalian cell DNA can be achieved. The most studied is referred to as excision or "cut and patch" repair. The chemical region in the DNA is recognized by a complex enzyme system that excises the modified base from the DNA, degrades it, resynthesizes a section to reconstitute the original DNA strand, and then inserts this section into the preexisting DNA. Evidence for this form of repair has come from measurments of the loss of mutagen-induced substituents from DNA and from the detection of nonsemiconservative DNA synthesis, sometimes called "repair synthesis" in alkylated cells. The uptake of $[^3H]$-thymidine into cells that are not in S-phase is generally taken as an indicator of unscheduled DNA synthesis.

Following treatment with the mutagen methylmethane sulfonate (MMS), thymidine incorporation can be demonstrated not only in spermatogonia but also in the leptotene, zygotene, pachytene, and diplotene cells. In contrast, the spermatogenic cells, spermatids and sperm, do not demonstrate thymidine incorporation following MMS exposure, suggesting an inability to repair damaged DNA. DNA repair capacity appears to be finite and may become saturated with very high test doses of mutagens. This overloading of the repair system could result in increased toxicity. Thus, repair rates need to be quantified (Dixon and Lee 1980).

Damage inflicted on the DNA templates, unless repaired, may interfere with transcription and replication resulting in lethal mutations (cell death), mutations which develop into transformed cells, or genetic mutations which, in the case of germ cells, can be amplified by generations of genetic recombinations.

Current Laboratory Assessment of Reproductive Hazards

The ability of rodents to become fertile and produce offspring is the most common indicator of reproductive capacity. Multigenerational breeding tests are often applied to food additives and environmental chemicals. However, these tests are time consuming, require large numbers of animals, are very expensive, and are relatively insensitive (Dixon and Hall 1982).

Serial mating studies have been used to determine genetic effects and to construct "fertility profiles" which offer important clues regarding mechanisms of action (Lee and Dixon 1972a, b). Using this method, toxic effects can be associated with specific spermatogenic cell types. By knowing the general cellular biology of spermatogonia, spermatocytes, spermatids, and sperm, mechanisms of toxicity are suggested. In addition, the reversibility of the toxic effect can also be studied. Attempts are being made to associate recovery time with the percentage of stem cells damaged. This will allow investigators to quantify more accurately the cell-killing potential of selected drugs and environmental agents.

Thus, the following question must be asked. Is there an appropriate laboratory animal model to identify chemicals affecting human male reproduction? In comparison with the human, spermatogenesis is relatively more efficient in laboratory rodents. A larger number of sperm with fewer abnormal forms are produced. More sperm are stored in the epididymides and almost all conceptuses implant successfully and result in live offspring. A rodent's sperm count must be reduced by as much as 80% before fecundity is altered. In contrast, man with a lower count of poorer quality sperm lives much nearer an apparent "threshold of sterility." Greater efforts are needed to refine our ability to assess chemically-induced reproductive effects. Genetic selection and prenatal treatment with radiation and drugs might be used to develop strains of rodents with a reproductive capacity more like that of man. Biochemical, morphological, and functional indicators need to be better correlated. However, an even more important approach is to define better the basic mechanism of action and the pharmacodynamics of chemicals altering reproductive processes and causing reproductive dysfunction.

Newer Test Procedures

It is obvious that improved laboratory and clinical tests must be developed to assess the impact of chemicals on male reproductive capacity. Two general areas will be discussed here. The first concerns monitoring changes in the sperm surface that are either a part of the maturational process or accompany it. The second involves an effort to test human sperm functionality by studying sperm penetration of ova obtained from laboratory animals. The search for improved test methods is an active one.

Sperm Surface Changes. In this laboratory, as well as others, efforts are underway to define changes in the sperm surface which accompany epididymal maturation. Because this seems a promising direction, various approaches are being tried. Two of these are the binding of plant lectins to the sperm surface and the interaction of monoclonal antibodies with sperm surface antigens. Although interesting, the plant lectins have lacked specificty and sensitivity. Thus, attention is now focused on the application of monoclonal antibodies.

Hybridoma cells can be produced by fusing myeloma cells with splenocytes from male mice immunized with sperm from the same strain of mice (Feuchter et al. 1981). Clonally-derived cell lines which secrete monoclonal antibodies against sperm surface components can then be selected. Each of the sperm monoclonal antibodies binds to a specific region of the sperm surface. Vernon et al. (1982) have demonstrated that sperm retained in the efferent ducts following ligation do not acquire the antigen. This suggests that the antigen is not due to changes intrinsic to the sperm, but that these proteins are acquired in the epididymis. Indirect immunofluorescence studies have indicated that the antigen is a secretory product of the epididymal epithelium and is produced in a short segment of the distal caput epididymis. Sperm maturation is age-dependent. The antigen is not identified until mice are between 2 and 44 weeks old (Vernon 1982). Looking to the future, it can be anticipated that antibodies will be selected which will be indicators of sperm maturation. Applied to ejaculated human sperm, specific antibodies might identify "immature" sperm and aid in relating this condition to chemical exposure. It should be kept in mind that the process of sperm maturation not only presents many targets for chemically-induced toxicity but also offers unexplored avenues for developing effective male contraceptives.

Sperm Penetration Assays. Another intriguing avenue of study is the fertilizing capacity of human sperm using ova of laboratory animals. Because the clinical detection of human reproductive capacity is generally unreliable, a number of investigators have sought to develop a heterologous (interspecies) in vitro fertilization test system which utilizes human sperm and ova of laboratory animals. It is of interest to note that because ejaculation is non-invasive, it is relatively easier to obtain a sample of semen than of blood.

Ongoing research seeks to answer the question of whether or not the heterologous in vitro fertilization test system utilizing human sperm is a reliable

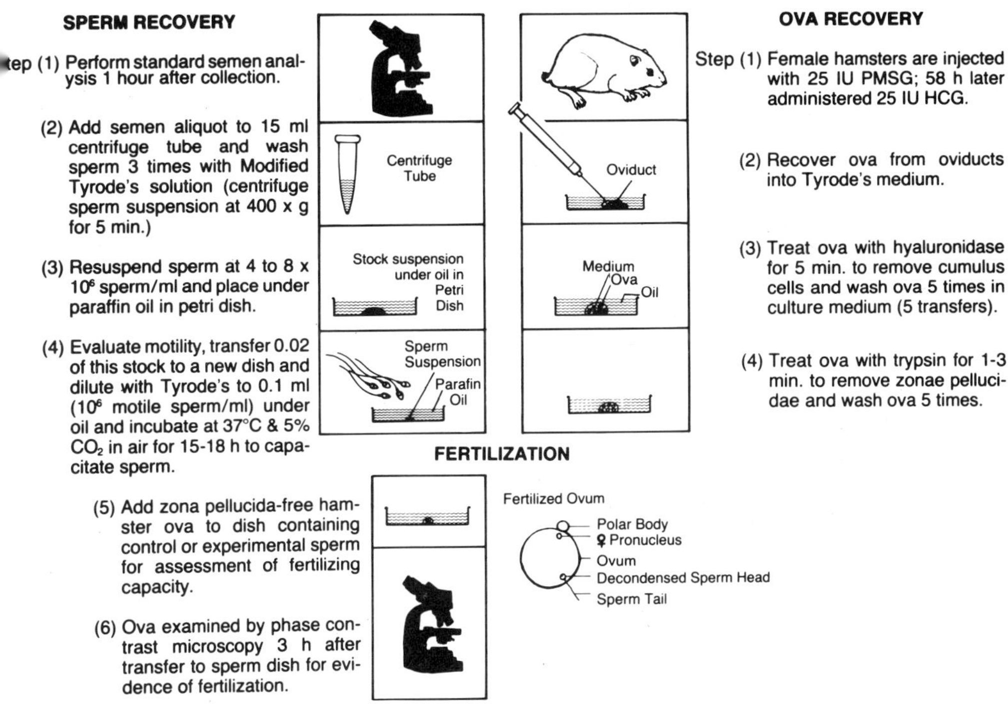

Fig. 2. Experimental steps involved in the interspecies (human/hamster) sperm penetration assay

indicator of reproductive capacity. At the NIEHS, heterologous (human sperm/hamster ova) in vitro fertilization is being used to assess the fertilizing capacity of human males (Hall 1981). These studies identified certain individuals as subfertile who have a routinely determined normal sperm number, motility, and morphology. This approach demonstrated that the usual parameters for semen analyses are unsure predictors of male fertility; only the most extreme semen abnormalities are reliable indicators. Thus, the in vitro penetration of laboratory animal ova by human sperm appears to be an improved technique in assessing human fertilization potential.

The steps involved in the heterologous (interspecies) in vitro fertilization technique are presented in Fig. 2. Zona pellucida-free hamster ova are added to a dish containing control or experimental sperm. Fertilizing capacity is assessed by measuring sperm binding to the ova, decondensed sperm heads, and the pronucleus or both with the corresponding sperm tail in the ovum's cytoplasm. Although sometimes referred to as "fertilization," the process under investigation is the penetration of the sperm into the ovum with subsequent decondensation of the sperm. Further events of normal fertilization, such as genetic union of the cells, do not occur under these controlled artificial conditions.

Summary

The complicated biological interactions upon which succesful mammalian reproduction depends, present many targets for toxic chemicals. During the past decade, laboratory and clinical efforts to more readily identify and describe those chemicals in the environment which perturb essential molecular and cellular processes and result in morphological and functional alterations have increased greatly. However, understanding of the underlying biological mechanisms of reproductive toxicity remains incomplete and the predictability of these current test approaches is unsure. But advances have been made. A clearer understanding now exists of the biological properties of the various cells and tissues which comprise the male and female reproductive systems. There is a greater appreciation of their unique developmental and chemical susceptibilities. Likewise, understanding of the events involved in fertilization and implantation phenomena continues to increase. More is known about the pharmacokinetic factors which determine the amount of active chemical which reaches its site of toxicity and more is understood of how the organism adapts to chemicals and recovers from damage. Even the molecular dynamics of the toxic event and its direct and indirect consequences are beginning to be understood.

Acknowledgements. The author wishes to acknowledge the assistance of Vickie Englebright and Susan Donn Schrag in the preparation of this paper.

References

Barlow SM, Sullivan FM (1982) Reproductive hazards of industrial chemicals. Academic Press, London

Council on Environmental Quality (1981) Chemical hazards to human reproduction. US Government Printing Office, Washington DC

Dixon RL (1980) Toxic responses of the reproductive system. In: Doull J, Klaassen CD, Amdur MO (eds) Casarett and Doull's toxicology, 2nd edn. Macmillan Publishing Co., New York, pp 332–334

Dixon RL, Hall JL (1982) Reproductive toxicology. In: Hayes AW (ed) Principles and methods of toxicology. Raven Press, New York, pp 107–140

Dixon RL, Lee IP (1980) Pharmacokinetic and adaptation factors in testicular toxicity. Fed Proc 39: 66–72

Dixon RL, Lee IP (1981) Pharmacokinetic and adaptive factors as modifiers of testicular toxicity and risk estimation. In: Richmond CR, Walsh PJ, Copenhaver ED (eds) Proceedings of third life sciences symposium on health risk analysis. Franklin Institute Press, pp 196–212

Feuchter FA, Vernon RB, Eddy EM (1981) Analysis of the sperm surface with monoclonal antibodies: Topographically restricted antigens appearing in the epididymis. Biol Reprod 24: 1099–1110

Hall RL (1981) Relationship between semen quality and human sperm penetration of zona-free hamster ova. Fertil Steril 35: 457–463

Lee IP, Dixon RL (1972a) Antineoplastic drug effects on spermatogenesis studied by velocity sedimentation cell separation. Toxicol Appl Pharmacol 23: 20–41

Lee IP, Dixon RL (1972b) Effects of procarbazine on spermatogenesis studied by velocity sedimentation cell separation and serial mating. J Pharmacol Exp Ther 181: 219–226

Mukhtar H, Lee I, Foureman GL, Bend JR (1978a) Epoxide metabolizing enzyme activities in rat testes: Postnatal development and relative activity in interstitial and spermatogenic cell compartments. Chem Biol Interact 22: 153–165

Mukhtar H, Philpot RM, Lee IP, Bend JR (1978b) Developmental aspects of epoxide-metabolizing enzyme activities in adrenals, ovaries and testes of the rat. In: Mahlum D, Sikov U, Hackett P, Andrew F (eds) Developmental toxicology of energy-related pollutants. US Department of Energy Technical Information Center, Washington DC, pp 89–104

Okumura K, Lee IP, Dixon RL (1975) Permeability of selected drugs and chemicals across the blood-testis barrier of the rat. J Pharmacol Exp Ther 194: pp 89–95

Pruett JG, Winslow SG (1982) Health effects of environmental chemicals on the adult human reproductive system. Toxicology Information Response Center, Oak Ridge, Tennessee (NLM/TIRC-82-1)

Vernon RB, Muller CH, Herr JC, Feuchter FA, Eddy EM (1982) Epididymal secretion of a mouse sperm surface component recognized by a monoclonal antibody. Biol Reprod 26: 523–535

Disease, Metabolism and Reproduction in the Toxic Response to Drugs and Other Chemicals
Arch. Toxicol., Suppl. 7, 128–139 (1984)

Toxic and Mutagenic Influences on Spermatogenesis

M. Parvinen, J. Lähdetie, and L.-M. Parvinen

Institute of Biomedicine, Department of Anatomy, University of Turku, 20520 Turku 52, Finland

Abstract. Cells at various stages of spermatogenesis show remarkable differences in their sensitivities to toxic and mutagenic agents. For accurate analyses of toxicity and mutagenicity, the most sensitive cell types should be obtained for studies soon after treatment before development of disturbing secondary alterations. The transillumination phase contrast microscopic technique has proved to be useful for this purpose. It allows recognition of rat and mouse seminiferous tubules in living unstained conditions for accurate selection of the desired stages of the cycle of the seminiferous epithelium for morphological and biochemical studies. Specific cell damage can be frequently recognized by transillumination only, whereas in most cases phase contrast microscopy is useful in screening the early stage-specific toxic alterations. A summary is presented of the results obtained by treatment with heat and with anticancer drugs.

A meiotic micronucleus method has been developed for direct estimation of the severity of mutagenic insult on rat spermatogenesis. The segment that contains the second meiotic division and the early postmeiotic cells (stages XIV and I) is selected for study. Chromosome damage induced by mutagens may result in the formation of acentric fragments that after meiotic divisions are seen in early spermatids as separate micronuclei. They can be quantitated in squash preparations; the sensitivity of this method is comparable with that of the meiotic metaphase scoring.

Recently, an in vitro technique has been developed for stage and cell specific measurements of replicative and repair syntheses of DNA during rat spermatogenesis after mutagen treatments.

Key words: Rat – Spermatogenesis – Toxic effects – Mutagenic effects

Introduction

Spermatogenesis is a complex process of cell differentiation that ultimately leads for formation of the spermatozoon, a cell with a haploid number of chromosomes, condensed chromatin and a flagellum that makes independent movements possible. The differentiation occurs in the seminiferous tubules of the testis. They are surrounded by interstitial tissue, a source of testosterone. Together with pituitary follicle stimulating hormone, testosterone is the main endocrine regulator of spermatogenesis. These hormones act on Sertoli cells, the only somatic component of the seminiferous epithelium. Recent observations have demonstrated that Sertoli cells play a key role in the local regulation of spermatogenesis (Ritzén et al. 1981; Mather et al. 1983), obviously through secreting factors that have a paracrine type of action on the germ cells.

Spermatogenesis has three main phases: spermatogonial multiplication by mitoses, meiosis and spermiogenesis. These phases show a multitude of alterations in cellular metabolism which obviously is a cause of their variable susceptibility to toxic agents. DNA synthesis occurs only in spermatogonia and at the onset of meiosis in preleptotene spermatocytes and these cells are the most sensitive to toxic influences. This is facilitated by their location close to the basal lamina of the seminiferous epithelium; the substances entering spermatogonia do not have to pass the barrier formed by Sertoli cells. During spermatogenesis, extensive selection of germ cells occurs through physiological degeneration at several critical points that diminishes the probability of the damage of spermatogonia to be transferred to mature spermatozoa. Therefore, it is important to study the toxic and mutagenic effects in meiotic and particularly postmeiotic cells. It is important to recognize the early effects of treatment on specific cell types, since they most sensitively reflect the characteristic toxic and mutagenic action of each agent before the development of disturbing secondary effects. The results are summarized of a series of experiments that have been designed to meet these requirements.

Selection of Sensitive Cells for Analyses

In the rat and most other mammalian species, spermatogenesis proceeds in the seminiferous tubules in a wave-like fashion (Perey et al. 1961), where various generations of spermatogonia, spermatocytes and spermatids are arranged in defined cell associations with constant composition. Based on the morphology of the acrosomic system and of the nuclei of the early spermatids, fourteen different cell associations have been defined in the rat (Leblond and Clermont 1952). When a freshly isolated living unstained seminiferous tubulus of the rat is transilluminated under a stereomicroscope, a characteristic light absorption pattern permits recognition of the stages of the cycle of the seminiferous epithelium (Parvinen and Vanha-Perttula 1972). The exact stage of spermatogenesis can be identified by phase contrast microscopy of cell squashes (Söderström and Parvinen 1976), where the morphology of the spermatogenic and Sertoli cells become very clearly observable. The early cell injury can be recognized in these freshly isolated unstained cells; the resolution is in many instances better than in fixed and sectioned material. Sensitive cells localized by this rapid screening method can subsequently be isolated and processed further for analyses by morphological, cytochemical and biochemical methods.

Early Toxic Effects of Increased Temperature

The testis is sensitive to increased temperature. In Finland this problem is of great concern owing to the popularity of sauna bathing; it is known to reduce sperm counts in extreme conditions (Procopé 1965). The early effects of heat treatment have been studied by subjecting the rat testes to local heating in a 43° C water bath for 15 min (Chowdhury and Steinberger 1970). Seminiferous tubules were examined after 1.5 and 3 h under stereomicroscope. A zone of increased light absorption covered stages XI-I of the cycle after 3 h, and light microscopic analysis indicated that late pachytene primary spermatocytes, cells at meiotic reduction divisions and very early spermatids degenerated first (Parvinen 1973). For a more detailed analysis of the cell degeneration process, a more moderate heat treatment, experimental cryptorchidism was suggested (Plöen 1972). Very early spermatids proved to be the most susceptible cells. Before the appearance of any signs of morphological damage, these cells became phagocytosed by Sertoli cells (Fig. 1). The squash technique makes practicable analyses of the phagocytosing activity of the Sertoli cells, which is important for both early detection of damaged cells in experimental animals and particularly in human testicular biopsies.

The experiments with heat and experimental cryptorchidism showed that very early alterations during particular stages of meiosis and spermiogenesis can be analyzed by living cell techniques. They are rapid and accurate screening techniques; no fixation or staining are needed during selection of the appropriate doses and the spermatogenic stages for demonstration of stage-specific early toxic effects.

Early Effects of Anticancer Drugs

The increasing efficiency of anticancer chemotherapy and the prolongation of life have brought up the problems of fertility. Hence, the mechanism of action of anticancer drugs have become important. The early effects have been analyzed of four main classes of anticancer drugs on rat spermatogenesis, namely alkylating agents (thiotepa and nitrogen mustard), vinca alkaloids (vincristine and vinblastine), anticancer antibiotics (adriamycin and actinomycin D) and procarbazine. All of these drugs were investigated using transillumination, phase contrast microscopy, light microscopy and electron microscopy. In addition, the alkylating agents and adriamycin were evaluated by their effects on DNA and RNA syntheses.

All the drugs caused degenerative changes in cells that are most active in RNA synthesis, i.e. the mid-pachytene spermatocytes (Fig. 2). Another phase

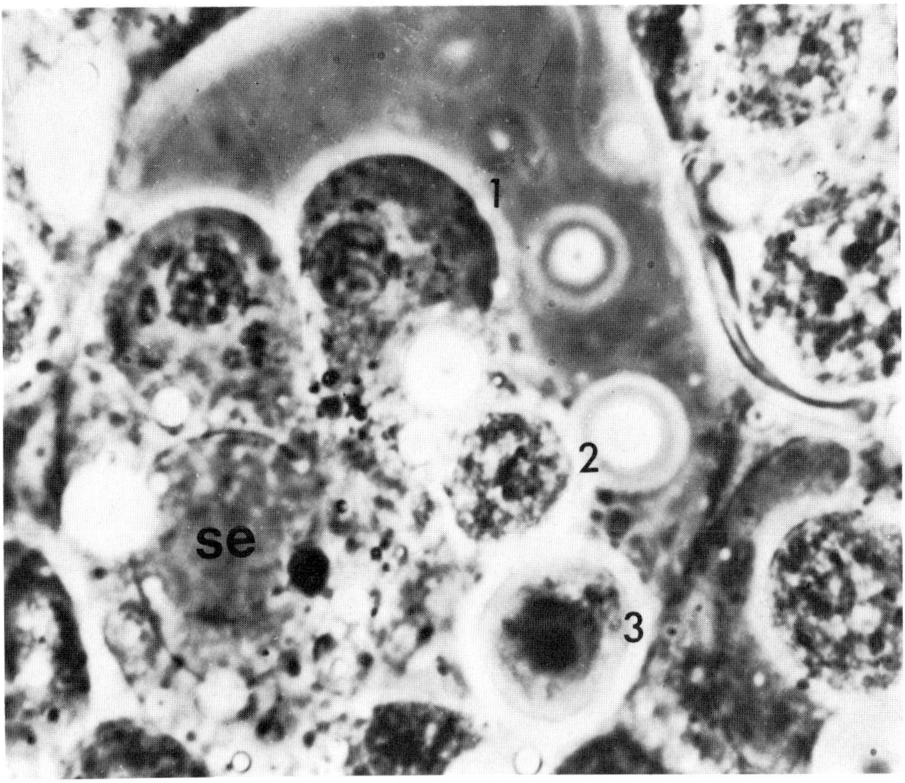

Fig. 1. Effects of heat (12 h of experimental cryptorchidism) on early spermatids of the rat. The cells are phagocytosed by the Sertoli cell *(Se)* and show various degrees of degeneration (*1:* close to normal, *3*: complete degeneration with strongly altered phase contrast characteristics). Phase contrast. × 700. (Reproduced with permission from the publisher)

that was affected by several drugs was the meiotic reduction division. This effect was prominent with the vinca alkaloids that inhibit the microtubule polymerization (Parvinen et al. 1978a). In addition, these drugs had a pronounced effect on the morphology of the Sertoli cells. The effects on the meiotic chromosomes indicate an ability of vinca alkaloids to penetrate the barrier formed by Sertoli cells and act directly on the germ cells.

Alkylating agents caused multiple alterations on the germ cells. Particularly those in active nucleic acid synthesis become affected. Spermatids in nuclear protein transition stages seemed to be very sensitive to alkylating agents as well; they showed early engulfment in Sertoli cells and decondensation of their chromatin (Fig. 3). Clear effects were also induced on both premitotic and premeiotic DNA syntheses in stages IV–VI and VII–IX, respectively (Parvinen and Parvinen 1978a).

Adriamycin had probably the most specific action among the drugs investigated. It very selectively and rapidly killed preleptotene spermatocytes, mid-pachytene primary spermatocytes and cells performing the meiotic

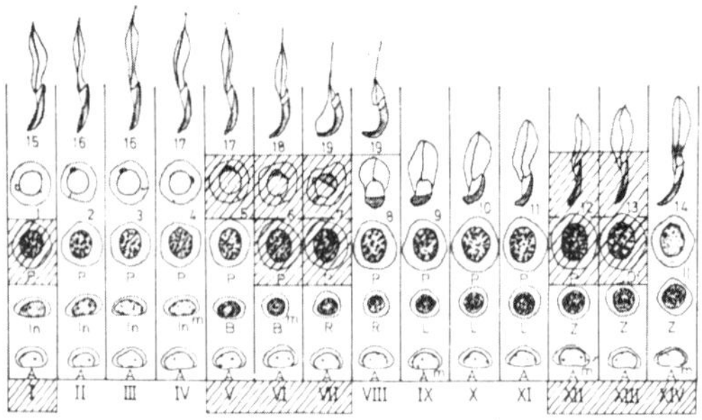

Alkylating agents nitrogen mustard and thiotepa

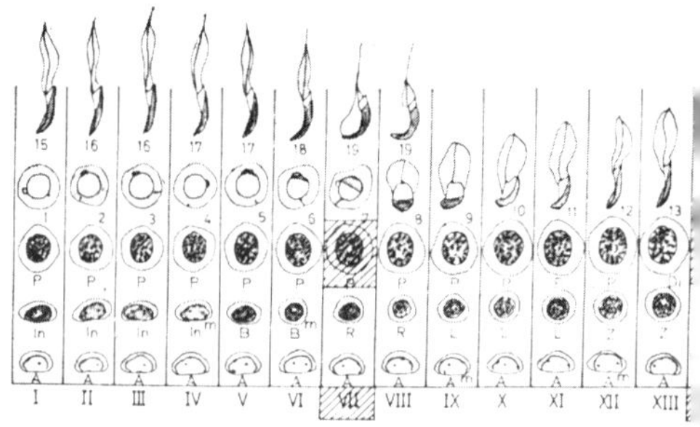

Vinca alkaloids vinblastine and vincristine

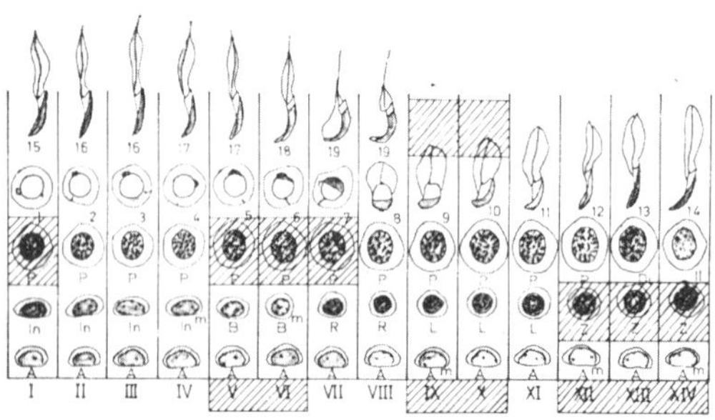

Procarbazine

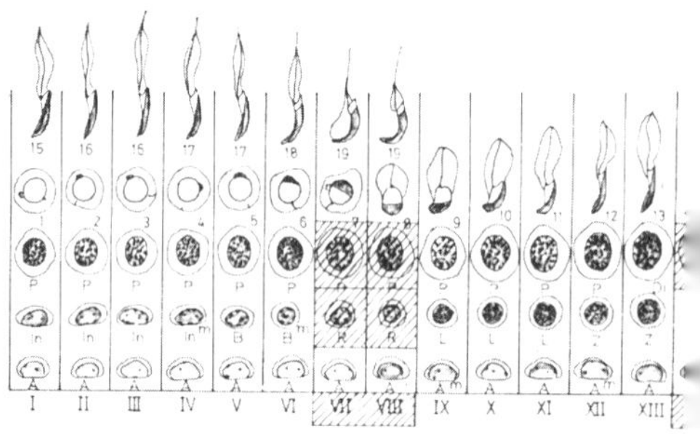

Adriamycin

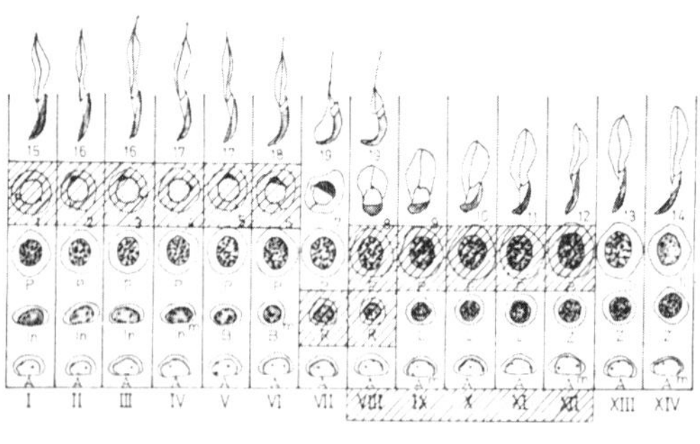

Actinomycin D

Fig. 2. Early effects of anticancer drugs on rat spermatogenesis. The shaded areas superimposed on the map of spermatogenesis (Perey et al. 1961) represent the most sensitive stages on cell types

reduction divisions. DNA and RNA synthesis were inhibited; the premitotic synthesis seemed to be more sensitive than the premeiotic one. A peculiar characteristic of adriamycin action was induction of micronuclei during the meiotic reduction divisions (Parvinen and Parvinen 1978b; Lähdetie et al. 1984).

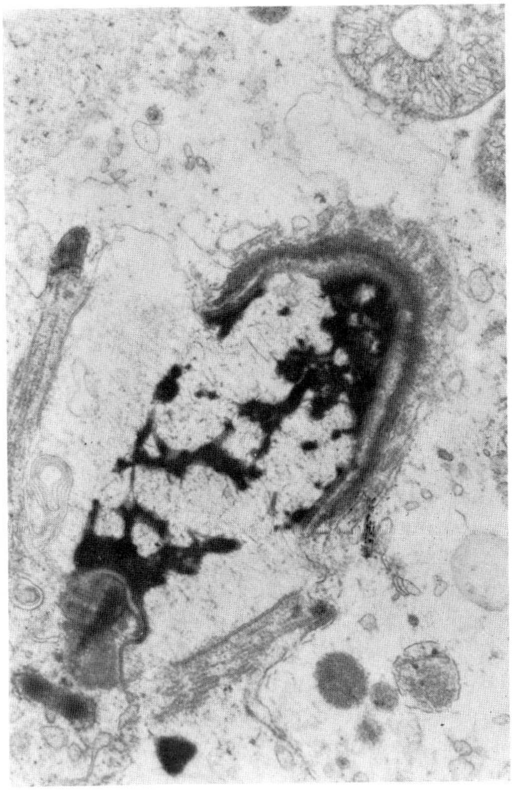

Fig. 3. The disintegrating effect of nitrogen mustard on rat step 12–13 spermatid. The nuclear envolope is disrupted and the chromatin decondensed resulting in deliberation of the DNA fibres. Electron micrograph. × 20,000. (Reproduced with permission from the publisher)

Actinomycin D, a specific inhibitor of RNA polymerase II similarly had an effect on RNA synthesizing cells during meiosis and spermiogenesis. Mid-pachytene spermatocytes degenerated first. In early spermatids during haploid chromosome activity, the chromatoid body showed morphological changes (Parvinen et al. 1978b) and a lack of labelling with [^{3}H]-uridine (Söderström 1978) that suggest a dependence of this organelle on postmeiotic RNA transcription.

Procarbazine, an important anticancer drug in the treatment of Hodgkin's disease has a mechanism of action different from other anticancer drugs. During spermatogenesis, it affected cells in zytogene stage of meiotic prophase, cells that have a minimal amount of RNA transcription or DNA synthesis, but where the meiotic chromosomes pair. Another clearly affected site was the early spermiogenesis, where the young spermatids became fused together at their acrosomes and formed multinuclear giant cells. Procarbazine also had an effect on mid-pachytene primary spermatocytes that suggests its activity on meiotic RNA transcription (Parvinen 1978).

Figure 2 summarizes the early cytotoxic effects of different anticancer drugs on rat spermatogenesis. As is known, a multitude of biochemical events are located in various cell types, the principal mechanism of action can be estimated for each anticancer drug using this model system. This is of potential value in the design of effective combinations of drugs in anticancer chemotherapy. Parameters for studying the Sertoli cell function are few, but are increasing rapidly after recognition of the primary importance of the Sertoli cells in supporting the germ cell differentiation. The mechanisms involved may be very sensitive to the action of noxious treatments.

Meiotic Micronucleus Test

The analysis of spermatogonial and meiotic metaphase chromosomes has been mostly used for analyses of mutagenic effects on male germ cells. However, the meiotic metaphase figures are difficult to assess, and alternative methods are questioned for screening purposes. Encouraged by the usefulness and simplicity of the micronucleus test of polychromatic erythrocytes in the bone marrow (Schmid 1975), it was decided to try an analogous method during meiotic reduction division.

Mutagens induce principally two types of damage that lead to altered chromosome distribution during cell division. Breaks in the DNA chain lead to formation of acentric chromosome fragments that lag behind the moving chromosomes during anaphase and become surrounded by their own nuclear envelope during telophase. They are subsequently recognized as micronuclei beside the main nucleus of the cell. During erythropoiesis, the main nucleus is expelled from the cell, but micronuclei remain in the polychromatic erythrocytes and can be scored. Micronuclei are also induced by compounds that disrupt the spindle function.

The meiotic reduction divisions are located in a distinct segment of the seminiferous tubule at stage XIV (Leblond and Clermont 1952) in the rat. Early postmeiotic cells are found in stage I of the cycle. These stages can be accurately found by a combined transillumination-phase contrast microscopic technique (Fig. 4; Lähdetie and Parvinen 1981).

The meiotic micronucleus induction was analyzed after X-irradiation (Fig. 5). The spontaneous induction rate was very low (0.1%). A slight increase

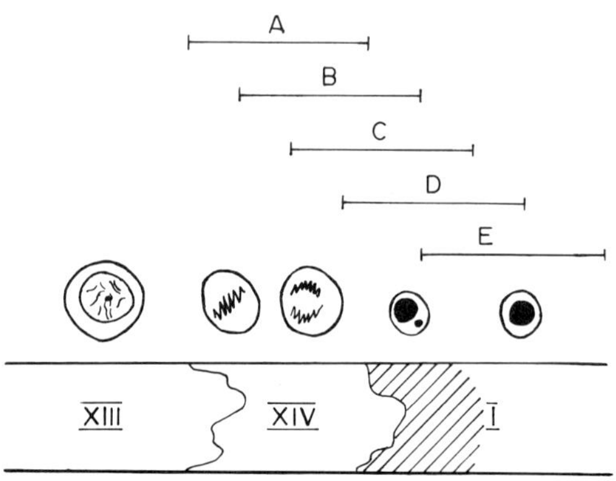

Fig. 4. Selection of the segment of rat seminiferous tubulus at stages XIV–I of the cycle for micronucleus scoring. Shaded area depicts the zone where most enrichment of the micronuclei is found, and the segment should be selected at the bars *c* or *d*. (Reproduced with permission from the publisher)

was observed after anaesthesia with Hypnorm (0.3%), whereas 10 rads X-rays elevated it significantly (to 0.5%). Thereafter, the increase was linear up to 600 rads; above that a decrease occurred obviously due to cytotoxicity. Small doses typically induced only one micronucleus per spermatid, and frequently, the micronuclei were of small size and had a condensed chromatin.

Some mutagenic chemicals induced micronuclei obviously by different mechanisms compared with X-irradiation. The micronuclei induced by adriamycin often remained in contact with the main nucleus through narrow bridges (Lähdetie et al. 1984). Vincristine did not induce micronuclei in the spermatogenic cells (Lähdetie and Parvinen 1982).

The meiotic micronucleus method is useful for estimation of the relative sensitivity of different stages of the meiotic prophase to chemical mutagens. Since the rate of the development of the germ cells is constant (Clermont et al. 1959), the micronuclei reflect the sensitivity of particular stages when analyzed at appropriate time intervals after exposure to the mutagen. Cells at the preleptotene stage of meiotic prophase and at mid-pachytene were most

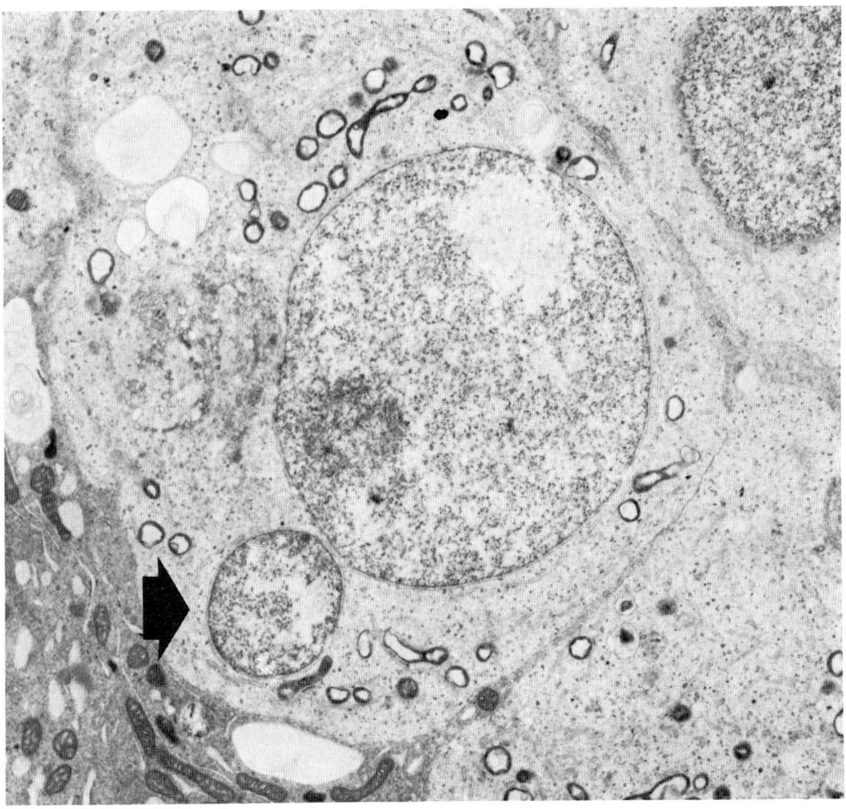

Fig. 5. A meiotic micronucleus induced by 500 rads of X-rays during the meiotic reduction divisions *(arrow)*. The structure of the step 1 spermatid is otherwise without any detectable alterations. Electron micrograph. × 7,000

susceptible to the action of adriamycin (Lähdetie 1983a) whereas preleptotene was the most susceptible stage to the action of cyclophosphamide and dimethylbenzanthracene (Lähdetie 1983b). This technique makes it possible to analyze the mechanisms of mutagen action at meiosis. The majority of mutagens require DNA synthesis to cause an increase of micronucleus induction, and therefore, preleptotene is the most sensitive stage. Chromatin, active in RNA synthesis, may be susceptible to certain mutagens, such as adriamycin which affected mid-pachytene spermatocytes.

Present experience indicates that the meiotic micronucleus method has a sensitivity comparable with the analysis of the meiotic metaphase chromosomes. It is simple to perform; the recognition and scoring of the meiotic micronuclei does not require specific skills. A particular improvement is the use of a fluorochrome (H 33258) that selectively stains the DNA-protein complexes. The meiotic micronucleus method gives direct information about the genetic defects of the haploid cells, the most likely candidates for fertilizing the oocytes.

In vitro DNA Synthesis During Spermatogenesis

Although the in vivo measurement of testicular DNA synthesis is an important method for assays of the effects of the mutagens on genetic material (Friedman and Staub 1976), it is subject to errors caused by non-specific mutagen effects such as decreased body temperature or diminished blood flow (Donatsch et al. 1982). Therefore, development of an in vitro method became pertinent.

The DNA replication occurs during spermatogenesis only in spermatogonia and in preleptotene primary spermatocytes. The former is considered as premitotic DNA replication, whereas the latter precedes the prophase of the meiotic reduction division. These DNA replications can be accurately located in discrete stages of the cycle of the seminiferous epithelium. Several stages have DNA synthesis of spermatogonia (Monesi 1962), whereas the premeiotic DNA replication only occurs in a very limited segment of the seminiferous tubule, i.e., in stages VII and VIII of the cycle in rat (Hilscher 1967). More accurately, the beginning of the long stage VII (substages VIIa, b and c) has the lowest DNA replication rate during the whole spermatogenesis, and preleptotene spermatocytes only start their premeiotic DNA synthesis at late stage VII (VIId) to be continued maximally at stage VIII and ending during stage IX of the cycle of the seminiferous epithelium (Lähdetie et al. 1983).

Ethyl methanesulfonate (EMS) induced a significant reduction of in vitro DNA replication in both premitotic and premeiotic phases; however, the possible repair type of DNA synthesis in substages VIIa–c could not be detected after exposure to EMS, as had been suggested after exposure to nitrogen mustard (Parvinen and Parvinen 1978a). X-rays did not affect DNA replication in the model system used, where the interval between the irradiation (in vivo) and the assay of DNA synthesis (in vitro) was 1–3 h.

The transillumination-phase contrast microscopic method provides the means for cell-specific analyses of repair synthesis of DNA. Rats were either exposed to X-irradiation in vivo, or segments of their seminiferous tubules were

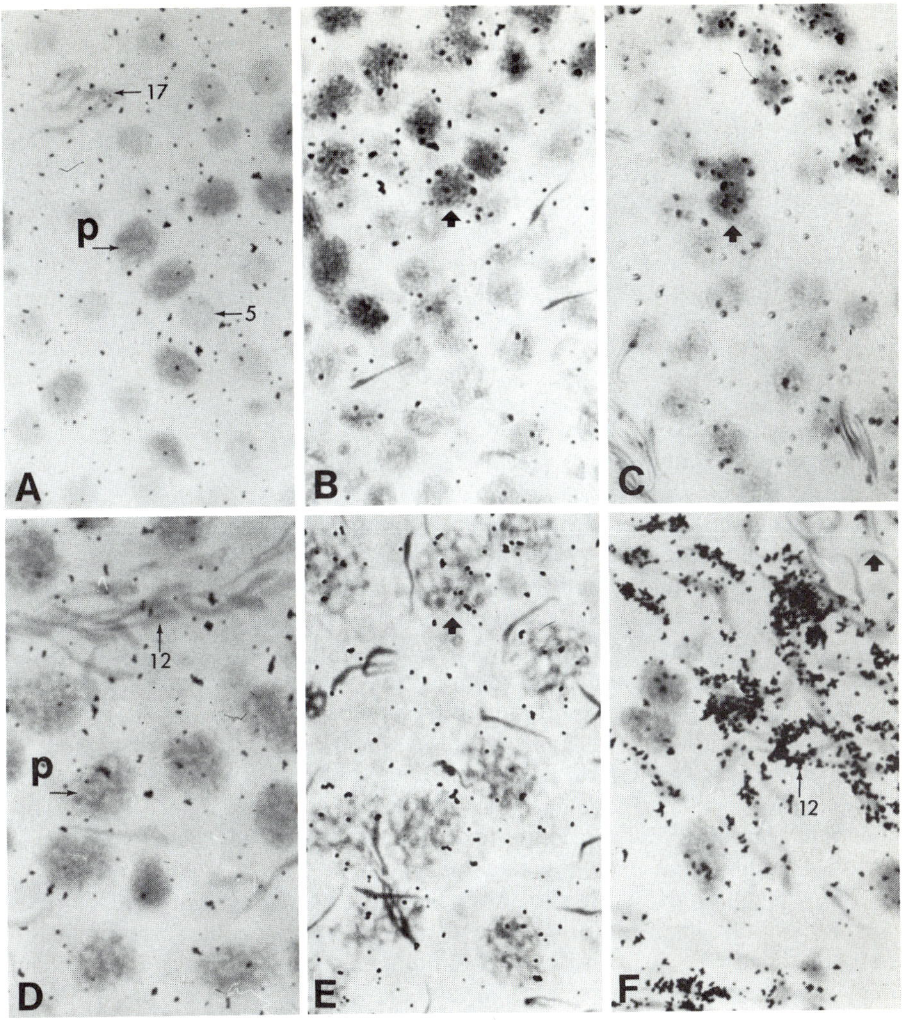

Fig. 6. Repair synthesis of DNA at stages V **(A–C)** and XII–XIII **(D–E)** of the cycle of the rat seminiferous epithelium. **A** and **D** are controls, **B** and **E** are irradiated with 600 rads of X-rays and **C** and **F** are exposed to EMS (5 and 1 mg/ml, respectively) in vitro. Pachytene spermatocytes *(p)* are labelled in **B, C** and **E** *(thick arrows)* whereas step 12 spermatids *(12)* show heavy labelling after EMS treatment **(F).** Note that step 13 spermatids are not labelled (*thick arrow* in **F**). 5 and 17: Steps 5 and 17 spermatids. Light micrographs of hematoxylin stained autoradiograms from squash preparations. × 1,000

incubated in vitro in the presence of EMS for one hour, and then labelled with [^{3}H]-thymidine for 2 h. Then, cell squashes were made using the method described earlier (Lähdetie and Parvinen 1981). After cell recognition by phase contrast microscopy, the sample was frozen by liquid nitrogen and the coverslip was removed. In the frozen state, the preparation was fixed and then covered by autoradiographic emulsion. After exposure for 2 weeks or 2 months, the photographic processing was completed and the preparation was stained with hematoxylin and eosin. The grain counts above the appropriate nuclei indicated the stage-specific repair synthesis of DNA, compared with the control preparations. Cells in RNA transcription (mid-pachytene and early spermatids) showed the most active DNA-repair synthesis (Fig. 6). Surprisingly, the highest rate of repair type of DNA synthesis was found in stage XII, where particularly the elongating spermatids seemed to be the most active cells (Fig. 6F). These cells are in the process of nucleoprotein transition (Grimes et al. 1977), and it is possible that these cells repair their damage induced in DNA at the last moment before the final inactivation and condensation of their chromatin (Lähdetie et al. 1983).

Conclusions and Possibilities of Analyses of Human Male Germ Cell Toxicity

Rapid screening methods for analyses of stage-specific early cell injury of male rat meiotic and postmeiotic germ cells have been summarized. Physical (heat and X-irradiation) and chemical toxic and mutagenic treatments induce very stage-specific early effects that can be selected for analyses by light and electron microscopic techniques using transillumination and phase contrast microscopic analyses of isolated seminiferous tubules and isolated germ cells at defined stages of the cycle of the seminiferous epithelium. Grossly altered phase contrast microscopic morphology of damaged cells is a sensitive and rapid assay method for spermatogenic cytotoxicity. It is also reflected early by the phagocytic activity of the Sertoli cells that can be easily evaluated in squash preparations. This phenomenon also gives possibilities for analyses of phagocytic activity in human Sertoli cells obtained from testicular biopsies.

The evaluation of mutagenic and toxic effects in human testicular biopsies may be valuable in the future, and after development of the accuracy of the methods, it may be an indicator of the mutagenic influence in addition to the analysis of the semen sample, where new techniques are also under development.

Acknowledgement. This work has been supported by The Academy of Finland (Project no. 200 at the Medical Research Council).

References

Chowdhury AK, Steinberger E (1970) Early changes in the germinal epithelium of rat testes following exposure to heat. J Reprod Fertil 22: 205–212

Clermont Y, Leblond CP, Messier B (1959) Durée du cycle de l'épithélium séminal du rat. Arch Anat Microsc Morphol Exp 48: 37–56

Donatsch P, Gürtler J, Matter BE (1982) Critical appraisal of the mouse testicular DNA-synthesis inhibition test for the detection of mutagens and carcinogens. Mutat Res 92: 265–273

Friedman MA, Staub J (1976) Inhibition of mouse testicular DNA synthesis by mutagens and carcinogens as a potential simple mammalian assay for mutagens. Mutat Res 37: 67–76

Grimes SR Jr, Meistrich ML, Platz RD, Hnilica LS (1977) Nuclear protein transitions in rat testis spermatids. Exp Cell Res 110: 31–39
Hilscher W (1967) DNA synthesis: Proliferation and regeneration of the spermatogonia in the rat. Arch Anat Microsc Morphol Exp [Suppl] 56: 75–84
Lähdetie J (1983a) Meiotic micronuclei induced by adriamycin in male rats. Mutat Res 119: 79–82
Lähdetie J (1983b) Micronuclei induced during meiosis by ethyl methanesulfonate, cyclophosphamide, and dimethylbenzanthracene in male rats. Mutat Res 120: 257–260
Lähdetie J, Parvinen M (1981) Meiotic micronuclei induced by X-rays in early spermatids of rats. Mutat Res 81: 103–115
Lähdetie J, Parvinen M (1982) Meiotic micronuclei as indicators of mutagenesis. In: Prevention of Occupational Cancer – International Symposium. Occupational Safety and Health Series No. 46, International Labour Office, Geneva, pp 483–487
Lähdetie J, Kaukopuro S, Parvinen M (1983) Genotoxic effects of ethyl methanesulfonate and X-rays at different stages of rat spermatogenesis, studied by inhibition of DNA synthesis and induction of DNA repair in vitro. Hereditas 99: 269–278
Lähdetie J, Parvinen LM, Parvinen M (1984) Meiotic micronuclei in male rats – Ultrastructural studies about their induction by mutagens. In: Hemminki K, Vainio H, Sorsa M (eds) Occupational hazards and reproduction. Hemisphere, Washington DC, pp 145–154
Leblond CP, Clermont Y (1952) Definition of the stages of the cycle of the seminiferous epithelium in the rat. Ann NY Acad Sci 55: 548–573
Mather JP, Gunsalus GL, Musto NA, Cheng CY, Parvinen M, Wright WW, Margioris A, Liotta T, Becker R, Krieger DT, Bardin CW (1983) The hormonal and cellular control of Sertoli cell function. J Steroid Biochem 19: 41–51
Monesi V (1962) Autoradiographic study of DNA synthesis and the cell cycle in spermatogonia and spermatocytes of mouse testis using tritiated thymidine. J Cell Biol 14: 1–18
Parvinen LM (1979) Early effects of procarbazine (N-isopropyl-L-(2-methyl-hydrazino)-p-toluamide hydrochloride) on rat spermatogenesis. Exp Mol Pathol 30: 1–11
Parvinen LM, Parvinen M (1978a) A "living cell method" for testing the early effects of antispermatogenic compounds: Model experiments with two alkylating agents thiotepa and nitrogen mustard. Int J Androl [Suppl] 2: 523–540
Parvinen LM, Parvinen M (1978b) Biochemical studies of the rat seminiferous epithelial wave: DNA and RNA synthesis and effects of adriamycin. Ann Biol Anim Biochim Biophys 18: 585–594
Parvinen LM, Jokelainen PT, Parvinen M (1978a) Chromatoid body and haploid gene activity: Actinomycin D induced morphological alterations. Hereditas 88: 75–80
Parvinen LM, Söderström KO, Parvinen M (1978b) Early effects of vinblastine and vincristine on the rat spermatogenesis: Analyses by a new transillumination-phase contrast microscopic method. Exp Pathol 15: 85–96
Parvinen M (1973) Observations on freshly isolated and accurately identified spermatogenic cells of the rat. Early effects of heat and short-time experimental cryptorchidism. Virchows Arch [Cell Pathol] 13: 38–47
Parvinen M, Vanha-Perttula T (1972) Identification and enzyme quantitation of the stages of the seminiferous epithelial wave in the rat. Anat Rec 174: 435–450
Perey B, Clermont Y, Leblond CP (1961) The wave of the seminiferous epithelium in the rat. Am J Anat 108: 47–77
Plöen L (1972) An electron microscope study of the immediate effects on spermateleosis of a short-time experimental cryptorchidism in the rabbit. Virchows Arch [Cell Pathol] 10: 293–309
Procopé BJ (1965) Effect of repeated increase of body temperature on human sperm cells. Int J Fertil 10: 333–340
Ritzén EM, Hansson V, French FS (1981) The Sertoli cell: In: Burger H, deKretser D (eds) The testis. Comprehensive endocrinology. Raven Press, New York, pp 171–194
Schmid W (1975) The micronucleus test. Mutat Res 31: 9–15
Söderström KO (1977) Effect of actinomycin D on the structure of the chromatoid body in rat spermatids. Cell Tissue Res 184: 411–421
Söderström KO, Parvinen M (1976) RNA synthesis in different stages of rat seminiferous epithelial cycle. Mol Cell Endocrinol 5: 181–199

Disease, Metabolism and Reproduction in the Toxic Response to Drugs and Other Chemicals
Arch. Toxicol., Suppl. 7, 140–145 (1984)

Gonadal Damage in Hodgkin's Disease from Cancer Chemotherapeutic Regimens

G. Bonadonna[1], A. Santoro[1], S. Viviani[1], C. Lombardi[2], and G. Ragni[2]

[1] Istituto Nazionale Tumori, Via Venezian 1, 20133 Milan, Italy
[2] IV Clinica Ostetrica Ginecologica, University of Milan, Via Melloni 52, 20129 Milan, Italy

Abstract. The paper re-emphasizes that intesive prolonged anticancer chemotherapy containing alkylating agents or procarbazine or both produces a high-incidence of gonadal failure, particularly in males. This evidence has been documented mostly in patients with Hodgkin's disease. On the contrary, effective combination regimens, such as ABVD, not including the above mentioned drugs induce a comparatively less and transient germ cell toxicity. In devising chemotherapy for potentially curable neoplastic diseases in young patients efforts should be made to avoid or minimize the potential risk of drug-induced gonadal failure.

Key words: Gonadal failure – Chemical castration – MOPP chemotherapy – ABVD chemotherapy – Hodgkin's disease

Thanks to modern treatment (Bonadonna 1982; Bonadonna and Santoro 1982) about 70% of patients with Hodgkin's disease are curable and about 85% survive 5 years. Current research efforts are also attempting to decrease treatment complications. In fact, the days of minimizing the potential long-term toxicity of treatment programs are past, and in devising therapy for all stage subgroups the increased risk for relapse must be weighed against the increased risk of iatrogenic morbidity involving single or multiple organs (Perry 1982). This statement also applies to other neoplasms, such as most pediatric tumors, breast cancer, and testicular cancer in which the addition of intensive chemotherapy to local-regional modalities has consistently increased total survival or cure rate or both. Late complications which are relevant to the chemotherapy strategy of potentially curable neoplasms are treatment-induced secondary neoplasms, sterility, cardiotoxicity and lung fibrosis. This paper will summarize the effects of different forms of intensive chemotherapy on the gonadal function of patients with Hodgkin's disease which is the neoplasm where the endocrine studies were more systematically carried out.

Although drug-induced azoospermia and amenorrhea were known side effects for a number of years, until recently the impact of gonadal toxicity on the quality of life has received little attention. Infertility in Hodgkin's disease is of particular concern because many patients are young. The assessment of gonadal function before and after chemotherapy usually includes semen analysis (density, count, motility), testicular or ovarian biopsy, serum testosterone (total and free), serum 17-β estradiol, follicle-stimulating hormone (FSH), luteinizing hormone (LH), prolactin and 17-OH progesterone. Recently, is has been confirmed that gonadal abnormalities similar to those produced by intensive and prolonged chemotherapy are present in some men with Hodgkin's disease before therapy (Vigersky et al. 1982). The most important findings can be summarized as follows: basal serum testosterone levels in 19 young men with Hodgkin's disease was 27% lower than in 19 normal men of similar age but 26% greater than in 13 men with primary testicular failure; free testosterone levels were lower in patients with stage III–IV compared with patients with stage I–II lymphoma; total serum testosterone levels in stage III–IV and in patients with systemic symptoms were indistinguishable from those of patients with primary testicular failure; serum FSH levels were lower compared with those of 11 men with malignancies other than Hodgkin's disease; serum LH levels were normal both in patients with Hodgkin's disease and other malignancies; serum 17-OH progesterone levels were lower in stage III–IV and in patients with systemic symptoms compared with stage I–II and no systemic symptoms; serum prolactin levels were significantly higher than normal in men with Hodgkin's disease but not in men with other malignancies; the results of semen analysis showed that 33% of men with Hodgkin's disease had abnormal sperm density and 40% had abnormal total sperm counts. Both men with Hodgkin's disease (69%) and those with other malignancies (66%) had diminished sperm motility. The authors concluded that gonadal dysfunction may be specific for Hodgkin's disease and the hypogonadism consists of a constellation of findings rather than simple primary testicular failure. This suggests a complex abnormality of hypothalamic-pituitary-testicular axis while the results of semen analysis indicate seminiferous tubular dysfunction.

In men treated with cytotoxic chemotherapy, when spermatogenesis is impaired FSH blood levels rise, while in complete Leydig cell failure, levels of LH rise and testosterone levels fall (Chapman et al. 1979). Combination chemotherapy regimens including procarbazine alkylating agents or both such as in combined mechlorethamine, vincristine, procarbazine, and prednisone therapy (MOPP) or its variants, have a profound effect on spermatogenesis as first reported in Hodgkin's disease by the National Cancer Institute group (Sherins and De Vita 1973). Table 1 summarizes the incidence of gonadal failure following MOPP or MOPP-like combinations as derived from representative case series. It is evident that at least 90% of the men become azoospermic or severely oligospermic. Recovery of spermatogenesis is unpredictable and, through retrospective studies it has been reported to vary from 10 to 20%. This appears to be mostly partial, delayed (up to 10 years), related to age (i.e., greater in patients < 30 years), directly related to the length of time off therapy and indirectly related to the total dose of chemotherapy. Testicular biopsy shows

Table 1. Oligo-azoospermia following MOPP or MOPP-like combinations

Author or institution	Number of patients	Oligo-spermia (%)	Azoo-spermia (%)	Recovery (%)
De Vita (1981)	45	4	89	Unknown
Chapman (1979)	64	23	77	Unknown
Whitehead (1982)	49	10	86	Unknown
Andrieu (1981)	10		100	12
Waxman (1982)	46		88	20 (< 30 years)
Milan (1983)	27	0	96	8

atrophy of germinal epithelium while follicle-stimulating hormone (FSH) and luteinising hormone (LH) levels are increased. The damage of germinal epithelium and Leydig cells is particularly evident in adults, but recent observations have also emphasized the vulnerability of pubertal and prepubertal testis to alkylating agents and procarbazine or both. Pubertal boys treated with MOPP have in addition to impairement of spermatogenesis, a high frequency of gynecomastia. Libido tends to decrease after the diagnosis of Hodgkin's disease and treatment with chemotherapy.

The sterility problem appears to be less common in adult females than males, probably because the low germ cell proliferative rate of the ovary is less sensitive to cytotoxic drugs compared with the testicular epithelium and Leydig cells. When ovarian failure occurs, there are greatly increased levels of FSH and LH with abnormally low estradiol and progesterone levels. The available data (Table 2) would indicate that 40–50% of younger women treated with regimens containing procarbazine or alkylating agents or both will become amenorrheic. The premature ovarian failure appears dependent upon age (> 30 years, about 85%; < 30 years, about 20%); it is most probably related to the total dose of drugs, and is progressive from 1 to 10 years after chemotherapy rather than an all-or-none phenomenon (Schilsky et al. 1981). Reestablishment of menses and the possibility of pregnancy in a treated woman is also correlated with the age and the cumulative drug exposure as shown in the adjuvant treatment of breast cancer (Bonadonna et al. 1981). However, pregnancy does not prove lack of ovarian damage. The ovaries of prepubertal and pubertal girls are relatively insensitive to anticancer drugs unless very high and prolonged doses are administered.

In contrast to the above reported findings there seems to be consistent evidence that the administration of anticancer drugs other than alkylating agents or procarbazine or both produces only a limited and transient germ cell toxicity, both in males and females. Table 3 summarizes the main characteristics of patients evaluated for gonadal dysfunctions and which were taking part in a prospective randomized study testing MOPP plus radiotherapy versus combined adriamycin, bleomycin, vinblastine, and dacarbazine therapy (ABVD) plus radiotherapy (Bonadonna 1982). The comparative analysis of gonadal failure was limited to patients less than 45 years of age with no pelvic irradiation. The updated results are reported in Tables 4 and 5. In males, ABVD affected

Table 2. Ovarian failure following MOPP or MOPP-like combinations

Author or institution	Number of patients	Amenorrhea > 6 months (%)	Irregular menses (%)	Patients with pregnancy
Schilsky (1981)	24	46	Unknown	7
Horning (1981)	34	15	29	8
Chapman (1979)	41	34	49	3
Waxman (1982)	28	79	Unknown	Unknown
Milan (1983)	36	17		3

Table 3. Characteristics of patients studied after chemotherapy plus radiotherapy

	MOPP + RT[a]	ABVD + RT[a]
Sex		
Males	27	18
Females	36	24
Median age (years)		
Males	30 (19–45)	28 (16–41)
Females	27 (17–41)	26 (15–41)
No. of cycles	6	6

[a] Subtotal nodal radiotherapy, i.e., pelvic nodes excluded from radiation fields

Table 4. Comparative percent of gonadal failure in males following MOPP vs ABVD

	MOPP (27 cases)	ABVD (18 cases)
Azoospermia	96	33
Oligospermia	0	17
Recovery, total	8 (1/12)	100 (8/8)
Median time (months)	36	11 (2–18)

Table 5. Comparative percent gonadal failure in females following MOPP vs ABVD

	MOPP (36 cases)	ABVD (24 cases)
Amenorrhea		
> 6 months	17	0
< 30 years	0 (0/23)	
> 30 years	46 (6/13)	
Recovery, total	17 (1/6)	
Median time (months)	6	
Patients with pregnancy	3	3

spermatogenesis in a considerably less percentage than MOPP. More important, the recovery of spermatogenesis, in patients in whom the sperm count was so far repeated, occurred in all instances in the ABVD-treated group (8 of 8) compared with only one of 12 cases treated with MOPP. Also the median time to recovery was definitely in favor of ABVD chemotherapy. Post treatment serum FSH levels were determined in 30 patients (MOPP 19, ABVD 11). Markedly elevated values were observed in 16 males treated with MOPP compared with three patients given ABVD. Although in women the follow up time remains an important factor in the evaluation of ovarian failure secondary to cytotoxic chemotherapy, Table 5 indicates that prolonged amenorrhea in MOPP-treated women is definitely higher compared with ABVD-treated women.

The above reported findings are in keeping with the results of a limited series of sarcoma patients treated with drugs other than procarbazine or alkylating agents (Shamberger et al. 1981). Since gonadal function is also related to the intensity of drug-treatment, it will be useful to document in future evaluations whether the incidence of azoospermia and of permanent amenorrhea will be decreased by alternating MOPP with ABVD, particularly when half-cycles of either regimen will be delivered within a 1-month period (Bonadonna 1982). In conclusion, to circumvent chemotherapy-induced gonadal dysfunction and therefore minimize the psychological and physical impact of chemical castration the following procedures are recommended: semen cryopreservation prior to therapy in males, the administration of oral contraceptives in premenopausal women (Chapman and Sutcliffe 1981), appropriate trials with an analogue of gonadotrophin-releasing hormone (Glode et al. 1981) and, whenever possible, the use of effective alternative drug regimens not containing either procarbazine or alkylating agents.

References

Andrieu JM, Masson D, Fiet J, Gourmel B, Czyglik F, Bernard J (1981) La fertilité des jeunes hommes atteints de la maladie de Hodgkin avant et aprés chimiothérapie. Nouv Presse Med 10: 2085–2088

Bonadonna G (1982) Chemotherapy strategies to improve the control of Hodgkin's: The Richard and Hinda Rosenthal Foundation Award Lecture. Cancer Res 42: 4309–4320

Bonadonna G, Santoro A (1982) Drug selection in the treatment of Hodgkin's disease. Haematol Oncol 1: 3–12

Bonadonna G, Valagussa P, De Palo GM (1981) The results of adjuvant chemotherapy in breast cancer are predominantly due to the hormonal change such therapy induces: the view against. In: Van Scoy-Mosher MB (ed) Controversies in medical oncology. Hall KG, Boston, pp 100–109

Chapman RM (1979) Cyclical combination chemotherapy and gonadal function. Lancet 1: 285–289

Chapman RM, Sutcliffe SB (1981) Protection of ovarian function by oral contraceptives in women receiving chemotherapy for Hodgkin's disease. Blood 58: 849–851

Chapman RM, Sutcliffe SB, Malpas JS (1979) Cytotoxic-induced ovarian failure in women with Hodgkin's disease: I Hormone function. JAMA 242: 1877–1881

De Vita VT (1981) The consequences of the chemotherapy of Hodgkin's disease: The 10th David A. Karnofsky Memorial Lecture. Cancer 47: 1–13

Glode LM, Robinson J, Gould SF (1981) Protection from cyclophosphamide-induced testicular damage with an analogue of gonadotrophin-releasing hormone. Lancet 1: 1132–1134

Horning SJ, Hoppe RT, Kaplan HS, Rosenberg SA (1981) Female reproductive potential after treatment for Hodgkin's disease. N Engl J Med 304: 1377–1382

Perry MC (ed) (1982) Toxicity of chemotherapy. Semin Oncol 9: 1–149

Shamberger RC, Rosenberg SA, Seipp CA, Sherins RJ (1981) Effect of high-dose methotrexate and vincristine on ovarian and testicular functions in patients undergoing postoperative adjuvant treatment of osteosarcoma. Cancer Treat Rep 65: 739–746

Schilsky RL, Sherins RJ, Hubbard SM, Wesley MN, Young RC, De Vita VT (1981) Long-term follow-up of ovarian function in women treated with MOPP chemotherapy for Hodgkin's disease. Am J Med 71: 552–556

Sherins RJ, De Vita VT (1973) Effects of drug treatment for lymphoma on male reproductive capacity. Ann Intern Med 79: 216–220

Vigersky RA, Chapman RM, Berenberg J, Glass AR (1982) Testicular dysfunction in untreated Hodgkin's disease. JAMA 73: 482–486

Waxman JHX, Terry YA, Wrigley PFM, Malpas JS, Rees LH, Besser GM, Lister TA (1982) Gonadal function in Hodgkin's disease: long-term follow-up of chemotherapy. Br Med J 285: 1612–1613

Whitehead E, Shalet SM, Blackledge G, Todd I, Crowther D, Beardwell CG (1982) The effects of Hodgkin's disease and combination chemotherapy on gonadal function in the adult male. Cancer 49: 418–422

Disease, Metabolism and Reproduction in the Toxic Response to Drugs and Other Chemicals
Arch. Toxicol., Suppl. 7, 146 (1984)

Approaches to the Suppression of Testicular Function for Male Fertility Control

E. Nieschlag[1] and Th. Schürmeyer[2]

[1] Max-Planck-Gesellschaft, Klinische Forschungsgruppe für Reproduktionsmedizin, Steinfurter Strasse 107, 4400 Münster, Federal Republic of Germany
[2] Department of Health, Human Services, Public Health Services, National Institutes of Health, Bldg. 10, Room 10 B 12, Bethesda, MD 20205, USA

Abstract. The development of chemical methods for male fertility control is only partially based on a systematic search and depends to a large extent on serendipity. An untoward and often unexpected side effect of a great number of substances is their influence on spermatogenesis. This applies to several pesticides, herbicides and nematocides as well as to indazoles, thiophenes, dinitropyrroles and chlorinated sugars. Some pharmaceutical agents such as nitrofuranes, cytotoxic agents and psychopharmacological drugs have fertility suppressing effects. In most instances these substances are either so toxic or have other side effects that they must be excluded as agents for male fertility control. Some registered drugs however, have side effects on the male reproductive system but low toxicity and may therefore be considered seriously for male fertility control. One such example is sulphasalacine, used for inflammatory bowel disease for several decades, which is now under consideration for male fertility control because of its interference with sperm function. More recently, antifungal imidazoles, well tolerated after oral application, have been recognized to suppress testicular testosterone production and may thus interfere with fertility.

The endocrine approach to male fertility control is based on more rational investigations. Since FSH and testosterone are of prime importance for maintenance of spermatogenesis, means of interfering either with FSH or testosterone action or both are being sought. However, experiments in monkeys demonstrated that the specific neutralization of FSH by antibodies may not be sufficient for fertility control. Clinical trials with testosterone alone or in combination with progestins, antiandrogens or other steroids such as danazol demonstrated that suppression of spermatogenesis can be achieved in humans, but have not yet resulted in a specific "male pill". More recently, the pituitary and testis suppressing effects of LHRH agonists in high doses have provided a promising new approach to male fertility control.

Key words: Male fertility – Suppression of spermatogenesis – Follicle stimulating hormone

Disease, Metabolism and Reproduction in the Toxic Response to Drugs and Other Chemicals
Arch. Toxicol., Suppl. 7, 147–150 (1984)

Morphological Changes Produced in Rat Testis by Anticancer Drugs

C. Hodel[1], R. A. Ettlin[1], and A. Zschauer[2]

[1] F. Hoffmann-La Roche & Co. Ltd., 4002 Basel, Switzerland
[2] Sandoz Ltd., 4002 Basel, Switzerland

Abstract. Testicular side effects of procarbazine (Proc: 50 or 200 mg/kg i.p.), vincristine (Vin: 0.15 or 0.6 mg/kg i.p.) or busulfan (Bu: 10 mg/kg p.o.) were examined by morphological methods 3 days, 1 week and weekly thereafter until week 10 after a single exposure. With Proc a degeneration of the germ cells, particularly of mid primary spermatocytes, was seen first. Morphogenesis of early spermatids was disturbed, especially of those subcellular elements depending on an intact RNA metabolism. Later, giant cells were frequent. Vin led first to a malformation of late spermatids and arrest of cell division of spermatocytes and especially of spermatogonia, indicating microtubule dysfunction. After 2 and 4 weeks Bu showed a disappearance of spermatogonia and early spermatocytes leading to a depletion of the germinal epithelium by maturation. Late effects were rather similar in all the groups.

Key words: Testicular toxicity – Histopathology – Semi-thin sections – Anticancer Drugs – Busulfan – Procarbazine – Vincristine

Introduction

Within the last 20 years it became apparent that the testis is a very sensitive target organ for certain toxins especially anticancer agents. The present investigation was undertaken in order to detect early toxic changes of the germinal epithelium and to assess the sequence of morphological events after a single exposure to three anticancer drugs.

Material and Methods

Sprague Dawley rats (10 weeks old) were treated with Proc (50 or 200 mg/kg body weight intraperitoneally [i.p.]), Vin (0.15 or 0.6 mg/kg body weight i.p.) or

Abbreviations. Proc: procarbazine; Vin: vincristine; Bu: busulfan

Bu (10 mg/kg body weight orally [p.o.]). These doses are in the range of the cumulated dose per therapeutic course in man. Two to five animals per dose were killed at sequential time intervals after 3 days, 1 week and then weekly up to 10 weeks. Body weights were taken, as well as the organ weights of the testes, epididymides, accessory sex organs and other endocrine glands including the pituitary. Testicular tissue was fixed by perfusion with 5% glutaraldehyde (Proc, Vin) or immersion in Bouin's solution (Bu), it was embedded in Epon or paraffin, sectioned at 1 or 4 μm and stained with toluidine blue or He, PAS.

Results

All the compounds tested lowered testicular and, to a lesser degree, epididymal weight in a dose-dependent fashion. With the exception of a slight increase in pituitary weight, the organ weights and histology of the endocrine and accessory sex organs remained normal. The testicular effects were dose dependent; only the high dose effects will be summarized.

Three days after i.p. administration of 200 mg Proc per kg body weight particularly zygotene and younger pachytene spermatocytes were degenerating in considerable number. Special and particularly interesting features in the spermatids were acrosomal abnormalities such as nuclear indentation by some abnormally big acrosomic granules and retarded development. The latter lead to a desynchronization of the spermatogenic cycle. The normally irregularly shaped chromatoid body was rounded as were some nucleoli. Spermatogonia are rare in semi-thin sections and no definite changes could be observed. However, extrapolation from cellular gaps at later time points indicated that spermatogonia were destroyed to a considerable extent. One week after treatment and later, some of the late spermatids were found to be phagocytized. Giant cells with multiple nuclei covered by acrosomes were found. The diameters of the affected tubules were reduced. After 2 weeks spermatocytes and spermatids began to disappear. Spermatid heads were partly malformed or displaced. In the following weeks, regeneration of the germinal epithelium was evident to various degrees in different tubules and animals. About 20% of the tubules became partly or completely atrophic. A few Sertoli cells were found between week 1 and 3 with signs of degeneration such as coarse nucleoplasm. Leydig cells appeared normal under the light microscope. In the epididymis of animals treated with the high dose of Proc, many cellular elements, some multinucleated were detected and the concentration of sperm was decreased.

Three days following Vin treatment many spermatogonia were seen in mitosis, some in stages of the cycle at which they do not divide normally, thus indicating a mitotic arrest. The spermatogonia and preleptotene spermatocytes were already missing in some tubules. The frequency of necrotic meiotic figures in spermatocytes was clearly increased too. Some elongated spermatids showed unusual configurations of their heads. The movement of late spermatids towards the surface was partly retarded. Some Sertoli cells showed degenerative changes. Loosening of cell contact and sloughing of germ cells were also noted.

Some animals examined at 2 weeks and later, after treatment, had up to 80% of tubules with only Sertoli cells. No changes could be detected in the Leydig cells.

A fairly extensive regeneration followed testicular damaged induced by Proc and Vin in the majority of animals.

For animals treated with Bu a striking feature was the disappearance of young spermatocytes following a direct cytotoxic effect on spermatogonia. After 4 weeks a depletion of the germinal epithelium by maturation became apparent; regeneration was slow and incomplete. No changes were apparent in the Sertoli or Leydig cells.

Discussion

Proc acts in a unique manner on young to mid term spermatids probably by interfering with RNA metabolism thus inducing alterations in acrosomes, chromatoid bodies and nucleoli. Other compounds inhibiting RNA synthesis show similar changes (Parvinen et al. 1978). Furthermore, mitotic (spermatogonia) and meiotic (spermatocytes) cell division necessitating intensive DNA, RNA and protein synthesis are affected by Proc as was described by Lee and Dixon (1978).

Vin is a microtubule disrupting agent. Microtubules are important elements for cell division which was found to be disturbed. Meiosis was less affected than mitosis possibly because spermatocytes are protected better than spermatogonia which are closest to the blood vessels containing the toxin and outside the protective barrier formed by inter-Sertoli cell tight junctions. Microtubules seem to have some importance in the elongation of spermatid heads which were found to be disturbed. The effects were similar to those observed after vinblastine (Russell et al. 1981). The action of Bu seems more orientated towards the spermatogonia. As far as was interpretable in the paraffin sections after Bouin's fixation, the later stages of the cycle were primarily not affected. The full effect on fertility is apparent only after 5–7 weeks (Gomes 1970). It is obvious that morphological changes cannot give definite clues as to the mechanism of action or the functional impact (Ettlin et al. 1984). However, they give indications of the site and might help in understanding the mode of action, particularly if more refined histopathological methods are used, mainly adequate fixation and embedding.

The results show that though the initial effects related closer to the pharmacological action of each compound investigated are different, the later effects, depending on the dose applied, may be very similar.

Acknowledgements: We thank Dr. Burckhardt for proof-reading.

References

Ettlin RA, Bechter R, Lee IP, Hodel C (1984) Aspects of testicular toxicity induced by anticancer drugs. Arch Toxicol (this supplement): 151–154

Gomes WR (1970) Chemical agents affecting testicular function and male fertility. In: Johnson AD, Gomes WR, Vandemark NL (eds) The testis, vol 3. Academic Press, New York, pp 483–554

Lee IP, Dixon RL (1978) Mutagenicity, carcinogenicity and teratogenicity of procarbazine. Mutat Res 55: 1–14

Parvinen LM, Jokelainen PT, Parvinen M (1978) Chromatoid body and haploid gene activity: Actinomycin D induced morphological alterations. Hereditas 88: 75–80

Russell LD, Malone JP, MacCurdy DS (1981) Effect of the microtubule disrupting agents, colchicine and vinblastine, on seminiferous tubule structure in the rat. Tissue Cell 13: 349–367

Disease, Metabolism and Reproduction in the Toxic Response to Drugs and Other Chemicals
Arch. Toxicol., Suppl. 7, 151–154 (1984)

Aspects of Testicular Toxicity Induced by Anticancer Drugs

R. A. Ettlin[1], R. Bechter[2], I. P. Lee[2], and C. Hodel[1]

[1] F. Hoffmann-La Roche & Co. Ltd., 4002 Basel, Switzerland
[2] National Institute of Environmental Health Sciences, LRDT, Research Triangle Park, NC 27709, USA

Abstract. Newer histopathologic techniques were used in combination with sperm head counts (SHC) and serial mating (SM) studies to assess different aspects of testicular toxicity. Adult male rats were treated once intraperitoneally (i.p.) with vincristine (Vin: 0.15 and 0.6 mg/kg) or procarbazine (Proc: 50 and 200 mg/kg). Investigations were performed at weekly intervals until 10 weeks after treatment. SHC are a good parameter for cytotoxicity (Vin, Proc) assessed in great detail by morphological examination. Optimal fixation after perfusion and high optical resolution of semi-thin sections also allow the study of early and subtle specific alterations. However, they do not replace SM studies for the assessment of genotoxicity (Proc). In turn, SM studies are poor indicators of cytotoxicity.

Key words: Testicular toxicity – Histopathology – Sperm head counts – Serial mating – Anticancer drugs – Vincristine – Procarbazine

Introduction

Mating studies are relatively insensitive tests of reproductive problems (Schwetz et al. 1980) and interpretation of histological sections of testes is limited because of major artifacts after routine fixation and embedding. As compounds are tested by repeated administration of high doses, testicular side-effects are generally pronounced enough to be detected by these standard procedures. However, more refined methods and experimental protocols have to be used for a detailed investigation of testicular toxicity including the dynamics of toxic injury and response. Different and significant types of testicular toxicity were induced by anticancer drugs. Some Vin and Proc effects will be discussed here.

Abbreviations: Proc: procarbazine; Vin: vincristine; spg: spermatogonia; spc: primary spermatocytes; spt: spermatids; spz: spermatozoa; SHC: sperm head counts; SM: serial mating

Animals and Methods

Groups of 31 Sprague-Dawley male rats 10 weeks of age were injected once i.p. with Vin (0.15 and 0.6 mg/kg), Proc (50 and 200 mg/kg) or the water vehicle. 2 animals per dose and compound were examined after 3 days and 1 week and thereafter at weekly intervals for 10 weeks. Organ weights (testes, accessory sex organs and other endocrine organs) were recorded and specimens were obtained for morphological evaluation (including liver, kidney and tissues with rapid cell turnover) and for sperm head count (SHC). One testis was perfused with 5% buffered glutaraldehyde, postfixed with osmium tetroxide and embedded in Epon (Ettlin et al. 1982). Semi-thin sections (1 μm) were examined under the light microscope and selected thin sections were subjected to electron microscopy.

SHC were performed in the other testis and epididymis using a method described by Robb et al. (1978) modified by digestion of the tissue by collagenase 1 (0.2%) and trypsin (0.2%) in phosphate buffered saline at pH 7.4 prior to homogenization. Seven males per dose and compound were used for serial mating (SM). For 10 weeks, each male was caged individually with one virgin female and the females were replaced at weekly intervals and sacrificed one week later. The uteri were examined for number of implants, their growth, viability and for resorptions.

Results and Comments

The morphological effects produced by Vin and Proc were described by Hodel et al. (1984). Early and subtle alterations observed after optimal fixation in semi-thin sections are most characteristic for the type of damage induced and the mode of toxicity involved. As the duration of each step of spermatogenesis is known, effects observed during the course of the study can be related back to the initial event occurring at the time of treatment (Fig. 1). This is particularly important for detection of effects on spermatogonia (spg) which are too rare to be evaluated accurately by direct observation. In contrast to the present belief, development of certain cell types can be retarded as was shown for young spt after treatment with Proc (Ettlin et al. 1982). This has to be taken into account when plotting findings in Fig. 1. Sequential analysis of testicular tissue allowed one to follow the development of cellular damage and to recognize and characterize regeneration early.

The number of tubules damaged correlated well with testicular weight and with the number of immature germ cells in the epididymal lumina (Table 1).

In contrast to the damaged tubules, qualitatively normal tubules also had normal diameters and normal epithelial height. The SHC correlated well with semiquantitative histological analyses (Table 1) and confirmed that the cytotoxic action was particularly marked in mid and early spt (Vin) and in spc (Proc).

Fertility was low in weeks 1 and 2 after Vin treatment and in weeks 3 and 4 as well as 9 and 10 after Proc treatment, indicating an effect of Vin on spermatozoa

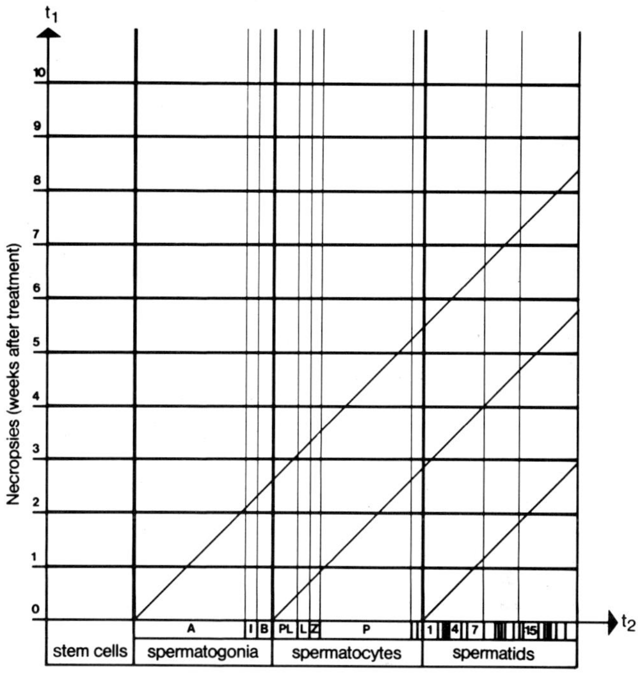

Fig. 1. t_1 time course of a study with weekly investigations. t_2 spermatogenesis at same time scale as used for t_1. *Oblique lines:* development of three selected germ cells in relation to time after start of study. This diagram allows the comparison of the toxicological effects on spermatogenesis observed at different intervals after a single exposure to a toxin and provides a means to relate later findings to the cell type initially exposed to the toxin

Table 1. Correlation coefficients (cc) between different parameters describing morphological changes, SHC and results of SM after treatment with Vin and Proc

Parameter 1	Parameter 2	Correlation coefficient	
		Vincristine (0.6 mg/kg i.p.)	Procarbazine (200 mg/kg i.p.)
Weight of testis	Tubules damaged	– 0.79[a]	– 0.61[a]
Tubules damaged[b]	Immature germ cells in epididymis[b]	– 0.82[a]	0.56
Tubules with decreased numbers of late spermatids	Testicular "sperm" count	– 0.50[a]	– 0.61[a]
Epididymal sperm count	Fertility	– 0.03	– 0.08
Normal tubules	Normal litters	0.67[a]	– 0.62

[a] cc statistically different from 0

[b] Testicular and epididymal findings during the initial 4 weeks after treatment only, when important destruction of the germinal epithelium takes place

(spz) (tail paralysis) and of Proc on spt and spg. The SHC did not correlate with fertility (Table 1) demonstrating that SM studies are relatively insensitive for cytotoxicity because of the abundance of sperm produced by animals. Following treatment with Proc but not with Vin, retarded growth and resorptions of implants were frequent, especially during the first half of the study and again towards the end indicating a genotoxic effect on spz, spt and partly on spg. Unscheduled DNA synthesis after Proc treatment is absent in spz and low in spt (Bürgin et al. 1979), indicating that these cells have no or only minor capacity to repair chemical damage in DNA. Genotoxic effects of Proc on spg which are outside the inter-Sertoli cell tight junctions, seem to be particularly severe. As there are no unequivocal morphological parameters for genotoxicity, correlation of morphological and SM results are not reliable (Table 1). This indicates that different approaches have to be used to assess the main aspects of testicular toxicity.

Acknowledgements. We thank Dr. Theiss and Dr. Hummler for their critical reading of the text and discussion and Dr. Burckhardt for proof-reading.

References

Bürgin H, Schmid B, Zbinden G (1979) Assessment of DNA damage in germ cells of male rabbits treated with isoniazid and procarbazine. Toxicology 12: 251–257

Ettlin RA, Bechter R, Dixon RL (1982) Assessment of testicular toxicity associated with anticancer agents: I. Histopathology. Proc West Pharmacol Soc 25: 381–384

Hodel C, Ettlin RA, Zschauer A (1984) Morphological changes produced in rat testis by anticancer drugs. Arch Toxicol (this supplement)

Robb GW, Amann RP, Killian GJ (1978) Daily sperm production and epididymal sperm reserves of pubertal and adult rats. J Reprod Fertil 54: 103–107

Schwetz BA, Rao KS, Park CN (1980) Insensitivity of tests for reproductive problems. J Environ Pathol Toxicol 3: 81–98

Disease, Metabolism and Reproduction in the Toxic Response to Drugs and Other Chemicals
Arch. Toxicol., Suppl. 7, 155–158 (1984)

Changes in Germinal Tissue and Leydig Cells Correlated with Ethanol Consumption in Males with and without Liver Disease

P. J. Karhunen[1], A. Penttilä[1], K. Liesto[1], A. Männikkö[1], M. Välimäki[2], M. Möttönen[1], and R. Ylikahri[2]

[1] Department of Forensic Medicine, University of Helsinki, Kytösuontie 11, 00280 Helsinki, Finland
[2] Research Laboratories of State Alcohol Monopoly (ALKO), 00280 Helsinki, Finland

Abstract. The weight of testicles and morphometric changes in testicular germinal tissue and Leydig cells were correlated with chronic consumption of ethyl alcohol and liver diseases in 44 consecutive autopsies. The mass and volume of seminiferous tubules decreased with the increase in alcohol consumption ($p < 0.05$). The atrophy and fibrosis of testicles were most advanced in males with liver cirrhosis ($p < 0.005$) and in males with moderate or heavy fatty liver ($p < 0.01$) whereas these parameters were only slightly decreased in alcoholic males with normal liver despite the greater amount of ethanol consumed. The changes in Leydig cells were mainly inconspicuous. These results indicate that the most sensitive tissue to chronic alcohol-induced injury in testis is the germinal tissue and point out the role of liver diseases in testicular damage found in alcoholics.

Key words: Alcoholism, pathology – Testis – Liver disease, alcoholic – Leydig cells

The role of alcohol-induced liver damage in the pathogenesis of reduced plasma levels of testosterone and increased concentrations of plasma oestrone and prolactin is emphasized by the finding that among chronic male alcoholics similarly exposed to the toxic effects of alcohol the changes in sex hormones are more marked in cirrhotics than in non-cirrhotic patients (Välimäki et al. 1982).

Morphologically, chronic use of alcohol is connected with diminished spermatogenesis, tubular atrophy and fibrosis (Strauss 1982), leading ultimately to extensive sclerosis of seminiferous tubules. Reports on the effect of chronic use of alcohol on Leydig cells are controversial (Edmondson 1980; Boiesen et al. 1979; Kuller et al. 1980). In earlier histological studies either no relationship (Boiesen et al. 1979) or only a weak association (Kuller et al. 1978) between liver and testicular pathology has been noted.

In this preliminary study findings on the effect of chronic alcohol consumption on testicular structure in males with and without liver disease are reported.

Following 60 autopsies of sudden death in males of 35–69 years in Helsinki city, further information on the consumption of alcohol and drugs was obtained by interviewing their relatives or friends. Cases with insufficient information, users of neuroleptic drugs or corticosteroids, as well as one male with cardiac cirrhosis and an other with parkinsonism, were excluded. The testicles were weighed without the epididymis and cases with unilateral atrophy were excluded. The final material consisted of 44 males. Standard formalin-fixed, Van Gieson stained, paraffin sections were analyzed by a point counting method with a microscope equipped with a ocular grid at a magnification of 40×. On each testicle 400 representative points were calculated randomly between the septa of spermatic cords to obtain the proportion of the glandular tissue and Leydig cells. The relative amount of glandular tissue was calculated. Liver specimens were stained for collagen and assessed as having normal, slightly changed, fatty or cirrhotic, including early cirrhotic, structure. The statistical analysis was made using Student's *t*-test and linear regression.

Fourteen of 44 men studied had been sober or had consumed only small amounts of alcohol and they served as controls. The value of 30 l absolute alcohol in a year was chosen as the limit for heavy consumers (Liesto et al. 1981). The mean weight of testicles (Table 1) in non-alcoholic males (42.1 g) was about the same as the normal testicular weights reported in other studies (Tillinger 1957). The absolute weight of testicles tended to be decreased in males with liver damage. The decrease of relative glandular mass correlated with the increase of the amount of alcohol consumed in a year ($r = -0.32$, $n = 44$, $p < 0.05$) indicating loss of glandular tissue following chronic alcohol consumption. Histologically this was evident as an increase of the peritubular and interstitial fibrous tissue (Fig. 1). The correlation with age was poor. In heavy drinkers (79 ± 39 l alcohol/year, $n = 13$) with normal liver the relative glandular mass (0.25 ± 0.11) was slightly decreased (Fig. 2) as compared with controls (0.29 ± 0.08, 6 ± 6 l alcohol/year, $n = 14$), whereas in males with moderate or severe fatty liver (0.21 ± 0.06, 34 ± 31 l alcohol/year, $n = 10$) the decrease was significant ($p < 0.01$) despite of the smaller amount alcohol consumed ($p < 0.05$). The testicular atrophy was most advanced in cirrhotic males (0.17 ± 0.06, $n = 7$, $p < 0.005$).

Table 1. Age, consumption of alcohol (liters of absolute alcohol/year) and weight of testicles in males with and without liver disease

Liver structure	Age	Alcohol consumption	Weight of testicles (g)
Normal or slightly altered ($n = 14$) (< 30 l absolute alcohol/year)	56.2 ± 7.1	6 ± 6	42.1 ± 12.1
Normal or slightly altered ($n = 13$) (> 30 l absolute alcohol/year)	54.3 ± 9.1	79 ± 39	38.9 ± 12.9
Moderate or severe fatty change ($n = 10$)	56.1 ± 8.9	34 ± 31	36.3 ± 11.2
Cirrhosis ($n = 7$)	50.8 ± 10.5	96 ± 55	35.0 ± 8.0

The values are mean ± 1 SD

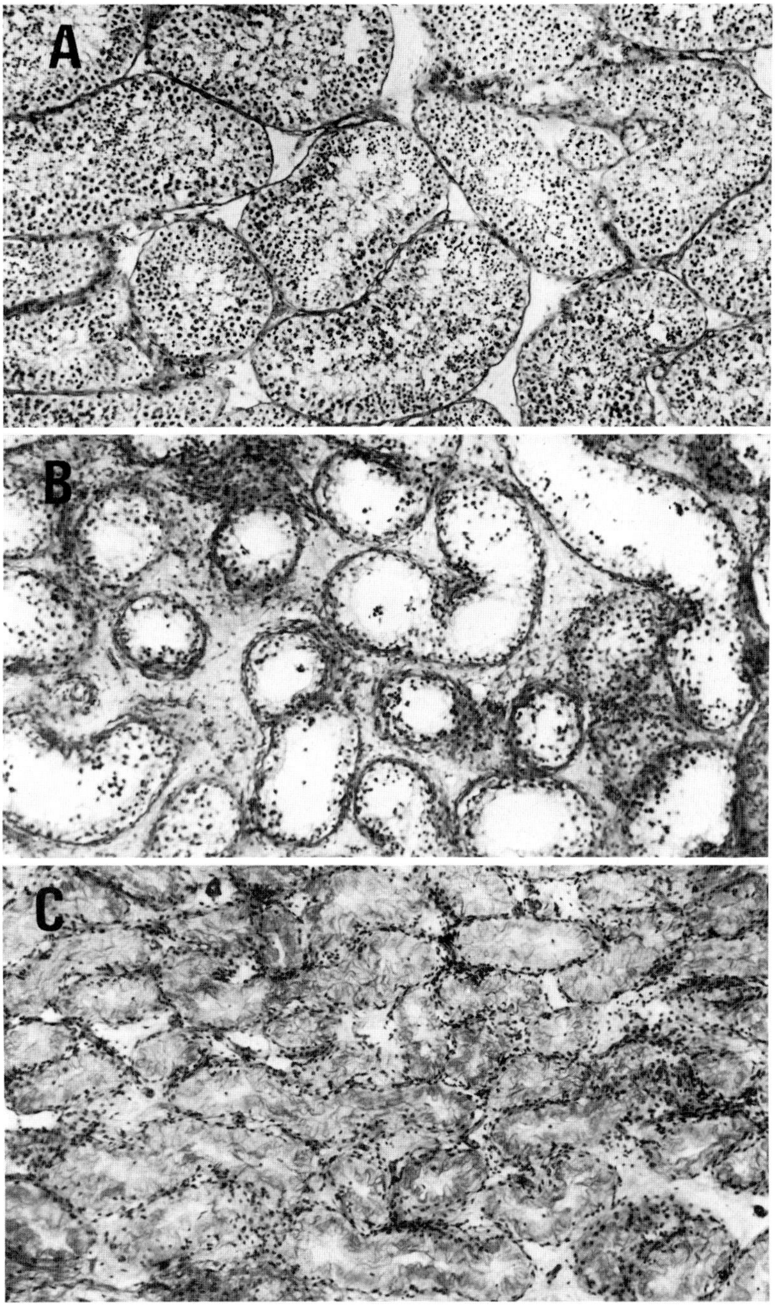

Fig. 1. A Normal seminiferous tubules showing intense spermiogenesis and high germinal epithelium in a non-alcoholic male. **B** Thin germinal epithelium, nearly complete absence of spermatogenesis, tubular and peritubular fibrosis with diminution of the diameter of seminiferous tubules in a chronic alcoholic with normal liver. **C** Obliterative tubular fibrosis of the seminiferous tubules associated with liver cirrhosis

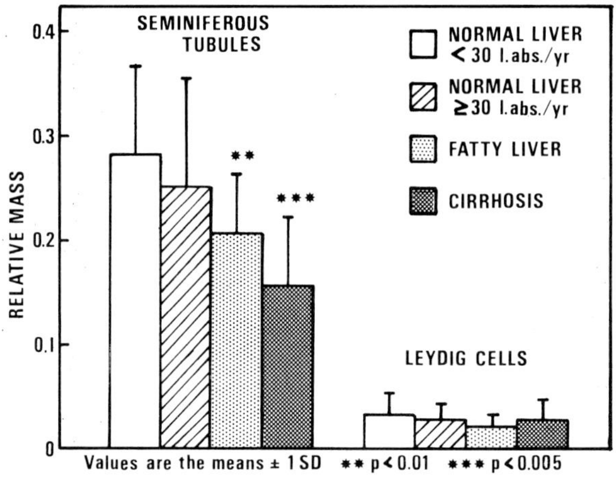

Fig. 2. Changes in the relative mass of seminiferous tubules and Leydig cells in males with normal or slightly altered, fatty and cirrhotic liver

The changes in Leydig cells (Fig. 2) were inconspicious as also reported by Boiesen et al. (1979) but more detailed study is needed because of the difficulties in differentiating morphologically between the atrophic Leydig cells and the fibroblasts in fibrotizing interstitial tissue.

These preliminary results indicate that the site most sensitive to chronic alcohol-induced injury in the testis is the germinal tissue. The frequency of testicular atrophy associated with liver cirrhosis and the progressing peritubular fibrosis in patients with moderate or severe fatty liver point out the important role of liver diseases in the pathogenesis of hypogonadism.

Acknowledgement. This research was supported by the Finnish Foundation for Alcohol Studies.

References

Boiesen PT, Lindholm J, Hagen C, Bahnsen M, Fabricius-Bjerre N (1979) Histological changes in testicular biopsies from chronic alcoholics with and without liver disease. Acta Pathol Microbiol Scand [A] 87: 139–142

Edmondson HA (1980) Pathology of alcoholism. Am J Clin Pathol 74: 725–742

Kuller LH, May SJ, Perper JA (1978) The relationship between alcohol, liver disease and testicular pathology. Am J Epidemiol 108: 192–199

Liesto K, Männikkö A, Möttönen M, Penttilä A, Karhunen P (1981) Alcohol consumption and sudden cardiac death – preliminary results. J Forensic Sci Soc 21: 127

Strauss FH (1982) The testis. In: Riddell RH (ed) Pathology of drug-induced and toxic diseases. Churchill Livingstone, New York, pp 279–295

Tillinger K-G (1957) Testicular morphology. Acta Endocrinol [Suppl 30] 24: 1–191

Välimäki M, Salaspuro M, Härkönen M, Ylikahri R (1982) Liver damage and sex hormones in chronic male alcoholics. Clin Endocrinol 17: 469–477

Van Thiel DH (1982) Endocrine function. In: Arias I, Popper H, Schachter D, Shafritz D (eds) The liver: biology and pathobiology. Raven, New York, pp 717–744

Van Thiel DH, Lester R, Sherins RJ (1974) Hypogonadism in alcoholic liver disease: Evidence for a double effect. Gastroenterology 67: 1188–1199

Van Thiel DH, Gavaler JS, Lester R, Loriaux DL, Braunstein GD (1975) Plasma estrone, prolactin, neurophysin and sex steroid-binding globulin in chronic alcoholic men. Metabolism 24: 1015–1019

Disease, Metabolism and Reproduction in the Toxic Response to Drugs and Other Chemicals
Arch. Toxicol., Suppl. 7, 159–163 (1984)

Testicular Effects of Some Xanthine Derivatives in the Rat

M. Dahlbäck and Å. Ryrfeldt

AB Draco, Research and Development Laboratories, Box 1707, 2201 01 Lund, Sweden

Abstract. Testicular toxicity as well as effects on body weight gain and food consumption of four xanthine derivatives were studied in the Sprague-Dawley rat. The influence on toxicity by variation of the substituent at positions 1 and 3 on the xanthine skeleton was tested. The compounds were administered orally once a day for 1 month. The 1-methylated xanthines seemed to be more toxic than the non-methylated compounds.

Key words: Xanthines – Testicular toxicity – Rat

It is well known that xanthines, such as theobromine (Tarka et al. 1979), caffeine and theophylline (Friedman et al. 1979) can induce testicular atrophy in the rat at high doses. Recent investigations have shown that a xanthine derivative (D 4026) was almost 100 times more potent than the above mentioned compounds in inducing testicular damage (Dahlbäck et al. 1981). The aim of the present investigation was to elucidate the potency of some structural analogues of D 4026 in inducing testicular atrophy in the rat. Preliminary experiments indicated that substitutions at positions 1 and 3 on the xanthine skeleton were of special interest (Fig. 1). Xanthine derivatives are of potential interest as drugs, e.g., in the treatment of respiratory diseases, such as bronchial asthma.

Methods

Forty-five male Sprague-Dawley rats, weighing about 200 g, were used (Table 1). The substances (see Fig. 1), provided by Dr. G. Kjellin, AB Draco, were suspended in Kenacort vehicle (Tween 80 0.04%, NaCl 0.65%, CMC 0.75% in water) and administered orally (0.25 ml/100 g) by means of a gastric tube once a day for 1 month. Dose levels are given in Table 1 and they were chosen based on knowledge gained from pharmacological studies showing that the 1-methylated xanthines were more potent than their non-methylated

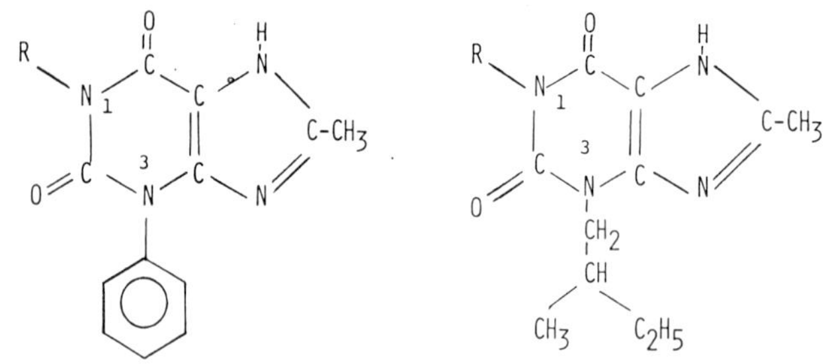

	R		R
D 4152	H⁻	D 4173	H⁻
D 4026	CH_3^-	D 4160	CH_3^-

Fig. 1. Molecular sturctures of xanthine derivatives

structural analogues. Food consumption and body weights were recorded three times a week. At the end of the study, the animals were anaesthetized with ether and blood was withdrawn from the orbital plexus (2 h) or from the abdominal aorta (24 h). Plasma was extracted and stored (−30° C) until time for analysis for concentrations of unchanged drug by the use of high performance liquid chromatography [column: Nucleosil C18; mobile phase: sodium phosphate buffer 0.01 mol/l, pH 6.0/acetonitrile 80/20 (v/v)]. The left testis was preserved in buffered neutral formaldehyde solution. After paraffin embedding, 7 μm sections were prepared and stained with Harris hematoxylin and eosin.

Results and Discussion

The animals seemed to tolerate the treatment with the substances well, with the exception of the rats receiving the high dose of D 4160 (100 μol/kg). Two of the five treated animals died after 2 days of treatment and another animal died after 3 days. At autopsy these animals showed severe irritation and ulceration of the gastric mucosa. Dose related decreases in body weight gain relative to the control animals were found in all animals (Table 1). The animals receiving the high doses of D 4160, D 4173, and D 4026 showed the most pronounced effects. A reduced food intake in comparison with the control animals was noted during the first days of treatment, especially with the high doses of D 4160, D 4173, and D 4026 (60−80%). From the second week of treatment, the food intake was considered to be normal (20−25 g/animal/day). At the end of the study histopathological examination revealed that testicular atrophy was caused by high doses of D 4026, D 4152, and D 4173. However, frequency and degree of damage varied considerably between D 4026 and the other two substances. All animals receiving the high dose of D 4026 (100 μol/kg) showed pronounced testicular atrophy with degeneration and necrosis of the germinal epithelium (Fig. 2). These effects were generally more pronounced in the periphery of the

Table 1. Terminal body weights, testes weights, and plasma concentrations (nmol/ml) of unchanged compound after oral administration of xanthine derivatives to male Sprague-Dawley rats after the last dose in the 1 month toxicity study

Substances	n	Doses (µmol/kg)	Body weights (g)	Testes weights (g)	Plasma concentrations			
					2 h after administration		24 h after administration	
					Low dose	High dose	Low dose	High dose
Vehicle	5	–	375 ± 10	3.99 ± 0.13				
D 4026	5	25	328 ± 14*	4.01 ± 0.08	13.6 ± 1.1		1.2 ± 0.1	
(MW 256)	5	100	296 ± 7**	4.17 ± 0.50		70.3 ± 5.6		11.8 ± 2.0
D 4152	5	100	344 ± 12	3.60 ± 0.08	14.7 ± 1.1		< 0.4	
(MW 242)	5	400	360 ± 9	3.86 ± 0.04		14.8 ± 1.8		1.0 ± 0.5
D 4160	5	25	325 ± 4*	4.05 ± 0.25	24.7 ± 2.4		0.6 ± 0.2	
(MW 250)	2	100[a]	316 ± 26	3.56 ± 0.42		38.4 ± 2.4		1.8 ± 1.4
D 4173	5	100	350 ± 10	3.94 ± 0.22	119.5 ± 7.0		14.5 ± 4.9	
(MW 236)	5	400	314 ± 13**	3.77 ± 0.25		343.4 ± 10.2		124.2 ± 10.3

Given values are means ± SEM

* $p < 0.5$, ** $p < 0.01$

[a] After 3 days of treatment, the dose was decreased to 50 µmol/kg

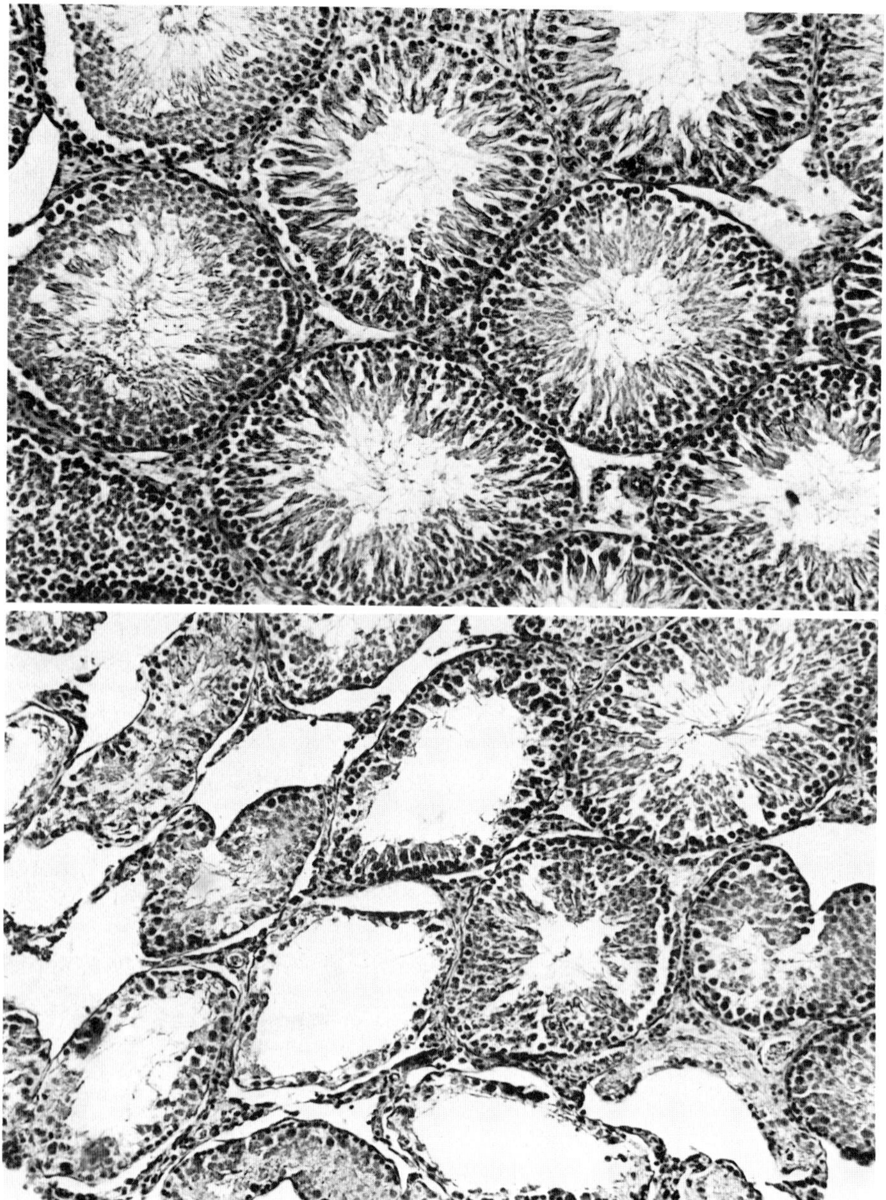

A

B

Fig. 2. Light micrographs of a testis from a control rat **(A)** and from a testis of a rat treated with D 4026 (100 μmol/kg) for 1 month **(B).** Note degeneration and necrosis of seminiferi tubuli. (H/E, × 32)

testes. Occasionally, multinucleated giant cells were found. Out of the five animals treated with either D 4152 or D 4173 only one showed a slight atrophy. The remaining four animals were unaffected.

The surviving animals receiving the high dose of D 4160 had normal testes. No effects on the testes of all the low dosed animals or the control animals were found. The analyses of plasma samples showed that dose related plasma concentrations were achieved with the exception of compound D 4152 where unexpected low concentrations were found. These low concentrations may be due to either firstpass metabolism poor absorption from the gastrointestinal tract or both. This may explain the low toxicity found with D 4152. Among these compunds, the 1-methylated derivatives (D 4026 and D 4160) seemed to be more toxic (testicular atrophy general toxicity or both) than their non-methylated analogues. The mechanism behind the testicular atrophy found after treatment with xanthines is not known. However, it is considered not to be due to decreased food consumption (Tarka et al. 1979). The relevance of the testicular atrophy found in the rat for man may be argued, since the rat may be exceptionally sensitive (Tarka et al. 1979; Gans et al. 1980).

References

Dahlbäck M, Karlberg IB, Ryrfeldt Å, Sörenby L, Havu N (1981) General toxicity in rats of D 4122 and D 4026 with special reference to testicular effects – a preliminary study. Data on file at Draco

Friedman L, Weinberger M, Farber T, Moreland F, Peters E, Gilmore C, Kahn M (1979) Testicular atrophy and impaired spermatogenesis in rats fed high levels of methylxanthines caffeine, theobromine or theophylline. J Environ Pathol Toxicol 2: 687–706

Gans J, Kordson R, Cater M, Ackerly C (1980) Effects of short-term and long-term theobromine administration to male dogs. Toxicol Appl Pharmacol 53: 481–496

Tarka S, Zoumas B, Gans J (1979) Short-term effects of graded levels of theobromine in laboratory rodents. Toxicol Appl Pharmacol 49: 127–149

Disease, Metabolism and Reproduction in the Toxic Response to Drugs and Other Chemicals
Arch. Toxicol., Suppl. 7, 164–166 (1984)

Effects of Daily High Doses of Paracetamol Given Orally During Spermatogenesis in the Rat Testes

A. Jacqueson, H. Semont, M. Thevenin, J.-M. Warnet, R. Prost, and J. R. Claude

Laboratoire de Recherches de la DASS,
27, rue Lacordaire, 75015 Paris and Inserm Paris, France

Abstract. Daily treatment of male rats with high doses of Paracetamol (500 mg/kg) during spermatogenesis provokes a significant decrease of testes weight ($p < 0.001$), a significant increase of testicular cytosol glutathione transferase activity ($p < 0.02$) and of lipid peroxides in the whole homogenate ($p < 0.01$) but not in the microsomes. These alterations could be related to a stimulation of testicular metabolism but cannot produce a biochemical lesion such as glutathione depletion since its testicular content is not modified in these experimental conditions.

Key words: Glutathione – Glutathione S-transferase – Paracetamol – Peroxides – Rat – Testes

Introduction

The effect of continuous daily intake of large doses of analgesic drugs on fertility is still a problem (Boyd 1970). Chronic administration of Paracetamol (4′-hydroxyacetanilide; acetaminophen) produces loss of testicular weight and impaired spermatogenesis in the rat. Since rat testes are the most important source of glutathione S-transferase (GST) after the liver (Dierickx 1982), the detoxification by GST was investigated to see if it could be involved, as in the liver of rats poisoned by high doses of Paracetamol.

Material and Methods

Animals and experimental procedure. Male Sprague-Dawley rats weighing 300–320 g were used (10 in each group). Paracetamol was suspended in 1% carboxymethyl-cellulose (CMC) and administered by gastric intubation at doses of 500 mg/kg/day for 70 days. The controls received only 1% CMC.

The controls and the treated rats were killed by mebubarbital injection and the testes were quickly excised, washed with iso-osmotic NaCl, dried with filter paper and weighed. One was used for histological examination and the second was used to prepare a 20% (w/v) testis homogenate in 1.15% KCl; the cytosol and microsomes were separated by differential sedimentation.

Analytical Methods. Reduced glutathione (GSH) was determined by the 5,5′-dithiobis(2-nitrobenzoic acid) reaction (Jollow et al. 1974) in the total homogenate.

GST activity was assayed using 1-chloro-2,4-dinitrobenzene as substrate (Carmagnol et al. 1981) in the cytosol.

The lipid peroxides were determined by the thiobarbituric reaction (Ohkawa et al. 1979) in the total homogenate and in the microsomes.

Protein. All the results were expressed relative to proteins measured with a modified Lowry method (Markwell 1978).

Statistical Analysis. All the results were statistically analysed, the significance of the differences between the controls and the treated rats was assayed by Student's *t*-test and a *p*-value of 0.05 or less was considered significant.

Results

Daily treatment of male rats with high doses of Paracetamol during spermatogenesis provokes a significant decrease in the weight of the testes (Table 1). Testicular GST activity is significantly increased, but GSH is not affected (Table 1). The results of the effect of Paracetamol on lipid peroxides are summarized in Table 2.

Table 1. Effect of paracetamol (500 mg/kg/day) on rat testes: weight and glutathione metabolism (Mean ± SD)

	Testes weight (g)	GSH (nM/mg protein)	GST (μM/mg protein)
Controls	3.567 ± 0.253	26.1 ± 12.3	1.38 ± 0.14
Paracetamol	2.699 ± 0.627	28.8 ± 20.9	1.62 ± 0.26
p-Value	< 0.001	NS	< 0.02

Table 2. Effect of paracetamol (500 mg/kg/day) on testicular peroxides in the rat

	Lipid peroxides (nM of malondialdehyde/mg protein)	
	Whole homogenate	Microsomes
Controls	1.38 ± 0.34	0.84 ± 0.19
Paracetamol	1.96 ± 0.36	0.95 ± 0.17
p-Value	< 0.01	NS

Lipid peroxides of the whole homogenate are significantly increased; on the other hand, the slight increase in microsomal peroxides is not statistically significant.

Discussion

The testicular GST increase after continuous oral treatment with high doses of Paracetamol (500 mg/kg/day for 70 days) may reflect a detoxification of electrophilic metabolites of Paracetamol, whose formation involves an oxidative pathway, if testicular metabolism is similar to hepatic metabolism. The increase of lipid peroxides is in agreement with this hypothesis. However, this peroxidation seems to be a slight and transitory phenomenon, since it can only be seen at the total homogenate level, whereas the microsomes, the first target of lipoperoxidation, do not show any sign of lipid peroxidation. This study corroborates the work of Boyd (1970) on the morphological changes in rat testes produced by Paracetamol (Boyd 1970). These alterations could be related to a stimulation of the testicular metabolism of the drug but they cannot produce a biochemical lesion such as GSH depletion since its testicular content is not modified in the conditions of this experiment.

Acknowledgements. The authors thank Y. Save and P. Claude for their technical assistance.

References

Boyd EM (1970) Testicular atrophy from analgesic drugs. J Clin Pharmacol (New Drugs) 10 : 222–227

Carmagnol F, Sinet PM, Rapin J, Jerome H (1981) Glutathione S-transferase of human red blood cells. Clin Chim Acta 117 : 209–217

Dierickx PJ (1982) Soluble glutathione S-transferase from rat testes: isoenzyme pattern and lack of inducibility by drug metabolizing enzyme inducers. Toxicol Eur Res 4 : 47–51

Jollow DL, Mitchell JR, Zampaglione N, Gillette JR (1974) Bromobenzene-induced liver necrosis. Protective role of glutathione and evidence for 3,4-bromobenzene oxide as the hepatotoxic metabolite. Pharmacology 11 : 151–169

Markwell MAK (1978) A modification of the Lowry procedure to simplify protein determination in membrane and lipoprotein samples. Anal Biochem 87 : 206–210

Ohkawa H, Ohishi N, Yagi K (1979) Assay for lipid peroxides in animal tissues by thiobarbituric acid reaction. Anal Biochem 95 : 351–358

Disease, Metabolism and Reproduction in the Toxic Response to Drugs and Other Chemicals
Arch. Toxicol., Suppl. 7, 167–170 (1984)

The Effects on the Rat Testis of Single Inhalation Exposures to Ethylene Glycol Monoalkyl Ethers, in Particular Ethylene Glycol Monomethyl Ether

D. M. Samuels, J. E. Doe, and D. J. Tinston

Central Toxicology Laboratory, Imperial Chemical Industries PLC,
Alderley Park, Macclesfield, Cheshire, Great Britain

Abstract. The effects of a single inhalation exposure to the rat of the saturated vapours derived from four ethylene glycol monoalkyl ethers have been investigated. No effects on the testis were observed following exposure to ethylene glycol isopropyl ether (EG ISOPE) and ethylene glycol butyl ether (EGBE), but there were marked reductions in testicular weight 14 days after exposure to ethylene glycol monomethyl ether (EGME) and ethylene glycol monoethyl ether (EGEE). Further studies were designed to establish the effect of a single exposure to EGME. Mature male albino rats were exposed to various levels of EGME vapour for a single 4-h period and killed 14 days later. Following this single exposure a dose-related decrease in testis weight was observed in rats exposed to 5,000, 2,500 or 1,250 ppm EGME. Histopathological examination revealed disordered spermatogenesis and tubular atrophy in these animals. Minimal degenerative changes were seen in the testis of rats exposed to 625 ppm EGME. When rats were examined at various time intervals after exposure to EGME vapour for 4 h, testis weight was reduced in rats examined 2 days after exposure to 2,500 and 1,000 ppm EGME and remained depressed when compared with control values for up to 19 days following exposure. Histopathological examination of the testis revealed disordered spermatogenesis in exposed animals evident at 1 day following exposure to either 2,500 or 1,000 ppm EGME.

Key words: Reproduction toxicity – Rat – Inhalation exposure – Testis – Solvents – Glycol ethers – Ethylene glycol monomethyl ether

Ethylene glycol monoalkyl ethers are used extensively as co-solvents for various resins, lacquers, paints, varnishes, dyes, inks, printing pastes, cleaning compositions, liquid soap and cosmetics. They are also widely used as chemical intermediates. Attention has been focussed recently on the glycol ethers as a result of studies demonstrating adverse effects on the reproductive processes of animals, namely testicular atrophy and abnormal foetal development.

EGME has been shown to cause testicular atrophy in rats following exposure to 300 ppm for either 90 days (Miller et al. 1982) or 10 days (Doe et al. 1983; Miller et al. 1981). Subsequently the effects of a single inhalation exposure in the rat to the saturated vapours derived from four ethylene glycol monoalkyl ethers have been investigated. No effects on the testis were observed following exposure to EG ISOPE or EGBE. Marked reductions in testis weight were seen 14 days after exposure to the saturated vapours of EGME or EGEE. Further studies were designed to characterise the effect on the testis of a single exposure to EGME in terms of the dose response and the time course of the histopathological changes accompanying the testicular weight reduction.

In the first study groups of 20 eight-week-old specific pathogen-free (SPF) Alderley Park (Alpk/AP) male albino rats were exposed for 4 h to a saturated vapour (5,000 ppm), 2,500, 1,250, 625, 300, or 150 ppm EGME. A further group of 40 rats was sham exposed to air. On the day before the exposure period the rats were transferred to whole body exposure chambers. Following exposure they were returned to their holding cages for 13 days without further exposure to EGME vapour. Atmosphere concentrations were monitored using an infra red analyser (MIRAN IA). Individual body weights were recorded on the day before the day of exposure and on days 6 and 13. On day 14 rats were killed with an overdose of halothane BP (Fluothane ICI). At autopsy the testes were weighed separately and preserved in Bouin's fixative for subsequent processing and microscopic examination. Cauda epididymides were also weighed and preserved for processing and microscopic examination. The accessory sex glands, seminal vesicle and ventral prostate, were weighed and later examined histopathologically.

In the second study groups of 90 eight-week-old SPF Alderley Park albino rats were exposed to either 2,500 ppm or 1,000 ppm EGME for a single 4-h period. A further group of 90 rats was sham exposed to air. Ten rats in each group were killed on each of days 1, 2, 3, 4, 5, 8, 10, 15 and 19 following exposure. Individual body weights were recorded on the day before exposure and subsequently on days 4, 8, 15 and 19. Testes, cauda epididymides and accessory gland weights were recorded for each rat at autopsy. Samples of these tissues were preserved in Bouin's fixative prior to processing and microscopic examination. On days 1, 2, 3, 4, 5 and 19 prior to fixation samples of testis were fixed in glutaraldehyde phosphate buffer and sections of resin-embedded material were examined with the electron microscope.

In the first study significant reductions in testis weight, compared with the control values, were seen in rats exposed to 1,250, 2,500, and 5,000 ppm EGME (Fig. 1). Epididymal weight was also significantly reduced in rats exposed to 5,000 ppm EGME. Histological examination of the testis revealed severe bilateral tubular atrophy with disordered spermatogenesis in rats exposed to 5,000 ppm EGME for 4 h with many tubules showing only stem cells and Sertoli cells. Similar, though less marked changes were seen in rats exposed to 2,500 and 1,250 ppm EGME. Although testis weight was not reduced when compared with the control values at 625 ppm EGME exposure, maturing spermatids showed evidence of damage.

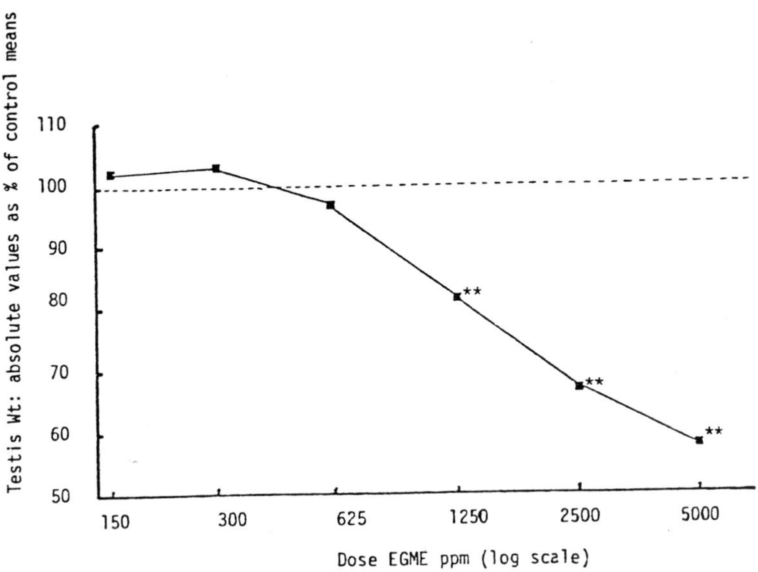

Fig. 1. Log dose response for the effect on testis weight of exposure to EGME 14 days after a single exposure

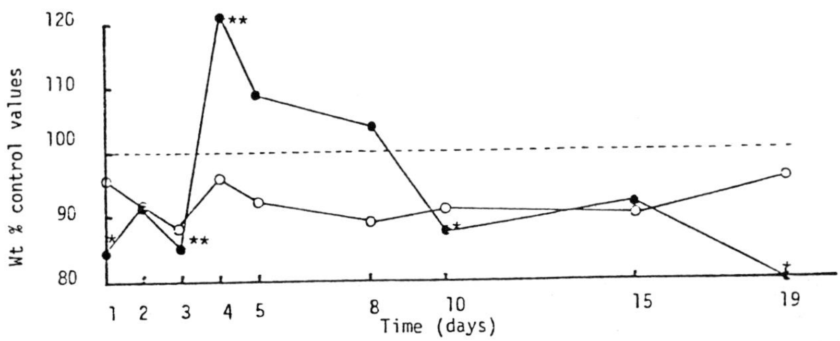

Fig. 2. Cauda epididymal weight in rats-exposure to 2,500 ppm and 1,000 ppm EGME for 4 h. ●——● 2,500 ppm; ○——○ 1,000 ppm; * $P < 0.05$; ** $P < 0.01$ Students *t*-test

In the second study testis weight reduction was seen in exposed rats 48 h after exposure to either 2,500 or 1,000 ppm. Testis weights were lower than control values in both exposed groups at subsequent time points and the degree of reduction was related to dose. Histological examination of the testis of exposed animals revealed damage to the germinal epithelium 24 h post exposure with primary spermatocytes apparently the target cells for EGME. Recovery was not evident 19 days following exposure to 2,500 ppm and the germinal epithelium remained disordered. Electron microscopy revealed changes in Sertoli cells with cytoplasm retraction and swollen mitochondria evident 4 days after exposure to EGME. There was a biphasic response in exposed animals with regards to epididymal weight (Fig. 2). The increased weight at day 4 probably reflects the passage through the epididymis at this point of large numbers of immature germ cells shed from the testis following the initial insult. Subsequently epididymal weights were reduced when compared with the control values again reflecting the situation in the testis where there was a marked reduction in the number of spermatozoa produced following exposure.

EGME would appear to be exerting its effect primarily on rapidly dividing cells with primary spermatocytes being initially affected. Subsequently Sertoli cells show signs of damage and this may account for the subsequent marked loss of immature germ cells.

These studies indicate that even a relatively brief exposure to EGME vapour can cause marked testicular atrophy, albeit at high concentrations. Even at concentrations comparable with these causing testicular atrophy over a 90 day period there were subtle effects on spermatogenesis highlighting the need for further studies.

References

Doe JE, Samuels DM, Tinston DJ, Wickramaratne GA de S (1983) Comparative aspects of the reproductive toxicology by inhalation in rats of ethylene glycol monomethyl ether and propylene glycol monomethyl ether. Toxicol App Pharmacol 69 : 43–47

Miller R, Ayres J, Calhoun L, Young J, McKenna M (1981) Comparative short term inhalation toxicity of ethylene glycol monomethyl ether and propylene glycol monomethyl ether in rats and mice. Toxicol Appl Pharmacol 61 : 368–377

Miller R, Ayres J, Young J, McKenna M (1982) Ethylene glycol monomethyl ether subchronic inhalation study in rats and rabbits. Toxicologist 2 : 11

Disease, Metabolism and Reproduction in the Toxic Response to Drugs and Other Chemicals
Arch. Toxicol., Suppl. 7, 171–173 (1984)

Effects of an Indenopyridine Derivative, Compound 20-438, on Spermatogonial Stem Cells of the Rat

K. E. Suter

Preclinical Research, Sandoz Ltd., 4002 Basel, Switzerland

Abstract. Single high doses of the antitesticular compound 20-438 caused pronounced testis weight loss in rats. Treatment of adult testes containing fully populated tubules led to irreversible weight losses, indicative of damage to the spermatogonial stem cells. On the other hand, treatment of lightly populated tubules in either juventile testes or adult, cryptorchid testes also caused weight losses, but these were followed by substantial recovery. The fact that the damage induced by 20-438 in spermatogonial stem cells is related to the germ cell density points to the possibility that this compound acts by reducing the availability of an essential substrate.

Key words: Antispermatogenic compound – Rat

Sandoz compound 20-438, an indenopyridine derivative, exhibits strong antitesticular activity in dogs, rats and mice (Hodel et al. 1978; Matter et al. 1979; Suter et al. 1981). It causes inhibition of testicular fluid production, hyperemia, and, most pronounced, depletion of the seminiferous epithelium resulting in testis weight reduction. In mice at high dose levels germ cell renewal is incomplete, leading to permanent damage to at least some of the spermatogonial stem cells, as demonstrated by histological examination (Matter et al. 1979). Since the cause for this action is not known, the present study assesses the effects of 20-438 on the stem cells of Sprague Dawley rats, using the weight recovery of treated testes as a functional test.

In the first part of the experiment, adult rats were treated with single oral doses of either 30 or 100 mg/kg. As shown in Table 1, marked testis weight reductions were observed at both dose levels within 2 weeks following treatment. Whereas partial recovery occurred at the low dose level, starting 4 weeks after treatment, no recovery was seen at the high dose level even after 56 weeks. These findings confirmed earlier mice studies (Matter et al. 1979) which showed that at low doses spermatids, spermatocytes and intermediate spermatogonia were primarily affected, whereas spermatogonial stem cells were not. At high doses, however, the stem cells were also severely affected.

Table 1. Testes weights of adult rats after single oral treatment with 20-438. All values represent % of the corresponding controls. Three animals were used per time interval and dose

Weeks after treatment	Dose (mg/kg)	
	30	100
2	57*	43*
4	53*	36*
6	95	40*
12	81	43*
24	78*	36*
36	68	38*
56	89	33*

* $p < 0.05$

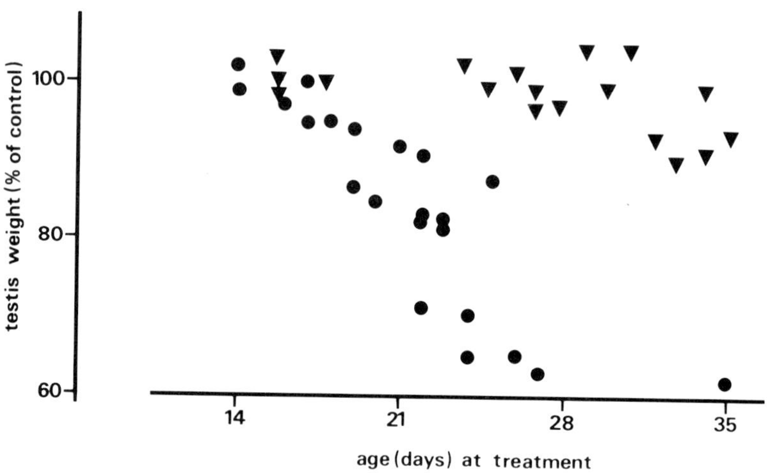

Fig. 1. Testes weights of juvenile rats treated with a single oral dose (100 mg/kg) of 20-438 at different ages. Each point represents the mean of one litter ($n = 2-5$). *Circles:* weight measurements 2 weeks after treatment; *Triangles:* weight measurements 8 weeks after treatment

Table 2. Long term effect of 20-438 (100 mg/kg) on the testes of adult rats which had been partially depleted by artificial cryptorchidism

Treatment	Pretreatment	Weight measurements (days after treatment)	n	Testis weight (mg/100 g BW)	
				Cryptorchid testis	Normal testis
Controls	14 days unilateral cryptorchidism	0	7	169 ± 18	524 ± 47
20-438	14 days unilateral cryptorchidism	75 105	4 5	215 ± 94 307 ± 22	153 ± 23 169 ± 25

In the second part of the experiment, juvenile rats aged from 14 to 35 days were treated orally with a single dose of 100 mg/kg (Fig. 1). No testis weight reductions were observed two weeks after administration to animals younger than 19 days; the testes of the older rats were, however, progresssively more sensitive with age. When testes weights were measured 8 weeks after administration, recovery had taken place, and the weights had returned to the normal range. Thus, in juvenile rats, in contrast to adult rats, spermatogonial stem cells are insensitive to a high dose of 20-438. From these results it was not clear whether the reduced sensitivity was due to special characteristics of juvenile metabolism or to the low germ cell density in the testis tubules of rat pups. Therefore, in the third part of the experiment, testis tubules of adult animals were artificially depleted of germ cells except for the spermatogonia. This was achieved by rendering the animals unilaterally cryptorchid 2 weeks prior to treatment (Clegg 1963). The intact testes served as controls. For reinitiation of spermatogenesis the cryptorchid testes were released into the scrotums immediately after the administration of a single dose of 100 mg/kg. As shown in Table 2, the weights of the originally intact testes were still drastically reduced after 75 and 105 days. In the cryptorchid testes, on the other hand, substantial recovery had taken place within the same periods, as demonstrated by the testis weight increase.

The results of this experiment provide evidence that the damage inflicted by high doses of 20-438 to spermatogonial stem cells is related to the density of the germ cell population in the testis tubules. In lightly populated tubules of either juvenile rats or adult, cryptorchid rats these cells retain their capacity for recovery, whereas in the densely populated tubules of intact, adult, rats they suffer permanent damage. This points to the possibility that the action of 20-438 may be due to the reduced availability of an essential substrate. In conditions where competition for such a substrate is most intense, i.e., in fully populated tubules, the effects of 20-438 are more pronounced.

References

Clegg EJ (1963) Studies on artificial cryptorchidism: Degenerative and regenerative changes in the germinal epithelium of the rat testis. J Endocrinol 27: 241–251

Hodel C, Suter KE (1978) Reversible inhibition of spermatogenesis with an indenopyridine derivative (20-438). Arch Toxicol [Suppl] 1: 323–326

Matter BE, Jaeger I, Suter W, Tsuchimoto T, Deyssenroth H (1979) Actions of an antispermatogenic, but non-mutagenic indenopyridine derivative in mice and salmonella typhimurum. Mutat Res 66: 113–127

Suter KE, Donatsch P (1981) Effect of the antitesticular compound 20-438 on testicular fluid production and blood volume in rats. Teratology 24: 50A

Disease, Metabolism and Reproduction in the Toxic Response to Drugs and Other Chemicals
Arch. Toxicol., Suppl. 7, 174–176 (1984)

Monitoring Chemically Induced DNA Damage in the Germ Cells of Male Mice

R. R. Racine and B. P. Schmid

Sandoz Ltd., Preclinical Research, Toxicology, 4002 Basel, Switzerland

Abstract. Unscheduled DNA synthesis (UDS) was assayed by measuring the uptake of ^{3}H-dT into the nucleic DNA of sperm cells of mice during the meiotic and postmeiotic stages of spermatogenesis. Incorporation of the radioactive compound into the DNA was measured by liquid scintillation counting. UDS was indicated by the statistically significantly higher incorporation of ^{3}H-dT observed in the treated groups after administration of the mutagens methylmethane sulfonate, cyclophosphamide and the immunosuppressive drug azathioprine. Cyclosporin A, also an immunosuppressive drug, caused no effects in this assay, nor did the two hydrazine derivatives endralazine and hydralazine.

Key words: Drug effects – In vivo mutagenicity test system – Germ cells – Unscheduled DNA synthesis – Azathioprine – Cyclosporin A – Cyclophosphamide – Hydralazine – Methylmethane sulfonate – Endralazine

DNA damage is one of the initial events in both mutagenesis and carcinogenesis; it can lead to mutations, transformations, or cell death.

The occurrence of repair processes is an indicator of possible DNA damage. Repair enzyme systems can be assessed by measuring the incorporation of radioactive material into the DNA by means of unscheduled DNA synthesis (UDS). The method of Sega (1974) was used in the present study.

The purest available grades of the following substances were tested: MMS (Eastman), CP (Serva), AT (Sigma), CS A (Sandoz), EN (Sandoz) and HY (Ciba-Geigy). The radioactive material, ^{3}H-dT (Amersham), had a specific activity of 48–52 Ci/mmol.

Male CD-1 mice (Charles River), 8–12 weeks old, were administered the test substances once. CS A and AZ were applied by stomach tube in a 2%

Abbreviations: UDS, unscheduled DNA synthesis; ^{3}H-dT, radioactive thymidine; AZ, azathioprine; CP, cyclophosphamide; HY hydralazine; MMS, methylmethane sulfonate; EN, endralazine; CS A, cyclosporin A

Table 1. Unscheduled DNA synthesis evaluated in sperm of the cauda epididymidis

Days after treatment		dpm/2 · 10^6 sperm cells					
		MMS[a] 25*	CP[a] 200*	AZ[a] 100*	CS A 507*	EN 100*	HY 70*
14	C	5.27	8.60	33.45	0.21	14.99	30.09
	T	261.14	27.73	35.80	1.33	21.21	24.19
16	C	12.96	13.61	42.66	8.77	48.25	32.83
	T	354.41	60.35	84.38	21.32	30.72	29.85
18	C	22.81	25.06	57.78	34.21	39.01	31.82
	T	926.73	29.12	94.21	34.69	38.23	50.44
21	C	8.08	49.98	52.65	39.61	43.98	55.15
	T	639.27	62.51	76.17	84.67	60.44	97.76

C = Two control animals; T = three treated animals
* mg/kg
[a] Statistically different ($2\,p < 0.05$)

gelatine solution, the other substances were injected intraperitoneally (i.p.) in a 0.9% NaCl solution. One hour after administration, 30 µl of ^{3}H-dT, amounting to 30 µCi, was injected into each testis. The control animals received the corresponding vehicles alone. The doses of the following substances were selected from the literature: MMS (Sega et al. 1976), AZ (IARC 1981) and CP (Sotomayor et al. 1978). The following doses were determined in this laboratory. The CS A dose corresponded to the LD_5 value, the EN dose was one third of the LD_5 value. The HY dose was equimolar to the EN dose. Sperm heads were isolated from the cauda epididymidis 14, 16, 18, and 21 days posttreatment. They were lysed and the DNA of the sperm heads was monitored for ^{3}H-dT incorporation by liquid scintillation counting. Statistical analysis of the results, by means of both the U-test and a regression analysis, showed differences between the control values and those from MMS, CP and AZ treated animals ($2\,p < 0.05$), as seen in Table 1.

The positive results indicate that these compounds were able to damage the DNA. This damaged DNA initiated a series of repair processes which led to an incorporation of the ^{3}H-dT into the DNA. The negative results obtained with CS-A and with both hydrazine derivatives, EN and HY suggest that these three substances did not interfere with germ cell DNA.

References

IARC monographs on the evaluation of the carcinogenic risk of chemicals to humans (1981). Some antineoplastic and immunosuppressive agents. WHO (Switzerland) 26: 47–78

Sega GA (1974) Unscheduled DNA synthesis in the germ cells of male mice exposed in vivo to the chemical mutagen ethyl methynesulfonate. Proc Natl Acad Sci USA 71: 4955–4959

Sega GA, Owens JG, Comming RB (1976) Studies on DNA repair in early spermatid stages of male mice after in vivo treatment with methyl-, ethyl- propyl-, and isopropyl methanesulfonate. Mutat Res 36: 193–212

Sotomayer RE, Sega GA, Comming RB (1978) Unscheduled DNA synthesis in spermatogenic cells of mice treated in vivo with the indirect alkylating agents cyclophosphamide and mitomen. Mutat Res 50: 229–240

Disease, Metabolism and Reproduction in the Toxic Response to Drugs and Other Chemicals
Arch. Toxicol., Suppl. 7, 177–180 (1984)

Accumulation of Toxic Metals in Male Reproduction Organs

B. R. G. Danielsson, L. Dencker, A. Lindgren, and H. Tjälve

Department of Toxicology, Uppsala University, Box 573, 751 23 Uppsala, Sweden

Abstract. Occupation exposure to metals has been related to impaired reproduction in males. This report summarizes autoradiographic studies on the distribution of cadmium (Cd), chromium (Cr) and arsenic (As) in the testis and epididymis of rodents. Cd and Cr strongly accumulated in the interstitial tissues, indicating an effect on hormone production (Leydig cells) and blood supply or both. Arsenic accumulated in the lumen of the duct of epididymis causing long-term exposure of the semen.

Key words: Autoradiography – Reproduction – Male – Mouse – Hamster – Cadmium – Chromium – Arsenic

Occupational exposure to metals has sometimes been related to impaired reproduction in males, and several metals have been shown to produce degenerative changes in the testis of experimental animals. This report summarizes autoradiographic studies on the distribution in the male reproductive system of cadmium (Cd), chromium (Cr) and arsenic (As). The techniques employed have been whole-body autoradiography (Ullberg 1954), dry mounting microautoradiography (Hammarström et al. 1965) and conventional microautoradiography after fixation of the tissues in formaldehyde (Kopriwa and Leblond 1962). $^{109}CdCl_2$, $^{51}CrCl_3$ (Cr^{3+}), $Na_2{}^{51}Cr_2O_7$ (Cr^{6+}), and ^{74}As-arsenic acid were obtained from the Radiochemical Centre, Amersham, England. ^{74}As-arsenic acid was oxidized or reduced to produce ^{74}As-arsenate (As^{5+}) and ^{74}As-arsenite (As^{3+}), respectively (Vahter and Nordin 1980).

Cd may produce complete testicular necrosis after single doses (Parizek and Záhor 1956), which has been proposed to be due either to a damage to the blood vessels followed by irreversible circulatory collapse, or to a primary effect on the spermatogenetic epithelium (SE). Radioactive Cd was found almost exclusively in the interstitial tissues, where radioactivity appeared to be localized in Leydig cells as well as blood vessels (Fig. 1). This indicates that the effect on the SE is indirect. A direct effect on the capillary system is a likely mechanism for the

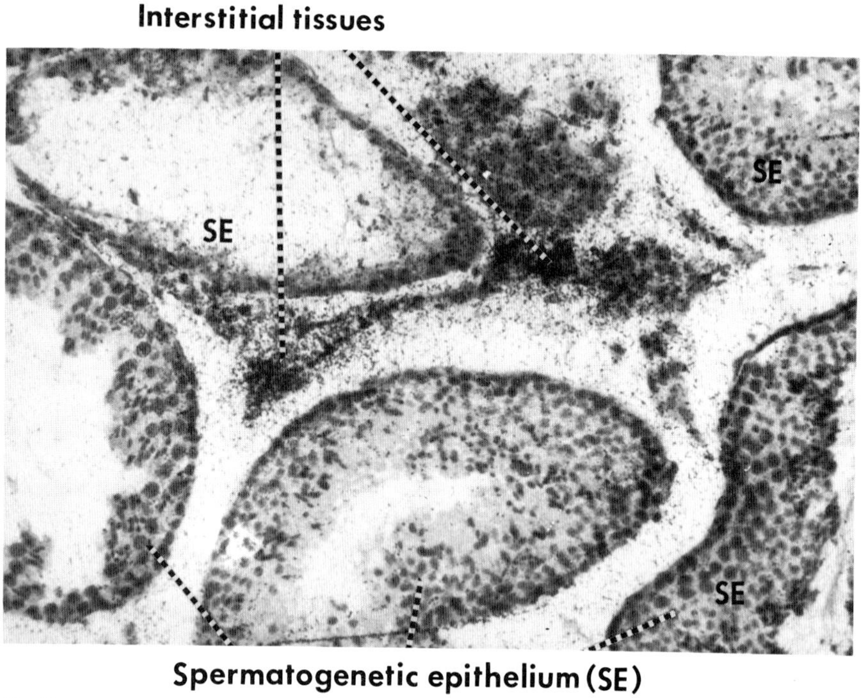
Interstitial tissues
SE
SE
SE
Spermatogenetic epithelium (SE)

Fig. 1

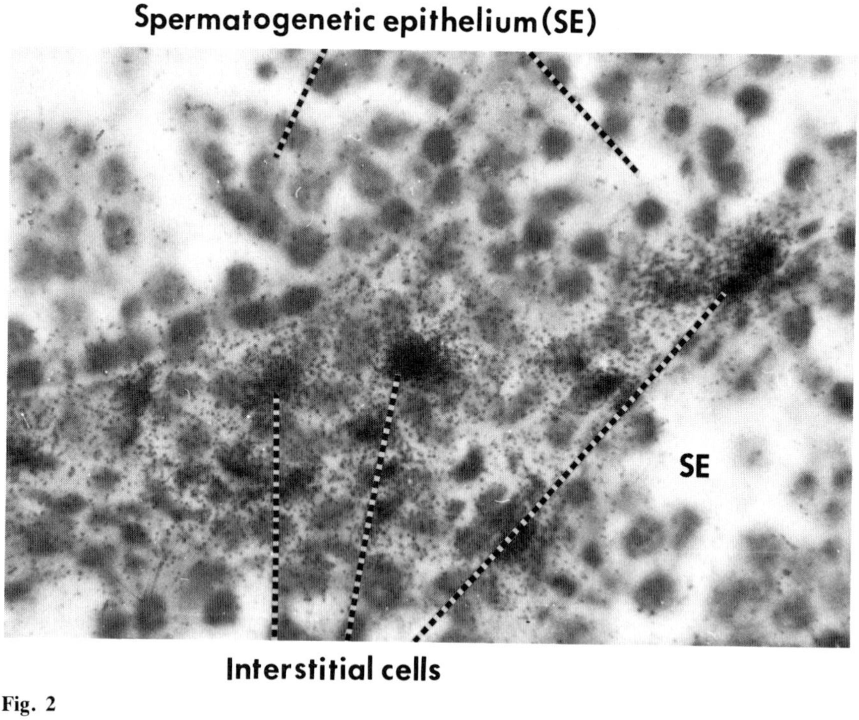
Spermatogenetic epithelium (SE)
SE
Interstitial cells

Fig. 2

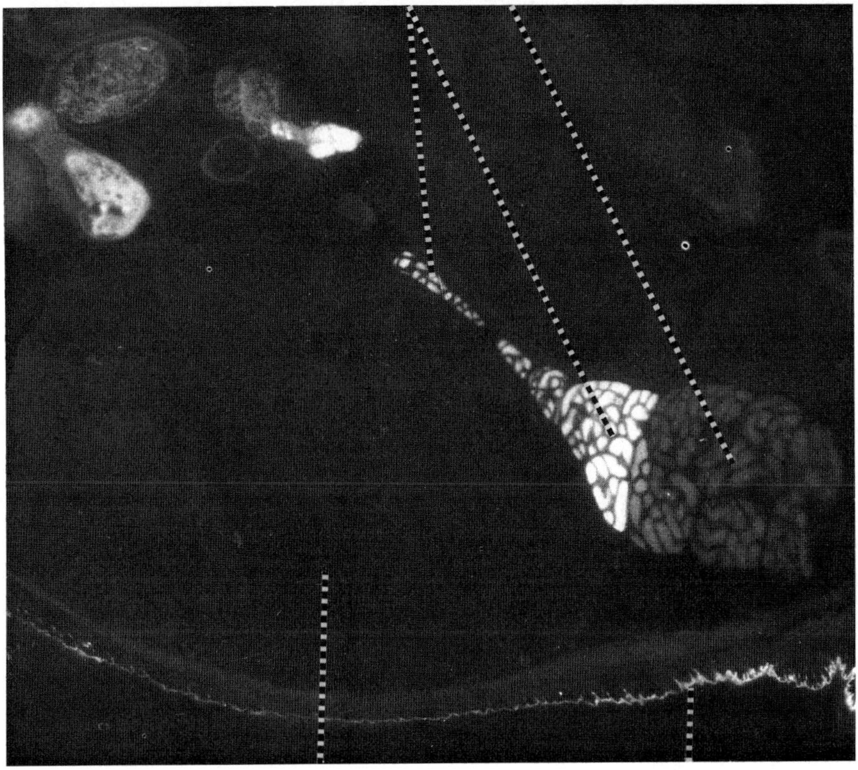

Fig. 3. Detail of whole-body autoradiogram of golden hamster, showing testis and epididymis. It is 24 h after i.v. injection of ^{74}As-arsenate. Note strong luminal accumulation *(white areas)* especially in the corpus epididymidis

acute cadmium toxicity to the testes. Upon chronic exposure, the accumulation of cadmium in the Leydig cells may well result in impaired reproductive function.

Cr has been shown to cause degeneration of the SE and interstitial edema, followed by interruption of the spermatogenesis after repeated doses in rabbits (Behari et al. 1978). These microautoradiographic studies revealed a large uptake of radioactive Cr (especially Cr^{3+}) in the interstitial tissues, probably localized to the Leydig cells (Fig. 2). Blood vessels were nonlabelled and no

---

Fig. 1. Microautoradiogram of freeze-dried testicular tissues (dry-mounted section) of mouse 24 h after i.v. injection of $^{109}CdCl_2$. Note accumulation *(black grains)* in the interstitial tissues

Fig. 2. Microautoradiogram of formalin-fixed testicular tissues from mouse 72 h after i.v. injection of $^{51}CrCl_3$. Note the specific labelling *(black grains)* of scattered cells in the interstitial tissues, probably Leydig cells

radioactivity could be detected in the SE. It is possible, therefore, that the Leydig cells are the primary target for the Cr in the testis.

Arsenic has been suspected to cause reproductive failure in male workers at a smelter in Sweden (Beckman 1978). In rodents, radioactive As was found to be taken up only slightly in the testis, with a similar level in all cells. In the epididymis, on the other hand, a high accumulation was seen in the lumina of the ducts of the epididymis, especially in corpus epididymidis (Fig. 3). This was true for arsenite as well as for arsenate. High activity was subsequently seen in the seminal ducts 1–2 weeks after exposure. This means that the semen will be exposed to As for a long period of time, which indicates a risk of decreasing sperm viability and of impaired reproduction.

Acknowledgement. This work was supported by grants from the Swedish Work Environment Fund.

References

Beckman L (1978) The Rönnskär smelter – occupational and environmental effects in and around a polluting industry in northern Sweden. Ambio 7: 226–231

Behari J, Chandra SV, Tandon SK (1978) Comparative toxicity of trivalent and hexavalent chromium to rabbits. III. Biochemical and histological changes in testicular tissue. Acta Biol Med Ger 37: 463–468

Hammarström L, Appelgren L-E, Ullberg S (1965) Improved method for light microscopy autoradiography with isotopes in a watersoluble form. Exp Cell Res 37: 608–613

Kopriwa MB, Leblond CP (1962) Improvements in the coating technique of radioautoradiography. J Histochem Cytochem 10: 269–284

Parizek J, Záhor (1956) Effect of cadmium salts on testicular tissue. Nature 177: 1036

Ullberg S (1954) Studies on the distribution and fate of 35-S-labelled benzylpenicillin in the body. Acta Radiol [Suppl] (Stockh) 118: 1–110

Vahter M, Nordin H (1980) Metabolism of ^{74}As-labeled trivalent and pentavalent inorganic arsenic in mice. Environ Res 21: 446–457

Metabolism and Toxicity

Disease, Metabolism and Reproduction in the Toxic Response to Drugs and Other Chemicals
Arch. Toxicol., Suppl. 7, 183–192 (1984)

Active Metabolites in Toxicology: The Role of Cytochrome P-448 and Flavoprotein Oxidases

D. V. Parke and C. Ioannides

Department of Biochemistry, University of Surrey, Guildford, Surrey, GU2 5XH, Great Britain

Abstract. The activation of toxic chemicals and carcinogens into reactive intermediates involves oxygenation in hindered positions of the molecule, by cytochrome P-448 (LM_4), flavoprotein oxidoreductases, or transoxygenation during prostaglandin biosynthesis. Cytochrome P-450 (LM_2) does not oxygenate in hindered positions and therefore generally detoxicates carcinogens and toxic chemicals. Cytochrome P-448 has a different active site from cytochrome P-450, which enables it to oxygenate substrates in conformationally-hindered positions.

Key words: Reactive intermediates – Proximate carcinogens – Free radicals – Cytochrome P-450 – Cytochrome P-448 – Oxygenation at hindered positions – Flavoprotein oxidoreductases

Introduction

It is now realised that many toxic and carcinogenic chemicals manifest their toxicity only after undergoing metabolism to highly electrophilic reactive intermediates, which may generate free radicals or become covalently bound to critical intracellular macromolecules, such as enzymes or DNA. Carcinogens, such as the polycyclic aromatic hydrocarbons, and aromatic amines, as well as drugs such as paracetamol have been shown to express their toxicity only after metabolism by the mixed-function oxidases or flavoprotein oxidoreductases (Nelson 1982). The cytochrome P-450-dependent mixed-function oxidases have thus been considered to participate in both the detoxication of chemicals and in their activation into reactive intermediates. It is evident, therefore, that the balance between detoxication and activation is frequently the determining factor in the expression of toxicity, although it is difficult to understand how such opposing consequences may result from the action of the same enzyme or group of enzymes. This balance is determined by genetic factors and by age, and may be altered by nutrition, and the selective induction of cytochrome P-450 isoenzymes following exposure to environmental chemicals. However in general, when the amount of ingested xenobiotic is small and tissue levels are low, pathways of detoxication are the most dominant, and activation of environmental chemicals to reactive intermediates is minimal. Furthermore, these low levels of reactive intermediates are usually effectively deactivated by interaction with protective intracellular nucleophiles, such as glutathione.

Many reactive intermediates are free radicals, formed from xenobiotics such as paracetamol, nitrofurantoin, adriamycin, halothane and paraquat, often by oxidative metabolism catalysed by the cytochrome P-450 system or by flavoprotein oxidoreductases (Nelson 1982; Trush et al. 1982). These free readical intermediates may directly cause tissue damage, interact with tissue oxygen to generate superoxide ($O_2^{\overline{\cdot}}$) and hydroxyl radicals ($OH^{\cdot}$), oxidize cellular molecules, or interact with these to generate secondary radicals in a propagative mechanism resulting in a cascade of autoxidative damage, similar to that which occurs on exposure to ionizing radiation, leading to tissue necrosis, mutations, malignancy and death (Trush et al. 1982; Parke 1983).

Until recently it had been generally considered that the multiple forms of cytochrome P-450 were all equally concerned with both the detoxication and activation of environmental chemicals, and that toxicity and carcinogenicity were principally consequences of the chemical structures of the environmental chemicals concerned. However, the pioneering work of Nebert (1982) showed that certain genetic differences, at least in mice, could result in profound differences in activities of the mixed-function oxidase enzymes and, consequently, in chemical toxicity. Furthermore, studies on the mechanism(s) of action of carcinogenic polycyclic hydrocarbons have shown that oxygenation in certain conformationally-hindered positions (bay-regions) may lead to the formation of epoxides which are not acceptable substrates for subsequent detoxication by epoxide hydrase and other enzymes (Levin et al. 1977); as a result, these bay-region epoxides react more readily with essential intracellular nucleophiles, such as DNA, and have been shown to be ultimate carcinogens. It has further been postulated that this is a general phenomenon, and that the toxicity and carcinogenicity of environmental chemicals is frequently due to their oxygenation in hindered positions, thereby impeding any possible subsequent detoxication (Parke and Ioannides 1982). One difficulty with this hypothesis is that, if the conformationally hindered oxygen is inaccessible to detoxicating enzymes, how is the inital oxygenation effected? Three possible mechanisms have been considered, namely, (i) non-enzymic oxygenation by hydroxyl radicals, including transoxygenation during prostaglandin formation (Anderson et al. 1982) (ii) oxygenation by flavoprotein oxidoreductases not involving binding of the carbon substrate to the enzyme, and (iii) oxygenation by a form of cytochrome P-450 that has an active site which can accommodate the required conformation of the xenobiotic substrate, and is fundamentally different from the active site of most cytochromes P-450.

Cytochrome P-450 has been solubilised, and the various isoenzymes isolated and purified to apparent homogeneity from rat, rabbit, mouse, pig and man pretrated with inducing agents, or from untreated animals. These isozymes differ in their physicochemical properties, immunological characteristics, amino acid sequencing, substrate specificity, and enzyme kinetics (Lu and West 1980). The LM_2 and LM_4 forms of rabbit liver P-450 have been among the most extensively studied; LM_4 (P-448) is induced by carcinogens such as 3-methylcholanthrene, and by β-naphthoflavone and 2,3,7,8-tetrachlorodibenzo-p-dioxin (TCDD) and metabolizes polycyclic aromatic hydrocarbons and other substrates by oxygenation in hindered positions (Levin et al. 1977; Parke and Ioannides 1982); LM_2 (P-450) is induced by phenobarbitone, and metabolizes substrates such as benzphetamine, but not polycyclic aromatic hydrocarbons. Similarly, the P-450 and P-448 forms of rat and mouse liver have been extensively studied in respect of their differences in substrate specificity and the position of oxygenation in the substrate. Among all the forms of the cytochrome isolated from different tissues, and animals species, these two, namely P-450 (LM_2) and P-448 (LM_4) appear to possess the most widely contrasting substrate specificities making them relatively easy to distinguish. Furthermore, whereas P-450 is able to insert oxygen only into unhindered positions of the xenobiotic, P-448 can also oxygenate conformationally-hindered or "bay regions". In addition, P-448, more than P-450, tends to activate carcinogens and other toxic chemicals; P-448 predominates in malignant tissue and its predominance is an early event in malignant transformation (Parke and Ioannides 1982).

The contrasting roles of these forms of the cytochrome in the metabolism of chemicals was first recognised when the pathways of benzo(a)pyrene metabolism were elucidated (Levin et al. 1977). The activation of benzo(a)pyrene to mutagens is catalysed preferentially by P-448 in all animals studied (Ioannides et al., 1981a); and solubilised preparations of P-448 were more efficient than P-450 in forming mutagenic products from this carcinogen and in converting the (±)-trans-benzo(a)pyrene-7,8-dihydrodiol to the 7,8-dihydrodiol-9,10-epoxide, the ultimate carcinogen (Levin et al. 1977). Paracetamol is also preferentially metabolised to its reactive intermediate(s) by P-448, probably through N-hydroxylation (Ioannides et al. 1983; Steele et al. 1983). Other substrates that are preferentially activated by P-448 include other polycyclic hydrocarbons, the aminoazo dyes (Igarashi et al. 1982), 2-acetamidofluorene (Hara et al. 1981), and the protein pyrolysis products Trp-P-1, Trp-P-2, etc. (Nebert et al. 1979) (see Table 1).

The enzymic activities of cytochromes P-450 and P-448 have not been adequately distinguished because of the use of non-specific substrates and the use of suspect methodology, as in the case of aryl hydrocarbon hydroxylase (Yang et al. 1978). The 2-hydroxylation of biphenyl has also been used as an assay reflecting P-448 activity but, although specific, is relatively insensitive. A substrate which exhibits high specificity and adequate sensitivity for the determination of cytochrome P-448 is ethoxyresorufin, and with purified, solubilised preparations from livers of rats it has been demonstrated that the deethylation of this substrate to resorufin is exclusively catalysed by cytochrome P-448 (Burke and Mayer 1975). Moreover, this activity of cytochrome P-448 is selectively inhibited by 9-hydroxyellipticine (Delaforge et al. 1982). As it has been shown that P-448, rather than P-450, catalyses the activation of many toxic chemicals and carcinogens, it seemed pertinent to (i) examine the effects of various enzyme inducing agents, (ii) determine if P-448 is induced only by

Table 1. Selective activation of carcinogens and toxic chemicals by cytochrome P-448

4-Ipomeanol	3-Methylcholanthrene (P-448) increases covalent bound compounds in liver, and shifts toxicity from lung to liver. Phenobarbitone (P-450) increases glucuronide conjugation, decreases overall toxicity	Statham and Boyd (1982)
Benzo(a)pyrene	P-448 but not P-450 oxygenates benzo(a)pyrene-7,8-diol to the 9,10-epoxide ultimate carcinogen	Levin et al. (1977)
2-Acetamidofluorene	Antibodies to P-448, but not P-450, decreased N-hydroxylation (90%) and covalent binding (80%)	Hara et al. (1981)
	LM_4 (P-448) of rabbit liver catalyses N-hydroxylation faster than did the other three isoenzymes (P-450)	Johnson et al. (1980)
N-Dimethylaminoazobenzene	Antibody to P-448, but not P-450, decreased Ames' mutagenicity (90%)	Igarashi et al. (1982)
Trp-P-1	Mutagenicity in Ames' test is proportional to purified P-448 added	Nebert et al. (1979)
Paracetamol	Covalent binding to microsomal proteins catalysed by P-448 but not by P-450	Steele et al. (1983)

carcinogens, and (iii) study these aspects in extrahepatic tissues as well as liver.

Materials and Methods

3-Methylcholanthrene, 2-anthramine, 2-acetamidofluorene, benzo(e)pyrene, benzo(a)pyrene, antipyrine, rifampicin, and all confactors (Sigma, Poole, Dorset, U.K.), resorufin and ethoxyresorufin (Pierce Chemicals, Rockford, Illinois, USA) and DDT (BDH, Poole, Dorset, U.K.) were purchased. Arochlor 1254 and 7,12-dimethylbenzanthracene were generous gifts from Monsanto Chemical Co. (St. Louis, Michigan USA) and IIT Research Institute (Chicago, Illinois, USA).

Male Wistar albino rats (150–200 g) were from the Animal Breeding Unit, University of Surrey. They received the compound dissolved in either saline or corn oil by intraperitoneal injection, and were killed 24 h later. Liver, lung, and kidney microsomes (105,000 *g* pellet resuspended) were prepared (Ioannides and Parke 1975) and O-deethylation of ethoxyresorufin (Burke and Mayer 1975), benzphetamine N-demethylase activity (Lu et al. 1972), cytochrome P-450 (Omura and Sato 1964), and protein (Lowry et al. 1951) were determined.

Results

In untreated adult male rats, ethoxyresorufin O-deethylase activity was detected not only in the liver (75–300 pmol resorufin/min/mg microsomal protein) but

Table 2. The effects of enzyme inducing agents on rat liver mixed-function oxidase activities[a]

Treatment	Benzphetamine N-demethylase (nmol HCHO/min/mg protein)	Ethoxyresorufin O-deethylase (nmol/min/mg protein	Total cytochromes P-450 (nmol/mg protein)
Control	3.4	0.3	0.23
Phenobarbitone	10.1	0.1	0.87
3-Methylcholanthrene	3.3	2.0	0.45
Benzo(a)pyrene	1.9	1.7	0.31
Benzo(e)pyrene	4.6	0.2	0.20
Arochlor 1254	4.7	2.1	0.90

[a] Rats (three per group) were given three single daily i.p. injections of 3-methylcholanthrene (20 mg/kg), phenobarbitone (80 mg/kg), benzo(a)pyrene (50 mg/kg), benzo(e)pyrene (50 mg/kg), or Arochlor 1254 (500 mg/kg) and were killed 24 h after the last injection

Table 3. Induction of cytochrome P-448 activity in rat liver and extrahepatic tissues by carcinogenic and non-carcinogenic chemicals[a]

Chemical	Carcino-genicity	Ethoxyresorufin O-deethylase activity in (% control values)		
		Liver	Kidney	Lung
3-Methylcholanthrene	+	1,100	3,200	–
7,12-Dimethylbenzanthracene	+	560	200	350
2-Anthramine	+	970	880	160
DDT	±	130	175	–
Rifampicin	–	30	80	40
Antipyrine	–	20	20	10

[a] Male Wistar albino rats were given a single i.p. dose of the chemicals (50 mg/kg) and were killed 24 h later. Liver, kidney, and lung microsomal preparations were obtained (Ioannides and Parke 1975) and ethoxyresorufin O-deethylase activity determined by the procedure of Burke and Meyer (1974)

also in the kidney (10–20 pmol/min/mg) and lung (20–40 pmol/min/mg), the liver being by far the most active tissue.

3-Methylcholanthrene was seen to increase ethoxyresorufin O-deethylase activity (P-448) but not benzphetamine N-demethylase activity (P-450). Phenobarbitone, as expected increased P-450 activity and decreased P-448 activity; the high dose of Arochlor 1254 markedly increased both. The carcinogenic benzo(a)pyrene markedly increased P-448 activity but decreased P-450 activity, while the non-carcinogenic benzo(e)pyrene showed the converse effect (Table 2).

The deethylation of ethoxyresorufin was enhanced in microsomal preparation of liver, kidney and lung by the carcinogens, 3-methylcholanthrene, 7,12-dimethylbenzanthracene and 2-anthramine (see Table 3). The extent of stimulation ranging from 100% for 7,12-dimethylbenzo(a)anthracene in kidney and for 2-anthramine in lung, to 10-fold for 3-methylcholanthrene in liver and

30-fold in kidney. When activities are expressed per nmole of haemoprotein, instead of per mg of microsomal protein, the increase in activity is generally higher indicating than the increased enzymic activity is due not only to an increased synthesis of enzymic haemoprotein, but also to the formation of a new form of the cytochrome (P-448) exhibiting high affinity to ethoxyresorufin. DDT, a doubtful carcinogen, and non-genotoxic, gave rise to no significant increase in ethoxyresorufin deethylase activity in liver and kidney. The non-carcinogenic, enzyme-inducing drug, rifampicin, and the drug, antipyrine, resulted in decreases in P-448 activity in all three tissues studied.

Discussion

The marked differences in substrate specificity and the position of hydroxylation, between cytochrome P-450 and P-448 may reflect dissimilar substrate binding sites, which have been studied by difference spectroscopy. Pretreatment with phenobarbital, which increases microsomal P-450, also increased the magnitude of the type I substrate interaction, but pretreatment with benzo(a)pyrene or 3-methylcholanthrene decreased the type I spectral change with substrates such as hexobarbitone, benzphetamine or perhydrofluorene, or even abolished it (Phillipson et al. 1982). In contrast, microsomes from control, phenobarbital- and benzo(a)pyrene-treated animals all exhibited the same type II interaction with substrates such as aniline, indicating that the haem of the newly formed cytochromes did not differ from that of control in their ability to interact at the 6th ligand (Schenkman 1970; Phillipson et al. 1982). These findings constituted the first experimental evidence that P-450 and P-448 possessed binding sites of different substrate specificity.

Initially it was considered that these two forms of the cytochrome do not represent two distinct proteins, but that cytochrome P-448 was formed following the binding of either the inducing agent, e.g., benzo(a)pyrene and 3-methylcholanthrene, or one of their metabolites, to the constitutive cytochrome, thus blocking the substrate site, or causing a conformational change which prevented type I substrate interaction (Jefcoate and Gaylor 1969; Hashimoto and Imai 1976). When hepatic microsomes from 3-methylcholanthrene-pretreated rats were incubated with biphenyl, which displaces ligands from the haem (Ioannides et al. 1981b), there was in increase in the amount of cytochrome determined as the CO-reduced cytochrome complex (Delaforge et al. 1982); no such effect was observed when microsomes from phenobarbital-pretreated rats were employed. These observations indicate that 3-methylcholanthrene, or a metabolite, is attached to the 6th ligand of the haem, preventing its interaction with CO. This ligand-binding of the inducing agent could affect the substrate binding site and be partly responsible for the different substrate specificities exhibited by these two cytochromes. However, cytochrome P-448 is undoubtedly induced by de novo synthesis following treatment of animals with 3-methylcholanthrene and similar substrates. Furthermore, a cytosolic binding protein for 3-methylcholanthrene and similar inducing agents has been identified (Poland et al. 1976) and the intracellular appearance of an inducer-receptor complex has been shown to correlate with induction of cytochrome P-448 mRNA (Tukey et al. 1982).

The successful solubilization and purification to homogeneity of cytochromes P-448 and P-450 has allowed a more precise study of the substrate binding sites of these isoenzymes, and spectral studies of the binding of various substrates has shown that cytochrome P-450 possesses one substrate binding site of broad specificity which can accommodate a diversity of substrates, while P-448 possesses a different binding site exhibiting narrow specificity (Phillipson et al. 1982). The possibility that P-448 may also have a binding site, similar to that of P-450 blocked by the inducer or one of its metabolites cannot be excluded. This is however unlikely, as type I substrates exhibiting high affinity towards P-450 do not displace the blocking material. This difference in binding site between P-450 and P-448 substantiates the findings of Dus (1982) that the cytochromes P-450 exhibit homology especially in the haemopeptide, which is associated with the haem catalytic site and the substrate-binding site, but that this is much less in evidence for cytochrome P-448 (rabbit liver LM_4).

Two other possible mechanisms may account, at least partly, for the substrate specificity of cytochrome P-448. In the first mechanism, the bound oxygen could be activated to form superoxy anion or hydroxyl radicals which then hydroxylate carbon and nitrogen substrates non-enzymically (Cohen and Cederbaum 1979), as has been proposed for the novel cytochrome P-450 induced by ethanol and benzene (Ingelman-Sundberg and Hagbjörk 1982). In the second mechanism, the cytochrome could become decoupled from the flavoprotein reductase, when the latter could function as a hydroxyl radical generator (Lai et al. 1979).

A variety of chemical carcinogens, including Arochlor 1254, and the aromatic amine, 2-anthramine, in addition to the polycyclic hydrocarbons, 3-methylcholanthrene, benzo(a)pyrene, and 7,12-dimethylbenzanthracene were shown to markedly enhance hepatic ethoxyresorufin O-deethylase activity, presumably by induction of P-448; activity was also enhanced in the lung and kidney, but to a much lesser extent. Furthermore, the non-polycyclics, 2-acetamidofluorene, safrole, and N-methyl-N-nitro-nitroguanidine (MNNG) have also been shown to induce P-448 activity (Ioannides et al. 1983). However, the specificity of this assay is best evaluated using known pairs of carcinogen and non-carcinogen analogues, as has been demonstrated with benzo(a)pyrene and benzo(e)pyrene (Table 2).

Cytochrome P-448 has been shown to selectively activate a variety of carcinogens and toxic chemicals into reactive intermediates, mutagens and proximate carcinogens, including the carcinogenic polycyclic hydrocarbons (Ioannides et al. 1981a) the aminoazo dyes (Igarashi et al. 1982), 2-acetamidofluorene (Hara et al. 1981), the protein pyrolysis products, Trp-P-1 and Trp-P-2 (Nebert et al. 1979), as well as the drug, paracetamol (Ioannides et al. 1983; Steele et al. 1983) and the toxic chemical ipomeanol (Statham and Boyd 1982) (Table 1). In many cases, solubilized and purified, reconstituted cytochrome P-448, but not purified P-450, have been shown to selectively oxygenate and activate these chemicals.

As cytochromes P-450 and P-448 have widely different substrate binding sites, and show markedly different substrate specificities, they may be considered as two distinct enzyme proteins rather than as isozymes of the same enzyme. The fact that appearance of one form does not occur at the expense of the other lends support to this hypothesis. Phenobarbitone and 3-methylcholanthrene, administered simultaneously, led to additive induction of the cytochromes (Bidelman and Mannering 1970), and the DBA/2N strain of mice although unable to respond to 3-methylcholanthrene by induction of P-448 does show induction of P-450 in response to treatment with phenobarbital (Nebert et al. 1972; Thorgeirsson et al. 1975), indicating that the two enzymes are under separate regulatory control.

In addition to the oxygenation of xenobiotics by cytochromes P-450 and P-448, flavoprotein oxidoreductases such as the flavin-containing monooxygenase of porcine liver are known to catalyse the N-oxygenation of amines, amides (Frederick et al. 1982) and oxygenation at carbon and sulphur groups in many chemicals. Flavoprotein oxidoreductases may also catalyse the one-electron reduction of tissue oxygen to superoxide, and the reduction of quinones and quinoneimines to semiquinone radicals (Parke 1983). Generation of superoxide occurs during many biochemical reactions including the autoxidation of flavins and ferridoxins, the action of cytochrome P-450 systems, and the flavoprotein-catalysed reduction and coupled cyclic autoxidation associated with chemicals such as adriamycin, paracetamol, and paraquat, or their quinone and quinoneimine metabolites. This autoxidative formation of superoxide leads to cellular damage, mediated by the hydroxyl radical, only where its rate of formation exceeds the rate of metabolic deactivation by the protective enzymes superoxide dismutase, catalase and glutathione peroxidase (Parke 1983; Reiter and Wendel 1983).

References

Andersson B, Nordenskjöld M, Rahimtula A, Moldeus P (1982) Prostaglandin synthetase-catalysed activation of phenacetin metabolites to genotoxic products. Mol Pharmacol 22 : 479–485

Bidelman K, Mannering GJ (1970) Induction of drug metabolism. V. Independent formation of cytochrome P-450 and P_1-450 in rats treated with phenobarbital and 3-methylcholanthrene simulatenously. Mol Pharmacol 6 : 697–701

Burke MD, Mayer RT (1975) Inherent specificities of purified cytochromes P-450 and P-448 towards biphenyl hydroxylation and ethoxyresorufin deethylation. Drug Metab Dispos 3 : 245–253

Cohen G, Cederbaum AI (1979) Chemical evidence of production of hydroxyl radicals during microsomal electron transport. Science 204 : 66–68

Delaforge M, Ioannides C, Parke DV (1982) Selective inhibition of the safrole-induced mixed-function oxidase activities by 9-hydroxyellipticine. Chem Biol Interactions 42 : 279–289

Dus KM (1982) Insights into the active site of the cytochrome P-450 haemoprotein family – a unifying concept based on a structural considerations. Xenobiotica 12 : 745–772

Frederick CB, Mays JB, Ziegler DM, Guengerich FP, Kadlubar FF (1982) Cytochrome P-450 and flavin-containing monooxygenase-catalysed formation of the carcinogen N-hydroxy-2-aminofluorene and its covalent binding to nuclear DNA. Cancer Res 42 : 2671–2677

Hara E, Kawajiri K, Gotoh O, Tagashira Y (1981) Immunochemical study on the contributions of two molecular species of microsomal cytochrome P-450 to the metabolism of 2-acetylaminofluorene by rat liver microsomes. Cancer Res 41 : 253–257

Hashimoto C, Imai Y (1976) Purification of a substrate complex of cytochrome P-450 from liver microsomes of 3-methylcholanthrene-treated rabbits. Biochem Biophys Res Commun 68 : 821–827

Igarashi S, Yonekawa H, Kawajiri K, Watanabe J, Kimura T, Kodama M, Nagata C, Tagashira Y (1982) Participation of the microsomal electron transport system in mutagenic activation of 4-dimethylaminoazobenzene, 4-methylaminoazobenzene, and their 3′-methyl derivatives. Biochem Biophys Res Commun 106: 164–169

Ingelman-Sunberg M, Habjörk AL (1982) On the significance of the cytochrome P-450-dependent hydroxyl radical-mediated oxygenation mechanism. Xenobiotica 11 : 673–686

Ioannides C, Parke DV (1975) Mechanism of induction of hepatic microsomal drug metabolizing enzymes by a series of barbiturates. J Pharm Pharmacol 27: 739–746

Ioannides C, Parkinson C, Parke DV (1981a) Activation of benzo(a)pyrene and 2-acetamidofluorene to mutagens by microsomal preparations from different animal species: Role of cytochrome P-450 and P-448. Xenobiotica 11 : 701–708

Ioannides C, Delaforge M, Parke DV (1981b) Safrole: Its metabolism, carcinogenicity and interactions with cytochrome P-450. Food Cosmet Toxicol 19 : 657–666

Ioannides C, Steele CM, Parke DV (1983) Species variation in the metabolic activation of paracetamol to toxic intermediates: Role of cytochromes P-450 and P-448. Toxicol Lett 16 : 55–61

Jefcoate CR, Gaylor J (1969) Ligand interactions with hemoprotein P-450. II Influence of phenobarbital and methylcholanthrene induction processes on P-450 spectra. Biochemistry 8 : 3464–3472

Johnson EF, Levitt DS, Muller-Eberhard U, Thorgeirsson SS (1980) Catalysis of divergent pathways of 2-acetylaminofluorene metabolism by multiple forms of cytochrome P-450. Cancer Res 40 : 4456–4459

Lai C-S, Grover TA, Piette LH (1979) Hydroxyl radical production in a purified NADPH-cytochrome c (P-450) reductase system. Arch Biochem Biophys 193 : 373–378

Levin W, Wood AW, Lu AYH, Ryan D, West S, Conney AH, Thakker DR, Yagi H, Jerina DM (1977) Role of purified cytochrome P-448 and epoxide hydrase in the activation and detoxication of benzo(a)pyrene. In: Jerina DM (ed) ACS symposium, Drug metabolism concepts. American Chemical Society, Washinton, DC, pp 99–125

Lowry OH, Rosebrough NJ, Farr AL, Randall RJ (1951) Protein measurement with the Folin phenol reagents. J Biol Chem 193 : 265–275

Lu AYH, West SB (1980) Multiplicity of mammalian microsomal cytochromes P-450. Pharmacol Rev 31 : 277–295

Lu AYH, Kuntzman R, West S, Jacobson M, Conney AH (1972) Reconstituted liver microsomal enzyme that hydroxylates drugs, other foreign compounds and endogenous substrates. II Roles of the cytochrome P-450 and P-448 fractions in drug and steroid hydroxylations. J Biol Chem 247 : 1727–1734

Nebert DW, Negishi M (1982) Multiple forms of cytochrome P-450 and the importance of molecular biology and evolution. Biochem Pharmacol 31 : 2311–2317

Nebert DW, Goujon GM, Gielen JE (1972) Aryl hydrocarbon hydroxylase induction by polycyclic hydrocarbons: simple autosomal dominant trait in the mouse. Nature (New Biol) 236 : 107–110

Nebert DW, Bigelow SW, Okey AB, Yahagi T, Mori Y, Nagao M, Sugimura T (1979) Pyrolysis products from amino acids and protein: Highest mutagenicity requires cytochrome P_1-450. Proc Natl Acad Sci USA 76 : 5929–5933

Nelson SD (1982) Metabolic activation and drug toxicity. J Med Chem 25 : 753–765

Omura T, Sato R (1964) The carbon monoxide pigment of liver microsomes. I. Evidence for its haemoprotein nature. J Biol Chem 239 : 2370–2378

Parke DV (1983) Mechanism of chemical toxicity – A unifying hypothesis. Regul Toxicol Pharmacol 2 : 267–286

Parke DV, Ioannides C (1982) Role of mixed-function oxidases in the formation of biological reactive intermediates. Adv Exp Med Biol 136A : 23–38

Phillipson CE, Ioannides C, Delaforge M, Parke DV (1982) Studies on the substrate-binding sites of liver microsomal cytochrome P-448. Biochem J 207: 51–56

Poland AP, Glover E, Kende AS (1976) Stereospecific, high-affinity binding of 2,3,7,8-tetrachlorodibenzo-p-dioxin by hepatic cytosol. Evidence that the binding species is the receptor for the induction of aryl hydrocarbon hydroxylase. J Biol Chem 251: 4936–4946

Reiter R, Wendel A (1982) Chemically-induced glutathione depletion and lipid peroxidation. Chem Biol Interact 40: 365–374

Schenkmann JB (1970) Studies on the nature of the type I and type II spectral changes in liver microsomes. Biochemistry 9: 2081–2091

Statham CN, Boyd MR (1982) Effects of phenobarbital and 3-methylcholanthrene on the in vivo distribution, metabolism and covalent binding of 4-ipomeanol in the rat; implications for target organ toxicity. Biochem Pharmacol 31: 3973–3977

Steele CM, Masson HA, Battershill JM, Gibson GG, Ioannides C (1983) Metabolic activation of paracetamol by highly purified forms of cytochrome P-450. Res Commun Chem Pathol Pharmacol 40: 109–119

Thorgeirsson SS, Felton JS, Nebert DW (1975) Genetic differences in the aromatic hydrocarbon-inducible N-hydroxylation of 2-acetylaminofluorene and acetaminophen-produced hepatotoxicity in mice. Mol Pharmacol 11: 159–165

Trush MA, Mimnaugh EG, Gram TE (1982) Activation of pharmacologic agents to radical intermediates. Implications for the role of free radicals in drug action and toxicity. Biochem Pharmacol 31: 3335–3346

Tukey RH, Hannah RR, Negishi M, Nebert DW, Howard JE (1982) The Ah locus: Correlation of intranuclear appearance of inducer-receptor complex with induction of cytochrome P_1-450 mRNA. Cell 31: 275–2854

Yang CS, Strickhart FS, Kicha LP (1978) Analysis of the aryl hydrocarbon hydroxylase assay. Biochem Pharmacol 27: 2321–2326

Disease, Metabolism and Reproduction in the Toxic Response to Drugs and Other Chemicals
Arch. Toxicol., Suppl. 7, 193 (1984)

The Role of Pharmacokinetics in the Design and Interpretation of Toxicological Studies

J. W. Daniel

Life Science Research Eye, Suffolk, England

Abstract. Despite recent advances in experimental techniques, the use of laboratory animals for assessing the risk to health from exposure to potentially toxic chemicals presents considerable problems. While some of the uncertainty can be attributed to the empirical nature of conventional toxicity tests a major contributory factor is the difference in sensitivity of individual species and even between strains of the same species. Toxicity is a dynamic process the intensity of which is determined by the dose, the rate at which the test material reaches the target-organ and its affinity for specific receptors. The situation is made more complex when the response is mediated by a metabolite rather than by the parent compound. Pharmacokinetic and metabolic data can assist in both the design and the interpretation of toxicological studies and, when supplemented by studies in human volunteers, they provide a more reliable basis for safety evaluation.

Key words: Dose dependent kinetics – Safety evaluation risk assessment

Disease, Metabolism and Reproduction in the Toxic Response to Drugs and Other Chemicals
Arch. Toxicol., Suppl. 7, 194–207 (1984)

Structural Characteristics of Compounds That can be Activated to Chemically Reactive Metabolites: Use for a Prediction of a Carcinogenic Potential

W. K. Lutz

Institute of Toxicology, ETH and University of Zurich, 8603 Schwerzenbach, Switzerland

Abstract. Many mutagens and carcinogens act via covalent interaction of metabolic intermediates with DNA in the target cell. This report groups those structural elements which are often found to form the basis for a metabolism to such chemically reactive metabolites. Compounds which are chemically reactive per se and which do not require metabolic activation form group 1. Group 2 comprises of olefins and aromatic hydrocarbons where the oxidation via an epoxide can be responsible for the generation of reactive species. Aromatic amines, hydrazines, and nitrosamines form group 3 requiring an oxidation of a nitrogen atom or of a carbon atom in alpha position to a nitrosated amine. Group 4 compounds are halogenated hydrocarbons which can either give rise to radicals or can form an olefin (group 2) upon dehydrohalogenation. Group 5 compounds depend upon some preceding enzymatic activity either not available in the target cell or acting on positions in the molecule which are not directly involved in the subsequent formation of electrophilic atoms. Examples for each group are taken from the "List of Chemicals and Industrial Processes Associated with Cancer in Humans" as compiled by the International Agency for the Research on Cancer, and it is shown that 91% of the organic carcinogens would have been detected on the basis of structural elements characteristic for group 1–5. As opposed to this very high sensitivity, the specificity (the true negative fraction) of using this approach as a short-term test for carcinogenicity is shown to be bad because detoxification pathways have so far not been taken into account. These competing processes are so complex, however, that either only very extensive knowledge about pharmacokinetics, stability, and reactivity will be required or that in vivo systems have to be used to predict, on a quantitative basis, the damage expected on the DNA. DNA-binding experiments in vivo are presented with benzene and toluene to

Abbreviations. CBI, Covalent Binding Index = (μmol substance bound per mol DNA nucleotides)/(mmol substance administered per kg body weight); HCH, hexachlorocyclohexane

demonstrate one possible way for an experimental assessment and it is shown that the detoxification reaction at the methyl group available only in toluene gives rise to a reduction by at least a factor of forty for the binding to rat liver DNA. This quantitative approach available with DNA-binding tests in vivo, also allows evaluation as to whether reactive metabolites and their DNA binding are always the most important single activities contributing to the overall carcinogenicity of a chemical. With the example of the liver-tumor inducing hexachlorocyclohexane isomers it is shown that situations will be found where reactive metabolites are formed and DNA binding in vivo is measurable but where this activity cannot be the decisive mode of carcinogenic action. It is concluded that the lack of structural elements known to become potentially reactive does not guarantee the lack of a carcinogenic potential.

Key words: Structure-activity relationship – Reactive intermediates – Metabolic activation – DNA Binding – Covalent binding index – Carcinogens – Benzene – Toluene – Hexachlorocyclohexane – Lindane

It has always been a dream of chemists to predict, on the basis of structure, the activity of chemicals in living systems. One is not aware though of any example where this approach would not have ended at some point with an exception to a rule so carefully established.

In the last decade, a new wave of optimism swept over the biologically interested chemists after the exciting finding that many well-known strong carcinogens belonging to a number of different chemical classes were shown to be metabolized via electrophilic, i.e., chemically reactive intermediates (Miller 1970) and that their covalent binding to DNA seemed to be an important early event in the chemical induction of a tumor (Lutz 1979). No wonder that many chemists tried to find ways to predict the carcinogenicity on the basis of critical structural elements. The most elaborate try came from Cramer et al. (1978) who developed a decision tree system where organic chemicals could be placed into one of three classes I, II, or III, on the basis of 33 questions. These classes were meant to reflect a presumption of low, moderate, or serious toxicity, and the authors claimed that so far the procedure had not resulted in any underestimation of toxicity. The analysis reported by Ashby (1978) and by Oesch (1982) revealed a much more complicated situation as soon as quantitative assessments are attempted.

The following report will try to answer three questions. How sensitive is a short-term test for carcinogenicity based exclusively on critical structural elements? How good is the specificity for this type of test, i.e., how large is the fraction of non-carcinogens lacking a critical structural element? If a reactive metabolite can be formed, is this activity always the most important for its over-all carcinogenic activity?

Question 1: How Sensitive is a Test Based on Critical Structural Elements?

In order to answer the question of sensitivity, there must be some base list of chemicals that have been shown to be carcinogenic. In this case, rather arbitrarily, the "List of Chemicals and Industrial Processes Associated with Cancer in Humans" as compiled by the International Agency for the Research on Cancer (IARC 1980) was chosen. It has to be mentioned that the evidence for carcinogenicity is admittedly inadequate for a number of the 54 compounds listed there, but the list still seemed appropriate for an evaluation of critical structural elements.

A comparison of the chemical structures revealed five groups where a formation of reactive intermediates has to be envisaged. These will be presented in the following sections.

Group 1: Chemically Reactive per se

Figure 1 shows a number of structural elements known to the chemist to be electrophilically reactive. The list comprises of the strained three-membered rings containing oxygen (a, epoxides), nitrogen (b, aziridines), and sulfur (c, epithio derivatives); halogenated alkanes (d and e) where the chloride becomes a favourable leaving group in a nucleophilic attack because of neighbouring effects by nitrogen (d, mustards) or oxygen (e, ethers): some alkylating and

Table 1. Group 1 of IARC 1980 list of carcinogens: chemically reactive per se (13 of 54)

a) Epoxides	27. Epichlorohydrin 28. Ethylene oxide 23. Dieldrin (also group 4)
b) Aziridines	52. Triaziquone 53. Thiotepa
c) Epithio derivatives	* Epithiobutyronitrile
d) 2-Chloroethyl derivatives	12. Chlornaphazine 16. Chlorambucil 21. Cyclophosphamide (also group 5) 37. Melphalan 38. Mustard gas
e) Chloromethyl derivatives	13. Bis(chloromethyl) ether
f) Sulfates, sulfonates	26. Dimethyl sulfate
g) Acid halides	25. Dimethyl carbamoylchloride
h) Aldehydes	* Formaldehyde
i/j) N-Nitroso derivatives	* Methylnitrosourea * Nitrosation products of primary amines

Numbering according to IARC (1980)
* Additional carcinogens

acylating agents (f and g); formaldehyde as most reactive representative of the class of carbonyl compounds and potential crosslinking agent (h); and two derivatives of the important class of N-nitroso derivatives, some of which, like ureas and primary amines are known to undergo spontaneous decay to alkylating agents. A reaction with a primary amine is depicted in Fig. 1, as one possible nucleophile present in protein and nucleie acids.

Although group 1 chemicals do not require metabolic activation to become reactive, this group has been included here and even put first because 13 out of the 54 IARC carcinogens belong to this class (Table 1). About half of these are cytostatic agents where a reactivity towards DNA is a prerequisite for its therapeutic effectiveness. Aldehydes and N-nitroso derivatives have been added because of their wide occurrence.

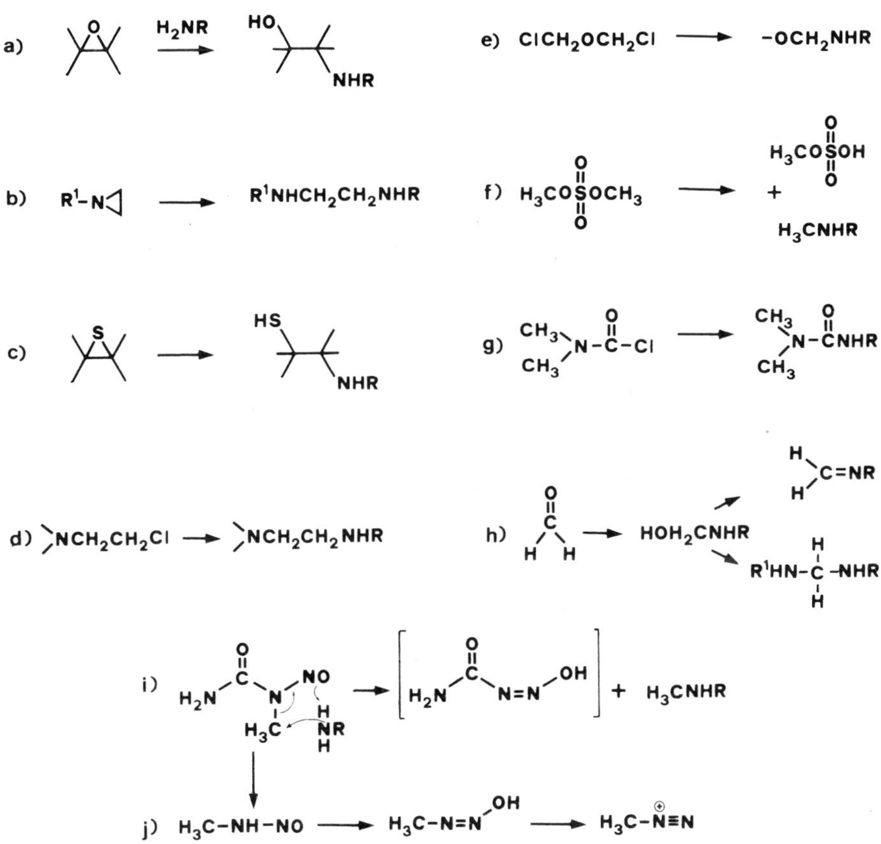

Fig. 1a–j. Structures of chemically reactive carcinogens selected from the IARC (1980) list of carcinogens. A primary amine H_2NR is shown as the nucleophilic reaction partner. **a** Epoxides, **b** aziridines, **c** epithio derivatives, **d** 2-chloroethyl derivatives (mustards), **e** chloromethylderivatives, **f** sulfates, sulfonates, **g** acid halides (dimethyl carbamoylchloride), **h** aldehydes (formaldehyde), **i/j** N-nitroso-derivatives of a urea and of a primary amine; **i**→**j** hydrolysis of the labilized amide bond

Group 2: Substituted Olefins

A large group is formed by those compounds which contain a carbon-carbon double bond (Fig. 2), including aromatic systems such as those found in polynuclear aromatic hydrocarbons. It is interesting to note that all the respective representatives taken from the IARC 1980 list of carcinogens (Table 2) have their double bond conjugated (c, d) or unsymmetrically substituted with electrophilic atoms (a, b). The reactive metabolite derived therefrom is an epoxide formed by the monooxygenase system which is discussed in more detail in subsequent presentations. Among the standard list of 54, 13 compounds would have been perceived as potential carcinogens (Table 2).

Group 3: Oxidation of Nitrogen or of an alpha-Carbon of a Nitrosamine

Aromatic amines have been responsible for the high incidence of bladder cancer in humans exposed to such compounds in the work place. The enzymatic activation involves first a N-hydroxylation which is followed by a conjugation reaction, potentially leading to a good leaving group and the generation of a

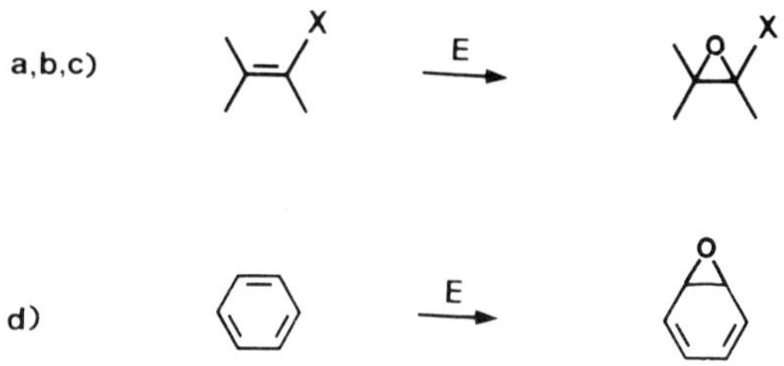

Fig. 2a–d. Part structures of carcinogens which can form an epoxide as reactive metabolite. **a, b, c** Activated olefins, **d** aromatic hydrocarbons; *X* electrophilic substituent

Table 2. Group 2 of IARC 1980 list of carcinogens: substituted olefins (13 of 54)

Substitution	
a) With chloride	18. Chlordane 47. Polychlorinated biphenyls 51. Trichloroethylene 54. Vinyl chloride
b) With oxygen	2. Aflatoxins
c) Unsaturation	1. Acrylonitrile 19. Chloroprene 24. Diethylstilbestrol 50. Styrene
d) In aromatic system	9. Benzene 44. Phenobarbitone 46. Phenytoin 49. Soots and tars

Numbering according to IARC (1980)

nitronium ion (Fig. 3a). Upon delocalization of electrons, the positive charge can move into the aromatic system and the analysis of the reaction products with DNA indeed revealed adducts formed via exocyclic nitrogen and ortho-carbon. The IARC 1980 list of carcinogens contains as much as seven aromatic amines (Table 3). They are probably overrepresented with respect to their importance for the general population but they are so numerous in this list because industrial exposure to a carcinogen is much more easily detectable by an epidemiological analysis.

Alkyl hydrazines are not only experimental carcinogens but are found as drugs and dietary constituents, especially in mushrooms. A postulated enzymatic pathway involving both N- and C-hydroxylations can lead to the generation of alkyl diazohydroxide (Fig. 3b). The same type of proximate carcinogen is formed in the metabolic degradation of nitrosamines derived from secondary amines (Fig. 3c). For this reason these environmentally important carcinogens have been included in group 3 (Table 3).

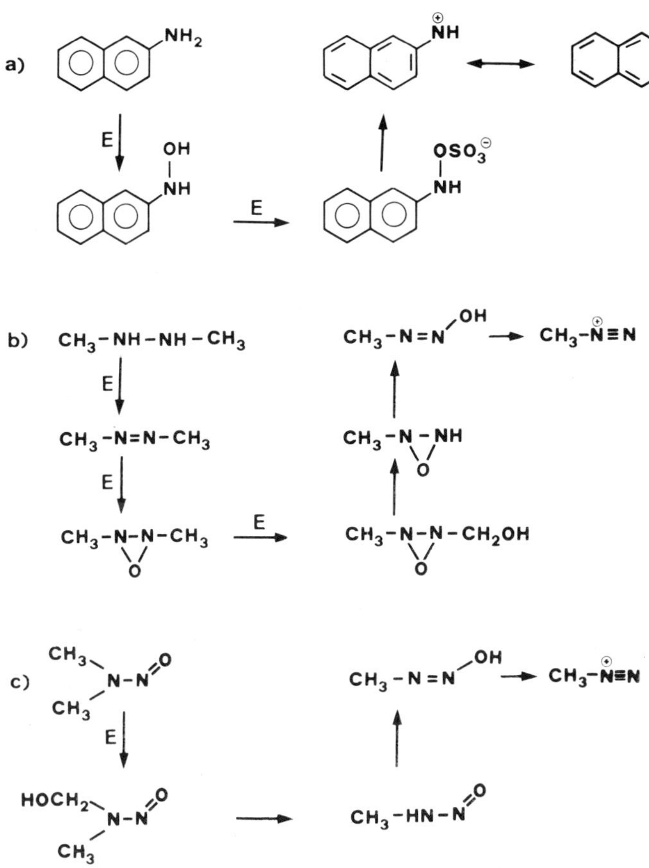

Fig. 3a–c. Metabolic activation of carcinogens via oxidation of nitrogen or of an alpha carbon to a nitrosated amine. **a** Beta-naphthylamine as an aromatic amine, **b** 1,2-dimethylhydrazine; the epoxide stands also for the azoxy resonance structures, **c** dimethylnitrosamine

Table 3. Group 3 of IARC 1980 list of carcinogens: aromatic amines, hydrazines, nitrosamines. Activation by oxidation of nitrogen or alpha-carbon to nitrogen (9 of 54)

a) Aromatic amines	3. 4-Aminobiphenyl 4. Amitrole 7./8. Auramine and its manufacture 10. Benzidine 39. 2-Naphthylamine 43. Phenacetin 45. N-Phenyl-2-naphthylamine
b) Hydrazines	33. Isoniazid
c) Nitrosamines	* Dimethylnitrosamine

Numbering according to IARC (1980)
* Additional carcinogen

Group 4: Halogenated Hydrocarbons

This is a highly complex class of carcinogens. Some can be dehydrohalogenated to an olefin (Fig. 4a; to a group 2 compound), some are known to undergo homolytic cleavage of a halogen-carbon bond and thus give rise to radicals able to react with critical target molecules or to lead to the generation of even more dangerous radicals (Fig. 4b). In addition to this potential formation of reactive intermediates, most of the halogenated hydrocarbons are well-known inducers of drug-metabolizing enzymes so that they have often been attributed, without experimental backup though, some type of co-carcinogenic activity. To make the situation even more complex, a number of these compounds have been shown to stimulate cell division and to act as tumor promoters in two-stage carcinogenicity tests (see Schulte-Hermann 1981). Some carcinogens of this class may therefore act on a variety of levels and it will be most challenging to determine the relative importance of the particular activities. However, one should not forget that the overall carcinogenic potency is low for this class of compounds and that many aspects may turn out to be species specific. It is therefore not surprising to see that the evidence for carcinogenicity in humans of the four members of this class, listed among the 54 (Table 4), has been termed inadequate by IARC (1980).

a)

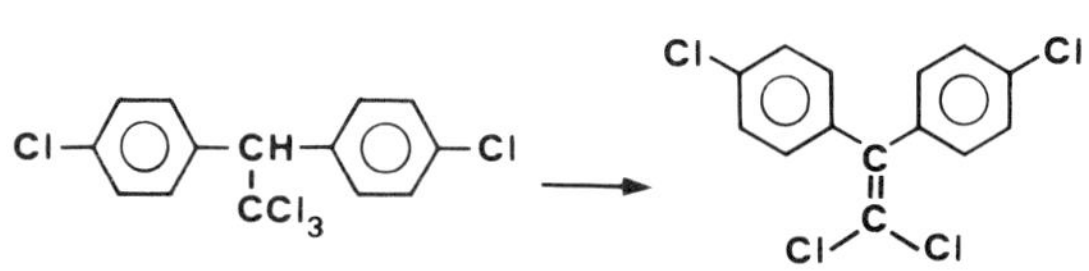

(2)

b) $CCl_4 \longrightarrow {}^{\bullet}CCl_3 + {}^{\bullet}Cl$

Fig. 4a, b. Possible steps in the metabolic activation of halogenated hydrocarbons. **a** DDT dehydrohalogenated to an olefin, **b** homolytic cleavage of carbon tetrachloride to radicals

Table 4. Group 4 of IARC 1980 list of carcinogens: aliphatic halogenated compounds (4 of 54)

a) Dehydrohalogenation to olefin (group 2)	22. DDT 31. Hexachlorocyclohexane
b) Homolytic cleavage of C-Cl bond to radical	15. Carbon tetrachloride 23. Dieldrin (also group 1)

Numbering according to IARC (1980)

Group 5: Preceding Reactions Required

This group of compounds requires some enzymatic modification of the molecule which is either not normally performed in the mammalian cell (nitro reduction or beta-glucosidase activity) or which does not center around the atom to become reactive (phosphoramide cleavage of a non-reactive mustard to liberate a reactive mustard or aromatization of a pyrrolizidine alkaloid to generate "benzylic" $-CH^+-$ and CH_2^+). These reactions are depicted in Fig. 5 (a and c, b and d, respectively). Only two such examples have been found in the IARC 1980 list of carcinogens (Table 5, a and b) and two have been added for the sake of

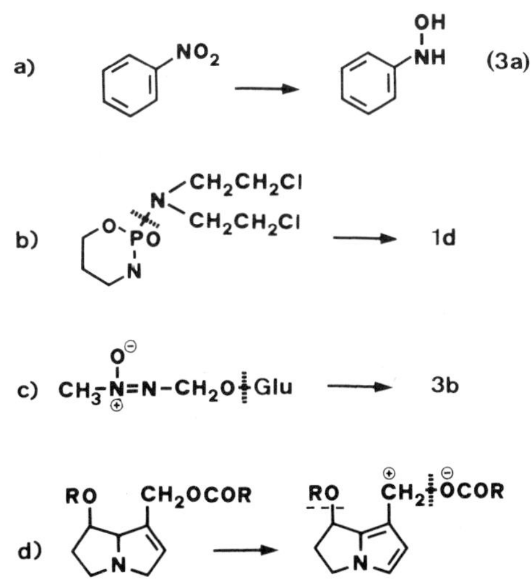

Fig. 5a–d. Selection of carcinogens known to require a preceding reaction not normally performed in the target cell (**a,** nitroreductase; **c,** beta-glucosidase) or not at the atom to become electrophilic (**b,** phosphoramide cleavage of cyclophosphamide to release a reactive mustard; **d,** aromatization of pyrrolizidine alkaloid to generate benzyl analogues)

Table 5. Group 5 of IARC 1980 list of carcinogens: preceding reactions required (2 of 54)

a) Nitroreduction	17. Chloramphenicol (to aromatic amine)
b) Phosphoramide cleavage	21. Cyclophosphamide (to reactive mustard)
c) Glucoside cleavage	* Cycasin (to group 1)
d) Aromatization	* Pyrrolizidine alkaloids

Numbering according to IARC (1980)
* Additional carcinogens

completeness. Nitroreductase and beta-glucosidase both are activities present in microorganisms, and it cannot, therefore, be surprising that the genotoxicity of dinitrotoluene is no longer observed in germ-free animals (Mirsalis et al. 1982). It is also conceivable that the diet can have an indirect influence on the carcinogenicity of this type of compound by changing the number and composition of the gut microflora.

Answer to Question 1: Sensitivity for Organic Compound is Very High

Table 6 shows that it would be possible to identify as much as 72% of the 54 carcinogens of the IARC list and even 91% if only organic chemicals are considered. This sensitivity is even slightly better than with the Ames test if applied to this selection of carcinogens, because of the well-documented problems of the Ames test with halogenated compounds and hydrazines (Rinkus and Legator 1979).

Table 6. Carcinogens of IARC 1980 list which could have been detected on the basis of structural elements

Group 1: Chemically reactive	13
Group 2: Substituted olefins	13
Group 3: Aromatic amines/hydrazines	9
Group 4: Aliphatic halogenated compounds	3 new
Group 5: Nitroaromatics and miscellaneous	1 new
Total	39 of 54 (72%)
If only organic carcinogens are taken	39 of 43 (91%)

The compounds of the IARC 1980 list which would not have been detected on the basis of structural elements as presented in groups 1–5 are primarily inorganic and include derivatives of arsenic (no. 5 of the IARC list), beryllium (11), cadmium (14), chromium (20), lead (36), nickel (40 and nickel refining, 41), as well as asbestos (6) and hematite (29 and its mining, 30). One possible mechanism of carcinogenic action might involve an interaction with the DNA polymerase system and a resulting decrease of template fidelity but such activity is obviously not amenable to an analysis of electrophilicity. Only four organic chemical are missed, i.e., iron dextran (32), isopropyl oils and their manufacture (34 and 35), oxmetholone (42) and reserpine (48). The latter two are known to interfere with the endocrine system. They could therefore be carinogenic along the line of hormones and are detectable in chronic toxicity studies by their respective activities.

Question 2: How Good is the Specificity?

The question of specificity deals with the problem of how many from a selection of non-carcinogens do not have structural elements placing them into one of

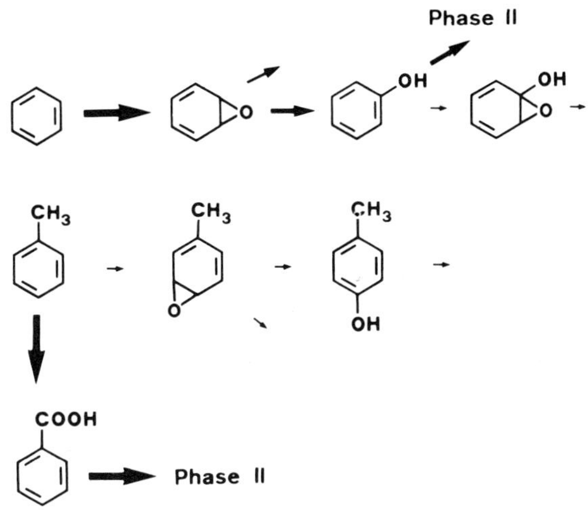

Fig. 6. Schematic metabolism of benzene, phenol, and toluene

groups 1–5. A simple example shown in Fig. 6 illustrates the main problem. Benzene, toluene, and phenol would all have to be termed potential carcinogens, if the rules set out above are adopted and they are placed in group 2. Only benzene is a detectable systemic carcinogen (Dean 1978). This is mainly because the metabolism of the other two compounds goes primarily via true detoxication reactions, such as the oxidation of the side chain of toluene and conjugation reactions with phenol. The oxidation in the ring does occur with both but represents only a minor pathway.

One could think of introducing this type of knowledge into the evaluation and to state that alkylated or phenolic aromatic hydrocarbons are less dangerous than their parent compounds. This approach would not be of much quantitative value because of two main points.

Firstly, in some instances, such as with benz(a)anthracene derivatives, many methylated analogues are much more potent carcinogens (Oesch 1982), or, the conjugation reaction can even be a prerequisite for the formation of the ultimate reactive carcinogen, such as with the aromatic amines or with 1,2-dibromoethane, where the reaction with glutathione leads to a reactive brominated sulfur mustard.

Secondly, on a quantitative basis, all the modulations are not taken into account which ultimately determine the concentration of reactive metabolite at the target and the reactivity with DNA. The competing activation and inactivation processes are highly complex and controlled on many possible levels some of which are discussed in later presentations.

It therefore seems that only in vivo studies can possibly give a quantitative answer on the level of DNA damage exerted by reactive metabolites. The difference between benzene and toluene for instance becomes very clear when a DNA-binding assay is performed in rats. The binding to liver DNA was found to be at least 40 times higher for benzene (Lutz and Schlatter 1977) if compared with toluene (Table 7).

Table 7. Covalent binding of [^{14}C]benzene and [p-^{3}H]toluene to rat liver DNA after exposure in a closed inhalation system

Compound	Benzene		Toluene
Dose			
(mg/kg)	62	63	64
(10^9 dpm/kg)	6.5	6.6	182
Period of exposure (h)	9	11.5	5
Formation of tritiated water (% of dose)	–	–	0.6
Liver DNA			
In vial (mg)	2.3	2.2	2.5
Spec. act. (dpm/mg)	42	37	25
(CBI units)[a]	1.7	1.5	<0.04

[a] Specific activity of DNA normalized by the dose administered and converted to molar units as defined in the list of abbreviations

Answer to Question 2: Bad Specificity

Therefore, it must be concluded that a large number of false positive answers will be generated if structure-activity considerations are used as a short-term test for carcinogenicity. Only in vivo experiments would accurately take account into the inactivation reactions which can be responsible for drastic reductions in the concentration of reactive metabolites at the target molecule. The specificity will therefore be bad, worse than with the Ames test where some inactivation processes, albeit distorted, are still taken into account. Because of the ready availability of the Ames test as a highly sensitive screening test for the production of metabolites damaging bacterial DNA, it would not seem that a sophisticated decision tree as set forth by Cramer et al. (1978) would be an alternative.

Question 3: What is the Role of Reactive Metabolites in Over-all Carcinogenicity?

Table 8 gives an outline of the possible modes of action of chemical carcinogens, divided into mutagenic and non-mutagenic events, each group being subdivided into possible specific activities. A compound exhibiting any one single activity could be found to increase the tumor incidence in a long-term bioassay on carcinogenicity if it is accepted that mutational events are to some extent unavoidable (Lutz 1982), and that the respective mutations can also form the basis for spontaneous tumor formation.

The reactive metabolites, discussed here, seem to act primarily by DNA binding. In addition, and as mentioned for the group of the halogenated hydrocarbons, there is the possibility of radical-induced damage also in other classes of compounds which might act via oxygen radical formation. Other papers in this volume will deal more thouroughly with this aspect. Besides these

Table 8. List of possible modes of action of chemical carcinogens

Mutagenicity	Non-mutagenicity (modulation of mutational events)
Derived from – DNA binding of test compound – Indirect DNA damage e.g., via oxygen radicals Other mutagenic mechanisms	At the level of – *Pre*-mutagenicity more DNA binding, more oxygen radicals – *Co*-mutagenicity more rapid fixation of DNA damage (stimulation of cell division) – *Post*-mutagenicity better expression of critical mutation towards tumor growth (= promotion?)

two modes of obvious genotoxicity, a number of additional mechanisms on the chromatid and chromosome levels will lead to mutations in a broadest sense.

On the non-mutational side, modulations have to be dealt with on many levels. Enzyme induction is often referred to as a possible co-carcinogenic mechanism of action although all reports seem to show the opposite: a pretreatment of animals with enzyme inducers of any kind, so far, has always led to a reduction in the incidence of tumors induced by a subsequent dose of a DNA-binding carcinogen (Wattenberg 1978).

The step between DNA damage and mutation is dependent on the repair of the critical DNA damage, the mutagenicity of the various adducts, and on the rate of DNA synthesis, i.e., of the rate of cell division. Any influence which increases the cell division rate reduces the time available for repair and increases the probability for a fixation of the damage in the form of mutation. Hormones might therefore be found to be carcinogenic in an animal bioassay on the basis of their stimulatory effect on target cell division.

Some compounds listed among the 54 IARC carcinogens are known to lead to liver growth in rodents, such as hexachlorocyclohexane (HCH) or phenobarbital. Both have also been mentioned before because of their critical structural elements. It is therefore possible that these compounds act by more than one mode. The third question raised here will deal with the quantitative importance of a single activity like DNA binding.

HCH includes a group of isomers of which the gamma-isomer, called lindane, has useful pesticidal activities. The alpha-isomer is a moderately strong hepatocarcinogen, much stronger than the gamma-isomer for which the evidence for carcinogenicity is inconclusive. The tumor induction in mice is strongly dependent on the strain used. Both isomers could give rise to reactive metabolites via dehydrohalogenation to an olefin and epoxidation. A DNA binding assay in mouse liver was performed with oral administration of tritiated HCH and isolation of the DNA after 10 h (Sagelsdorff et al. 1983). The results support the view that DNA-binding cannot be the decisive mode of tumorigenic activity in that Covalent Binding Indices, CBI (see list of abbreviations for definition), of ⩽ 0.26 and ⩽ 0.18 were determined for the gamma- and the alpha-isomer, respectively. The alpha-isomer therefore did not give rise to a higher CBI although it is the much more potent carcinogen. Furthermore, it was shown that the CBI of gamma-HCH for mouse liver DNA was ⩽ 0.28, ⩽ 0.26, and ⩽ 0.17 in the NMRI, CF1, and B6C3F1 strain, i.e., similar DNA binding was found in all strains of mice tested although the CF1 mice are more susceptible than the others. In addition, the absolute level of DNA binding determined for the alpha-isomer is by a factor of about three orders of magnitude lower than with typical DNA-binding carcinogens of similar carcinogenic potency (Lutz 1982).

HCH isomers therefore seem not to belong to that population of carcinogens where DNA binding is the most important mode of action although DNA binding is possible from structure-activity considerations and measurable in vivo.

In conclusion, the carcinogenicity of a chemical must be considered to be the result of the sum of a variety of single contributing factors. The example given above with hexachlorocyclohexane is only one of a probably large number of cases where the reactive metabolites and the respective DNA binding cannot be the main mode of carcinogenic activity. Conversely, this means that the lack of structural elements known to become potentially reactive dose not guarantee the lack of a carcinogenic potential and it will be important to establish biological activities common to representatives of the non-reactive carcinogens.

Answer to Question 3: Reactive Metabolites and Their DNA-Binding are not Always Decisive for a Carcinogenic Activity of a Chemical

References

Ashby J (1978) Structural analysis as a means of predicting carcinogenic potential. Br J Cancer 37 : 904–923

Cramer GM, Ford RA, Hall RL (1978) Estimation of toxic hazard – a decision tree approach. Food Cosmet Toxicol 16 : 255–276

Dean BJ (1978) Genetic toxicology of benzene, toluene, xylenes and phenols. Mutat Res 47 : 75–97

IARC Working Group (1980) An evaluation of chemicals and industrial processes associated with cancer in humans based on human and animal data: IARC monographs volumes 1 to 20. Cancer Res 40 : 1–12

Lutz WK (1979) In vivo covalent binding of organic chemicals to DNA as a quantitative indicator in the process of chemical carcinogenesis. Mutat Res 65 : 289–356

Lutz WK (1982) Constitutive and carcinogen-derived DNA binding as a basis for the assessment of potency of chemical carcinogens. Adv Exp Med Biol 136B : 1349–1365

Lutz WK, Schlatter C (1977) Mechanism of the carcinogenic action of benzene: Irreversible binding to rat liver DNA. Chem Biol Interact 18 : 241–245

Miller JA (1970) Carcinogenesis by chemicals: an overview – G. H. A. Clowes memorial lecture. Cancer Res 30 : 559–576

Mirsalis JC, Hamm Jr TE, Sherill JM, Butterworth BE (1982) Role of gut flora in the genotoxicity of dinitrotoluene. Nature 295 : 322–323

Oesch F (1982) Problems associated with the use of chemical class controls in absence of information on the underlying mechanism. In: Nicolini C (ed) Chemical carcinogenesis. Plenum, New York, p 67

Rinkus SJ, Legator MS (1979) Chemical characterization of 465 known or suspected carcinogens and their correlation with mutagenic activity in the Salmonella typhimurium system. Cancer Res 39: 3289–3318

Sageldorff P, Lutz WK, Schlatter C (1983) The relevance of covalent binding to mouse liver DNA to the carcinogenic action of hexachlorocyclohexane isomers. Carcinogenesis 4: 1267–1273

Schulte-Hermann R, Ohde G, Schuppler J, Timmermann-Trosiener I (1981) Enhanced proliferation of putative preneoplastic cells in rat liver following treatment with the tumor promoters phenobarbital, hexachlorocyclohexane, steroid compounds, and nafenopin. Cancer Res 41: 2556–2562

Wattenberg LW (1978) Inhibitors of chemical carcinogenesis. Adv Cancer Res 26: 197–226

Disease, Metabolism and Reproduction in the Toxic Response to Drugs and Other Chemicals
Arch. Toxicol., Suppl. 7, 208–218 (1984)

Covalent Binding to Proteins as a Mechanism of Chemical Toxicity

C. Pantarotto and C. Blonda

Istituto di Ricerche Farmacologiche "Mario Negri", Via Eritrea 62, 20157 Milano, Italy

Abstract. The capacity of chemicals to interact covalently with cellular macromolecules in in vitro systems was exploited to elucidate the structure of secondary metabolites, namely arene oxide derivatives, in the biotransformation of styrene. Covalent binding to proteins was also determined to check the presence and activity of enzymatic systems in subcellular compartments other than microsomes, e.g., nuclei. In experiments with cyclophosphamide as substrate it was shown that nuclear enzymatic activities might well be responsible for drug covalent binding to DNA.

Key words: Proteins – Covalent binding – Metabolism – Nuclei – Styrene – Cyclophosphamide

The capacity of chemicals to interact covalently with cellular macromolecules, either directly or through metabolic activation, has been studied in vitro and in vivo with different classes of compounds. Most of these studies were aimed at relating a chemical's carcinogenic potential with its alkylating capacity. However, it was found that the correlations were only good when in vivo DNA binding was determined. Binding to proteins was in fact never correlated with carcinogenicity (Lutz 1979; Gillette 1974; Tyndall 1979). Nevertheless, protein binding studies do show when a chemically reactive species is produced and, apart from this being a warning sign, these studies could prove useful tools for the structural elucidation of these species.

This paper reports some recent findings obtained in this laboratory on these aspects which illustrate the importance of also studying irreversible interactions with such cellular macromolecules.

Analytical Aspects

Because of the small amount of test compound found irreversibly bound, ^{14}C-labelled substrates were used in protein covalent binding studies. These studies are based on exhaustive extractions of the cell constituents (microsomal fraction, nuclei, total macromolecules, etc.) with different solvents or solvent mixtures, after their isolation and purification from tissues by a number of different procedures.

However, it is not the aim of this paper to go into these details and therefore readers are referred to other articles which explain these technical aspects (Ghezzi et al. 1981; Szczawinska et al. 1981). The amount of chemical or its metabolites or both irreversibly bound to cellular macromolecules is then determined by liquid scintillation counting.

Characterization of Minor Labile Metabolites

The capacity of exogenous compounds to bind covalently to proteins offer a good opportunity for structurally characterizing the chemical species involved in these interaction even if they are only present at the p-mole level and therefore represent a secondary metabolism. As an example some studies carried out in this laboratory on the biochemical mechanisms underlying styrene txocity will be reported (Pantarotto et al. 1980).

Figure 1 shows the known metabolism of this compound. The main pathway of biotransformation is styrene oxidation to phenylethylene glycol (through the intermediacy of the chemically reactive species styrene 7,8-oxide), mandelic acid, phenylglyoxylic acid, benzoic acid and hippuric acid (Leibman 1975; Pantarotto et al. 1978). The presence of an aromatic moiety in the styrene molecule suggests that metabolic intermediates of the arene oxide type could also be formed during a possible ring hydroxylation process (see Fig. 2). To investigate this, irreversible binding studies using ^{14}C-styrene as substrate were

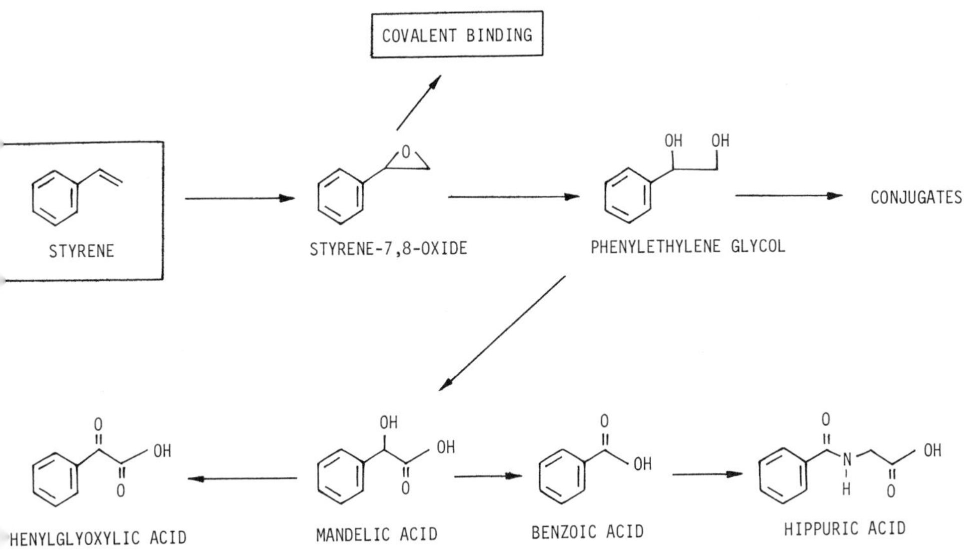

Fig. 1. Metabolism of styrene

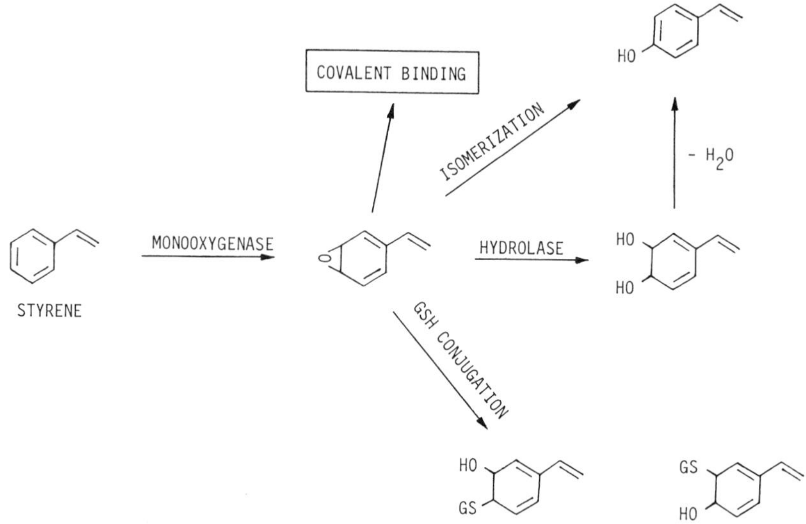

Fig. 2. Styrene metabolism through the intermediacy of arene oxides

performed in in vitro conditions, utilizing rat liver microsomal preparations as both the activating system and target.

Tables 1 and 2 summarize the results of these experiments. Styrene was found to bind irreversibly to proteins of the endoplasmic reticulum; however, binding was observed only when the drug was incubated in the presence of NADPH and O_2, this process being catalyzed by a cytochrome P-450 monooxygenase. In fact, CO and proadifen (SKF-525A), two specific inhibitors of microsomal mixed function oxidases, reduced ^{14}C-styrene covalent binding to microsomes whereas pretreatment of the animals with phenobarbital (PB) significantly enhanced it. Furthermore, the chemical species involved in this interaction is an electrophilic compound; it reacts with glutathione (GSH) and structurally is an epoxide since an increase in the extent of covalent binding was observed when incubations were carried out in the presence of non-competitive inhibitors of epoxide hydrolase such as trichloropropene oxide (TCPO) and cyclohexene oxide (CyO) (Oesch 1974). However these studies with styrene alone as substrate are difficult to interpret in establishing the relative roles of the 7,8-oxide and of any arene oxide intermediates in determining covalent binding.

An indirect demonstration of the intermediacy and chemical reactivity of arene oxide metabolites in styrene biotransformation was obtained in comparative experiments with ^{14}C-phenylethylene glycol which was tested under conditions similar to those described for styrene. The use of labelled phenylethylene glycol made it possible to distinguish between covalent binding resulting from epoxidation at the 7,8-double bond position and any binding due to oxidation of the aromatic ring. Tables 3 and 4 give the results of these experiments. Phenylethylene glycol also irreversibly binds to microsomal proteins following enzymatic activation. An epoxide intermediate may be

Table 1. Irreversible protein binding of ^{14}C-styrene (0.5 mM) catalyzed by rat liver microsomes in the presence of an NADPH generating system after 120 min of incubation. Effect of inducers of drug metabolizing enzymes

Animal pretreatment	Sample	Styrene metabolites irreversibly bound to 1 mg of microsomal protein (nmol ± SE)
Saline or corn oil	Boiled M + NADPH	0.46 ± 0.06
Saline or corn oil	M − NADPH	0.23 ± 0.04
Saline or corn oil	M + NADPH	2.56 ± 0.39[a]
PB (80 mg/kg i.p. × 3 days in saline)	M + NADPH	4.12 ± 0.16[b]
3-MC (40 mg/kg i.p. × 3 days in corn oil)	M + NADPH	2.60 ± 0.21[a]

Each figure is the mean ± SE of four determinations
M = microsomes; PB = phenobarbital; 3-MC = 3-methylcholanthrene
[a] $p < 0.01$. Compared with boiled control M + NADPH and control M − NADPH
[b] $p < 0.01$. Increased when compared with control M + NADPH and 3-MC M + NADPH

Table 2. Irreversible protein binding of ^{14}C-styrene (0.5 mM) catalyzed by liver microsomes from saline treated rats in the presence of an NADPH generating system after 120 min of incubation. Effect of inhibitors of drug metabolizing enzymes

Sample	Styrene metabolites irreversibly bound to 1 mg of microsomal protein (nmol ± SE)
M + NADPH	2.56 ± 0.39
M + NADPH + CO (95%)	0.68 ± 0.13[a]
M + NADPH + SKF-525A (1 mM)	0.92 ± 0.05[a]
M + NADPH + GSH (1 mM)	1.18 ± 0.01[a]
M + NADPH + TCPO (1 mM)	4.01 ± 0.11[b]
M + NADPH + CyO (1 mM)	3.63 ± 0.27[b]

Each figure is the mean ± SE of four determinations
M = microsomes; CO = carbon monooxide; SKF-525A – 2-dicthylaminocthyl-2,2 diphenylval erate; GSH = glutathione; TCPO = 1,1,1-trichloropropene oxide; CyO = cyclohexene oxide
[a] $p < 0.01$. Reduced when compared to M + NADPH; [b] $p < 0.01$. Increased when compared to M + NADPH

Table 3. Irreversible protein binding of ^{14}C-phenylethylene glycol (0.5 mM) catalyzed by rat liver microsomes in the presence of an NADPH generating system after 120 min of incubation. Effect of inducers of drug metabolizing enzymes

Animal pretreatment	Sample	Phenylethylene glycol metabolites irreversibly bound to 1 mg of microsomal protein (nmol ± SE)
Saline or corn oil	Boiled M + NADPH	0.026 ± 0.003
Saline or corn oil	M − NADPH	0.024 ± 0.001
Saline or Corn oil	M + NADPH	0.066 ± 0.003[a]
PB (80 mg/kg i.p. × 3 days in saline)	M + NADPH	0.077 ± 0.004[a]
3-MC (40 mg/kg i.p. × 3 days in corn oil)	M + NADPH	0.107 ± 0.008[b]

Each figure is the mean ± SE of four determinations
M = microsomes; PB = phenobarbital; 3-MC = 3-methylcholanthrene
[a] $p < 0.01$. Compared with boiled control M + NADPH and control M − NADPH
[b] $p < 0.01$. Increased when compared with control M + NADPH and PB M + NADPH

Table 4. Irreversible protein binding of ^{14}C-phenylethylene glycol (0.5 mM) catalyzed by liver microsomes from saline treated rats in the presence of an NADPH generating system after 120 min of incubation. Effect of inhibitors of drug metabolizing enzymes

Sample	Phenylethylene glycol metabolites irreversibly bound to 1 mg of microsomal protein (nmol ± SE)
M + NADPH	0.066 ± 0.003
M + NADPH + CO (95%)	0.030 ± 0.002[a]
M + NADPH + SKF-525A (1 mM)	0.032 ± 0.005[a]
M + NADPH + GSH (1 mM)	0.037 ± 0.002[a]
M + NADPH + TCPO (1 mM)	0.104 ± 0.006[b]
M + NADPH + CyO (1 mM)	0.091 ± 0.001[b]

Each figure is the mean ± SE of four determinations
M = microsomes; CO = carbon monooxide; SKF-525A = 2-diethylaminoethyl-2,2-diphenylvalerate; GSH = glutathione; TCPO = 1,1,1-trichloropropene oxide; CyO = cyclohexene oxide
[a] $p < 0.01$. Reduced when compared to M + NADPH
[b] $p < 0.01$. Increased when compared to M + NADPH

implicated in this interaction because binding was enhanced when incubation was carried out in the presence of the epoxide hydrolase inhibitors. However, contrarily to what was seen for styrene, the enzymatic process which activates phenylethylene glycol appears to be a cytochrome P-448 monooxygenase because an inductive effect has been demonstrated with microsomal preparations from 3-methylcholanthrene (3-MC) but not PB pretreated rats.

Thus, by combining radiochemical and enzymatic approaches considerable information has been obtained on the chemical structure of the reactive species involved in in vitro styrene covalent binding, i.e., styrene 7,8-oxide and possibly the arene oxide derivative. The formation of an arene oxide, styrene 3,4-oxide, represents a secondary metabolic pathway in the in vitro biotransformation of this monomer because it occurs at the p-mole level.

It is evident that traditional mass spectrometry cannot be applied for the characterization of a labile metabolite present at such very low concentrations. However having already postulated the structure of this reactive species on the basis of covalent binding studies, parallel mass fragmentographic evaluations of 4-vinylphenol, a styrene 3,4-oxide chemical rearrangement product, can now be made. This provides a basis for direct correlation between covalent binding to microsomes and concentrations of styrene phenolic metabolites in the incubation media, thus better supporting the intermediacy of a reactive arene oxide in styrene biotransformation.

The presence of 4-vinylphenol in the microsomal incubation mixture was shown up by mass fragmentography, this metabolite being present only at the level of a few nanograms (see Fig. 3). Good correlations were also found between ^{14}C-phenylethylene glycol covalent binding data and concentrations of 4-vinylphenol in conditions of metabolic induction and inhibition. In vivo this new minor metabolic pathway was confirmed by mass fragmentographic identification in rat urine of trace amounts of p-hydroxybenzoic acid, p-hydroxymandelic acid and p-hydroxyhippuric acid (see Fig. 4).

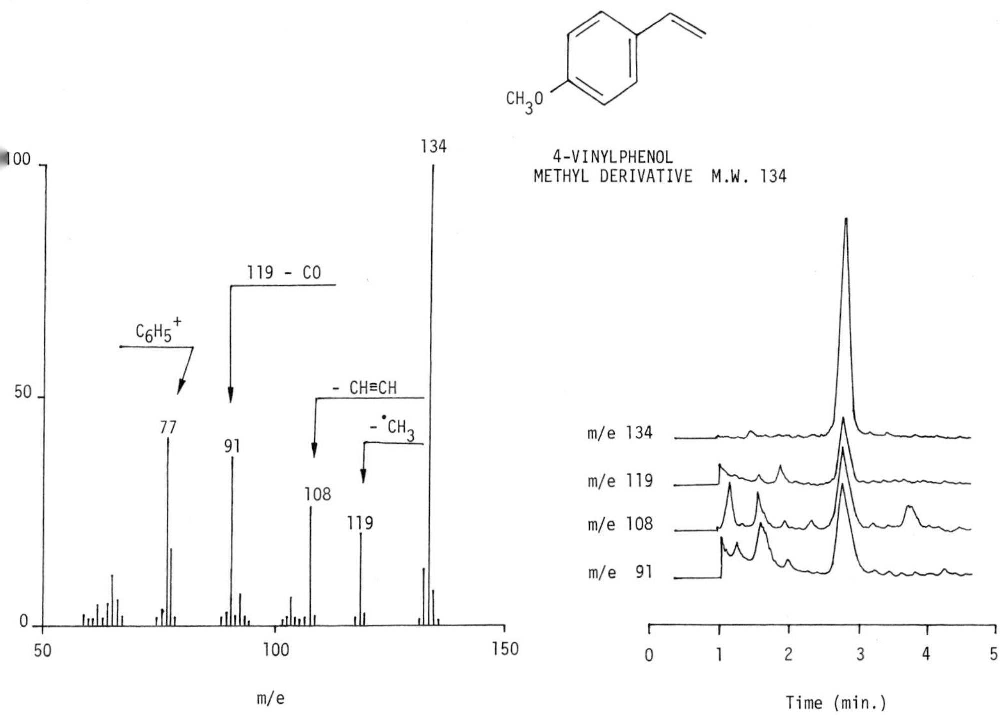

Fig. 3. Mass spectrum of 4-vinylphenol methyl derivative and its mass fragmentographic identification in the microsomal incubation mixture

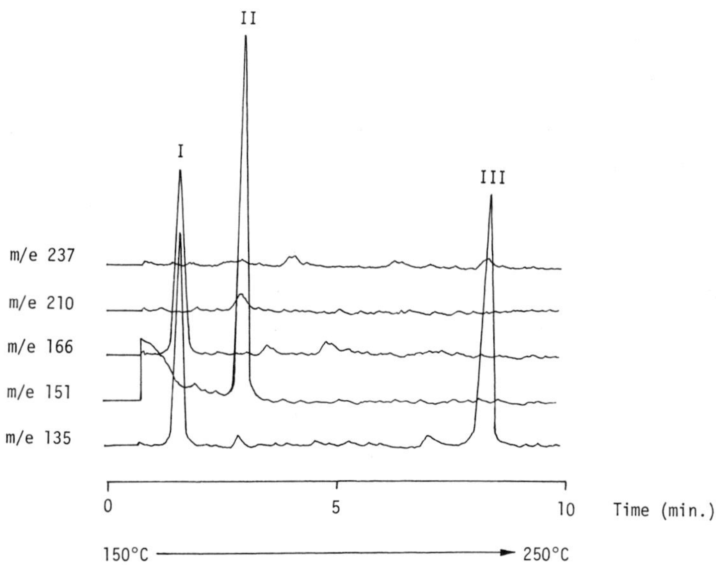

Fig. 4. Mass fragmentographic identification in rat urines of nanogram concentrations of p-hydroxybenzoic acid *(peak I)*, p-hydroxymandelic acid *(peak II)* and p-hydroxyhippuric acid *(peak III)* determined as their permethylated derivatives

Minor pathways may well play a crucial role as regards the toxicity of a compound. In mutagenicity tests by Watabe et al. (1978) styrene-3,4-oxide was shown to be far more toxic than the corresponding 7,8-oxide.

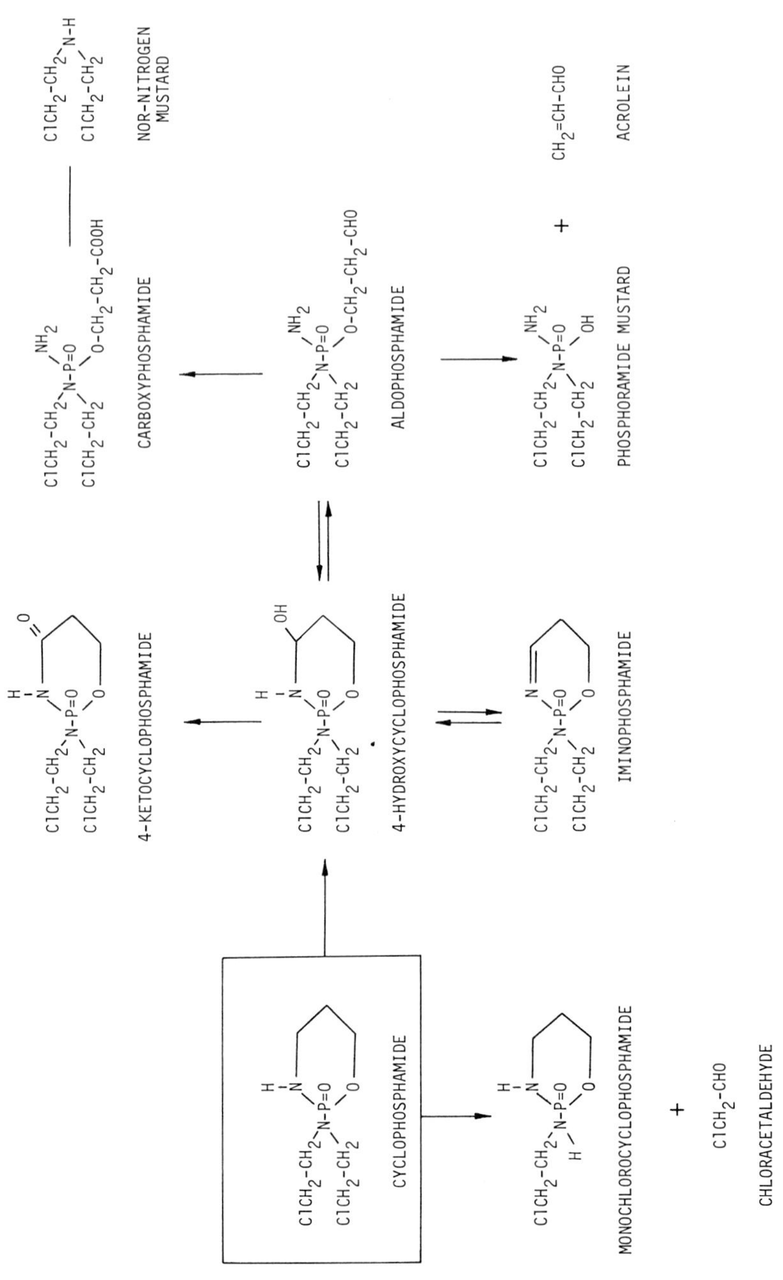

Fig. 5. Metabolism of cyclophosphamide

Metabolism Associated with Different Cell Compartments

The term "secondary metabolism" may be used to refer either to a metabolism which is quantitatively minor, or to a major metabolism present only to a limited extent in a subcellular compartment other than microsomes. During the last few years several articles have appeared in the literature concerning the capacity of the nuclear envelope to activate chemical carcinogens (Bereznzy et al. 1970; Bresnick et al. 1977; Garattini et al. 1980). Because of its spatial proximity to target DNA, the nuclear membrane may well be important in the onset of the genotoxic effects of these compounds. To approach the study of this kind of "secondary metabolism", cyclophosphamide was used as a model compound for these experiments; this anticancer agent is frequently used as a reference drug in mutagenesis tests.

The metabolism of cyclophosphamide is shown in Fig. 5. The initial activation process involves drug hydroxylation at the 4-position with formation of 4-hydroxycyclophosphamide, a compound in chemical equilibrium with iminophosphamide and aldophosphamide. Aldophosphamide in turn undergoes a β-elimination of acrolein with production of the highly cytotoxic species phosphoramide mustard (Torkelson et al. 1974). Table 5 shows the results of covalent binding experiments to microsomal proteins performed with ^{14}C-cyclophosphamide. It can be seen that the process of cyclophosphamide activation is catalyzed by a cytochrome P-450 monooxygenase since binding levels were higher with microsomes from PB pretreated rats. A parallel quantitative indication of cyclophosphamide conversion to phosphoramide mustard is given by the Km and Vmax values shown in Table 6. In vitro phosphoramide mustard production was also seen to be dependent on a PB inducible monooxygenase.

Table 5. Irreversible protein binding of ^{14}C-cyclophosphamide (25 μM) catalyzed by rat liver microsomes in the presence of an NADPH generating system after 120 min of incubation. Effect of inducers of drug metabolizing enzymes

Animal pretreatment	Sample	Cyclophosphamide metabolites irreversibly bound to 1 mg of microsomal protein (pmol ± SE)
Saline or corn oil	Boiled M + NADPH	5.3 ± 0.2
Saline or corn oil	M − NADPH	4.9 ± 0.1
Saline or corn oil	M + NADPH	113.3 ± 1.3[a]
PB (80 mg/kg i.p. × 3 days in saline)	M + NADPH	186.6 ± 4.0[b]
BNF (60 mg/kg i.p. × 2 days in corn oil)	M + NADPH	120.1 ± 1.6[a]
3-MC (40 mg/kg i.p. × 3 days in corn oil)	M + NADPH	93.3 ± 5.1[a]

Each figure is the mean ± SE of four determinations

M = microsomes; PB = phenobarbital; BNF = β-naphthoflavone; 3-MC = 3-methylcholanthrene

[a] $p < 0.01$. Compared with boiled control M + NADPH and control M − NADPH

[b] $p < 0.01$. Compared with control M + NADPH

Table 6. Apparent K_m and V_{max} values of the cyclophosphamide "activating" enzyme which is responsible for phosphoramide mustard formation. Effect of inducers on rat liver microsomal drug metabolizing enzymes

Animal pretreatment	$K_m \pm SE$ (mM)	$V_{max} \pm SE$ (ng/min × mg protein)
Saline or corn oil	3.15 ± 0.27	447 ± 12
PB (80 mg/kg i.p. × 3 days in saline)	1.34 ± 0.22[a]	632 ± 11[a]
BNF (60 mg/kg i.p. × 2 days in corn oil)	2.51 ± 0.23	452 ± 10
3-MC (40 mg/kg i.p. × 3 days in corn oil)	3.04 ± 0.38	435 ± 16

Determinations were made in quadruplicate
PB = phenobarbital; BNF = β-naphthoflavone; 3-MC = 3-methylcholanthrene
[a] $p < 0.01$. Compared with microsomes from the liver of control rats and rats pretreated with either BNF and 3-MC

Table 7. Irreversible binding of ^{14}C-cyclophosphamide (25 μM) to proteins and DNA from rat liver nuclei after 120 min of incubation

Sample	Cyclophosphamide metabolites irreversibly bound to 1 mg of nuclear proteins or DNA (pmol ± SE)	
	Nuclear proteins	DNA
Boiled nuclei + NADPH	1.2 ± 0.1	0.7 ± 0.1
Nuclei − NADPH	1.5 ± 0.3	0.7 ± 0.1
Nuclei + NADPH	7.9 ± 1.5[a]	2.6 ± 0.3[a]

Each figures is the mean ± SE of four determinations
[a] $p < 0.01$. Compared with boiled nuclei + NADPH and nuclei − NADPH

Table 8. Irreversible binding of ^{14}C-cyclophosphamide to proteins and DNA determined using different model systems[a]

Experimental model	Cyclophosphamide metabolites irreversibly bound to 1 mg of proteins or DNA (pmol ± SE)	
	Proteins	DNA
Microsomes + DNA	108.7 ± 2.1	8.6 ± 1.7
Nuclei	7.9 ± 1.5	2.6 ± 0.3
Hepatocytes	80.1 ± 10.2	1.1 ± 0.1
Isolated and perfused rat liver	21.8 ± 5.2	1.4 ± 0.2
Rat liver "in vivo"	12.3 ± 2.4	0.6 ± 0.1

Each figure is the mean ± SE of four determinations
[a] Microsomes, nuclei, and hepatocytes were incubated for 120 min with ^{14}C-cyclophosphamide at a concentration of 25 μM. Rat liver perfusion was carried out for 120 min with a ^{14}C-cyclophosphamide initial concentration in the perfusion medium of 25 μM. In vivo experiments were performed by injecting in the tale vein of rats ^{14}C-cyclophosphamide at a dose of 25 mg/kg; the animals were killed 120 min after treatment

If intact nuclei are tested for their "activating capacity" (see Table 7), they also show metabolizing activity, as can be observed from binding data to both nuclear proteins and DNA. The next question is thus: what is the nuclear membrane's real contribution in determining the covalent binding of an exogenous compound to nuclear DNA with respect to microsomal activities? This question is still unanswered, the main hindrance arising from the very different metabolic conditions in in vitro and in vivo systems. Table 8 shows the preliminary findings on cyclophosphamide covalent binding to proteins and DNA determined in different experimental conditions ranging from microsomes and DNA to the in vivo situation.

On the basis of these data it can be assumed that nuclei are active enough to metabolize cyclophosphamide, and in fact DNA binding was higher in nuclei than in hepatocytes, isolated perfused liver and liver tissue in vivo. However in the interpretation of these data account must be taken of the fact that the substrate availability for nuclear membranes in intact nuclei may differ considerably from that in hepatocytes and in intact organs because of different cell membrane permeability and because of the presence of the endoplasmic reticulum. The choice of an in vitro system closer to in vivo conditions is always a doubtful question, and is mainly related to the nature of the compound under testing. It may happen for example that, depending upon what substrate is used, different metabolic intermediates may be produced, with different chemical reactivity and stability. In the case of cyclophosphamide, the reactive species phosphoramide mustard is known to be stable enough to permit migration from the site of activation. The picture obviously changes when dealing with extremely reactive intermediates.

Conclusions

In the present work it has been shown that the study of how an exogenous substrate may interact irreversibly with cellular macromolecules (proteins and nucleic acids) in vitro and in vivo may prove useful in elucidating the structure of chemically reactive metabolic intermediates. The approach is to integrate traditional covalent binding experiments with characterization of the enzymatic activating processes and parallel quantitative determination of the metabolic pathways thought to be involved in these interactions.

Covalent binding studies might also prove useful in clarifying the relative capacity of single subcellular constituents to induce irreversible interactions between exogenous compounds and discrete biological molecules; this might give some indication of how much they contribute to the onset of toxic effects, be it cancer or any other toxicity. Such studies would be based on comparison of the in vivo situation with different in vitro model systems, but much more research is still needed, with a larger number and different classes of substances. In addition, this approach would need further refinement so as to select better "target" cellular macromolecules other than DNA and to characterize them for their biological function.

References

Bereznzy R, Funk LK, Crane FL (1970) The isolation of nuclear membrane from a large scale preparation of bovine liver nuclei. Biochim Biophys Acta 203: 531–546

Bresnick E, Vaught JB, Chuang AHL, Stoming TA, Bockman P, Mukhtar H (1977) Nuclear aryl hydrocarbon hydroxylase and interaction of polycyclic hydrocarbons with nuclear components. Arch Biochem Biophys 181: 257–269

Garattini E, Gazzotti G, Salmona M (1980) Is nuclear styrene monooxygenase activity a microsomal artifact? Chem Biol Interact 31: 341–346

Ghezzi P, Donelli MG, Pantarotto C, Facchinetti T, Garattini S (1981) Evidence of covalent binding of adriamycin to rat liver microsomal proteins. Biochem Pharmacol 30: 175–177

Gillette JR (1974) A perspective on the role of chemically reactive metabolites of foreign compounds in toxicity – I. Correlation of changes in covalent binding of reactivity metabolites with changes in the incidence and severity of toxicity. Biochem Pharmacol 23: 2785–2794

Leibman KC (1975) Metabolism and toxicity of styrene. Environ Health Perspect 11: 115–119

Lutz WK (1979) In vivo covalent binding of organic chemicals to DNA as a quantitative indicator in the process of chemical carcinogenesis. Mutat Res 65: 289–356

Oesch F (1974) Purification and specificity of a human microsomal epoxide hydratase. Biochem J 139: 77–88

Pantarotto C, Fanelli R, Bidoli F, Morazzoni P, Salmona M, Szczawinska K (1978) Arene oxides in styrene metabolism, a new perspective in styrene toxicity? Scand J Work Environ Health [Suppl 2] 4: 67–77

Pantarotto C, Salmona M, Szczawinska K, Bidoli F (1980) Gas chromatographic mass spectrometric studies on styrene toxicity. In: Albaiges J (ed) Analytical techniques in environmental chemistry. Pergamon, Oxford, pp 245–279

Szczawinska K, Ginelli E, Bartosek I, Gambazza C, Pantarotto C (1981) Caffeine does not bind covalently to liver microsomes from different animal species and to proteins and DNA from perfused rat liver. Chem Biol Interact 34: 345–354

Torkelson AR, LaBudde JA, Weikel JH Jr (1974) The metabolic fate of cyclophosphamide. Drug Metab Review 3: 131–165

Tyndall J (1979) Covalent binding and hepatotoxicity. Drug Metab Dispos 7: 451–453

Watabe T, Isobe M, Sawahata T, Yoshikawa K, Yamada S, Takabatake E (1978) Metabolism and mutagenicity of styrene. Scand J Work Environ Health [Suppl 2] 4: 142–155

Disease, Metabolism and Reproduction in the Toxic Response to Drugs and Other Chemicals
Arch. Toxicol., Suppl. 7, 219–231 (1984)

Species Differences in Oxidative Drug Metabolism: Some Basic Considerations

S. G. Al-Dabbagh[1] and R. L. Smith[2]

[1] Department of Pharmacology, College of Veterinary Medicine, University of Mosul, Iraq
[2] Department of Pharmacology, St. Mary's Hospital Medical School, London W 2 1PG, Great Britain

Abstract. Perhaps one of the single most important developments in the past 20 years in the understanding of chemical toxicity has been the realisation of the importance of metabolic transformation in this process. It is now widely appreciated that the toxic effects of many chemicals is a function of their metabolism rather than the substance itself. Of central interest to the toxicologist therefore is an understanding of the metabolism of a toxic chemical and the significance of this in the toxic process. The metabolic process itself however can be highly variable both between and within animal species. For this reason the toxicologist may have to consider both species and strain differences in metabolism when attempting to extrapolate findings to man in the safety evaluation process. For the past twenty years, work on species differences in metabolism has been largely of a descriptive nature and the cataloguing of differences. However, developments in the last few years in the understanding of the genetic diversity of species, including man, in terms of biotransformation and the nature and substrate preferences of the various multiple forms of the drug-metabolizing enzymes now give a better insight into the nature of species differences of metabolism. Furthermore, an understanding of this problem tempers expectations in terms of what may be hoped for in the extrapolation from other species. For example, the search for a species that metabolizes like man will be seen to be ill-conceived and ill-advised. The presentation deals with some of the fundamental aspects of species and strain differences in oxidative metabolism in particular and the implications that this has for the toxicologist in the safety evaluation process.

Key words: Drug metabolism – Monoxygenase enzymes – P-450 isozymes – Hydroxylation – Species differences – DA rat strain

The fact that species may vary in the way they metabolize foreign compounds has long been known. Probably one of the earliest observations in this respect was that of Jaffe (1877) who found that hens utilised ornithine for the metabolic conjugation of benzoic acid as opposed to glycine utilised by mammals. A marked species difference was also early observed with respect to the conjugation of phenylacetic acid; hens utilised ornithine while mammals utilise glycine except for humans and the chimpanzee, which uniquely appeared to utilise glutamine. A further interesting observation in this field was made by Parke and Williams in 1956 concerning species differences in the orientation of the aromatic hydroxylation of aniline. Although this chemical is hydroxylated by various species in both the *ortho* and *para* positions marked species differences occur of the relative orientation of hydroxylation. While *para* hydroxylation predominates in species such as the guinea pig, rabbit and rat the converse holds for the cat and dog. Thus, the fact of species variation with respect to the metabolism of foreign chemicals has been known for well over a century. However, the field received little consistent attention until the emergence of toxicology as a discipline which focussed the need to understand the relationship between metabolism and toxicity better and how this was influenced by species considerations.

The reviews that have appeared to date have largely been descriptive in nature describing and classifying various types of species differences in metabolism. Quite outstanding is the review by Williams (1967) while a second review by the same author published in 1974 is also of considerable interest.

Since that time however very considerable progress has been made in the understanding of the multiple form nature of the drug-metabolizing enzymes and the nature of the genetic diversity responsible for this that occurs both within and between species. This paper represents an attempt to address some of the basic issues underlying species differences in the metabolism of foreign chemicals. This has been done in the belief that when a better understanding of the nature of comparative differences in metabolism exists then expectations will become more realistic particularly with respect to issues of practical interest to the toxicologist such as whether a search for a species which metabolizes like man is an entirely realistic objective.

The General Pattern of Metabolism

As pointed out by Williams (1967) there is a basic general pattern of drug metabolism discernible in all species so far investigated. This concept bears the same sort of relationship to drug metabolism as does the Central Dogma to molecular biology. The general pattern can be written in the general form:

$$\text{Foreign compound} \xrightarrow[\substack{\text{Oxidation}\\ \text{reduction}\\ \text{hydrolysis}}]{\text{Phase I}} \begin{array}{c}\text{Phase I}\\ \text{metabolite}\end{array} \xrightarrow[\text{conjugation}]{\text{Phase II}} \text{Conjugate}$$

This general pattern is now well-known and does not bear repetition even in detail. What is remarkable however is that despite the various tendencies with respect to protein evolution, mammals as a whole have evolved and conserved a gene pool which in overall terms determines a basic pattern of metabolism irrespective of species (Table 1). Furthermore, the types of biochemical pathways which constitute the so called Phase I and II reactions are generally common to mammalian species and once more underline the commonness of the genetic pool from which this derives.

However, at this point the similarity begins to end. With respect to the individual pathways, very considerable intra- and inter-species differences are found in the ability to effect these reactions particularly in relation to specific substrates. Herein lies the problem of species differences in metabolism. Although mammals share a common gene pool which determines a similar general pattern of metabolism considerable diversity has occurred within this pool determining different gene products with different functional activities. Presumably, the course of events in this process has been the duplication and multiplication of what may be termed 'ancestral genes'. These in turn have undergone independent mutations with the course of time giving rise to new gene products with similar but not identical functional properties. This phenomenon can be best illustrated by a consideration of the multiple form nature of the P-450 monoxygenases and their genetic regulation. In recent years very considerable progress has been made in the isolation and determination of the structure (amino acid sequence) of various P-450 forms. The complete primary structure of a form of cytochrome P-450 induced in rat liver by phenobarbital treatment has been elucidated using recombinant techniques (Fujii-Kuriyama et al. 1982). This work and that of others which have elucidated the partial sequences of various P-450 forms have established several important points namely: (i) the different forms of P-450 within a species can differ markedly with regard to primary structure yet still retain monoxygenase functional activity; they also represent different gene products; (ii) there occurs marked inter-species heterogeneity with respect to primary structure, (iii) various isozymes can exhibit marked differences with respect to substrate *preference*.

A good example of the heterogeneity of the P-450 forms that occurs within a species is shown in Fig. 1. This shows the N-terminal amino acid sequences for three rat liver P-450 isozymes. It can be seen that there is marked heterogeneity

Table 1. Species differences in metabolism

The mammalian genetic pool determines a biphasic pattern of foreign compound metabolism common to all species and the following types of reactions:	
Phase I	oxidation at C, N, S, P centres reductions hydrolysis
Phase II conjugation with	carbohydrates amino acids fatty acids miscellaneous

Rat	P-450a	Met-Leu-Asp-Thr-Gly-Leu-Leu-Leu-Val-Val-Ile-Leu-Ala-Thr-Val-Met-Leu-Leu
	P-450b	Glu-Pro-Thr-Ile-Leu-Leu-Leu-Leu-Ala-Leu-Leu-Val-Gly-Phe-Leu-Leu-Leu-Leu-Val-Ary
	P-450c	Ile-Thr-Val-Tyr-Gly-Phe-Pro-Ala-Phe-Glu-Thr-Ala-Ser-Glu-Leu-Leu-Leu-Leu-Val
Rabbit	P-450_{LM2}	Met-Glu-Phe-Sec-Leu-Leu-Leu-Leu-Leu-Ala-Phe-Leu-Ala-Gly-Leu-Leu-Leu-Leu-Leu

Fig. 1. Cytochrome P-450 heterogeneity: N-terminal amino acid sequences for P-450 isozymes isolated from rat and rabbit liver microsomes. (Bortello et al. 1979; Coon and Persson 1980)

between the three rat liver forms; perhaps the only common major feature is the relatively large proportion of hydrophobic amino acid residues such as leucine, isoleucine and valine. Besides this, major differences in the C-terminal amino acids for the three forms have also been established. Quite clearly, each P-450 isozyme is a separate gene product. Also shown in Fig. 1 is the partial N-terminal amino acid sequence for rabbit liver P-450_{LM2}. A marked inter-species heterogeneity is indicated from this partial sequence. A common factor once again however, is the relatively high proportion of leucine residues present.

Of the greatest importance is the fact that the various P-450 isozymes, despite marked structural differences, still function catalytically as monoxygenase enzymes but they do display striking differences with respect to substrate preference. In this sense they are discriminating, preferring one particular substrate against another. This is illustrated in Tables 2 and 3 which show the substrate preference characteristics of three reconstituted rat liver P-450 isozymes.

It is quite clear from these studies that although all four chemicals can function as substrates to a greater or less extent for the P-450 isozymes nevertheless overlapping and substrate preference occurs. Thus while aniline, as a substrate has overlapping specificity for the three isozymes, benzphetamine is the preferred substrate for cytochrome P-450b while benzo(a)pyrene is the preferred substrate for isozyme P-450c. Further preferences are seen if one considers the stereospecific aspects of oxidation catalyzed by various P-450 isozymes. Table 3 shows the preferred positions of hydroxylation of testosterone by three rat liver P-450 isozymes. Cytochrome P-450a isozyme preferentially hydroxylates in the 7α-position, P-450b in the 16α-position and P-450c in the 6β-position.

It is clear therefore that there is great genetic diversity in the regulation of the cytochrome P-450's and that the various gene products can exhibit marked differences both with respect to primary structure and to substrate preference. Herein lies the problem of species differences in metabolism, at least in respect of oxidative metabolism. According to standard genetic theory the primary cause of this genetic diversity would be mutation leading to point amino acid changes perhaps thereby changing substrate preference characteristics. One theory current in modern genetics which may help one to understand this genetic diversity with respect to cytochrome P-450 is the so-called neutralist hypothesis

Table 2. Substrate preference of cytochrome P-450 isozymes derived from rat liver

Substrate	Activity[a]		
	Cytochrome		
	P-450a	P-450b	P-450c
Aniline	5.1	6.7	9.3
Benzphetamine	3.2	176	5.1
Benzo(a)pyrene	0.1	0.5	19.2
Zoxazolamine	0.9	2.4	27.9

[a] nmol/min/nmol cytochrome P-450 (Ryan et al. 1979)

Table 3. Substrate preference of cytochrome-P450 isozymes derived from rat liver

Testosterone	Activity[a]		
	Cytochrome		
	P-450a	P-450b	P-450c
6 β-OH	<0.1	<0.1	0.3
7 α-OH	4.4	<0.1	<0.1
16 α-OH	<0.1	2.4	<0.1

[a] nmol/min/nmol cytochrome P-450 (Ryan et al. 1979)

of mutation. This argues that many mutations that occur are not necessarily deleterious and make little or no difference to the functional properties of protein enzyme molecule. They are effectively neutral or near neutral from the standpoint of natural selection. Such mutations may spread fortuitously and achieve relatively high frequencies.

In this way one might explain the large number of isoenzymic forms of P-450 that are encountered that still essentially retain monoxygenase function but which nevertheless manifest substrate preferences when challenged with xenobiotic substrates.

Genetic Diversity and Species Differences in Oxidation of Xenobiotic Substrates

The case has been developed that there exists considerable genetic diversity between species with respect to the nature and substrate preferences of the various P-450 isozymes. How does this manifest itself in terms of comparative in vivo differences in metabolism? Two situations may be discerned: (i) species differences in relative extents of competing reactions, (ii) occurrence with respect to specific substrates of apparent species defects of certain reactions.

Species Differences in Relative Extents of Competing Reactions

Species difference in the extent of occurrence of competing metabolic reactions is probably the most commonly encountered situation. Thus, a xenobiotic molecule may present a number of options with respect to oxidation at various centres (e.g., C, N, and S) and one may find that the relative balance of these options varies with species.

One of the most commonly encountered situations with respect to species differences in aromatic hydroxylation is that of orientation differences. Aryl functions may undergo hydroxylation in several positions but one finds that there occur major species differences with respect to the preferred positions of oxidation. This was made clear many years ago from a systematic study of the hydroxylation of aniline by several species to yield o- and p-amino-phenol (Table 4). In species such as the cat and dog of the two competing pathways, *ortho* oxidation was the preferred option whereas in the rat, rabbit and guinea pig, *para* oxidation was the preferred option (Parke and Williams 1956).

The problem of species differences in respect of competing options for oxidation is also well illustrated by the case of N-2-fluorenyl-acetamide (Table 5). This carcinogen undergoes oxidation at both C- and N-centres to yield mainly 7-hydroxy and N-hydroxy metabolites. However, there occur marked species differences with respect to the relative importance of C- and against N-hydroxylation.

The two pathways are of about equal significance in the rabbit and hamster whereas the 7-C-oxidation pathway dominates in man and mouse. In the steppe lemming and guinea pig the aromatic hydroxylation pathway appears to be completely dominant. The lack of carcinogenic activity of N-2-acetamidofluorene in these two latter species has been attributed to their failure, metabolically, to form the N-hydroxy metabolite, which is considered to be a proximate carcinogen.

Many drugs, are chemically quite complex and may contain within their structures several different types of cyclic structure and hetero atoms. In general the greater chemical complexity of the molecule clearly provides for an increased number of metabolic options. Here once again, one may encounter marked species differences with regard to preferred oxidation options. This situation is well illustrated by a consideration of the metabolism of viloxazine (Case et al. 1975; Case and Reeves 1975). This drug (2-(2-ethoxyphenoxymethyl)-2,3,4,6-tetrahydro-1,4-oxazine) structurally, offers a number of metabolic oxidation possibilities with regard to aromatic hydroxylation, oxidative de-ethylation, and metabolism of the morpholino function. One finds however with respect to the relative balance of these various competing options that marked species differences obtain (Table 6). Thus, in the rat the major pathway is by O-dealkylation, in the dog extensive metabolism of the morpholine function occurs whereas humans metabolize the drug dominantly by aromatic hydroxylation. Once again these species differences for the various options almost certainly have their origin in the genetic diversity of the P-450 isozymes and their preferred substrate and site characteristics.

Species Defects in Oxidative Reactions

This is a much less frequently encountered situation but is nevertheless of great interest. As to how far the defect is a real absolute one or whether it represents

Table 4. Species differences in oxidative metabolism: competing pathways-orientation effects

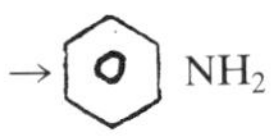

Species	Ratio p/o hydroxylation
Dog	0.5
Cat	0.4
Ferret	1.0
Mouse	3
Rat, rabbit, hamster, guinea pig	6–15

Table 5. Species difference in C- and N-oxidation of N-2-fluorenylacetamide. (Weisburger et al. 1964)

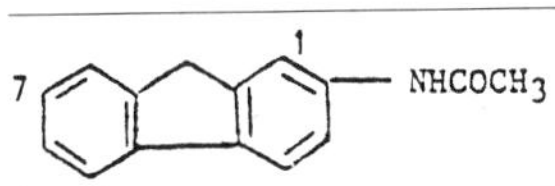

Species	N-Hydroxylated	7-C-Hydroxylated
Man	4–14	25–30
Rabbit	13–30	15–29
Hamster	15–20	35–39
Mouse	2	20
Steppe lemming	Trace	42
Guinea pig	0	72

Table 6. Species differences in preferred metabolic options. (Case et al. 1975)

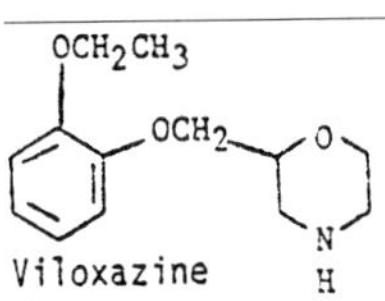

Viloxazine

Species	Preferred metabolic option
Rat	0-Dealkylation
Dog	Morpholine oxidation
Man	Aromatic hydroxylation

the minimal activity of a pathway against more active competing options is difficult to say at the present time. Some examples of apparent species defects in oxidative pathways are shown in Table 7. The defects are probably not absolute but probably reflect a particular species-substrate situation where the P-450 monoxygenases have low affinity for the substrate in question. In this situation marked species differences in metabolism may obtain, e.g., amphetamine, chlorphentermine, phenmetrazine and viloxazine.

Thus, amphetamine undergoes aromatic hydroxylation in most species to a greater or lesser extent, but not in the guinea pig where this reaction appears to be defective for this substrate (Dring et al. 1970). The guinea pig exhibits a similar defect of the aromatic hydroxylation pathway in the case of phenmetrazine. This drug is, however, extensively metabolized by this pathway by several other species including rat, the tamarin monkey and man (Franklin et al. 1977). The aliphatic N-hydroxylation of the anorectic drug chlorphentermine is defective in the rat whereas this is a major pathway of metabolism of the drug in the guinea pig, rabbit rhesus monkey and man (Caldwell et al. 1975). The commonly encountered metabolic pathway of O-dealkylation has been reported to be deficient in the dog for at least two substrates, namely, viloxazine (Case et al. 1975) and for 2-butylaminomethyl-8-ethoxy-1,4-benzodioxane (McMahon et al. 1960).

Genetic Polymorphism and the Origin of New Genes Controlling Drug Oxidation: the DA Rat – a Case Example

Although there is considerable discussion as to how new genes are maintained and change in frequency of occurrence within population groups there is widespread agreement that they first have their origin in the occurrence of a mutation which may become manifest as a genetic polymorphism. Discernment of a genetic polymorphism depends upon its frequency of occurrence and also that the variant gene product has properties discernable from those of the normal gene. Mutation, and hence genetic polymorphism, have been called the fuel of evolution, for it is through this process that new genes and diversity in a population can occur.

It is also the driving force in speciation – the development of new species. Darwin for example always insisted that a permanent variety should be viewed as a species in the making.

Table 7. Examples of apparent species defects with respect to certain oxidative pathways

Reaction	Substrate	Species
Aromatic hydroxylation	Phenmetrazine, amphetamine	Guinea pig
Aliphatic N-hydroxylation	Chlorphentermine	Rat
Acetamido-N-hydroxylation	N-2-Fluorenylacetamide	Guinea pig
Ø-Dealkylation	Viloxazine	Dog

In terms of the evolution of new genes controlling drug oxidation, the DA strain of rat affords an interesting case study.

Studies of the females of various rat strains, revealed that one of these lines, the DA, showed a genetically determined impairment with respect to the oxidation of a probe drug debrisoquine as well as a number of other compounds (Table 8; Al-Dabbagh et al. 1981; Al-Dabbagh 1982). The trait which is recessive in character, is manifest in the female of the line, and is transmitted by simple Mendelian inheritance. Nine other strains of rat investigated (Wistar, Lewis, Fischer, A/Gus, PVG, WAG, BN, Long Evans and Sprague-Dawley) were all normal with respect to oxidation capacity. Spectral binding studies also showed that the hepatic microsomes from the female DA did not show the normal type I spectral interaction with several oxidisable substrates such as debrisoquine, phenformin and sparteine (Küpfer et al. 1982). The observations are explicable on the basis that within the genus Rattus a variant gene has now evolved which occurs in the DA strain which determines a product with quite different functional properties. Whether or not the new gene product determines the metabolism of some substrates in the opposite direction (i.e., more rapid metabolism) has yet to be determined.

Genetic Polymorphism and Drug Oxidation in Man

In recent years several examples of polymorphic drug oxidation in man have been described which provide evidence of newly evolving genes regulating this process. The oxidation of a number of substrates in vivo has been shown to be discontinuous (bimodal) and at least two separate phenotypes (extensive metabolizers [EM] and poor metabolizers [PM]) respectively, can be recognised. These polymorphic situations arise from the occurrence in the population of variant forms of normal genes regulating the oxidation process. The trait of impaired metabolism arises in individuals homozygous for the allele determining impaired oxidation. Most information is available for the debrisoquine polymorphism (Mahgoub et al. 1973; Smith and Idle 1981). However since then two other oxidation polymorphisms have been described, which appear to be independent of the debrisoquine situation, namely the polymorphic sulphoxidation of S-carboxymethyl-L-cysteine (Waring et al. 1982) and the aromatic

Table 8. Drug oxidation in the DA rat strain. (Al-Dabbagh 1982)

Substrates where oxidation is	
Impaired	Unaltered
Debrisoquine	Tolbutamide
Phenformin	Acetanilide
Sparteine	
Phenacetin	
Hexobarbitone	

hydroxylation of (S)-mephenytoin (Küpfer et al. 1979; 1981). The locus controlling debrisoquine oxidation has also been shown to regulate or influence the metabolic oxidation of many other drugs. The oxidative pathways affected include those of aromatic hydroxylation, alicyclic hydroxylation, O-dealkylation and aliphatic oxidation. Of the greatest interest is that individuals who show impaired metabolism (PM phenotype) constitute a distinct subgroup with respect to propensity to develop adverse drug reactions. Three types of situation can be recognised:

(a) The individual shows excessive pharmacological reactions to normal doses of the drug. This is a consequence of impaired first-pass hepatic oxidation so that the bioavailability is higher in the affected individual. Indeed the bioavailability of a drug may be 3–5 times greater in an individual of the PM phenotype than in EM subjects because of impaired oxidative metabolism. Examples of this are seen with debrisoquine (Ritchie et al. 1980), metoprolol (Lennard et al. 1982) and encainide (Wang et al. 1982; Woosley et al. 1981).

(b) For drugs where oxidative metabolism is a prerequisite for elimination, accumulation may occur when this process is impaired as in subjects of the PM phenotype. An example of this is provided by the anti-anginal drug perhexiline. This drug undergoes metabolic mono- and dihydroxylation as an essential prerequisite to elimination (Wright et al. 1973). However, in PM subjects this process is impaired and as a consequence the drug accumulates. It has been observed that PM subjects are disproportionately much more likely to develop peripheral neuropathy following chronic use of the drug than are patients who are extensive metabolisers (EM)(Shah et al. 1982).

(c) In some cases impairment of the normal oxidative pathway of metabolism may lead to the metabolism of the drug along what are usually secondary and minor pathway. The O-dealkylation of phenacetin for example is sluggish in poor metabolizers (PM) and as a consequence more of the drug is handled by the normally minor pathways of aromatic hydroxylation and deacetylation leading to toxic 2-hydroxyphenetidine formation. This is haemotoxic and as a consequence one finds that a small dose (1 g) of phenacetin to PM's will result in the formation of significant amounts of MetHb due to 2-hydroxyphenetidine formation whereas this is not seen in subjects of the EM phenotype (Kong et al. 1982). Thus, discontinuity of oxidative metabolism in man is very important from the point of view of determining phenotypes with a propensity to develop untoward reactions to drugs. Some examples of adverse effects of drugs in subjects of the PM phenotype are shown in Table 9.

The implications of the polymorphic sulphoxidation reactions of carboxymethylcysteine and the aromatic hydroxylation of (R)-mephenytoin have yet to be explored. The recognition of poor sulphoxidisers of drugs may provide an insight into why some individuals experience toxic reactions when given certain sulphur containing drugs such as thioureas, thioamides and phenothiazines.

The present data emphasizes the discontinuity of several forms of metabolic oxidation in man. Furthermore, the recognition of discrete phenotypes with respect to drug oxidation underlines the inappropriateness of a search for a

Table 9. Impaired drug hydroxylation in man and adverse drug reactions. Adverse drug responses seen in subjects of the poor-metabolizer phenotype

Drug	Effect
Debrisoquine	Exaggerated postural hypotension
Phenformin	Lacticacidosis
Perhexiline	Peripheral neuropathy; cirrhosis
Metoprolol	Excessive and prolonged β-blockade
Sparteine	Diplopia, blurred vision
Bufuralol	Nausea, vomiting
Phenacetin	MetHb

Table 10. Polymorphic oxidation of drugs in man

Polymorphism	Recessive trait and incidence[a]	Other drugs affected
4-Hydroxylation of debrisoquine	Poor metabolizers (PM); 8–9%	Sparteine, phenformin, guanoxan, phenacetin, nortriptyline, metoprolol, bufuralol
Sulphoxidation of carboxymethyl-cysteine	Poor sulphoxidizers; ≈ 10%	Penicillamine?
Aromatic hydroxylation of (S)-mephenytoin	Deficient hydroxylators; ≈ 5%	Unknown

[a] Data for Caucasian

species that oxidatively metabolises like man. The question must be, which man or rather which human phenotype. This brings back the question again of looking for models of human diversity in drug oxidation. An argument could be made that it would be more valuable to look at strain differences within a single species as a guide to what may be the human situation rather than looking at quite separate species. In this connection it is striking that the polymorphic drug oxidation phenomenon described for the DA strain of rat closely parallels the human debrisoquine hydroxylation polymorphism. Thus a study of various rat strains, including the DA, could be revealing as to the latitude likely to be encountered in man.

Some Conclusions

This article has dwelt upon two basic biological considerations with respect to species diversity and oxidative drug metabolism. These themes have been firstly, the very marked diversity that occurs both between and within species with respect to the genetic regulation of oxidative metabolism. The second is the consequential, marked heterogeneity of the multiple P-450 isozymes which, although characterisable functionally as monoxygenases, nevertheless display marked differences with respect to substrate preferences. These differences can determine marked inter- and intra-species differences in oxidative metabolism which manifest themselves externally in terms of in vivo metabolism as follows: species differences in the relative extents of competing oxidative options or apparent species defects with respect to certain substrates.

Of importance to the practising toxicologist is the question of whether or not species differences in oxidative metabolism are predictable? In the opinion of the authors and in view of what has been said of genetic diversity and substrate preferences they are not and probably will remain so. This is particularly true of the most commonly encountered situation of species differences in competing metabolic options. In some cases it will be found that a species, or a particular strain of a species does resemble man in terms of metabolic profile but in general this has to be determined empirically. Probably, the most important contribution that a study of the metabolism of a chemical in a particular species can make is to help us interpret an effect and allow an assessment, on the basis of comparative species studies, as to whether or not the observed toxic effect is likely to be species dependent.

Of the greatest theoretical and practical importance is the recognition of intra-species variations with respect to the genetic regulation of oxidative drug metabolism. The uncovering of genetic polymorphisms of drug oxidation both in the rat and man point to the manner by which new genes regulating oxidative metabolism may evolve. The recognition of human phenotypes with regard to drug oxidation is important particularly now that it is known that one of these, the PM phenotype, is particularly prone to a number of adverse drug reactions as a consequence of impaired metabolism. From the point of view of modelling for man it may be that more attention paid to intra-strain differences in metabolism as opposed to inter-species differences could be more revealing for the reality of the human situation.

References

Al-Dabbagh SG (1982) Genetic polymorphism of drug oxidation in the rat. PhD thesis, University of London

Al-Dabbagh SG, Idle JR, Smith RL (1981) Animal modelling of human polymorphic drug oxidation – the metabolism of debrisoquine and phenacetin in rat inbred strains. J Pharm Pharmacol 33 : 161–164

Botelho LH, Ryan DE, Levin W (1979) Amino acid compositions and partial amino acid sequences of three highly purified forms of liver microsomal cytochrome P-450 from rats treated with polychlorinated biphenyls, phenobarbital or 3-methylcholanthrene. J Biol Chem 254 : 5635–5640

Caldwell J, Köster V, Smith RL, Williams RT (1975) Species variations in the N-oxidation of chlorphentermine. Biochem Pharmacol 24 : 2225–2332

Case DE, Reeves PR (1975) The disposition and metabolism of I.C.I. 58,834 (viloxazine) in humans. Xenobiotica 5 : 113–129

Case DE, Illiston H, Reeves PR, Shuker B, Simons P (1975) The disposition and metabolism of I.C.I. 58,834 (viloxazine) in animals. Xenobiotica 5 : 83–111

Coon MJ, Persson AV (1980) Microsomal cytochrome P-450: A centre catalyst in detoxication reactions. In: Jakoby WB (ed) Enzymatic basis of detoxication vol 1. Academic Press, New York, pp 117–134

Dring LG, Smith RL, Williams RT (1970) The metabolic fate of amphetamine in man and other species. Biochem J 116: 425–435

Franklin RB, Dring LG, Williams KT (1977) The metabolism of phenmetrazine in man and laboratory animals. Drug Metab Dispos 5: 223–233

Fujji-Kuriyama Y, Mizukami Y, Kawajiri K, Sogawa K, Muramatsu M (1982) Primary structure of a cytochrome P-450: Coding nucleotide sequence of phenobarbital-inducible cytochrome P-450 cDNA from rat liver. Proc Natl Acad Sci USA 79: 2793–2797

Jaffe M (1877) Ber Dtsch Chem Ges 10: 1925

Kong I, Devonshire JW, Cooper M, Sloan TP, Idle JR, Smith RL (1982) The influence of oxidation phenotype on phenacetin metabolism and haemotoxicity. Br J Clin Pharmacol 13: 275–276P

Küpfer A, Desmond P, Schenker S, Branch P (1979) Family study of a genetically determined deficiency of mephenytoin hydroxylation in man. Pharmacologist 21: 173

Küpfer A, Dick B, Preisig R (1981) Polymorphic mephenytoin hydroxylation in man: a new phenotype in the genetic control of hepatic drug metabolism. Hepatology 1: 524

Küpfer A, Al-Dabbagh SG, Ritchie JC, Idle JR, Smith RL (1982) Spectral binding studies of the polymorphically metabolized drugs debrisoquine, sparteine and phenformin by cytochrome P-450 of normal and hydroxylation deficient rat strains. Biochem Pharmacol 31: 3193–3199

Lennard MS, Silas JH, Freestone S, Ramsay LE, Tucker GT, Woods HF (1982) Oxidation phenotype – a major determinant of metoprolol metabolism and response. N Engl J Med 307: 1558–1560

Mahgoub A, Idle JR, Dring LG, Lancaster R, Smith RL (1977) Polymorphic hydroxylation of debrisoquine in man. Lancet 2: 584–586

McMahon RE, Welles JS, Lee HM (1960) The metabolism of benzodioxane derivatives. II Ethoxybutamoxane-^{14}C. J Am Chem Soc 82: 2864–2866

Parke DV, Williams RT (1956) Species differences in the o- and p-hydroxylation of aniline. Biochem J 63: 12P

Ritchie JC, Sloan TP, Idle JR, Smith RL (1980) Toxicological implications of polymorphic drug metabolism. In: Environmental chemicals, enzyme function and human disease. Ciba Foundation Symposium 76. Excerpta Medica, Amsterdam, pp 219–244

Ryan DE, Thomas PE, Korzeniowski D, Levin W (1979) Separation and characterisation of highly purified forms of liver microsomal cytochrome P-450 from rats treated with polychlorinated biphenyls, phenobarbital and 3-methylcholanthrene. J Biol Chem 254: 1365–1374

Shah RR, Oates NS, Idle JR, Smith RL, Lockhart JDF (1982) Impaired oxidation of debrisoquine in patients with perhexiline neuropathy. Br Med J 284: 295–299

Smith RL, Idle JR (1981) Genetic polymorphism in drug oxidation. In: Davis M, Tredger JM, Williams R (eds) Drug reactions and the liver. Pitman Medical, London, pp 95–104

Wang T, Roden DM, Wolfenden HT, Woosley RL, Wilkinson GR, Wood AJJ (1982) Pharmacokinetics of encainide and its metabolites in man. Clin Pharmacol Ther 31: 278

Waring RH, Mitchell SC, Shah RR, Idle JR, Smith RL (1982) Polymorphic sulphoxidation of S-carboxymethyl-L-cysteine in man. Biochem Pharmacol 31: 3151–3154

Weisburger JH, Grantham PH, Vanhorn E, Steigbigel NH, Ray DP, Weisburger EK (1964) Activation and detoxication of N-2-fluorenylacetamide in man. Cancer Res 24: 475–479

Williams RT (1967) Comparative patterns of drug metabolism. Fed Proc 26: 1029–1039

Williams RT (1974) Inter-species variations in the metabolism of xenobiotics. Biochem Soc Trans 2: 359–377

Woosley RL, Roden DM, Duff HJ, Carey EL, Wood AJJ, Wilkinson GR (1981) Coinheritance of deficient oxidative metabolism of encainide and debrisoquine. Clin Res 29: 501A

Wright GJ, Leeson GA, Zeiger AV, Lang JF (1973) The absorption, excretion and metabolism of perhexiline maleate by the human. Postgrad Med J [Suppl 3] 49: 8–15

Disease, Metabolism and Reproduction in the Toxic Response to Drugs and Other Chemicals
Arch. Toxicol., Suppl. 7, 232–235 (1984)

Human Pharmacokinetics and Safety of Boric Acid

J. S. Schou[1], J. A. Jansen[1], and B. Aggerbeck[2]

[1] Department of Pharmacology, University of Copenhagen,
20 Juliane Maries Vej, 2100 Copenhagen, Denmark
[2] A/S Alfred Benzon, The Medical Department, 29 Halmtorvet, 1700 Copenhagen V, Denmark

Abstract. Using an in vitro technique it has been demonstrated that water-emulsifying and hydrophobic ointments containing boric acid liberate only minute amounts (1–6%) within 24 h compared with the nearly total liberation from a jelly. When an amount of boric acid containing ointment is swallowed, the absorption is only slightly delayed compared with a similar intake when dissolved in water, and in both cases nearly total excretion is found in the urine within 96 h. The halflife ($t_{1/2\beta}$) is 21 h (mean, 7 adult men). The pharmacokinetics rule out the risk of cumulative poisoning with topical preparations containing low amounts of boric acid. The use of water-emulsifying ointments containing up to 3% boric acid should be safe, even for repeated daily use in the napkin region.

Key words: Boric acid – Water-emulsifying ointments – Cosmetic safety – Pharmacokinetics – Skin absorption – Gastrointestinal absorption – Urinary excretion – Napkin area protection

Boric acid was introduced into medicine by Godlee (1873) as a mild antiseptic. As a medicine it has fallen into disrepute because of the occurence of fatal poisoning in babies after the application of undiluted powders to napkin areas affected by severe dermatitis, and also because of the availability of more effective antibacterial agents. A number of ointments of low boric acid content (up to 3%) is still in use, mainly for napkin region hygiene and to protect sensitive skin areas.

The safety of this use has been reported in two recent publications. Stüttgen et al. (1982) showed that the application of a water- emulsifying ointment even to abraded skin gave no rise in urinary boron excretion, and Friis-Hansen et al. (1982) demonstrated that the blood boron concentration in newborn infants was unaffected by daily use of the same ointment in the napkin region. Both investigations emphasized that the quality of the vehicle was the important factor affecting absorption of boric acid.

This has been further established by in vitro experiments, in which the boric acid released into distilled water in a dialysis chamber was determined. Water-emulsifying and hydrophobic ointments containing 1.2–3.0% boric acid have been investigated and compared with a methyl cellulose jelly containing 3% boric acid. The results for the jelly and for one of the water-emulsifying and one hydrophobic ointment are shown in Fig. 1. The findings explain why the boric acid in these types of ointments are not absorbed from the skin; it is retained in the ointment. The water-emulsifying ointment can even bind significant amounts of water or urine, and in this way further protects the skin against the abraision due to excretions.

In another series of experiments six adult male volunteers ingested, in a cross over design, 750 mg boric acid dissolved in water or as much as possible of the contents of a 50 g tube of water-emulsifying ointment containing 3% boric acid. The fractionated urinary excretion of boric acid was measured up to 96 h after ingestion (Table 1). The cumulated 96 h excretion for the six volunteers did not show any significant difference between the vehicles (solution 93.9 ± 3.7, water-emulsifying ointment 92.3 ± 3.2% of the doses ingested). However, there was a slight delay of excretion in the first two hour sampling periods after ingestion of the ointment, showing a somewhat delayed absorption rate in comparison with the water solution experiment.

To elucidate the risk of accumulation of boric acid if the alimentary daily intake should be supplemented by repeated uptake from a medicine or cosmetic product, there was a need to update the pharmacokinetic data for the compound. An intravenous dose of 600 mg boric acid was administered to seven

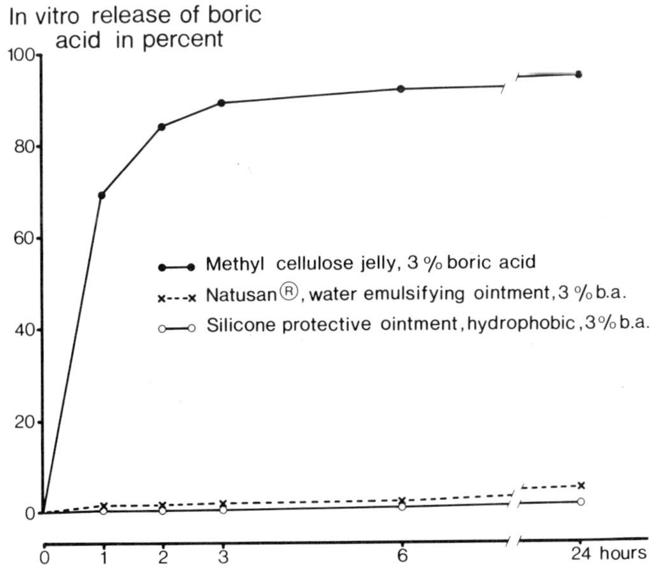

Fig. 1. Boric acid release into distilled water from two oily ointments and from a methyl cellulose jelly, all containing 3% boric acid. The dialysis method of Mutimer et al. (1950) was used, and the cumulated release was measured for 24 h

Table 1. Boric acid absorption from ointments[a]

Subject	Percent excreted		mg boric acid in ingested ointment
	Solution	Ointment	
A. P.	98.3	94.0	762
B. H.	95.1	93.0	832
J. S.	89.5	89.2	1,023
B. A.	89.1	97.5	1,473
J. J.	95.4	88.9	740
L. H.	95.7	91.3	1,275
Mean ± SD	93.9 ± 3.7	92.3 ± 3.2	

[a] Ninety-six hours urinary excretion of boric acid after oral intake by six male volunteers of a solution containing 750 mg boric acid or a water-emulsifying ointment (Natusan) containing amounts of boric acid from 740 to 1,473 mg. The figures indicate the amounts excreted in percent of the amount ingested

Table 2. Human pharmacokinetics of boric acid[a]

	V_1	V_2	V_3	$t_{1/2}$ (β)	Total clearance	
					V_1k_{10}	D/AUC
Mean	0.251	0.456	0.340	21.0	54.6	54.4
± SD	0.099	0.067	0.128	4.9	8.0	6.1

[a] Seven young male volunteers were infused intravenously with approximately 600 mg boric acid for 30 min. From the plasma concentration data the following pharmacokinetic parameters were calculated (mean of 7 values). The volumes of distribution in l/kg (V_1, V_2, V_3) and the final half life in hours $t_{1/2}$ (β) were obtained by fitting a three compartment model. Clearance values are given in ml/min/1.73 m^2

volunteers and the plasma concentration was followed for 120 h. Curve fitting of the results was performed by computer to test whether a two or a three compartment open model gave the best simulation. The Akaike's Information Criterion (AIC) was used for the comparative analyses (Yamaoka et al. 1978). The three compartment model gave the best fit. Now the pharmacokinetic parameters could be calculated for each person, and the figures in Table 2 show the means ± SD for the seven volunteers. The final half life ($t_{1/2\beta}$) of 21 h rules out the risk of any significant accumulation.

These results further establish the safety of the use of boric acid in water-emulsifying and hydrophobic ointments. The water-emulsifying ointment can take up considerable amounts of water and thereby protect the skin against maceration, while the boric acid exerts its mild antiseptic and buffering effect.

References

Friis-Hansen B, Aggerbeck B, Jansen JAa (1982) Unaffected blood boron levels in newborn infants treated with boric acid ointment. Food Chem Toxicol 20: 451–454

Godlee RJ (1873) On the antiseptic system. Lancet 1: 694–695

Mutimer MN, Riffkin C, Hill JA, Glickman ME, Cyr GN (1956) Modern ointment base technology II. Comparative evaluation of bases. J Am Pharm Assoc 45: 212–218

Stüttgen G, Siebel T, Aggerbeck B (1982) Absorption of boric acid through human skin depending on the type of vehicle. Arch Dermatol Res 272: 21–29

Yamaoka K, Nakagawa T, Uno T (1978) Application of Akaike's information criterion (AIC) in the evaluation of linear pharmacokinetic equations. J Pharmacokin et Biopharm 4: 165–177

Disease, Metabolism and Reproduction in the Toxic Response to Drugs and Other Chemicals
Arch. Toxicol., Suppl. 7, 236–239 (1984)

The Influence of Paracetamol on the Hepatic Biosynthesis of Lecithin

J. Lohmann[1], U. Lessing[1], H. Schriewer[1], M. Clemens[2], and U. Gerlach[1]

[1] Medizinische Universitätsklinik, Domagkstrasse 3, 4400 Münster, Federal Republic of Germany
[2] Chirurgische Universitätsklinik, Jungeblodtplatz 1, 4400 Münster, Federal Republic of Germany

Abstract. In paracetamol induced liver injury changes in the phospholipid components of microsomal membranes are usual. Direct incubation of paracetamol with subcellular fractions of human liver specimens did not alter the biosynthesis of lecithin. Preincubation of liver slices with paracetamol led to an increased synthesis of lecithin. The presence of intact cells and the integrity of hepatocellular function seem to be a prerequisite for the poisoning effects in vitro.

Key words: Paracetamol – Liver injury – Phospholipids

As yet the toxic intermediate metabolites of paracetamol have not been identified. In paracetamol-induced liver injury changes in the phospholipid components of microsomal membranes are believed to be due to increased methylation reactions, interactions with electrophilic metabolites and also lipidperoxidation (Toghill et al. 1969; McLean Day 1975; McLean and Nuttall 1978). These experiments were designed to study the influence of paracetamol on the biosynthesis of phosphatidylcholine. Portions of liver tissue taken from four patients for pathological examination and found to be without obvious liver disease were used. 200–300 mg was obtained in this way research. The liver tissue, 10,000 *g* supernatant fluid, cytosolic and microsomal fractions were incubated with paracetamol (3.3–8.0 mmol/l of total incubation volume). The tissue was incubated in a Warburg apparatus under 5% carbon dioxide in oxygen for 2 h at 37° C. The incubation medium consisted of 20 ml Krebs-Ringer solution: 95 parts 0.9% NaCl, 4 parts 1.15% KCl, 3 parts 1.62% $CaCl_2$, 1 part 2.11% KH_2PO_4, 1 part 3.82% $MgSO_4$, 3 parts 1.3% $NaHCO_3$, 3 parts Na-phosphate-buffer (0.1 mol/l Na_2HPO_4/0.1 mol/l NaH_2PO_4=4:1), 4 parts 0.16 mol/l Na-pyruvate, 7 parts 0.1 mol/l Fumarate, 4 parts 0.16 mol/l Na-glutamate, 5 parts 0.3 mol/l glucose. After the incubation the tissue was washed for 20 min in ice cold 0.9% NaCl solution, then homogenisation and ultracentrifugation was performed. The enzyme activity of cholinekinase was measured according to

Weinhold and Rethy (1974) (EC 2.7.1.32), the phosphocholinecytidyltransferase (EC 2.7.7.15) according to Weinhold et al. (1973) and the diacylglycerinecholinephosphotransferase (EC 2.7.8.2) according to Coleman and Bell (1977).

Results

Following direct incubation of paracetamol with the 10,000 g supernatant fluid radioincorporation of ^{14}C-(methyl)choline in lecithin slightly decreased, cholinekinase activity was slightly diminished whereas the activity of phosphocholinecytidyltransferase did not change. As is seen in Fig. 1 the enzyme activity of phosphocholinecytidyltransferase in the cytosolic fraction (100,000 *g* S) and in the microsomal fraction (100,000 *g* P) did not change significantly after direct incubation of these fractions with paracetamol. All experiments were done twice with double estimations. Figure 2 shows above, the radioincorporation of ^{14}C-(methyl)choline into lecithin of the 10,000 *g* supernatant fluid after preincubation of liver slices with paracetamol for a period of 2 h at 37° C. Here it

Paracetamol (mmol/l)	0	3.3	6.6
100,000 × gS nmol ^{14}C-CDP-choline/mg protein/min	0.26	0.24	0.24
100,000 × gP nmol ^{14}C-CDP-choline/mg protein/min	0.87	0.83	0.80

Fig. 1. Radioincorporation of ^{14}C-phosphocholine (as substrate for phosphocholinecytidyltransferase) in 100,000 *g* supernatant *(S)* and pellet *(P)* derived from human liver specimens during direct incubation with paracetamol

Paracetamol (mmol/l)	0	4	8
^{14}C-Choline as precursor pmol ^{14}C-Phospatidyl-choline/mg protein/15 min	35.4	54.2	58.6
^{14}C-CDP-Choline as precursor pmol ^{14}C-Phospatidyl-choline/mg protein/15 min	8.0	15.2	15.0

Fig. 2. Radioincorporation of ^{14}C(methyl)-choline and ^{14}C-CDP-choline in phosphatidylcholine of a 10,000 *g* supernatant after incubation of human liver tissue with paracetamol for a period of 2 h at 37° C

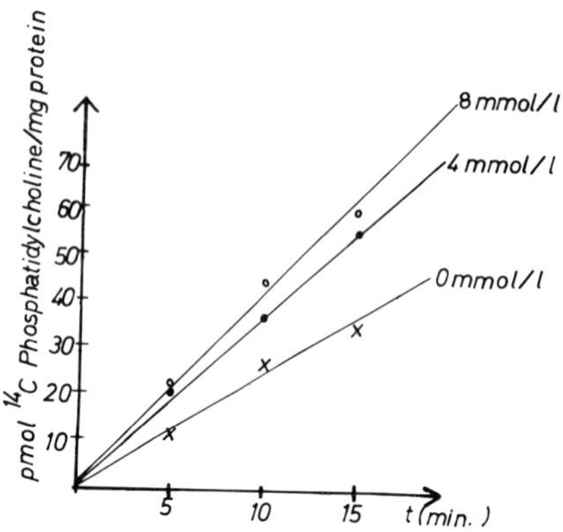

Fig. 3. Radioincorporation of ^{14}C(methyl)-choline in phosphatidylcholine of a 10,000 *g* supernatant after incubation of human liver slices with paracetamol for a period of 2 h at 37° C

was found that an increase of the overall synthesis of lecithin was connected with the concentration of paracetamol. Below in Fig. 2 is shown the incorporation of ^{14}C-CDP-choline into lecithin, as radioenzymeassay of diacylglycerine-cholinephosphotransferase, this is definitely increased. Figure 3 shows the kinetic pattern of the overall synthesis of lecithin at two concentrations of paracetamol after preincubation of liver slices with the toxic agent for 2 h.

Conclusion

These results suggest that not paracetamol itself but a metabolite of paracetamol catabolism may enhance lecithin biosynthesis in vitro. The presence of intact cells and the integrity of hepatocellular function seems to be a prerequisite for the poisoning effects.

In contrast with the findings of McLean (McLean and Nuttall 1978) of abnormal lipid metabolism in rat liver only after pretreatment with phenobarbital, metabolic disorders in human liver are demonstrable without pretreatment with phenobarbital.

References

Coleman R, Bell RM (1977) Phospholipid synthesis in isolated fat cells. J Biol Chem 252: 3050–3056

McLean AEM, Day PA (1975) The effect of dict on the toxicity of paracetamol and the safety of paracetamol-methionine mixtures. Biochem Pharmacol 24: 37–42

McLean AEM, Nuttall L (1978) An in vitro model of liver injury using paracetamol treatment of liver slices and prevention of injury by some antioxidants. Biochem Pharmacol 27: 425–430

Toghill P, Williams R, Stephens J (1969) Acute hepatic necrosis following an overdose of paracetamol. Gastroenterology 27: 773–776

Weinhold PA, Rethy VB (1974) The separation, purification and characterisation of ethanolamine kinase and choline kinase from rat liver. Biochemistry 13: 5135–5141

Weinhold PA, Skinner RS, Sanders RD (1973) Activity and some properties of choline kinase, cholinephosphate cytidyltransferase and choline phosphotransferase during liver development in the rat. Biochim Biophys Acta 326: 43–51

Disease, Metabolism and Reproduction in the Toxic Response to Drugs and Other Chemicals
Arch. Toxicol., Suppl. 7, 240–242 (1984)

Decreased Blood Levels of Ethanol and Acetaldehyde by S-Adenosyl-L-Methionine in Humans

C. Di Padova[1], R. Tritapepe[2], P. Rovagnati[1], M. Pozzoli[2], and G. Stramentinoli[3]

[1] 3rd Medical Clinic, University of Milan School of Medicine, Via Pace 15, 20122 Milan, Italy
[2] 3rd Surgical Clinic, University of Milan School of Medicine, Via F. Sforza 35, 20122 Milan, Italy
[3] BioResearch Co., Research Laboratories, Liscate, 20060 Milan, Italy

Abstract. In view of the protective effects of SAM on alcohol-induced fatty liver degeneration, an investigation has been carried out to see if this compound accelerates the clearance of ethanol and acetaldehyde in humans. Both parameters were significantly lower after SAM, indicating the capability of exogenous SAM to favour the inactivation of ethanol without increasing blood levels of acetaldehyde.

Key words: Acetaldehyde – Ethanol – S-adenosyl-L-methionine – Blood level

Recent experimental and clinical investigations have shown that the administration of S-adenosyl-L-methionine (SAM) prevents or reverses ethanol induced fatty liver degeneration (Pascale et al. 1982; Fiaccadori et al. 1982). However, little is known at present about the mechanism by which SAM gives protection against alcohol-induced steatosis. It might result from SAM-dependent phospholipid methylation, the biochemical event which is involved in the control of liver membrane fluidity and lipoprotein assembly (Pascale et al. 1982; Schreiber et al. 1983; Boelsterli et al. 1983). In addition the protective action of SAM (precursor of glutathione) could also be interpreted as a replacement for the alcohol induced depletion of thiol compounds (Shaw et al. 1981; Hirayama et al. 1983). Since it is still unclear whether SAM interferes with the metabolism of ethanol as well as of acetaldehyde, the toxic product of ethanol oxidation, the present study was performed.

Six adult non-obese female subjects in good general health and free from hepatic diseases were investigated after informed consent was obtained. Each subject consumed a standard diet without alcohol intake and received no drug throughout the investigational period. At 3-day intervals after overnight fasting, the subjects were given, according to a randomized sequence of treatments, either absolute ethanol (0.5 g/kg), diluted with 500 ml saline, or ethanol plus

---

Abbreviation: SAM, S-adenosyl-L-methionine

SAM (15 mg/kg), in the stable form of disulfate-di-p-toluene-sulfonate (BioResearch Co., Milan, Italy), through the antecubital vein over 60 min. One third of the administered SAM was injected intravenously 10 min prior to ethanol infusion and two thirds were added to alcohol solution. SAM (2 mg/kg) was also given intramuscularly three times during the day before the investigation. Each subject was monitored continuously during the study and blood samples were taken before ethanol, at the end of the infusion and every subsequent hour during the following 4 h. Blood ethanol was measured enzymatically (Di Padova et al. 1982). The method for evaluation of blood acetaldehyde was based on the transformation of the compound into 2,4-dinitrophenylhydrazones and by analysis of the derivative by high pressure liquid chromatography (HPLC), as described by Pezzoli et al. (1984). Since each subject served as her own control, the results have been analyzed for significance by the Student's paired *t*-test. All values represent the mean ± SE.

Figures 1 and 2 show blood ethanol and acetaldehyde concentrations measured at intervals after the administration of either ethanol or ethanol plus SAM. Both parameters were significantly lower after SAM indicating the capability of exogenous SAM to decrease alcohol concentrations without increasing blood levels of acetaldehyde. The possibility that SAM affected laboratory test results by directly interfering with ethanol was ruled out, since the intravenously infused ethanol-SAM mixtures gave normal analytical results for the ethanol content.

The reduced concentrations of ethanol and acetaldehyde cannot be related to increased activity of liver alcohol and aldehyde dehydrogenases since other authors (Feo, personal communication) have recently observed no interference of SAM with the main routes of alcohol metabolism.

On the other hand, as previously reported, the neutralizing action of SAM might be dependent on its proven capacity to accelerate synthesis of both membrane phospholipid and thiol compounds which are capable of forming adducts with ethanol and acetaldehyde (Kenney 1980; Hirayama et al. 1983). The difference between the decay curves of ethanol might be also related to an

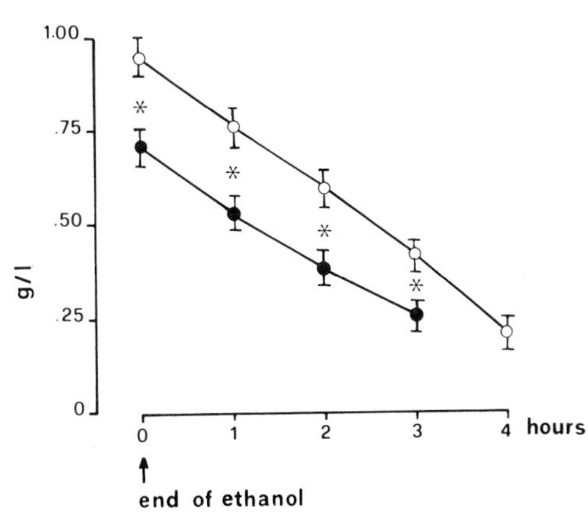

Fig. 1. Blood ethanol concentrations at various times after the intravenous administration of ethanol (○–○) or ethanol plus SAM (●–●). Each point represents the means ± SE.
*, $p < 0.01$

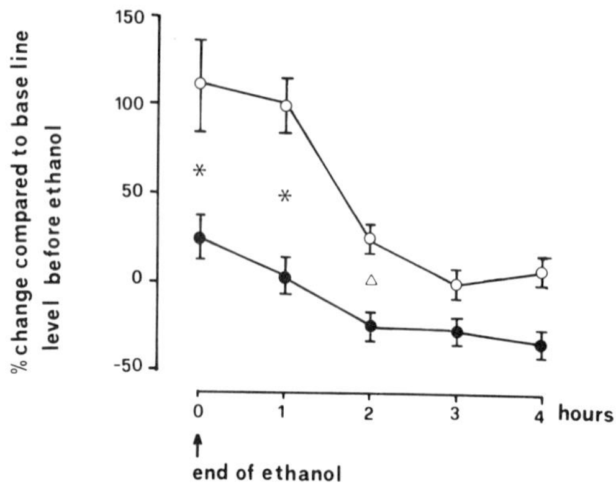

Fig. 2. Changes in blood acetaldehyde after the intravenous administration of ethanol (○–○) or ethanol plus SAM (●–●). The basal acetaldehyde concentrations (11.41 ± 2.32 μM) were assigned a value of 100%. Each point represents the mean ± SE. △, $p < 0.05$; * $p < 0.01$

increase in the relative volume of distribution of alcohol in SAM-treated subjects. These data, even if obtained in acute conditions, might explain in part the protective effect of SAM on alcohol-induced fatty liver degeneration.

References

Boelsterli UA, Rakhit G, Balazs T (1983) Modulation by S-adenosyl-L-methionine of hepatic Na^+, K^+-ATPase, membrane fluidity, and bile flow in rats with ethinyl estradiol-induced cholestasis. Hepatology 3: 12–17

Di Padova C, Tritapepe R, Rovagnati P, Bessone E, Di Padova F (1982) Effect of ethanol on biliary unconjugated bilirubin and its implication in pigment gallstone pathogenesis in humans. Digestion 24: 112–117

Fiaccadori F, Di Padova C, Ghinelli F, Magnani G, Pelosi G, Sacchini D (1982) Effects of S-adenosyl-L-methionine (SAM) on alcoholic liver disease in humans. Hepatology 2: 179

Hirayama C, Kishimoto Y, Wakushima T, Murawaki Y (1983) Mechanism of the protective action of thiol compounds in ethanol-induced liver injury. Biochem Pharmacol 32: 321–325

Kenney WC (1980) Interaction of acetaldehyde with phospholipids. Gastroenterology 79: 1030

Pascale R, Pirisi L, Daino L, Frassetto S, Zanetti S, La Spina V, Garcea R, Chiandussi L, Bartoli E, Feo F (1982) Role of transmethylase pathway in alcoholic liver steatosis. Gastroenterol Clin Biol 6: 823–824

Pezzoli C, Galli-Kienle M, Di Padova C, Stramentinoli G (1984) HPLC method for the evaluation of blood acetaldehyde without ethanol interference. L Liquid Chromatogr 7: 765

Schreiber AJ, Warren G, Sutherland E, Simon FR (1983) Enhancement of taurocholate secretory maximum: S-adenosyl-methionine (SAM)-induced cytoprotection. Clin Res 31: 86A

Shaw S, Jayatilleke E, Ross WA, Gordon ER, Lieber CS (1981) Ethanol-induced lipid peroxidation: potentiation by long-term alcohol feeding and attenuation by methionine. J Lab Clin Med 98: 417–424

Disease, Metabolism and Reproduction in the Toxic Response to Drugs and Other Chemicals
Arch. Toxicol., Suppl. 7, 243–248 (1984)

Metabolic Activation of 2-Aminofluorene in the Salmonella Mutagenicity Assay by Different S-9 Preparations

G. Cantelli Forti[1], M. E. Fracasso[2], P. Hrelia[1], R. Leone[2], M. S. Venturini[2], and M. C. Guerra[1]

[1] Institute of Pharmacology, University of Bologna, Via Irnerio 48, 40126 Bologna, Italy
[2] Institute of Pharmacology, University of Verona, Policlinico Borgo Roma, 37100 Verona, Italy

Abstract. Before exerting a carcinogenic or mutagenic effect, many chemicals must undergo metabolic activation. The most widely used activation system is the 9,000 *g* supernatant fraction (S-9) of rat liver homogenate, prepared from male rats pretreated with Aroclor 1254 (AC). The present study compares the capabilities to induce metabolic activation of 2-aminofluorene (2-AF), using different sources of S-9 preparations as a test-promutagen, both in the Ames test and in the minimal saline liquid medium (MSLM). In particular, S-9 preparations of liver and kidney fractions from male rats and guinea pigs, with or without AC or phenobarbital (PB) pretreatment, were used. The 2-AF was tested in *Salmonella typhimurium* TA 1538 strain (frame-shift mutation) at different level of concentrations. In the Ames test the enzymatic activation of liver fractions, induced by PB, shows a large increase of mutagenicity of 2-AF in both animal species studied. The AC pretreatment in rats significantly reduced the mutagenic activity of 2-AF, when compared with controls. With rat renal microsomes no differences were observed in mutagenicity as compared with controls. A significant increase was seen in the microsomes of guinea pigs pretreated with AC. The experiments carried out with MSLM confirmed the results in full.

Key words: 2-Aminofluorene – Mutagenicity – *Salmonella typhimurium* assay – Metabolic activation – Guinea pig – Rat – Liver – Kidney – S-9 Fraction

Aromatic amines, such as 2-acetylaminofluorene (2-AAF) and 2-aminofluorene (2-AF), are well known to be potent carcinogens and mutagens. In particular 2-AAF is generally used in genotoxicity tests as a standard compound of the aromatic amine group (Miller and Miller 1979). Since they are promutagens,

Abbreviations. 2-AF, 2-aminofluorene; 2-AAF, 2-acetylaminofluorene; PB, sodium phenobarbital; AC, Aroclor 1254; C, uninduced control; MSLM, minimal saline liquid medium

they require metabolic activation in vitro in order to show their activity (Guenthner and Oesch 1981). The first step in the metabolic activation involves the oxidation of the arylamino group to the N-hydroxy-derivative by cytochrome P-450-dependent mixed-function oxidase (Thorgeirsson et al. 1973). Several studies have shown that the ultimate carcinogen(s) is represented by one or more of the metabolites of the N-hydroxy-derivative, rather than the compound itself (Mulder and Hinson 1977). This metabolic process occurs mainly in the liver, where enzyme systems such as sulfotransferase(s), deacetylase(s), trans-acetylase(s) and UDP-glucuronyl-transferase(s) are involved in the conversion of the N-hydroxy-derivative to various reactive electrophiles (Mulder and Hinson 1977; Schut et al. 1978). However the nature of the ultimate carcinogen(s) is still unclear.

Durston and Ames (1974) have found in *Salmonella typhimurium* TA 1538, a frame-shift strain, that N-hydroxy-2-AF is 200–300 times more mutagenic than N-hydroxy-2-AAF. Schut et al. (1978) have indicated that deacetylation is the most important step in the mutagenic activation of N-hydroxy-2-AAF by liver and kidney fraction in mouse and rat. The arylnitrenium ion is the electrophilic species which interacts with the bacterial DNA, resulting in the frame-shift mutation (Schut et al. 1978).

By using the most mutagenic compound 2-AF, in this laboratory a comparative study has been carried out on the enzymatic activation capabilities, related to the genetic polymorphism of several mammalian species, including man. In the present work the differences between 9,000 *g* supernatant preparation (S-9) from liver and kidney of rats and guinea pigs, both with or without Aroclor 1254 (AC) or phenobarbital (PB) pretreatment have been determined.

Materials and Methods

Chemicals. 2-AF was obtained from Aldrich Chemical Co. (U.K.), AC from Analabs, Inc. (USA) and PB from Carlo Erba Pharmaceutical Co. (Italy). All chemicals and solvents were reagent grade.

Animals. Male Sprague-Dawley rats (200–220 g body weight; Nossan, Italy) and male guinea pigs (300–350 g b. w.; derived in our laboratories), were used in the preparation of liver and kidney S-9 fractions. Some animals were injected intraperitoneally (i.p.) once with AC suspended in corn oil (500 mg/kg b. w.) 5 days before the sacrifice (Thompson et al. 1980); others were injected i.p. with PB dissolved in 0.15 M NaCl (80 mg/kg b. w.) every 24 h for 3 days and killed 24 h after the last injection (Cantelli Forti and Trieff 1980).

Microbial Test System for Mutagenicity. The test procedures were performed as described by Ames et al. (1975), utilizing the *Salmonella typhimurium* strain TA 1538, the most sensitive strain to aromatic amines. The metabolic activation of 2-AF was performed by adding to the plate various S-9 fractions prepared according to Ames et al. (1975). The protein content of the S-9 preparations was determined colorimetrically (Lowry et al. 1951). Dose-response studies with varying concentrations of 2-AF (0.25, 0.5, 1, and 2 μg/plate) and a fixed S-9 protein concentration of 1 mg/plate were performed, using liver and kidney preparations from uninduced or induced male rats and guinea pigs. In addition, preliminary experiments had been performed in minimal saline liquid medium (MSLM) to determine the influence of the various S-9 fractions on the rate of the bacterial development. A 16 h fresh culture of *Salmonella typhimurium* strain TA 1538 (0.1 ml) was incubated in 5 ml of MSLM containing 4 μg of 2-AF and 0.5 ml (1 mg protein) of various S-9 preparations. At several intervals of time the rate of the bacterial development was determined by means of a spectrophotometer at 545 nm (Cantelli Forti et al. 1983, manuscript in preparation).

Results

The mutagenicity of 2-AF activated by liver microsomes (S-9 preparations) from rat and guinea pig, both uninduced (C) and induced with PB or AC, is demonstrated in Fig. 1. All S-9 preparations examined, in both animal species at all the tested concentrations, have produced metabolic activation of 2-AF. In particular, the PB treatment is able to induce, in the rat liver, enzymatic activities such as to increase the 2-AF mutagenicity up to that of C. This is especially true at doses of 0.5 and 1 μg/plate ($p < 0.05$) and 2 μg/plate

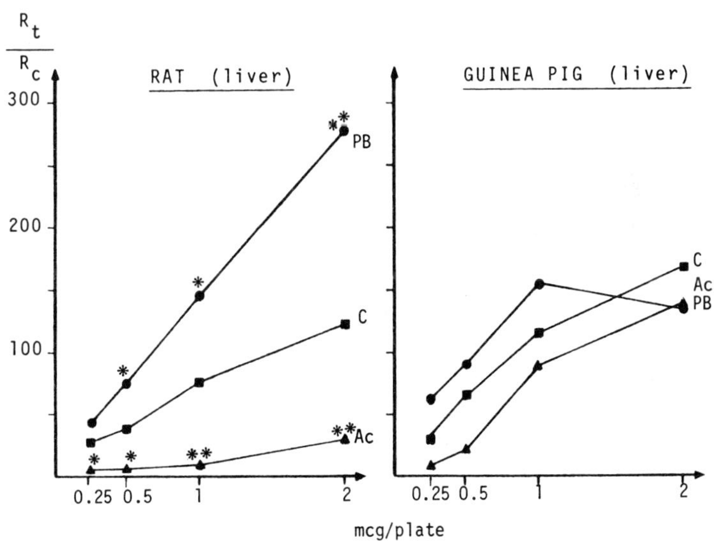

Fig. 1. Effect of several 2-aminofluorene concentrations on mutagenic response of the *Salmonella typhimurium* strain 1538 in the presence of uninduced (■–■ *C*), phenobarbital-induced (●–● *PB*), and Aroclor 1254-induced (▲–▲ *AC*) S-9 liver preparations from male rats and guinea pigs. R_t/R_c is the ratio of the number of revertants on treated plates to the number of spontaneous revertants on control plates. * Different ($p < 0.05$) from control value (independent *t*-test). ** Different ($p < 0.01$) from control value (independent *t*-test).

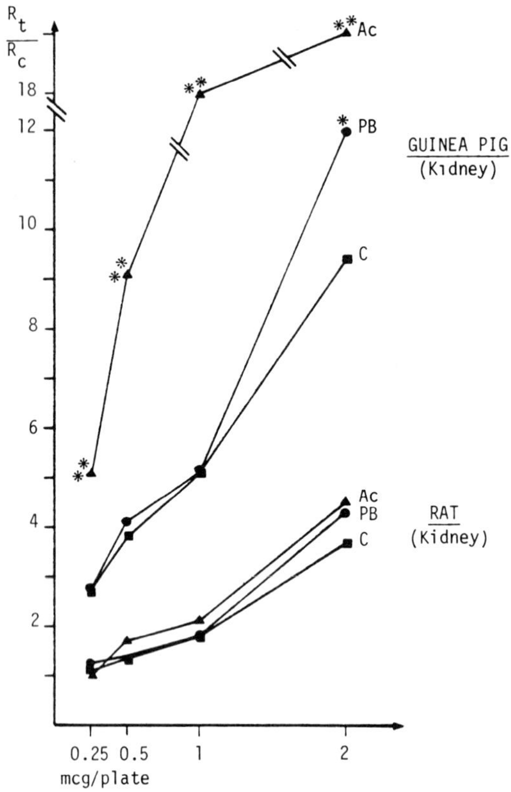

Fig. 2. Effect of several 2-aminofluorene concentrations on mutagenic response of the *Salmonella typhimurium* strain 1538 in the presence of uninduced (■–■ *C*), phenobarbital-induced (●–● *PB*), and Aroclor 1254-induced (▲–▲ *AC*) S-9 kidney preparations from male rats and guinea pigs. R_t/R_c is the ratio of the number of revertants on treated plates to the number of spontaneous revertants on control plates. * Different ($p < 0.05$) from control value (independent *t*-test). ** Different ($p < 0.01$) from control value (independent *t*-test)

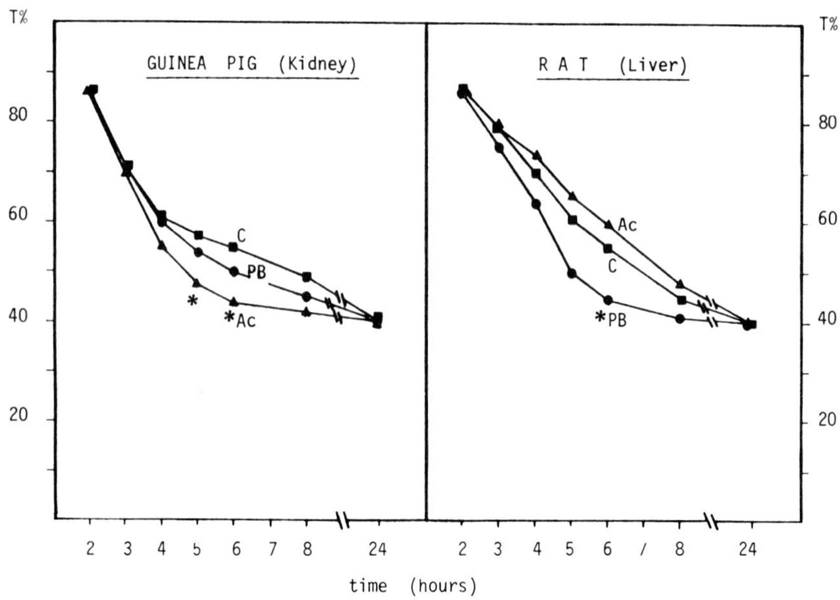

Fig. 3. Rate of development of *Salmonella typhimurium* strain 1538 (0.1 ml) in 5 ml MSLM in presence of 2-aminofluorene (4 μg) and uninduced (■–■ *C*), phenobarbital-induced (●–● *PB*), and Aroclor 1254-induced (▲–▲ *AC*) S-9 preparations (1 mg protein) from male rats and guinea pigs. * Different ($p < 0.05$) from control value (independent *t*-test)

($p < 0.01$). On the contrary the AC treatment significantly reduced the metabolic activation of the test compound.

The mutagenicity observed with guinea pig liver preparations seems to be also increased by PB treatment and decreased by AC treatment, but the results are not significantly different.

The data from the metabolic activation of 2-AF with kidney S-9 preparations are reported in Fig. 2. In rat, no difference in the mutagenic response is provoked by enzymatic induction with either PB or AC. In guinea pigs, PB was not different from C up to 1 μg/plate dose. On the other hand, there was a significant increase in mutagenic activity ($p < 0.01$), when kidney microsomes from AC treated animals were used. These results, obtained in the Ames test, were confirmed by experiments later performed on bacteria development rate in MSLM. Fig. 3 shows that kidney microsomes of guinea pigs treated with AC, and liver microsomes of rats treated with PB, increase significantly the rate of development of *Salmonella typhimurium* strain TA 1538, while a decrease is observed with liver microsomes of rats treated with AC.

Discussion

In Ames test 2-AF is a potent mutagen even at very low concentration (0.25 μg/plate), when it is incubated with microsomal preparations from liver and kidney of both rat and guinea pig, with or without PB or AC enzymatic induction. These results show that the metabolic activation of 2-AF to mutagenic product(s) is more evident with liver microsomes than that with kidney microsomes.

However, guinea pig kidney microsomes produce a greater mutagenic response than that from rat, especially after AC treatment. The toxicity of 2-AF is more enhanced by PB enzymatic induction in the liver rather than in the kidney. This result, moreover, is in agreement with the data of Rush and Hook (1981) and Kuo et al. (1982). On the other hand, AC induction seems to decrease the metabolic activation capability of liver microsomes, as also reported by Schut et al. (1978). All these results have been confirmed by means of a simple procedure in MSLM. In particular, the procedure gives the opportunity, during the incubation period, to follow the interaction between the activated metabolite(s) and the bacterial auxotroph cells. In fact, the rate of development depends upon the number of revertants which are able to grow in MSLM. At the present time, by combining this procedure and HPLC assay, the relationship between the metabolic fractions determined at selected times and the density of the bacterial cells are being studied.

Acknowledgments. This work was supported by the National Research Council of Italy (CNR) on the "Progetto Finalizzato Medicina Preventiva e Riabilitativa, sottoprogetto Rischio Tossicologico".

References

Ames BN, McCann J, Yamasaki E (1975) Methods for detecting carcinogens and mutagens with the Salmonella/mammalian microsome mutagenicity test. Mutat Res 31: 347–364

Cantelli Forti G, Trieff NM (1980) Kinetics of uptake and biliary excretion of Benzo(α)pyrene and mutagenic metabolites in isolated perfused rat liver. Teratog Carcinog Mutagen 1 : 269–282

Durston WE, Ames BN (1974) A simple method for the detection of mutagens in urine: studies with the carcinogen 2-acetylaminofluorene. Proc Natl Acad Sci USA 71 : 737–741

Guenthner TM, Oesch F (1981) Metabolic activation and inactivation of chemical mutagens and carcinogens. Trends in Pharmacological Sciences 2 : 129–132

Kuo CH, Rush GF, Hook SB (1982) Renal cortical accumulation of phenobarbital in rats and rabbits: lack of correlation with induction of renal microsomal monoxygenases. J Pharmacol Exp Ther 220 : 547–551

Lowry WO, Nira J, Rosebrough J, Lewis F, Randall JR (1951) Protein measurement with the Folin phenol reagent. J Biol Chem 193 : 265–275

Miller JA, Miller EC (1979) Risk evaluation and mechanisms. In: Emmelot P, Krien E (eds) Environmental carcinogenesis occurrence. Elsevier/North Holland, Amsterdam, pp 25–50

Mulder JC, Hinson AJ (1977) Role of sulfotransferase from rat liver in the mutagenicity of N-hydroxy-2-acetylaminofluorene in Salmonella typhimurium. Biochem Pharmacol 26 : 1356–1358

Rush G, Hook GB (1981) Differential induction of hepatic and renal cytochrome P-450 by β-naphtoflavone, phenobarbital and polybrominated biphenyls in the rat and rabbit. Pharmacologist 23 : 169

Schut HAS, Wirth PJ, Thorgeirsson SS (1978) Mutagenic activation of N-hydroxy-2-acetylaminofluorene in the Salmonella test system: the role of deacetylation by liver and kidney fraction from mouse and rat. Mol Pharmacol 14 : 682–692

Thompson CZ, Whitaker GW, McMahon RE (1980) Effect of Aroclor 1254 dose upon S-9 activation of aromatic amine bacterial mutagens. Mutat Res 77 : 361–366

Thorgeirsson SS, Jollow DJ, Sasame HA, Green I, Mitchell JR (1973) The role of cytochrome P-450 in N-hydroxylation of 2-acetylaminofluorene. Mol Pharmacol 9 : 398–404

Disease, Metabolism and Reproduction in the Toxic Response to Drugs and Other Chemicals
Arch. Toxicol., Suppl. 7, 249–252 (1984)

Reduction of Covalent Binding of Aflatoxin B_1 to Rabbit Liver DNA After Immunization Against this Carcinogen

M. Caviezel, A. P. Aeschbach, W. K. Lutz, and C. Schlatter

Institute of Toxicology, ETH and University of Zürich, 8603 Schwerzenbach, Switzerland

Abstract. The covalent binding of [^{3}H]aflatoxin B_1 (AF) to liver DNA was determined, 6 h after oral administration to male rabbits. A Covalent Binding Index, CBI (μmol AF/mol DNA-P)/(mmol AF/kg b. w.) = 8,500 was found. Pretreatment of rabbits with AF coupled to bovine serum albumin in Freund's adjuvant led to the production of AF-directed antibodies. Administration of [^{3}H]AF to such immunized rabbits resulted in a CBI of only 2,500, i.e., the immunization provided a protection by a factor of more than 3. Although this is encouraging evidence for the potential of active immunization against genotoxic carcinogens, a number of points will have to be clarified, such as the time course for the DNA binding and the question of a possible shift to other target cells.

Key words: Aflatoxin – Cancer prevention – Carcinogen – Covalent binding – DNA – Immunization

Introduction

Most genotoxic carcinogens are believed to exert their activity via covalent interaction with the DNA of the target cell (Lutz 1979). In addition to this reaction with nucleic acids, reaction with protein always occurs, in most cases to an even higher degree. Since protein-carcinogen adducts are potentially immunogenic, an immune response can result with the bound carcinogen acting as a hapten (Moolten et al. 1981). It was the aim of this study to determine whether immunization of rabbits against the hepatocarcinogen aflatoxin B_1 (AF) can result in a reduction of liver DNA binding exerted by a subsequent AF dose, due to a reduction by antibodies of carcinogen available for the uptake by liver cells.

Materials and Methods

Chemicals. Generally tritiated aflatoxin B_1 (AF), specific activity 16 Ci/mmol, was obtained from Moravek Biochemical (Brea CA, USA). The radiochemical purity was > 96% as checked by thin layer chromatography. All other chemicals were obtained from Merck (Darmstadt, F.R.G.) or Fluka AG (Buchs, Switzerland) and were of analytical grade.

Animals and Treatments. Adult male rabbits (Swiss rabbit, 3–3.5 kg, Hoffmann-La Roche, Basel) were immunized according to Nieschlag et al. (1975) with bovine serum albumin-AF conjugate prepared by the method described by Chu and Ueno (1977). [^{3}H]AF was administered orally in a gelatine capsule, filled by dropping 100 µl of an ethanol solution of AF onto lactose. After 6 h, the rabbits were killed by an overdose of Nembutal and the livers were excised.

Antibody Titer. Diluted serum taken from immunized rabbits and incubated with 2 nM [^{3}H]AF resulted in a 79% AF-binding at a titer of 1 : 500. Control serum used 1 : 10 gave rise to a background value of 1.7% [^{3}H]AF precipitation with anti-rabbit antiserum.

DNA Isolation. DNA was isolated immediately from 10 g of the left posterior lobe of the liver. A crude chromatin fraction was prepared at 4° C by a slightly modified method described by Yaneva and Dessev (1976). The further purification of the DNA from chromatin followed the standard method used in this laboratory which is based on a deproteination with phenol : chloroform : isoamyl alcohol and a hydroxyapatite column chromatography (Markov and Ivanov 1974). After dialysis against 0.2 M NaCl, DNA was precipitated with ethanol and dissolved in 10 mM Tris buffer pH 7.0. Repetitive redissolving of the DNA and precipitation with ethanol did not result in a decrease of the specific activity. Acid degradation of DNA and HPLC analysis of the purines revealed no measurable radioactivity co-eluting with the natural bases. It can therefore be assumed that no radiolabel was incorporated into DNA via biosynthesis. The amount of DNA was determined assuming an absorbance of 20 at 260 nm for a solution of 1 mg/ml (Viviani and Lutz 1978). An aliquot of the highly purified DNA (< 0.1% protein) was used for radioactivity counting in a Packard 460 CD after addition of 10 ml Insta-Gel (Packard).

Enzyme Assay. Cytochrome P-450 dependent mono-oxygenase in liver microsomes was determined with the gas chromatography (GC) assay of aldrin epoxidation as described by Wolff et al. (1979).

Results

Six hours after the oral administration of [^{3}H]AF to immunized and non-immunized rabbits, the concentration of the radiolabel was slightly lower in the livers of the immunized animals, but two to four times higher in the blood (Table 1). This difference could be due to antibodies keeping the AF molecules in the circulation for a longer period of time, thereby reducing the concentration of AF diffusible into liver cells.

Table 1. Covalent binding of aflatoxin B_1 to rabbit liver DNA, 6 h after oral administration of [^{3}H]labelled AF to AF-immunized and control animals

	Immunized		Control	
Body weight (kg)	2.90	3.40	3.40	3.08
AF Dose administered (ng/kg)	110	94	94	104
(10^7 dpm/kg)	1.25	1.07	1.07	1.18
[^{3}H] Activity in				
Blood[a] (% of dose)	7.4	4.2	2.0	1.9
Liver (% of dose)	0.5	0.5	0.9	0.9
Kidney (% of dose)	0.05	0.05	0.07	0.07
Liver DNA				
Total isolated (mg)	5.0	4.6	5.7	4.5
Amount in scint. vial (mg)	1.06	1.07	1.17	0.99
Total activity (cpm)	51.3	59.9	98.7	161.0
Specific activity[b] (dpm/mg)	71	113	204	428
Covalent binding index[c]	1,755	3,263	5,891	11,208
Mean	2,509		8,550	

[a] The amount of whole blood was assumed to represent 7% of the body weight

[b] The calculation of net radioactivity is based on background activities of 19.6 ± 1.54 cpm determined with DNA samples isolated from a control rabbit which had not been given radiolabels

[c] Conversion of the experimentally available data, CBI′ = (dpm/mg DNA)/(dpm/kg b.w.) to the CBI is done by multiplication with $3.09 \cdot 10^8$. CBI = (μmol chemical bound/mol DNA-P)/(mmol chemical applied/kg b.w.) (Lutz 1979)

This hypothesis is supported by the data on liver DNA binding (Table 1). On average, the immunization reduced the CBI by a factor of 3.4, i.e., provided a substantial protection from the genotoxicity exerted by AF, 6 h after oral administration.

A determination of the aldrin epoxidase activity in liver microsomes revealed no difference between the two groups of animals. The specific enzyme activities were 2.52 and 2.43 nmol dieldrin formed per min and per mg microsomal protein isolated from the immunized rabbits, whereas the control values were 2.14 and 2.22. This assay has been shown to measure cytochrome P-450-type activity (Wolff et al. 1979) which also generates the aflatoxin-2,3-oxide (Kawajiri et al. 1980) thought to be the most important electrophilic metabolite responsible for DNA binding (Lin et al. 1977). It is therefore unlikely that the immunization gave rise to changes in enzyme levels which, in turn, could have resulted in the observed difference in DNA binding.

Discussion

Covalent binding of aflatoxin B_1 to liver DNA of various animal species has been shown to reflect their susceptibility for liver tumor formation (Lutz et al. 1980). Since non-immunized rabbits gave rise to a CBI of almost 10,000 they could be about as susceptible as rats for which CBI of 10,000 has been reported (Lutz et al. 1980). The decrease of the CBI to 2,500 after immunization indicates some type of protection, but it would be premature to postulate this as a general phenomenon.

Firstly, the concentration of circulating antibody must be large enough to bind most of the dose administered. This condition was met in the present experiment by choosing a very low dose of AF.

Secondly, the scavenging of the AF molecules by antibodies obeys the laws of chemical complex formation equilibria and it is conceivable that AF is slowly released from the antibody binding site in parallel with the metabolism of the free fraction in the liver. It cannot, therefore, be excluded at present, that the damage to liver DNA is lowered only in the first hours and that the important damage $\times$ time integral will not be reduced by immunization.

Thirdly, it is possible that the DNA damage in the liver is indeed lower but that other cells take up more AF so that other tissue might become a target for AF-induced tumor formation.

Future work will have to elucidate whether the protection observed under the present experimental conditions will be real or whether it will be diminished by one or the other drawbacks mentioned above.

Acknowledgments: We thank Drs. A. von Däniken for the determination of antibody titers, and K. Frei for performing the aldrin epoxidase assay.

References

Chu FS, Ueno I (1977) Production of antibody against aflatoxin B_1. Appl Environ Microbiol 33: 1125–1128

Kawajiri K, Yonekawa H, Harada N, Noshiro M, Omura T, Tagashira Y (1980) Immunochemical study on the role of different types of microsomal cytochrome P-450 in mutagenesis by chemical carcinogens. Cancer Res 40: 1652–1657

Lin J-K, Miller JA, Miller EC (1977) 2,3-Dihydro-2-(guan-7-yl)-3-hydroxyaflatoxin B_1, a major acid hydrolysis product of aflatoxin B_1-DNA or -ribosomal RNA adducts formed in hepatic microsome-mediated reactions and in rat liver in vivo. Cancer Res 37: 4430–4438

Lutz WK (1979) In vivo covalent binding of organic chemicals to DNA as a quantitative indicator in the process of chemical carcinogenesis. Mutat Res 65: 289–356

Lutz WK, Jaggi W, Lüthy J, Sagelsdorff P, Schlatter C (1980) In vivo covalent binding of aflatoxin B_1 and aflatoxin M_1 to liver DNA of rat, mouse and pig. Chem Biol Interact 32: 249–256

Markov GG, Ivanov IG (1974) Hydroxyapatite column chromatography in procedures for isolation of purified DNA. Anal Biochem 59: 555–563

Moolten FL, Schreiber B, Rizzone A, Weiss AJ, Boger E (1981) Protection of mice against 7,12-dimethylbenz(a)anthracene-induced skin tumors by immunization with a fluorinated analog of the carcinogen. Cancer Res 41: 425–429

Nieschlag E, Kley HK, Usadel KH (1975) Production of steroid antisera in rabbits. In: Cameron EHD, Hillier SG, Griffiths K (eds) Steroid immunoassay. Alpha Omega, Cardiff, U.K., pp 87–96

Viviani A, Lutz WK (1978) Modulation of the binding of the carcinogen benzo[a]pyrene to rat liver DNA in vivo by selective induction of microsomal and nuclear aryl hydrocarbon hydroxylase activity. Cancer Res 38: 4640–4644

Wolff T, Deml E, Wanders H (1979) Aldrin epoxidation, a highly sensitive indicator specific for cytochrome P-450 dependent mono-oxygenase activities. Drug Metab Dispos 7: 301–305

Yaneva M, Dessev G (1976) Isolation and properties of structured chromatin from Guerin ascites tumor and rat liver. Eur J Biochem 66: 535–542

Disease, Metabolism and Reproduction in the Toxic Response to Drugs and Other Chemicals
Arch. Toxicol., Suppl. 7, 253–255 (1984)

Inactivation of 2-Amino-3-methyl-imidazo(4,5-f)quinoline by Horse Radish and Intestinal Peroxidase

P. Dolara, G. Caderni, and M. Lodovici

Institute of Pharmacology and Toxicology, University of Florence,
Viale Morgagni 65, 50134 Florence, Italy

Abstract. A dietary mutagen, 2-amino-3-methyl-imidazo(4,5-f)quinoline (IQ) was incubated with preparations of horse radish peroxidase and rat intestinal mucosa peroxidase, and the residual mutagenic activity was determined by means of the Salmonella-microsome assay, using strain TA 98 with metabolic activation. Horse radish peroxidase diminished but did not abolish the mutagenic activity. Preparations of intestinal mucosa completely abolished the mutagenic activity. Protein binding and metabolic inactivation are responsible for the variations of IQ mutagenic activity.

Key words: Dietary mutagens – Horse radish peroxidase – Intestinal peroxidase – Metabolism of mutagens – 2-amino-3-methyl-imidazo-(4,5-f)quinoline

A series of mutagenic and carcinogenic components are formed during the cooking of different protein foods (Shelby and Matsushima 1981). These compounds are potent mutagens after metabolic activation. However, neither the activation patterns nor the detoxification in vivo have been defined so far. A previous paper (Yamada et al. 1979) reported that many compounds of this group are inactivated by myeloperoxidase, lactoperoxidase, and horse radish peroxidase. The effect of horse radish peroxidase and of intestinal peroxidase on the mutagenic activity of 2-amino-3-methyl(4,5-f)quinoline (IQ), which is present in cooked fish and beef extract (Shelby and Matsushima 1981) was determined.

Horse radish peroxidase (type VII acidic isoenzyme) was obtained from Sigma. Rat intestinal preparations were obtained by scraping the mucosa from rat small intestines, suspending it 1 : 4 in 0.25 M sucrose and homogenizing it with a glass-teflon homogenizer. The homogenate was centrifuged at 2,000 $g \times$ 20 min, and the pellet, after resuspension, was again centrifuged at 2,000 $g \times 20$ min. The supernatants were pelleted at 22,000 $g \times 30$ min, and, after

---

Abbreviations. IQ, 2-amino-3-methyl-imidazo(4,5-f)quinoline

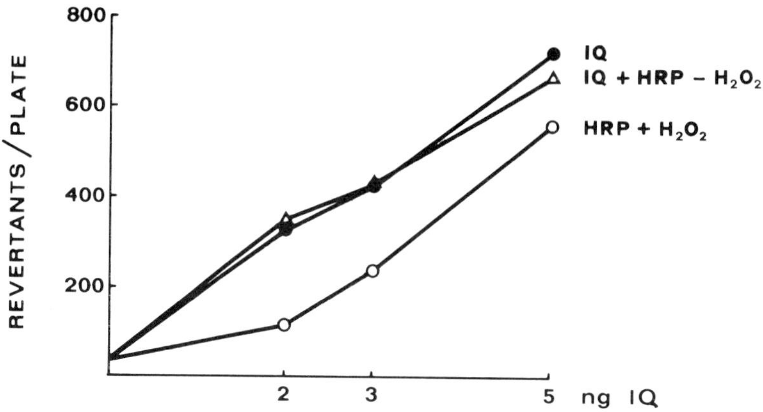

Fig. 1. Mutagenic activity of IQ on *Salmonella typhimurium* strain TA 98 with PCB induced rat liver S-9. Different concentrations of IQ were incubated for 1 h alone or with 16 mU of peroxidase

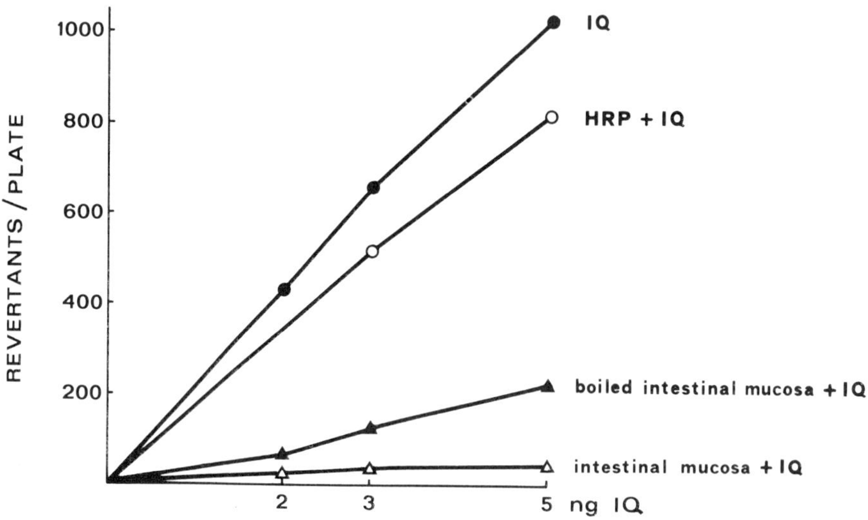

Fig. 2. Mutagenic activity of IQ on strain TA 98 with S-9 incubated alone or with 12 mU of horse radish peroxidase or 12 mU of peroxidase from the intestinal mucosa. One determination was obtained with boiled intestinal mucosa preparations

resuspension in an equal volume of 0.1 M Tris-HCl buffer pH 7.1, were kept for 2 h at pH 11, centrifuged at 38,000 $g \times 60$ min, finally brought back to pH 7.4, filtered through a millipore 0.45 μm for sterilization and used in the incubation experiments. Enzymatic activity was measured spectrophotometrically at 470 nm as described elsewhere (Sgaragli et al. 1980). After 1 h of incubation the samples containing IQ were tested with *Salmonella typhimurium* strain TA 98 with PCB induced rat liver S-9 fraction (Ames et al. 1975).

Figure 1 shows that horse radish peroxidase was capable of decreasing the mutagenic activity of IQ but not of abolishing it, and only in the presence of

H_2O_2. Figure 2 shows that intestinal mucosa preparations with an equivalent peroxidase activity were able to abolish the mutagenic activity of IQ at all doses tested. The addition of H_2O_2 was in this case not necessary; but H_2O_2 can be produced by intestinal mucosa. The inactivation in the absence of external hydrogen peroxide is therefore, not sufficient to exclude the importance of peroxidase in this process. However, Fig. 2 also shows that intestinal preparations boiled for 5 min with no residual peroxidase activity still cause a marked decrease of IQ mutagenic activity. This result shows that some protein components of the intestinal mucosa bind IQ so tightly that it is no longer available to exert all its mutagenic effects.

The observed inactivation of IQ by native preparations of intestinal mucosa seems to be a combined result of protein binding and enzymatic inactivation. Both processes are probably relevant in vivo, since these compounds are normally present in foods containing proteins and are absorbed through the intestinal mucosa.

Acknowledgements. This work was supported by a grant from MPI and from CNR (finalized project: Control of Toxicological Risk). We thank Dr. L. Della Corte for help and suggestions in the preparation of intestinal peroxidase, and Dr. T. Sugimura for the gift of IQ.

References

Ames BN, McCann J, Yamasaki E (1975) Methods for detecting carcinogens and mutagens with the Salmonella-mammalian/microsome mutagenicity test. Mutat Res 31: 347–364

Sgaragli G, Della Corte L, Puliti R, De Sarlo F, Francalanci R, Guarna A, Dolara P, Komarynsky M (1980) Oxidation of BHA by horse radish and mammalian peroxidase systems. Biochem Pharmacol 29: 763–769

Shelby MD, Matsushima T (1981) Mutagens and carcinogens in the diet and digestive tract. Mutat Res 85: 177–183

Yamada M, Tsuda M, Nagao M, Mori M, Sugimura T (1979) Degradation of mutagens from pyrolysates of tryptophan, glutamic acid and globulin by myeloperoxidase. Biochem Biophys Res Commun 90: 769–776

Disease, Metabolism and Reproduction in the Toxic Response to Drugs and Other Chemicals
Arch. Toxicol., Suppl. 7, 256–259 (1984)

The Influence of Two Histamine H_2-Receptor Antagonists, Cimetidine and Ranitidine, on the Plasma Levels and Clinical Effect of Nifedipine and Metoprolol

W. Kirch[1], K. Rämsch[1], H. D. Janisch[2] and E. E. Ohnhaus[1]

[1] Medical Department, University School of Medicine, 4300 Essen, Federal Republic of Germany
[2] Gastroenterological Department, Klinikum Charlottenburg, 1000 Berlin, Federal Republic of Germany

Abstract. In six healthy volunteers pharmacokinetic and pharmacodynamic interaction of metoprolol and nifedipine with cimetidine and ranitidine was investigated after 1 week of monotherapy with nifedipine and metoprolol and after 1 week each of combined treatment of these drugs with the H_2-receptor antagonists. Ranitidine led to a 50% increase in mean peak plasma levels and in the area under the plasma level time curve (AUC) of metoprolol ($p < 0.05$) and to an insignificant 30% rise in these parameters of nifedipine ($p > 0.05$). Cimetidine increased metoprolol's peak plasma levels of AUC by about 60% ($p < 0.05$) and those of nifedipine by 80% ($p < 0.05$). Compared to monotherapy with metoprolol beta blocking activity measured by exercise induced tachycardia was not significantly stronger inhibited under the combined treatment of metoprolol with each of the two H_2-receptor antagonists. On the other hand the antihypertensive effect of nifedipine was significantly increased during concurrent administration of cimetidine in seven hypertensive patients when compared with monotherapy.

Thus pharmacokinetic interaction between cimetidine and nifedipine leads to a clinically relevant pharmacodynamic interference.

Key words: Interaction – H_2-receptor antagonists – Metoprolol – Nifedipine

H_2-receptor antagonists like cimetidine or ranitidine both decrease liver blood flow by about 20%–30% but they differ in their effect on liver enzyme activity (Feely et al. 1981; Henry et al. 1981). Nifedipine and metoprolol are both drugs, which are mainly metabolized by the liver (Lederballe Pedersen et al. 1980; Kirch et al. 1981). Thus an interaction between these two drugs and H_2-receptor antagonists could be expected to occur, possibly leading to adverse effects of metoprolol and nifedipine.

Methods

Six healthy volunteers (mean age 30.2 ± 3.1 years, mean body weight 69.2 ± 4.7 kg ($\bar{X}$ ± SEM)) were treated for 1 week each with metoprolol 100 mg twice daily and nifedipine 10 mg four times daily respectively as monotherapy. Thereupon ranitidine (Zantic) 150 mg was given twice daily for one week concurrently with metoprolol 100 mg twice daily and after an adequate therapy free interval, with nifedipine (Adalat) 10 mg four times daily. The same procedure was performed for cimetidine (Tagamet) 1,000 mg a day combined with the same doses of nifedipine and of metoprolol (Lopresor) each administered for 1 week. Concentrations of metoprolol in plasma and urine were estimated by a fluorodensitometric method (Schäfer et al. 1979) and concentrations of nifedipine by gas chromatographic method (Lederballe Pedersen et al. 1980).

Beta blocking activity of metoprolol was determined by measuring exercise tachycardia, using a placebo, before the study and on the 6th treatment day of each therapy period with metoprolol. Seven hypertensives (WHO stage I and II, 53.4 ± 6.9 years; 71.9 ± 3.6 kg body weight) were treated for 4 weeks with nifedipine 10 mg four times daily as monotherapy, thereafter they were randomized to treatment with nifedipine and ranitidine 150 mg twice daily or nifedipine and cimetidine 1,000 mg a day, each therapy period lasting 2 weeks. All patients were pretreated with placebo for 2 weeks. Blood pressure and pulse frequency were measured in weekly intervals.

Results

H_2-Receptor Antagonists and Metoprolol

Metoprolol is a lipophilic betareceptor blocker which is biotransformed in the liver by more than 80%. Cimetidine increases mean peak plasma levels of metoprolol to 283 ng/ml, compared to 177 ng/ml under monotherapy with the beta blocker ($p < 0.05$). Also the AUC and elimination half life of metoprolol was increased by concurrent administration of cimetidine. Ranitidine leads to a rise of mean peak plasma levels of metoprolol to 266 ng/ml compared with 177 ng/ml under monotherapy with metoprolol. This difference between monotherapy and concurrent administration of ranitidine was not only observed on the first treatment day, but could be seen throughout the whole 1 week of the study period (Fig. 1).

Neither cimetidine, nor ranitidine significantly altered the beta blocking activity of metoprolol measured by exercise induced tachycardia.

H_2-Receptor Antagonists and Nifedipine

Cimetidine also increased mean peak plasma levels of nifedipine by about 80% ($p < 0.05$). An average of 43 ng/ml was reached with nifedipine alone and this

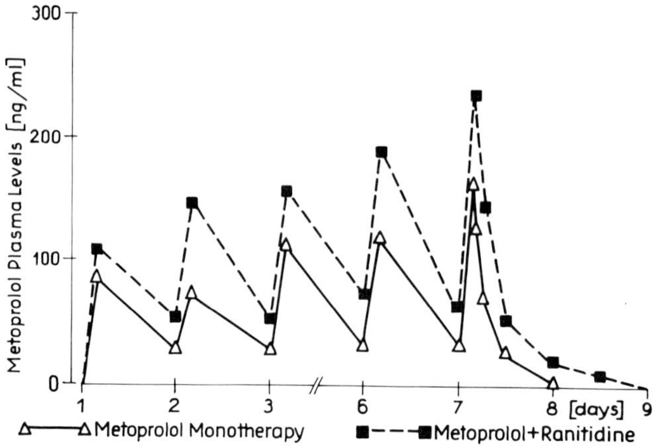

Fig. 1. Metoprolol plasma levels during 1 week monotherapy with 100 mg a day of the beta blocker and during combined treatment of 100 mg metoprolol with 300 mg ranitidine a day

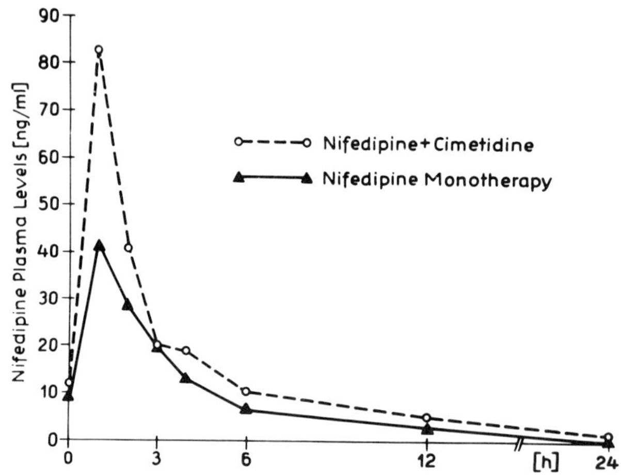

Fig. 2. Nifedipine plasma levels after the last 10 mg dose of this drug in the morning of the seventh monotherapy day and on the morning of the seventh day of treatment of nifedipine together with cimetidine

increased to 87 ng/ml when cimetidine was administered concurrently. The AUC showed similar behaviour: it was 153 ng/ml/h in monotherapy and rose to 245 ng/ml/h under cimetidine ($p < 0.05$; Fig. 2). Ranitidine increased the mean peak plasma levels of nifedipine from 43 ng/ml in nifedipine monotherapy to 53.6 ng/ml when combined with this H_2-receptor antagonists. The AUC was increased to 187 ng/ml/h from 153 ng/ml/h in nifedipine treatment alone ($p > 0.05$).

Mean arterial blood pressure values (MABP) after 4 weeks monotherapy with nifedipine were 109 ± 2.4 mm Hg and fell to 95 ± 3.1 mm Hg when cimetidine was added (MABP = diastolic blood pressure plus $^1/_3$ pulse pressure;

$P < 0.05$). Ranitidine augmented the blood pressure reduction of nifedipine compared with the monotherapy with this calcium channel blocker, but this reduction to 103 ± 3.8 mm Hg was not statistically significant ($p > 0.05$).

Discussion

Pharmacokinetic interaction of cimetidine with nifedipine and metoprolol could be expected, as the two last mentioned drugs are mainly biotransformed in the liver. This kinetic interaction did not, in the case of the beta blocker, result in a pharmacodynamic interaction as the dose response curve of beta blockers becomes very shallow in the upper plasma level ranges of these drugs. In the case of nifedipine, a pharmacodynamic interaction results due to the observed kinetic alterations caused by cimetidine. The blood pressure lowering activity of nifedipine given alone was significantly increased when the drug was administered in combination with cimetidine.

Surprising results were found for ranitidine. This H_2-receptor antagonist was not supposed to influence liver enzyme activity (Henry et al. 1981). However, it also produced a rise in the mean peak plasma levels and the AUC of metoprolol and nifedipine, but the degree of these increases was not as pronounced as with cimetidine. The effect of ranitidine on the plasma levels of both cimetidine or nitedipine did not reach any clinical relevance.

Adverse or toxic effects of the beta blocker or the calcium channel blocker due to concurrent administration of H_2-receptor antagonists could not be observed in this present study.

References

Feely J, Wilkinson GR, Wood AR (1981) Reduction of time blood flow and propranolol metabolism by cimetidine. N Engl J Med 304: 692–695

Henry BA, MacDonald IA, Kitelington G, Bill GD, Longman MJSC (1981) Cimetidine and ranitidine comparison of effects on hepatic drug metabolism. Br Med J 281: 775–777

Kirch W, Köhler H, Spahn H, Mutschler E (1981) Interaction of cimetidine with metoprolol, propranolol or atenolol. Lancet 2: 331–332

Lederballe Pedersen O, Christensen CJ, Mikkelsen E, Rämsch KD (1980) Relationship between the antihypertensive effect and steady-state plasma concentration of nifedipine given alone or in combination with a beta adrenoceptor blocking agent. Eur J Clin Pharmacol 18: 287–293

Schäfer M, Mutschler E (1979) Fluorimetric determination of oxprenolol and metoprolol in plasma by direct evaluation of thin layer chromatograms. J Chromatogr 64: 247–252

Disease, Metabolism and Reproduction in the Toxic Response to Drugs and Other Chemicals
Arch. Toxicol., Suppl. 7, 260 (1984)

Autoradiography of 2,4′,5-Trichlorobiphenyl Mercapturic Acid Indicates the Formation of Methyl Sulphone Metabolites with Selective Affinity for the Bronchial Mucosa

I. Brandt[1], J. Bakke[2], Å. Bergman[3], and P.O. Darnerud[1]

[1] Department of Pharmacology, SLU, Uppsala Biomedical Centre, Uppsala, Sweden
[2] MRRL, State University Station, Fargo, North Dakota, USA
[3] Organic Chemistry, Wallenberg Laboratory, University of Stockholm, Stockholm, Sweden

Abstract. Two isomeric methyl sulphone metabolites are formed from 2,4′,5-trichlorobiphenyl (triCB) in vivo; the 4-methylsulphonyl substituted metabolite is accumulated in the tracheo-bronchial mucosa in mice. The formation of the sulphones has been indicated to proceed via the mercapturic acid pathway (MAP) and involve biliary excretion and further metabolism of MAP metabolites by the intestinal microflora. To investigate whether the triCB mercapturic acid (MA-triCB) is precursor to the triCB methyl sulphones ($MeSO_2$-triCB), two series of female C57Bl mice were i.v. and intracaecally (i.c.) injected with MA-triCB-^{14}C. Autoradiograms obtained 90 min after i.c. injection revealed heavy labelling of the bile and a uniform distribution in the lung with no selective uptake in the bronchial mucosa. At 6 h, a slight accumulation in the tracheo-bronchial mucosa had taken place and at longer post-injection times (24 h to 9 days) the tracheo-bronchial mucosa showed the highest concentration in the body. Similar results were obtained after i.v. injection. Autoradiograms of mice, injected i.v. with 4-$MeSO_2$-triCB-^{14}C, were characterized by heavy labelling of the tracheo-bronchial mucosa at all post-injection times studied (4 h to 30 days). In contrast to MA-triCB-^{14}C, the administration of 4-$MeSO_2$-triCB-^{14}C resulted in low-activity in the bile and intestinal contents. Lung extracts from mice injected with MA-triCB-^{14}C contained radioactive substance, which, similar to PCB methyl sulphones, was soluble in concentrated, but not in diluted H_2SO_4, and it co-chromatographed with $MeSO_2$-triCB on capillary column. The results indicate biliary excretion and entero-hepatic circulation of the mercapturic acid alone or with its degradation products. The formation of sulphones implies cleavage of the mercapturic acid; due to similar distribution patterns in i.v. and i.c. injected mice the experiment does not allow conclusions on whether this took place predominantly in the intestinal microflora or not. Previous studies have shown, however, that the formation of $MeSO_2$-triCB from triCB in germfree mice is minute, although the biliary excretion is pronounced.

Key words: PCB marcapturic acid – PCB methyl sulphone – Bronchial mucosa

Acknowledgment. This research was supported by the Swedish Council for Planning and Coordination of Research and the National Swedish Environment Protection Board.

Disease, Metabolism and Reproduction in the Toxic Response to Drugs and Other Chemicals
Arch. Toxicol., Suppl. 7, 261–265 (1984)

Methadone Affects the Histochemical Pattern of Xenobiotic-Metabolizing Enzymes in the Liver of Pregnant Rats

P. Chieco[2], P. Hrelia[1], S. Candeletti[1], S. Ferri[1], and G. Cantelli Forti[1]

[1] Institute of Pharmacology, University of Bologna, Via Irnerio 48 40126 Bologna, Italy
[2] Institute of Oncology "F. Addarii", USL 28, Viale Ercolani 4/2, 40138 Bologna, Italy

Abstract. Enzyme histochemistry performed on the liver of pregnant and non pregnant rats indicates that methadone (ME) does not cause direct damage to the cells. On the other hand, the enzyme aldehyde dehydrogenase was decreased in the periportal tract of the liver lobule of pregnant rats treated with 10 mg/kg ME for 20 days. NADPH dehydrogenase was increased in the central areas of the liver lobule within 3 days of ME treatment. It is suggested that a derangement of xenobiotic metabolizing enzymes in the liver, as well as in other organs, may be contribute to some of the alterations observed in ME treated animals.

Key words: Methadone – Rat – Histo-cytochemistry – Liver – Aldehyde dehydrogenase – NADPH dehydrogenase – Tribromoethanol

It has been reported that ME slightly increases transaminases in the serum of experimental animals (Needham et al. 1981) and induces several neurological effects in human and animal offspring (Hutchings 1982). It would appear that the mechanisms underlying the toxic action of methadone (ME) are largely unknown and no morphological injury has been reported in organs of subjects exposed to this opiate. A modern histochemical approach has been used to examine the liver for changes in enzymic function.

Materials and Methods

Twenty pregnant and twelve non pregnant female Sprague-Dawley rats (250–300 g; Nossan, Italy), were used throughout this study. The animals received 10 mg/kg l-methadone-HCl (Wellcome) dissolved in distilled water or distilled water alone (controls), via a gastric cannula for 3, 8, and 20 days. The treatment schedule for pregnant animals was such that the last dose was given at

Abbreviations: ME, methadone; ALDH, aldehyde dehydrogenase; NADPH-DH, nicotinamide adenine dinucleotide phosphate dehydrogenase

Table 1. Sleeping time, liver weight, relative activities of ALDH and NADPH-DH in livers of ME treated pregnant rats and matched controls

Length of treatment	n	Sleeping time (min)		Liver weight[a]	ALDH[b] periportal/central	NADPH-DH[c] central/periportal
		Min	Max			
0: controls	6	70	85	3.7 ± 0.1	1.22 ± 0.1	1.4 ± 0.07
3 days	5	0	8	3.8 ± 0.5	1.21 ± 0.07	2.1 ± 0.05[d]
8 days	5	0	30	3.8 ± 0.1	1.27 ± 0.04	1.8 ± 0.3[e]
20 days	4	60	70	3.8 ± 0.1	0.94 ± 0.07[d]	2.5 ± 0.2[d]

[a] Grams/100 g body weight. Mean ± SD

[b] Values are the mean ± SD of the ratios between optical densities in the periportal and in the adjacent central zones of the liver lobule. Measuring diaphragma was 160 μm in diameter. Two wavelength method. For each animal at least 10 periportal tracts and adjacent central zones were measured

[c] As in [b], but the ratios are between central zones and adjacent periportal tracts

[d] Different ($p < 0.01$) from control value (independent t-test)

[e] Different ($p < 0.05$) from control value (independent t-test)

the 20th day of pregnancy. All the animals were anesthetized, 24 h after the last dose, with 10 mg/kg i.p. of tribromoethanol (Avertin, Winthrop) and sacrificed by abdominal aorta exsanguination at the end of the anesthesia. Small pieces of liver were quickly frozen in a mixture of Freon 22-dry ice and 8 μm thick serial sections were cut in a cryostat. Liver damage was checked for by haematoxylin-eosin stain. Intracellular calcium and lipid accumulation were examined respectively with red alizarin and oil red stain (Chieco et al. 1982).To evaluate the functional integrity of the cellular organelles and the oxidative metabolic pathways, a number of enzymatic histochemical reactions were performed on the frozen sections as previously described (Chieco et al. 1982). Aldehyde dehydrogenase (ALDH) and alcohol dehydrogenase activities were determinated at 25° C in a medium containing 1 mM acetaldehyde or 80 mM ethanol as substrate, 1.5 mM nitroblutetrazolium, 1.5 mM NAD, 50 mM phosphate buffer at pH 7.6 and 20% polyvinylalcohol (MW 30,000, Carlo Erba). Endoplasmic reticulum NADPH dehydrogenase (NADPH-DH) was determined in aqueous medium according to Chayen et al. (1973). After incubation, the tissues were fixed in 10% formalin, dehydrated in acetone, clarified in xylene and mounted in Canada balsam. Microdensitometric measurements were done with a Zeiss SF microphotometer. The two-wavelength method of Ornstein (1952) was adopted to correct distributional errors.

Results

The liver of all rats treated with ME was free of morphological damage and did not exhibit calcium or lipid accumulation. Moreover, no differences were observed between the liver of ME treated rats and that of controls for the following enzymes: cell membrane Mg^2 ATPase and 5′nucleotidase, lysosome acid phosphatase, endoplasmic reticulum glucose-6-phosphatase, mitochondria

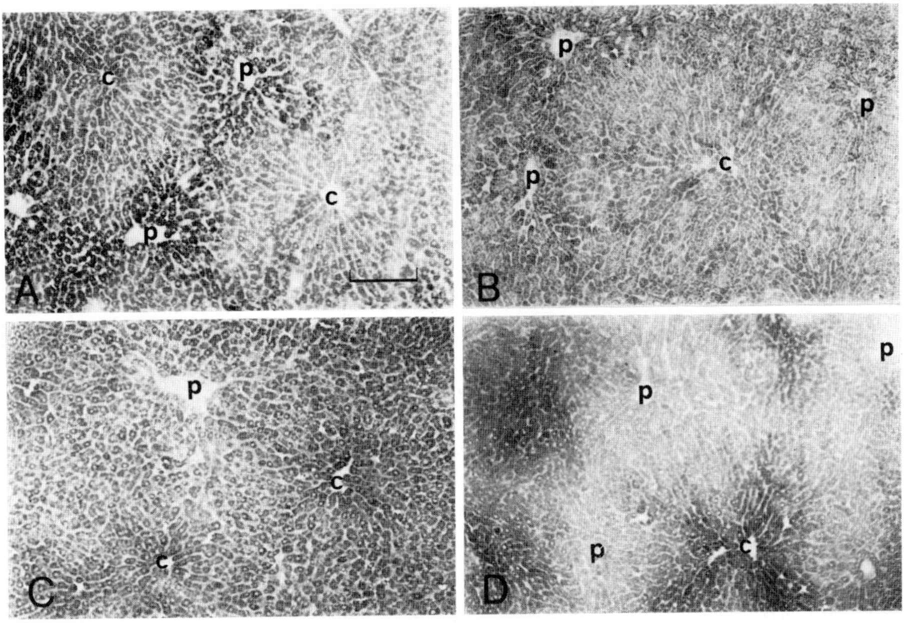

Fig. 1A–D. ALDH and NADPH-DH activities in the liver of 20 days ME treated pregnant rats and matched controls. **A** ALDH, controls; **B** ALDH, treated; **C** NADPH-DH, control; **D** NADPH-DH, treated. It is evident that ALDH is decreased in the periportal tract and that NADPH-DH is increased in the central areas of treated animals. *p* = portal branch; *c* = central vein. Bar = 200 μm. × 45

succinate, glutamate (NAD) and α-glycerophosphate dehydrogenase, cytochrome C and monoamine oxidase, cytosol lactate, malate, α-glycerophosphate (NAD), alcohol, glucose-6-phosphate and 6-phosphogluconate dehydrogenase.

The activities of ALDH and NADPH-DH were altered in the liver of ME treated pregnant rats. Table 1 reports the values obtained by comparing the optical densities of the final reaction product of zone 1 (periportal) and zone 3 (central) of the liver lobule. It is evident that the relative distribution of ALDH changed after 20 days ME treatment, while the relative distribution of NADPH-DH was already affected by a 3-day treatment with ME. It can be observed from Fig. 1 that these changes were due to a decrease in periportal ALDH and to an increase in centrolobular NADPH-DH activities.

An alteration in xenobiotic metabolism is also, suggested by a reduced sensitivity to tribromoethanol anesthesia shown by ME treated pregnant rats. In fact, as reported in Table 1, the sleeping time following tribromoethanol injection was greatly reduced after 3 and 8 days treatment.

Discussion

The reported evidence indicates that ME does not cause direct damage to the liver cells of both pregnant and non pregnant rats. On the other hand the activities of two xenobiotic metabolizing enzymes, ALDH and NADPH-DH, were clearly affected in pregnant rats.

In the histochemical model NADPH-DH has been shown to be a reliable indicator of the endoplasmic reticulum metabolic activity related to the mixed function oxidase (Chayen et al. 1973a). These data, therefore, agree with previous studies showing that ME induces xenobiotic metabolism in rodents (Bellward et al. 1977; Spaulding et al. 1974; Masten et al. 1974).

The stimulation of the mixed function oxidase system may well explain the diminished sensitivity to tribromoethanol anesthesia, shown by pregnant rats treated with ME for 3 and 8 days (Table 1). It is known, in fact, that alcohols can also be metabolized by the NADPH-dependent enzymes bound to the endoplasmic reticulum (Lieber and De Carli 1970). The re-established responsiveness to tribromoethanol after 20 days of ME treatment could be correlated with the concomitant decrease in periportal ALDH (Fig. 1). In fact, an impaired disposition of aldehydes resulting from alcohol oxidation may reverse the reaction equilibrium of cytoplasmic alcohol dehydrogenase and, consequently, decrease the alcohols oxidation rate (Crow et al. 1977).

Therefore, despite the higher activity of the mixed function oxidase system, tribromoethanol elimination from blood would decrease, re-establishing a normal sleeping time.

Acknowledgments. This work was supported by a grant from the Ministry of Education of Italy (MPI).

References

Bellward GD, Gontovnick LS, Otten M (1977) Induction of hepatic aryl hydrocarbon hydroxylase and epoxide hydratase in Wistar rats pretreated with oral methadone hydrochloride. Drug Metab Dispos 5: 211–218

Chayen J, Altman FP, Butcher RG (1973a) The effect of certain drugs on the production and possible utilization of reducing equivalents outside the mitochondria. In: Dikstein S (ed) Fundamentals of cell pharmacology. Thomas, Springfield, pp 196–230

Chayen J, Bitensky L, Butcher R (eds) (1973b) Practical histochemistry. John Wiley, London, pp 210–212

Chieco P, Moslen MT, Reynolds ES (1982) Histochemical evidence that plasma and mitochondrial membranes are primary foci of hepatocellular injury caused by 1,1 dichloroethylene. Lab Invest 46: 413–421

Crow KE, Cornell NW, Veech RL (1977) The rate of ethanol metabolism in isolated rat hepatocytes. Alcoholism: Exp Clin Res 1: 43–47

Hutchings DE (1982) Methadone and heroin during pregnancy: a review of behavioral effects in human and animal offspring. Neurobehav Toxicol Teratol 4: 429–434

Lieber CS, DeCarli LM (1970) Hepatic microsomal ethanol-oxidizing system. J Biol Chem 245: 2505–2512

Masten LW, Peterson GR, Burkhalter A, Way EL (1974) Effect of oral administration of methadone on hepatic microsomal mixed function oxidase activity in mice. Life Sci 14: 1635–1640

Needham WP, Shuster L, Kanel GC, Thompson ML (1981) Liver damage from narcotics in mice. Toxicol Appl Pharmacol 58: 157–170
Ornstein L (1952) The distributional error in microspectrophotometry. Lab Invest 1: 250–262
Spaulding TC, Minium L, Kotake AN, Takemori AE (1974) The effect of diazepam on the metabolism of methadone by the liver of methadone-dependent rats. Drug Metab Dispos 2: 458–463

Disease, Metabolism and Reproduction in the Toxic Response to Drugs and Other Chemicals
Arch. Toxicol., Suppl. 7, 266–267 (1984)

The Effects of Acetylcysteine on Liver Glutathione Depletion and Hepatic Necrosis Induced by Acetaminophen in Mice

M. Losa, L. Bonanomi, and A. Longo

Zambon Farmaceutici S.p.A., Via del Duca, 10, 20091 Bresso (MI), Italy

Abstract. The present study is a part of a large experiment designed to evaluate the protective role of N-acetyl-1-cysteine (NAC) against the toxicity of some xenobiotics. This report deals with the effects of NAC on the development of acetaminophen (NAPA) – induced hepatotoxicity. Adult mice were divided in three groups. Group A (n = 40) received NAPA, 700 mg/kg i.p.; group B (n = 40) received NAPA as group A, followed by 378 mg/kg given orally NAC 1 h later; group C (n = 16) received vehicle alone (control animals). At 6, 24, 48, 72 h after NAPA administration, the surviving mice of group A and B and four control animals were killed. The livers obtained at autopsy were examined grossly and by light microscopy. The tissues were prepared by fixation in Gendre's fluid, embedded in paraffin, sectioned and stained with Hematoxylin and Eosin (H&E) for general morphology. A portion of the right lobe was frozen in isopentane, cut in cryostat sections and stained for glutathione (GSH). Evaluation of GSH content in liver was also performed by HPLC. Liver necrosis was assessed morphologically on H&E sections by the quantitative method of Chalkley. Lethality was expressed as mean ± standard error of the mean. Statistical evaluation was made by χ^2 analysis. NAC administration produces a significant decrease in lethality when compared with animals treated with NAPA alone ($p < 0.005$). Deaths occurred between 4 and 9 h after NAPA administration. At these time intervals histological data clearly indicated that early hepatic lesions, including congestion and centrilobular necrosis, were completely abolished by NAC. These results suggest that the effect of NAC in preventing early mortality is due to the block of hepatic congestion, at least in part. As time goes on, all histological changes become exaggerated and NAC protects from hepatic damage only partially. The disappearance of GSH is strictly linked to the distribution and degree of hepatic necrosis, suggesting a relationship between histological damage and glutathione depletion.

Key words: Acetaminophen – Acetylcysteine – Glutathione – Liver necrosis

References

Boyd EM, Bereczky GM (1966) Liver necrosis from paracetamol. Br J Pharmacol 26: 606–614

Chalkley HW (1943) Method for the quantitative morphologic analysis of tissue. J Natl Cancer Inst 4: 47–53

Davidson DGD, Eastham WN (1966) Acute liver necrosis following overdose of paracetamol. Br Med J 2: 497–499

Hissin PJ, Hilf R (1976) A fluorometric method for determination of oxidized and reduced glutathione in tissue. Ann Biochem 74: 214–226

Mitchell JR, Jollow DJ, Potter WZ, Davis DC, Gillette JR, Brodie BB (1973a) Acetaminophen-induced hepatic necrosis. I. Role of drug metabolism. J Pharmacol Exp Ther 187: 185–194

Mitchell JR, Jollow DJ, Potter WZ, Gillette JR, Brodie BB (1973a) Acetaminophen-induced hepatic necrosis. IV. Protective role of glutathione. J Pharmacol Exp Ther 187: 211–217

Prescott LF, Illingworth RN, Critchley JAJH, Steward MJ, Adam RD, Proudfoot AT (1979) Intravenous N-Acetylcysteine: the treatment of choise for paracetamol poisoning. Br Med J 2: 1097–1100

Walker RM, Massey TE, McElligott TF, Racz WJ (1981) Acetaminophen-induced hypothermia, hepatic congestion, and modification by N-Acetylcysteine in mice. Toxicol Appl Pharmacol 59: 500–507

Disease, Metabolism and Reproduction in the Toxic Response to Drugs and Other Chemicals
Arch. Toxicol., Suppl. 7, 268–271 (1984)

Increased Microsomal Metabolism of n-Hexane in Rat Kidney and Liver After Inhalation of Isopropanol

K. Zahlsen, K. Aarstad, and O. G. Nilsen

Department of Pharmacology and Toxicology, University of Trondheim, 7000 Trondheim, Norway

Abstract. Inhalation of 200, 2,000, and 8,000 ppm isopropanol for 2 weeks enhanced the in vitro metabolism of n-hexane in microsomal preparations. The formation of the preneurotoxic metabolite 2-hexanol increased 9, 80, and 198%, respectively, in the kidney and 9, 22, and 132% in the liver. The concentration of cytochrome P-450 was also increased in a dose-dependent way with increases of 14, 40, and 43%, respectively, in the kidney and 6, 12, and 18% in the liver. The present investigation demonstrates similar effects of isopropanol after inhalation on kidney and liver microsomal enzymes. In both organs isopropanol was shown to potentiate the formation of neurotoxic metabolites from n-hexane. However, cytochrome P-450 appears to be more easily induced in kidney than in liver.

Key words: Isopropanol – Inhalation – Cytochrome P-450 – Metabolic activation – n-Hexane – Kidney – Liver – Rat

Most of the available data on the biological effects of isopropanol are based on intraperitoneal and oral administrations. However, occupational exposure to isopropanol is most likely to occur by inhalation. Owing to the fact that type and severity of a biological effect depends on the route and pattern of exposure, this investigation deals with the ability of inhaled isopropanol to enhance the metabolic activation of n-hexane in kidney and liver. This paper also focuses on differences between kidney and liver with respect to induction of the cytochrome P-450 enzyme system and the relation between the effect and the atmospheric concentration of isopropanol.

Male Sprague-Dawley rats (250–300 g) were exposed to 200, 2,000, and 8,000 ppm isopropanol for 2 weeks, 6 h each day. Exposure was performed

---

Abbreviations: NADH, nicotinamide-adenine dinucleotide (reduced); NADPH, nicotinamide-adenine dinucleotide phosphate (reduced)

Table 1. Metabolism of n-hexane in rat liver (L) and kidney (K) after inhalation of isopropanol for 2 weeks

Air concentration of isopropanol (ppm)	1-hexanol		2-hexanol		3-hexanol	
	L	K	L	K	L	K
200	119 ± 21	82 ± 34	109 ± 32	109 ± 1	110 ± 25	124 ± 71
2,000	121 ± 16	135 ± 10	122 ± 28	180 ± 3[b]	120 ± 23	144 ± 41
8,000	180 ± 25[b]	142 ± 24	232 ± 34[b]	299 ± 56[b]	261 ± 44[b]	206 ± 12[b]
Controls[a]	0.35 ± 0.11	0.92 ± 0.31	2.46 ± 0.38	0.73 ± 0.04	0.38 ± 0.10	0.17 ± 0.04

The results are given in percent of control values ± SD (control = 100%)

[a] Control absolute values ± SD given in nmol hexanol/min × mg microsomal protein and nmol hexanol/min × g kidney for liver and kidney respectively

[b] Results significantly different from control, $p < 0.05$, $n = 5$ in a two-tailed Student's *t*-test

Table 2. Cytochrome P-450, cytochrome b_5, NADPH cytochrome c reductase activity and microsomal protein content after 2 weeks of isopropanol exposure by inhalation given as per cent of control values ± SD (control = 100%)

Air concentration of isopropanol (ppm)	Cytochrome P-450		Cytochrome b_5		NADPH cytochrome c reductase		Microsomal protein content	
	L	K	L	K	L	K	L	K
200	106 ± 6	114 ± 14	105 ± 14	123 ± 21	98 ± 3	100 ± 8	94 ± 9	121 ± 7[b]
2,000	112 ± 12	140 ± 13[b]	117 ± 10[b]	134 ± 9[b]	102 ± 11	115 ± 8[b]	99 ± 16	133 ± 23[b]
8,000	118 ± 7	143 ± 17[b]	134 ± 8[b]	180 ± 11[b]	127 ± 16[b]	133 ± 6[b]	100 ± 12	125 ± 16[b]
Controls[a]	0.72 ± 0.13	0.96 ± 0.14	0.30 ± 0.04	0.53 ± 0.16	192.2 ± 6.6	153.2 ± 7.5	14.2 ± 1.1	17.5 ± 1.3

[a] Control absolute values ± SD given as nmol P-450/mg protein – nmol P-450/g kidney, nmol b_5/mg protein – nmol b_5/g kidney, nmol cytochrome c reduced/min × mg protein – nmol cytochrome c reduced/min × g kidney and mg microsomal protein/g liver – mg microsomal protein/g kidney respectively for liver and kidney

[b] Results significantly different from control, $p < 0.05$, $n = 5$ in a two-tailed Student's *t*-test

during day time in conical shaped inhalation chambers (0.75 m^3) made of steel and glass. Atmospheric concentrations of isopropanol were monitored by gas chromatography. Microsomal preparations from kidney and liver were made as described by Toftgård et al. (1980). Microsomal concentration of cytochrome P-450 was determined by the method of Omura and Sato (1964), and cytochrome b_5 was measured at 423 nm using NADH in kidney and dithionite in liver microsomes (Sato and Omura 1964). NADPH cytochrome c reductase activity was determined as described by Masters et al. (1967), while n-hexane metabolism was assayed according to Krämer et al. (1974). Protein concentration was measured by the method of Lowry (1951). Isopropanol with a purity of 99.9% was purchased from A/S Vinmonopolet. No stabilizers were added.

The results presented in Table 1 show that the metabolism of n-hexane increased 3 times in kidney and 2–2.5 times in liver after inhalation of isopropanol. In both organs the formation of 2- and 3-hexanol increased more than 1-hexanol, probably due to differential induction of cytochrome P-450 isoenzymes. The alteration in 2-hexanol formation was of comparable magnitude in both organs, although somewhat higher in kidney.

More pronounced differences between kidney and liver were observed in the microsomal concentration of cytochromes P-450 and b_5, as shown in Table 2. The kidney showed a net increase in the concentration of these enzymes which was twice that observed for liver. A possible explanation to this could be that liver holds a greater fraction of constitutive P-450 isoenzymes than kidney.

The most striking difference between liver and kidney after inhalation of isopropanol was the elevation of the total concentration of microsomal protein. The 20–30% increase observed in kidney at all concentrations of isopropanol (Table 2) was not seen in the liver. For all the microsomal parameters investigated, except for the concentration of liver microsomal protein, a positive correlation existed between the effect and the atmospheric concentrations of isopropanol. Although not significant for the lowest concentration, the data indicate that prolonged inhalation of isopropanol to concentrations near the threshold limit value (400 ppm) may enhance the metabolic activation and neurotoxicity of n-hexane if co-exposure occurs. These results indicate that the kidney, due to its greater inducibility of the cytochrome P-450 enzyme system and the high supply of blood, may contribute significantly to the total formation of neurotoxic metabolites from n-hexane.

The present study has shown that isopropanol by inhalation exerts induction of microsomal enzymes in liver and kidney which increase the formation of neurotoxic metabolites from n-hexane, most efficiently in the kidneys. The dose-dependent induction indicates that cytochrome P-450-mediated metabolic activation of n-hexane may have toxicological relevance at the present threshold limit value for isopropanol.

References

Krämer A, Staudinger H, Ullrich V (1974) Effect of n-hexane inhalation on the monooxygenase system in mice liver microsomes. Chem Biol Interact 8: 11–18

Lowry OH, Rosebrough NJ, Farr AL, Randall RJ (1951) Protein measurement with the Folin phenol reagent. J Biol Chem 193: 265–275

Masters BSS, Williams CH, Kamin H (1967) The preparation and properties of microsomal TPNH-cytochrome c reductase from pig liver. Methods Enzymol 10: 565–573

Omura T, Sato R (1964) The carbon monoxide-binding pigment of liver microsomes. I. Evidence for its hemoprotein nature. J Biol Chem 239: 2370–2378

Toftgård R, Nilsen OG, Ingelman-Sundberg M, Gustafson J-Å (1980) Correlation between changes in enzymatic activities and induction of different forms of rat liver microsomal cytochrome P-450 after phenobarbital, 3-methylcholanthrene and 16α-cyanopregnenolone treatment. Acta Pharmacol Toxicol 46: 353–361

Disease, Metabolism and Reproduction in the Toxic Response to Drugs and Other Chemicals
Arch. Toxicol., Suppl. 7, 272–277 (1984)

Dose-Dependent Pharmacokinetics of Clofibric Acid in the Non-human Primate

L. M. Walmsley

Huntingdon Research Centre, Huntingdon, Cambs, Great Britain

Abstract. The pharmacokinetics of clofibric acid (CPIB, the active metabolite of clofibrate) has been studied in two species of non-human primate after administration by two routes at three dose levels. Plasma CPIB concentrations were determined by HPLC. In both the cynomolgus monkey and the baboon, the systemic availability of orally administered CPIB did not differ significantly from 100%; the rates of bioavailability, however, showed a dose-related trend. At the lowest dose level (15 mg/kg), the plasma concentration-time profile appeared to follow first order kinetics, with an apparent $t_{1/2}$ of 1 h; at dose levels which might be used in toxicity studies (45 and 150 mg/kg) the apparent $t_{1/2}$ was longer, indicating dose-related trends by both routes of administration. The pharmacokinetics of CPIB are therefore non-linear over the dose range considered.

CPIB protein binding was concentration-dependent over the range 50–700 μg/ml. Re-estimation of kinetic parameters in terms of free drug concentration did not remove the non-linearity. It is concluded that the pharmacokinetics of CPIB in the non-human primate are dose-dependent but that the extent of absorption of an oral dose was independent of dose level over the range studied.

Key words: Clofibric acid, 2-(4-chlorophenoxy)-2-methylpropanoic acid (CPIB) – Clofibrate – Clofibride – Bioavailability – Half-life ($t_{1/2}$) – Kinetics – Plasma – Primate – Protein binding

Methods

Clofibric acid, 2-(4-chlorophenoxy)-2-methylpropanoic acid, (CPIB) is the active metabolite of the antihyperlipidaemic agent clofibrate (Cayen 1983). Its plasma concentrations and pharmacokinetics have been studied after single intravenous and oral doses of the sodium salt at dose levels of 15, 45, and 150 mg/kg to five cynomolgus monkeys and five baboons. Doses were administered as a six-way crossover in a Youden square design, with a two week wash-out period between successive doses.

Plasma concentrations of CPIB at each time interval were measured using high-performance liquid chromatography with ultraviolet absorption detection (Woodhouse et al. 1977). CPIB is extensively protein bound in plasma (Thorp 1962). Since this binding has been reported to be concentration dependent in humans (Gugler and Hartlapp 1978), protein binding was measured in both cynomolgus monkey and baboon plasma over the range 50–700 µg/ml using the equilibrium dialysis technique.

Results and Discussion

Protein binding of CPIB decreased with increasing concentration of the compound in plasma. A logarithmic transformation gave a linear plot (Fig. 1) from which the concentration of free (unbound) CPIB in plasma could be determined. Changes in protein binding, over the concentration range considered, were similar for both species examined. Plasma kinetics of CPIB were evaluated in terms of both free and total drug.

At the lowest dose level (15 mg/kg), the plasma concentration-time profile in both species of non-human primate appeared to follow first order kinetics with an apparent half-life ($t_{1/2}$) in the order of 1 h; at the highest dose level (150 mg/kg) this apparent $t_{1/2}$ had increased to 2 h. An analysis of variance of half-life data showed a significant effect of dose level. Pharmacokinetic parameters were

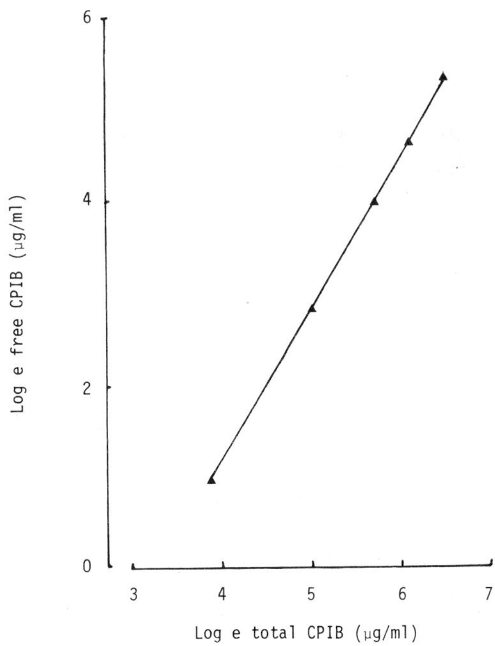

Fig. 1. Relationship between free (unbound) and total (free and bound) clofibric acid concentration over the concentration range 50–700 µg/ml

calculated by methods which are considered to be independent of a particular compartmental model, although these methods assume first order elimination from a "central" compartment. However, in a system where the magnitude of some or all pharmacokinetic parameters change with dose, non-linear pharmacokinetics are highly probable (Wagner 1975). This was confirmed by plotting plasma concentrations (normalised for dose) versus time; the resultant plots could not be superimposed (Fig. 2) indicating that some type of non-linearity was operative. Conventional pharmacokinetic compartmental models cannot be validly applied to a non-linear system.

Systemic availability of oral doses did not differ significantly from 100%; this is in agreement with the findings of other workers using a range of species

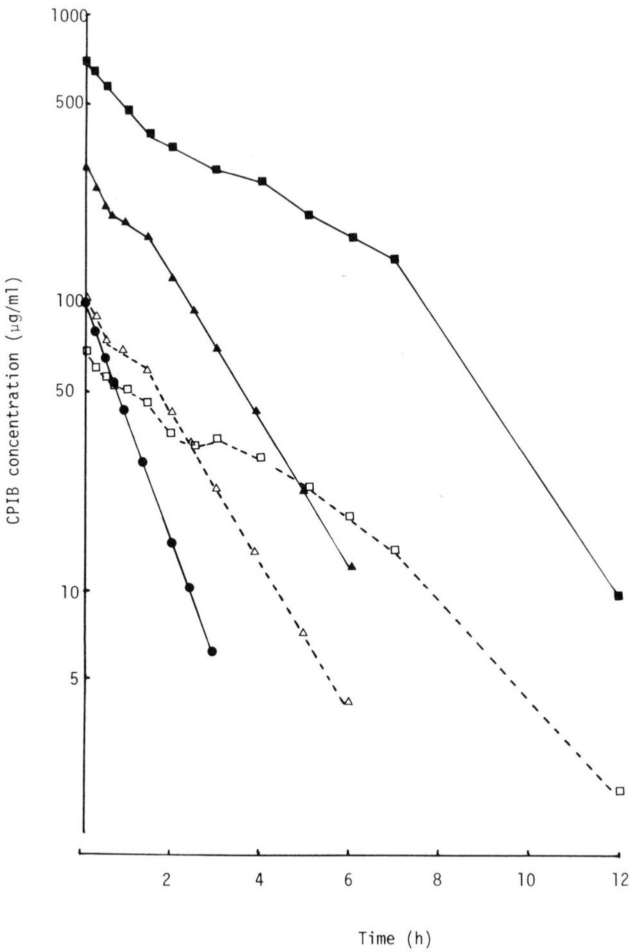

Fig. 2. Mean concentrations (µg/ml) of clofibric acid in the plasma of five cynomolgus monkeys after single intravenous doses of clofibric acid as the sodium salt. Semi-logarithmic plot; ■—■ = 150 mg/kg; ▲—▲ = 45 mg/kg; ●—● = 15 mg/kg; △---△ = 45 mg/kg normalised for dose; □---□ = 150 mg/kg normalised for dose

Pharmacokinetic parameter	Dose (mg/kg)					
	15		45		150	
	Oral	i.v.	Oral	i.v.	Oral	i.v.
Cynomolgus monkey						
AUC (bound + free) (μg · h/ml)	129 ± 20	122 ± 35	477 ± 114	636 ± 139	2,846 ± 694	2,736 ± 159
AUC (free) (μg · h/ml)	6 ± 2	6 ± 2	38 ± 9	69 ± 13	504 ± 183	504 ± 49
$t_{1/2}$ (h)	0.65 ± 0.11	0.80 ± 0.21	0.80 ± 0.18	1.11 ± 0.60	2.22 ± 0.65	1.91 ± 0.54
Peak concentration corrected for dose (μg/ml)	74 ± 23		55 ± 10		51 ± 12	
Time to peak (h)	1.0 ± 0.7		1.3 ± 0.6		1.7 ± 0.9	
Bioavailability (%)	118 ± 46		77 ± 15		104 ± 31	
Cl (bound + free) (ml/kg/h)	119 ± 21	130 ± 31	99 ± 23	74 ± 18	55 ± 10	55 ± 3
Cl (free) (ml/kg/h)	2,857 ± 925	2,794 ± 1,070	1,255 ± 353	673 ± 155	323 ± 91	300 ± 31
Vd area (bound + free) (ml/kg)		155 ± 55		133 ± 20		169 ± 58
Vd area (free) (ml/kg)		1,998 ± 1,255		763 ± 215		645 ± 130
VD ss (bound + free) (ml/kg)		147 ± 46		139 ± 29		207 ± 23
VD ss (free) (ml/kg)		2,001 ± 994		884 ± 244		818 ± 109
Baboon						
AUC (bound + free) (μg · h/ml)	199 ± 36	210 ± 70	517 ± 73	734 ± 264	2,257 ± 1,156	2,555 ± 518
AUC (free) (μg · h/ml)	11 ± 3	19 ± 9	45 ± 6	107 ± 49	361 ± 263	530 ± 126
$t_{1/2}$ (h)	1.46 ± 0.57	1.05 ± 0.21	1.74 ± 0.27	1.44 ± 0.23	1.95 ± 0.75	1.67 ± 0.33
Peak concentration corrected for dose (μg/ml)	56 ± 37		49 ± 13		31 ± 13	
Time to peak (h)	1.0 ± 0.5		2.3 ± 2.3		5.4 ± 0.9	
Bioavailability (%)	99 ± 37		74 ± 29		87 ± 38	
Cl (bound + free) (ml/kg/h)	77 ± 13	77 ± 20	88 ± 13	69 ± 28	76 ± 25	61 ± 4
Cl (free) (ml/kg/h)	1,446 ± 409	957 ± 373	1,014 ± 122	525 ± 291	544 ± 237	298 ± 81
Vd area (bound + free) (ml/kg)		113 ± 36		135 ± 58		143 ± 22
Vd area (free) (ml/kg)		890 ± 359		653 ± 406		457 ± 80
Vd ss (bound + free) (ml/kg)		117 ± 36		137 ± 55		188 ± 29
Vd ss (free) (ml/kg)		854 ± 357		615 ± 265		701 ± 184

AUC, Area under the plasma CPIB concentration – time relationship; $t_{1/2}$, Plasma half-life CPIB; Cl, Plasma clearance of CPIB; Vd, Volume of distribution of CPIB

(Cayen 1983). The rates of bioavailability of CPIB after administration of oral doses were assessed indirectly from the peak plasma concentrations of the drug and their times of occurrence. Analysis of these parameters showed a dose-related trend, with lower peak plasma concentrations of CPIB, corrected for dose, at higher dose levels; in the baboon this was associated with a trend of longer time to peak with increasing dose level (Table 1).

Plasma clearance of total CPIB decreased with increasing dose level in both cynomolgus monkey and baboon, by both routes of administration (Table 1); re-evaluation of the data in terms of free CPIB concentration magnified this trend. The volume of distribution of the free drug was reduced at higher dose levels in the cynomolgus monkey; this change was not apparent in the baboon, nor was it reflected in calculations based on total, bound and free, CPIB concentrations in either species (Table 1).

The findings from this study contrast sharply with much of the published work on clofibrate. The apparent half-life of 1–2 h, although not valid per se, is very much shorter than that reported in other species [5–8 h in rat, 18–22 h in man and 40–50 h in dog (Cayen 1983)]; it is however in good agreement with that of 1.8 h reported in rhesus monkey after oral doses of ca. 70 mg/kg CPIB (Waller et al. 1983). Loiseau (1980) reported a $t_{1/2}$ of 6 h in baboon after single oral doses of 500 mg/kg clofibride. An apparent $t_{1/2}$ of this order might be expected at this higher dose level if CPIB kinetics are indeed dose-dependent; alternatively the longer half-life may be associated with the different dosage form. Gugler and Hartlapp (1978) observed dose-dependent kinetics of clofibrate in human volunteers, with an increased (cf. current data) clearance at higher dose levels. These differences were attributed to changes in protein binding; when clearances were computed in terms of free drug concentration, clearance was independent of dose level. In the current non-human primate study, changes in protein binding did not account for the non-linearity in CPIB pharmacokinetics. CPIB clearance decreased significantly with increasing dose level, suggesting the possibility of saturation of one or more pathways of elimination. In the cynomolgus monkey there appeared to be associated changes in the volume of distribution of the free drug, but difficulties in estimating a true elimination rate constant reduce the reliability of the calculations of this parameter. It was concluded that the pharmacokinetics of CPIB in the non-human primate were dose-dependent but that the extent of absorption of an oral dose was independent of the dose level over the range studied.

References

Cayen MN (1983) Metabolism and pharmacokinetics of antihyperlipidaemic agents. In: Bridges JW, Chasseaud LF (eds) Progress in drug metabolism, vol 7. Wiley, London, pp 173–227

Gugler R, Hartlapp J (1978) Clofibrate kinetics after single and multiple doses. Clin Pharmacol Ther 24: 432–438

Loiseau GP, Millischer RJ, Lohier PY, Mardiguian JS, Gilede AP, Ginocchio AV (1980) On the metabolism of clofibride, a hypolipaemic drug. J Pharm Pharmacol 32: 483–488

Thorp JM (1962) Experimental evaluation of an orally active combination of aldosterone with ethyl chlorophenoxyisobutyrate. Lancet 1: 1323–1326

Wagner JG (1975) Fundamentals of clinical pharmacokinetics, 1st edn. Drug Intelligence, Hamilton, Ill., pp 247–283
Waller AR, Chasseaud LF, Taylor T (1984) Bioavailability studies of etofibrate in rhesus monkeys (in press)
Woodhouse RN, Cresswell DG, Chasseaud LF, Brodie RR (1977) Use of high performance liquid chromatography to measure plasma concentrations of p-chlorophenoxyisobutyric acid after administration of clofibrate to humans. J Chromatogr 137: 218–221

Disease, Metabolism and Reproduction in the Toxic Response to Drugs and Other Chemicals
Arch. Toxicol., Suppl. 7, 278–281 (1984)

Different Pathways of Chloroform Metabolism

E. Testai and L. Vittozzi

Department of Comparative Toxicology and Ecotoxicology, Istituto Superiore di Sanità, Viale Regina Elena, 299, 00161 Rome, Italy

Abstract. Chloroform metabolism can occur in liver, under physiological pO_2 conditions, with and without participation of O_2. Although, under anaerobic conditions the protein covalent binding of $CHCl_3$ metabolites is lowered, cytochrome P-450 decrease is more substantial. The loss of cytochrome P-450 cannot be accounted for either by heme destruction or lipid peroxidation under anaerobic conditions. It is not prevented by GSH. Different spectral changes occur between 400 and 500 nm, depending on the oxygen concentration; transition takes place at 1–6% pO_2.

Key words: Chloroform – Metabolism – Cytochrome P-450 – Rat liver – Microsomes – Oxygen concentration

It is largely accepted that $CHCl_3$ (Pohl et al. 1977; Mansuy et al. 1977) is metabolized by the microsomal cytochrome P-450-dependent monoxygenase system to trichloromethanol which spontaneously decomposes to phosgene. The process is dependent on reduced nicotinamide adenine nucleotide phosphate (NADPH) and requires molecular oxygen. Phosgene is the major metabolite responsible of $CHCl_3$ toxicity due to covalent binding to tissue macromolecules (Pohl et al. 1980; Ilett et al. 1973). Nonetheless, evidence such as chloride ion and CO formation and protein covalent binding (Pohl et al. 1980; Ahmed et al. 1977) suggests that $CHCl_3$ metabolism can occur without oxygen participation. The present results describe the behaviour of $CHCl_3$ metabolites produced under hypoxic conditions.

A standard incubation mixture (20 min, 37° C) contained 2 mg/ml microsomal protein from livers of phenobarbital-induced male Sprague-Dawley rats, together with glucose-6-phosphate (G6P) 2 mM, $MgCl_2$ 2 mM, glucose-6-phosphate dehydrogenase (G6PDH) 1 U, nicotinamide adenine nucleotide phosphate (NADP) 0.2 mM, in Tris-HCl 50 mM, 1 mM ethylene diamine tetraacetic acid (EDTA) (pH 7.4). Unless otherwise stated $CHCl_3$ was added as methanolic solution. Optical studies were carried out with a Hitachi Perkin

Elmer 557 spectrophotometer while stirring, and the pO_2 and temperature of the mixture was recorded.

Table 1 shows that under aerobic conditions enzyme activities dependent on cytochrome P-450 are greatly reduced and cytochrome P-450 decreases, especially the PB-inducible forms (data from induction experiments not shown).

Table 1. Effects of chloroform metabolism on rat liver microsomal cytochrome P-450 monoxygenase system

	Incubation conditions		
	Standard mixture variations	Aerobic	Anaerobic
Cytochrome P-450	–	70	52
Cytochrome P-450	+ GSH (3 mM)	89	52
Cytochrome P-450	+ Cys (2 mM)	80	–
Cytochrome P-450	+ SKF 525A (0.5 mM)	100	51
Cytochrome P-450 (metyrapone adduct)		46	35
Heme	–	90	86
Ethylmorphine N-demethylase[a]	–	29	60
Ethoxycoumarin O-deethylase	–	30	77

Results are expressed as percent of control values, obtained after similar incubations without $CHCl_3$

[a] Chloroform added as ethanolic solution

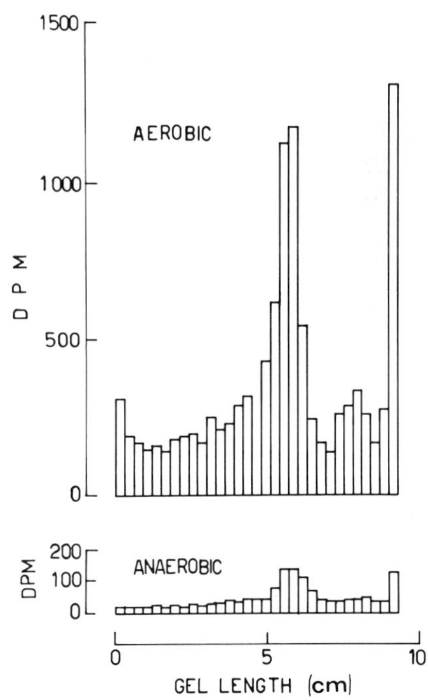

Fig. 1. Distribution of protein covalent binding of $^{14}CHCl_3$ metabolites after 10% poliacrylamide gel electrophoresis in the presence of 0.2% sodium dodecylsulphate

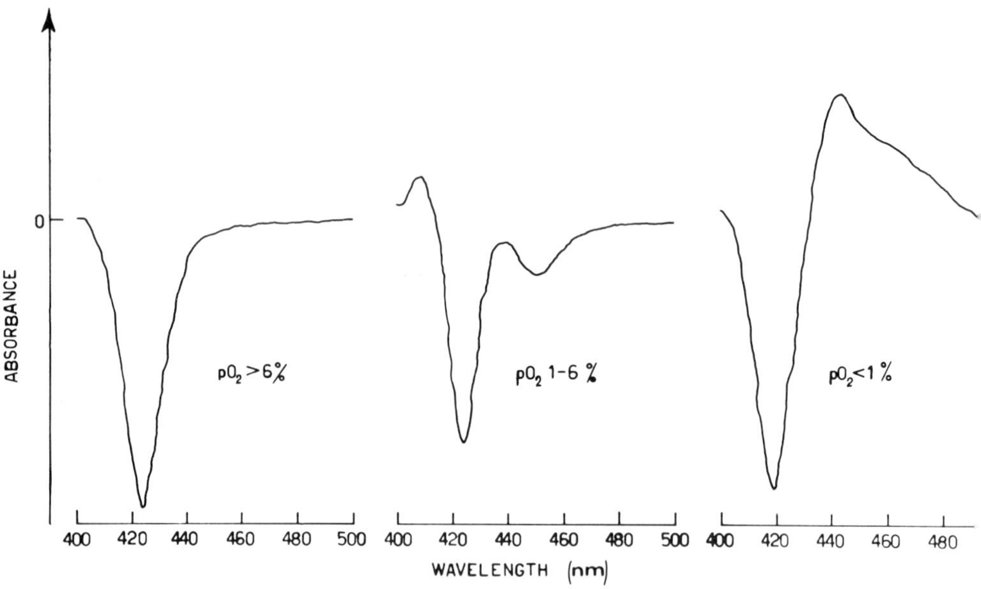

Fig. 2. Differential spectra of microsomes obtained upon $CHCl_3$ metabolism under different pO_2 conditions

Loss of cytochrome P-450 is prevented totally by SKF-525A (proadifen) and partially by 2 mM cysteine and glutathione (GSH). Under anaerobic conditions cytochrome P-450 inactivation is nearly doubled and GSH exerts no protective effect. The aerobic and anaerobic destructive events cannot be attributed only to a modification of the hemin structure. Qualitatively the electrophoretic covalent binding pattern is not altered in the absence of O_2 but the extent of binding is reduced to 30% (Fig. 1). $CHCl_3$ metabolism induces time dependent spectral changes between 400 and 500 nm. Optical studies under different O_2 concentrations showed that at $pO_2 > 6\%$ a trough at 423 nm is formed; at $1\% < pO_2 < 6\%$ a different spectrum is gradually obtained and at $pO_2 < 1\%$ a maximum at about 450 nm is formed (Fig. 2).

$CHCl_3$ is metabolized in liver under physiological pO_2 conditions (1–5% pO_2) with and without oxygen as cosubstrate, with production of different metabolites. Anaerobically-formed metabolites are very effective in producing cytochrome P-450 loss; they are not scavenged by GSH. Spectra obtained below 6% pO_2 are possibly due to the formation of a $CHCl_3$ metabolite-adduct with cytochrome P-450.

Acknowledgment. We wish to thank Miss Laura Moreschi for typing the manuscript.
This research was partly supported by a CNR grant within the frame of the applied Project "Preventive and Rehabilitative Medicine."

References

Ahmed AE, Kubic VL, Anders MW (1977) Metabolism of haloform to carbon monoxide. I. In vitro studies. Drug Metab Dispos 5: 198–204

Ilett KF, Reid WD, Sipes IG, Krishna G (1973) Chloroform toxicity in mice: correlation of renal and hepatic necrosis with covalent binding of metabolites to tissue macromolecules. Exp Mol Pathol 19: 215–229

Mansuy D, Beaune P, Cresteil T, Lange M, Leroux JP (1977) Evidence for phosgene formation during liver microsomal oxidation of chloroform. Biochem Biophys Res Commun 79: 513–517

Pohl RL, Bhooshan B, Whittaker NF, Krishna G (1977) Phosgene: a metabolite of chloroform. Biochem Biophys Res Commun 79: 684–691

Pohl RL, Martin JL, George W (1980) Mechanism of metabolic activation of chloroform by rat liver microsomes. Biochem Pharmacol 29: 3271–3276

Disease, Metabolism and Reproduction in the Toxic Response to Drugs and Other Chemicals
Arch. Toxicol., Suppl. 7, 282–285 (1984)

In Vitro Inhibition of Lysosomal Phospholipases by Aminoglycoside Antibiotics: A Comparative Study

M. B. Carlier, G. Laurent and P. Tulkens

Laboratoire de Chimie Physiologique and International Institute
of Cellular and Molecular Pathology,
Université Catholique de Louvain, Avenue Hippocrate, 75, 1200 Bruxelles, Belgium

Abstract. Aminoglycosides induce an early and characteristic phospholipidosis in the lysosomes of kidney tubular cells. Inhibition of lysosomal phospholipase activity by gentamicin has been demonstrated in vivo and in vitro. Ten aminoglycosides have been examined for their potency in inhibiting phospholipases A_1 and A_2. Similar IC_{50}'s and IC_{90}'s (concentrations causing 50 and 90% inhibition) were found for sisomicin, dibekacin, gentamicin, tobramycin, kanamycin B and netilmicin. Kanamycin A, HABA-dibekacin and amikacin showed increasingly higher IC's. Thus, both the number and the position of amino groups are important. Streptomycin had little effect on phosphatidylcholine hydrolysis. Kinetic studies with gentamicin suggest a competitive type of inhibition. This approach may help for the in vitro screening of less toxic aminoglycosides.

Key words: Aminoglycosides – Phospholipases – Phospholipidosis – Lysosomes – Liposomes – Nephrotoxicity

Aminoglycoside antibiotics are nephrotoxic and induce necroses in the proximal tubules. Histopathological alterations are preceeded by ultrastructural changes in the lysosomes (accumulation of "myeloid bodies") suggestive of a lysosomal phospholipidosis (Kosek et al. 1974). It has also been demonstrated that gentamicin accumulates inside the lysosomes of the proximal tubular cells (Just et al. 1977; Silverblatt et al. 1979). It has been shown that the activities of acid phospholipase A_1 and of sphingomyelinase, which catalyse the first steps of phospholipid breakdown in lysosomes (Brady et al. 1966; Kunze et al. 1982), are decreased in the renal cortex of rats treated with aminoglycosides. Inhibition of enzymatic activity depends, however, on the drug administered, since amikacin, an aminoglycoside showing less nephrotoxicity, also induces less inhibition of lysosomal phospholipase A_1 and sphingomyelinase (Carlier and Tulkens 1981; Laurent et al. 1982). Recently, an in vitro model has been developed to evaluate the inhibitory potency of aminoglycosides, under conditions mimicing those prevailing in lysosomes in vivo (Laurent et al. 1982). In the present study, 10 aminoglycosides (Fig. 1) of use in clinical practice or under clinical trials have been studied for their respective ability to inhibit lysosomal phospholipase activities.

Lysosomal phospholipases (EC 3.1.1.32; EC 3.1.1.4; EC 3.1.1.) were assayed using as substrate negatively charged bilayers of natural phospholipids (liposomes) at pH 5.4 (i.e., the intralysosomal pH in cells; Okhuma and Poole 1978). Liposomes (100 nmol phospholipid/test) contained egg yolk phosphatidylcholine, wheat-germ phosphatidylinositol, bovine brain sphingomyelin and cholesterol (4:3:4:5.5, molar ratio) and 140 μCi of 1-palmitoyl-2-[1-^{14}C] oleoylphosphatidylcholine per mmol of phosphatidylcholine. Incubation was carried out at 37° C for 30 min in the presence of 5,2 μg protein of highly purified liver lysosomes. Phospholipase A_1 was measured by the release of [^{14}C] lysophosphatidylcholine, and the sum of phospholipase A_2 and β-lysophospho-

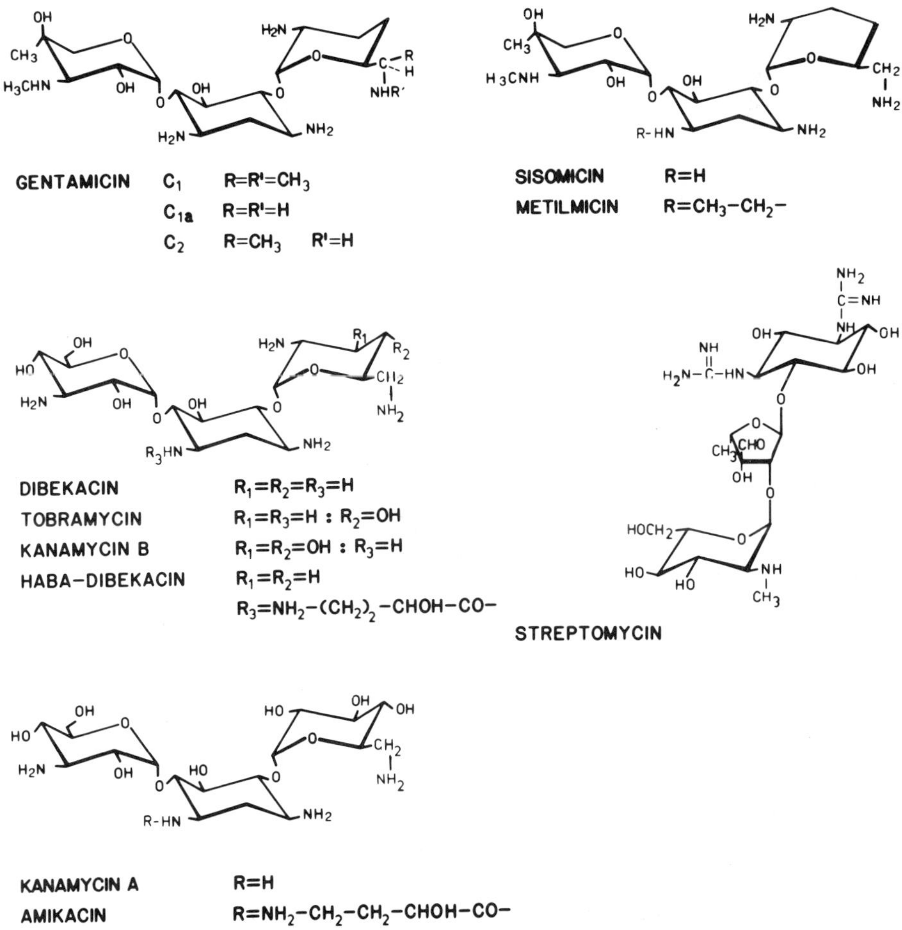

Fig. 1. Structural formulae of the aminoglycosides used in the present study

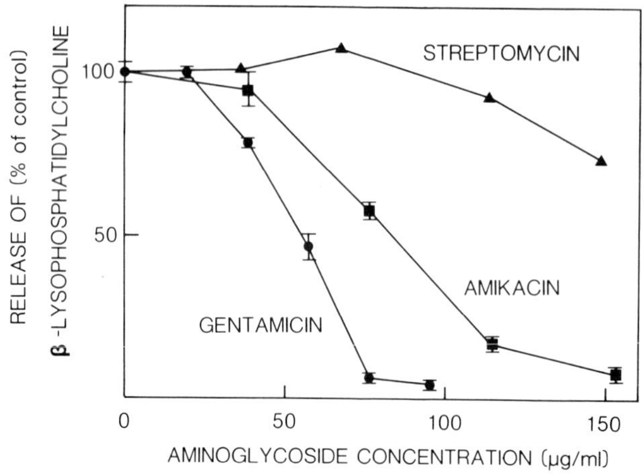

Fig. 2. Effect of gentamicin, amikacin, and streptomycin on phospholipase A_1 activity. *Abscissa:* Drug concentration in micrograms of free base per milliliter of reaction mixture. *Ordinate:* Release of β-lysophosphatidylcholine in percent of the value obtained in the absence of antibiotic. The bars indicate the SD ($n = 3$)

Table 1. Effect of aminoglycosides on phosphatidylcholine degradation

	Phospholipase Al		Phospholipase Al + β-lysophospholipase		No. of experiments
	IC_{50}	IC_{90}	IC_{50}	IC_{90}	
Dibekacin	44 ± 10[a]	65 ± 7	50 ± 8	74 ± 10	6
Sisomicin	48 ± 2	65 ± 3	43 ± 1	64 ± 3	3
Gentamicin	52 ± 9	73 ± 6	54 ± 6	77 ± 4	10
Tobramycin	53 ± 4	77 ± 8	49 ± 9	76 ± 16	4
Kanamycin B	54 ± 4	77 ± 5	56 ± 7	83 ± 3	4
Netilmicin	57 ± 4	78 ± 6	46 ± 5	84 ± 8	4
Kanamycin A	69 ± 11[b]	105 ± 14[c]	69 ± 6[c]	101 ± 9[c]	6
HABA-Dibekacin	79 ± 4[c]	83 ± 1[b]	79 ± 1[c]	93 ± 1[c]	3
Amikacin	85 ± 4[c]	143 ± 6[c]	96 ± 4[c]	137 ± 7[c]	4

For the $IC_{50\text{'s}}$ and $IC_{90\text{'s}}$ higher than those of gentamicin, the statistical difference was analyzed by the Student's *t*-test

[a] Means ± standard deviation

[b] $p < 0.05$

[c] $p < 0.001$

lipase activities were assayed by the release of $[^{14}C]$oleic acid (Laurent et al. 1982).

Figure 2 shows the dose response curves of phospholipase A_1 inhibition by gentamicin, amikacin and streptomycin. Although aminoglycosides were used as sulfate salts, the concentrations are expressed in free base equivalent. Above concentrations of approximately 75 and 150 µg/ml for gentamicin and amikacin respectively, the release of β-lysophosphatidylcholine is almost completely abolished. Streptomycin is a much less potent inhibitor.

Table I shows the compared IC_{50}'s and IC_{90}'s (concentrations causing 50 or 90% inhibition) for the 10 aminoglycosides investigated according to this protocol. Similarly, dose response curves were obtained for the oleic acid release, and the data are also shown in Table 1. For both the release of β-lysophosphatidylcholine and oleic acid, similar IC_{50}'s and IC_{90}'s were observed for dibekacin, sisomicin, gentamicin, tobramycin, kanamycin B and netilmicin. Kanamycin A, HABA-dibekacin and amikacin showed significantly higher IC_{50}'s and IC_{90}'s than gentamicin. In this group, amikacin was significantly different from kanamycin A. Significant differences were also found between kanamycin B and kanamycin A, as well as between dibekacin and HABA-dibekacin. Thus, both the number and the position of the amino groups are important. Streptomycin, which displays two guanidinium groups and only one amino group, had little effect.

The type of inhibition of phospholipase A_1 caused by gentamicin was investigated by kinetic studies. Both in the absence and presence of antibiotic, the rate of the release of β-lysophosphatidylcholine roughly followed an hyperbolic relationship with the liposome concentration. Analysis by double reciprocal plot ("Lineweaver-Burk plot") showed an apparent K_M of 3.1 mM (phosphatidylcholine) for control, and of 6.7 mM in the presence of 59 μg/ml gentamicin, but no difference in V_{max}. This result is compatible with a competitive inhibition.

Insofar as phospholidosis is an early sign of aminoglycoside nephrotoxicity, comparisons of derivatives in this system may help in the screening of less toxic compounds.

References

Brady RO, Kanfer JN, Mock MB, Fredrickson DS (1966) The metabolism of sphingomyelin, II Evidence of an enzymatic deficiency in Niemann-Pick disease. Proc Natl Acad Sci USA 55: 366–369

Carlier MB, Tulkens P (1981) Gentamicin induces a loss of activity of acid phospholipases A in rat kidney cortex. Arch Int Physiol Biochim 89: B5

Just M, Erdmann G, Habermann E (1977) The renal handling of polybasic drugs. 1. Gentamicin and aprotinin in intact animals. Naunyn-Schmiedebergs Arch Pharmacol 300: 57–66

Kosek JC, Mazze RI, Cousins MJ (1974) Nephrotoxicity of gentamicin. Lab Invest 30: 48–57

Kunze H, Hesse B, Bohn E (1982) Hydrolytic degradation of phosphatidylethanolamine and phosphatidylcholine by isolated rat-liver lysosomes. Biochim Biophys Acta 711: 10–18

Laurent G, Carlier MB, Rollman B, Van Hoof F, Tulkens P (1982) Mechanism of aminoglycoside-induced lysosomal phospholipidosis: In vitro and in vivo studies, with gentamicin and amikacin. Biochem Pharmacol 31: 3861–3870

Okhuma S, Poole B (1978) Fluorescence probe measurement of the intralysosomal pH in living cells and the perturbation of pH by various agents. Proc Natl Acad Sci USA 75: 3327–3331

Silverblatt FJ, Kuehn C (1979) Autoradiography of gentamicin uptake by the rat proximal tubule cell. Kidney Int 15: 335–345

Disease, Metabolism and Reproduction in the Toxic Response to Drugs and Other Chemicals
Arch. Toxicol., Suppl. 7, 286–290 (1984)

Erythrocyte-Dependent Metabolic Activation of Styrene and Induction of Sister Chromatid Exchange in Cultured Human Lymphocytes

H. Norppa[1], H. Vainio[1,2], M. Sorsa[1], and G. Belvedere[3]

[1] Institute of Occupational Health, Haartmaninkatu 1, 00290 Helsinki 29, Finland
[2] International Agency for Research on Cancer,
150 cours Albert-Thomas, 69372 Lyon Cedex 02, France (present address)
[3] Istituto di Ricerche Farmacologiche "Mario Negri", Via Eritrea, 62, Milan, Italy

Abstract. Human erythrocytes can oxidize styrene to styrene-7,8-oxide in the absence of the co-factors required for metabolic reactions catalysed by the microsomal cytochrome P-450 system. This probably explains the increased incidence of sister chromatid exchanges (SCEs) that was detected in whole blood lymphocyte cultures from 11 male donors after treatment in vitro (48 h) with styrene (2 mM). Styrene-7,8-oxide (0.15 mM) also induced SCEs in these cultures. Styrene (0.5–4.0 mM) increased the incidence of SCEs only slightly in cultures of isolated lymphocytes (2×10^4 erythrocytes/ml), but had a clear dose-dependent effect in whole blood cultures ($2-4 \times 10^8$ erythrocytes/ml). When erythrocytes were added to purified cultures, SCE incidence increased after treatment with styrene (2 mM). Cyclophosphamide elevated the incidence of SCEs almost equally efficiently in whole blood and in isolated lymphocytes. It is suggested that styrene induces SCEs after transformation to styrene-7,8-oxide by oxyhemoglobin in erythrocytes, whereas cyclophosphamide is activated by the lymphocytes themselves.

Key words: Cyclophosphamide – Erythrocytes – Human lymphocyte cultures – Metabolic activation – Reinforced-plastics factory workers – Sister chromatid exchange – Styrene – Styrene-7,8-oxide

Styrene has been reported to produce chromosomal aberrations, micronuclei and sister chromatid exchanges (SCEs) in human whole-blood lymphocyte cultures in the absence of exogenous metabolizing systems (Linnainmaa et al. 1978; Norppa et al. 1980). These findings suggested that the lymphocyte test system can activate styrene, since in other mutagenicity tests styrene has positive effects only when it is metabolically activated (Vainio et al. 1982). It is known that styrene-7,8-oxide, a potent mutagen, is formed in styrene-treated lymphocyte cultures, and that this metabolite induces SCEs (Norppa et al. 1980, 1981).

With regard to the question of which cell types in whole blood are responsible for the conversion of styrene into styrene-7,8-oxide, Belvedere and Tursi (1981) have reported that not only human lymphocytes, but also erythrocytes can catalyze this reaction. As the ratio of leucocytes to erythrocytes in normal blood is usually about one to a thousand, the oxidation of styrene in whole blood may be undertaken entirely by the red blood cells (Belvedere and Tursi 1981).

Whole blood lymphocyte cultures have been used widely to test the cytogenetic effects of chemicals; however, the possibility that erythrocytes mediate metabolic activation has not received much attention. Since some well-known premutagens, such as cyclophosphamide, have been shown to damage chromosomes in whole blood cultures in the absence of exogenous metabolizing systems (Waalkens et al. 1981), the possible role of erythrocytes in this process should be evaluated.

The present study was carried out to investigate whether or not erythrocytes are involved in the induction of SCEs by styrene and cyclophosphamide. Details of the methods used have been reported elsewhere (Norppa et al. 1983). Briefly, 72-h cultures of phytohemagglutinin-stimulated human lymphocytes (two per person for each treatment), containing 5 µg/ml 5-bromodeoxyuridine, were treated after a 24-h incubation period (37° C) and harvested after an additional 48 h.

Three separate experiments were performed. In the first, SCE induction by a single dose of styrene (2 mM; 50% solution, v/v, in acetone) or styrene-7,8-oxide (0.15 mM; 5% solution, v/v, in acetone) was studied in whole-blood lymphocyte cultures derived from 11 male donors. Six of the subjects were workers exposed to styrene in a reinforced-plastics factory, and five were unexposed control persons from a research institute.

A clear increase in the incidence of SCEs was seen in all cultures treated with styrene or styrene-7,8-oxide (Fig. 1), but there were significant differences (one-way analysis of variance of square-root-transformed data) in individual responses to the treatments, including the control series treated with acetone (6.8 mM). However, the mean numbers of SCEs/cell in the cultures from exposed workers did not differ from those for unexposed persons, except after acetone treatment ($p < 0.01$, one-tailed t-test). Three of the workers were smokers (Fig. 1), which probably explains this effect.

In the second experiment, SCE frequencies in whole-blood cultures and in isolated lymphocyte cultures were compared after treatment with different doses of styrene (0.5–4 mM) or cyclophosphamide (0.5–2 mM; 10 mg/ml in medium) (Table 1). Styrene induced a clear dose-dependent increase in the incidence of SCEs in whole-blood cultures (with $2-4 \times 10^8$ erythrocytes/ml), but had only a slight effect in isolated cultures (with about 2×10^4 erythrocytes/ml). Cyclophosphamide produced a distinct effect on the incidence of SCEs both in whole blood and in isolated cultures. The somewhat higher level of SCEs detected in purified lymphocytes reflects a basic increase that was probably brought about by the isolation process. Thus, the induction of SCEs by styrene depended on the presence of erythrocytes, whereas cyclophosphamide elevated the incidence of SCEs, irrespective of whether red blood cells were present.

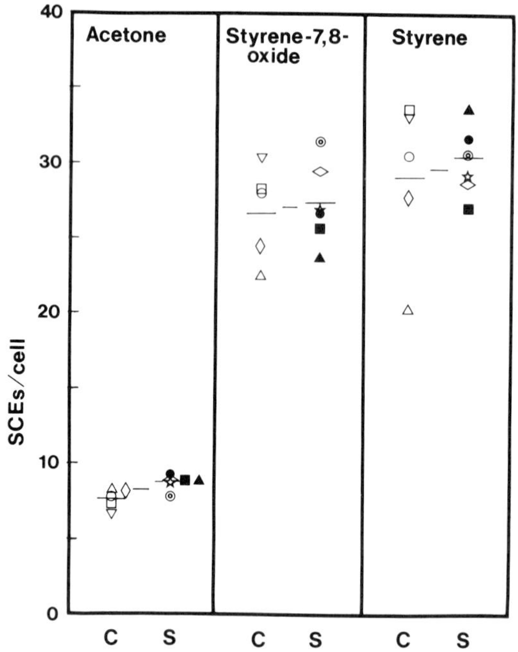

Fig. 1. Sister chromatid exchanges (SCEs) in cultured lymphocytes from eleven male donors after treatment in vitro (48 h) with acetone (6.8 mM, control cultures), styrene-7,8-oxide (0.15 mM), or styrene (2 mM). The symbols (one for each individual) represent means of 50 cells (25 from two parallel cultures) per person. *Black symbols* indicate smokers. *Horizontal lines* are group means; those between the two groups are means of the entire treatment. *C*, unexposed control persons; *S*, styrene-exposed reinforced-plastics workers

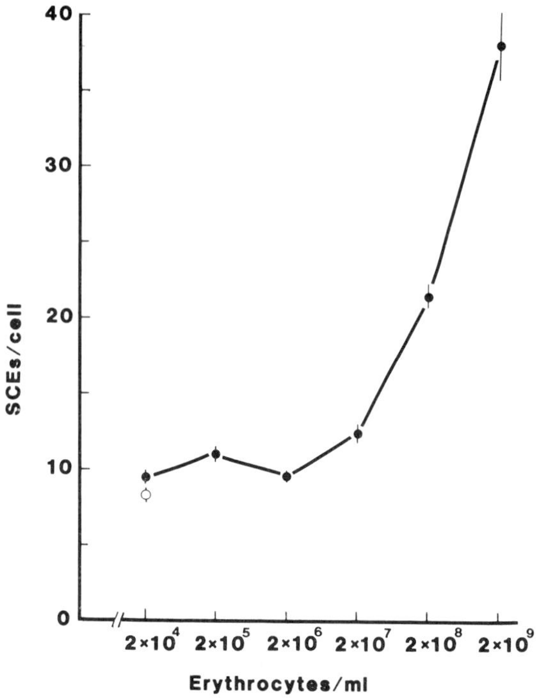

Fig. 2. The effect of the number of erythrocytes on the induction of sister chromatid exchanges (SCEs) in cultures of isolated lymphocytes treated for 48 h with styrene (2 mM). The points represent means (± SE) of 50 cells (25 from two parallel cultures); except that with 2×10^9 erythrocytes/ml only 10 cells were examined. ●, styrene treatment; ○, control treatment (acetone, 6.1 mM)

Table 1. Induction of sister chromatid exchanges (SCEs) in cultured human lymphocytes after 48-h treatment with styrene or cyclophosphamide. SCEs were counted in 50 cells per treatment per person (25 from two duplicate cultures), unless otherwise stated

Compound concentration (mM)	SCEs/cell ± SE			
	Whole blood cultures		Isolated cultures	
	Person A	Person B	Person A	Person B
Styrene				
0 (acetone, 12.9 mM)	6.9 ± 0.3[a]	9.0 ± 0.4	9.7 ± 0.3[a]	9.9 ± 0.3[a]
0.5	8.8[c] ± 0.4	11.0[b] ± 0.6	10.3 ± 0.5	10.9 ± 0.5
1.0	13.3[c] ± 0.7	17.4[c] ± 0.7	10.7 ± 0.6	10.0 ± 0.6
2.0	29.4[c] ± 1.0	26.9[c] ± 1.3	12.2[c] ± 0.6	10.8 ± 0.5
3.0	36.6[c] ± 2.3[d]	No 2nd division cells	11.9[b] ± 0.6	14.3[c] ± 0.6
4.0	43.5[c] ± 2.5[e]		No 2nd division cells	16.9[c] ± 1.4[d]
Cyclophosphamide				
0 (no treatment)	7.3 ± 0.4	–	8.2 ± 0.4	–
0.5	12.5[c] ± 0.6	–	13.2[c] ± 0.6	–
1.0	16.1[c] ± 0.7	–	21.6[c] ± 0.8	–
2.0	27.6[c] ± 1.0	–	28.2[c] ± 1.0	–

[a] 100 cells from four cultures analysed
[b] $p < 0.01$, one-tailed *t*-test
[c] $p < 0.001$, one-tailed *t*-test
[d] Only 10 cells analysed
[e] Only 15 cells analysed

In the third experiment, different numbers of erythrocytes ($2 \times 10^5 - 2 \times 10^9$/ml) were added to isolated lymphocyte cultures, which were then treated with styrene (2 mM). An increase in the incidence of SCEs was observed, which was dependent on the number of erythrocytes added (Fig. 2). The mean number of SCEs/cell started to rise with 2×10^7 erythrocytes/ml, although the difference from acetone-treated (6.1 mM) control cultures was already significant ($p < 0.01$, one-tailed *t*-test) with 2×10^5 erythrocytes/ml.

The results presented above suggest that styrene is activated by erythrocytes in the lymphocyte test system. Previous studies have indicated that the active metabolite is styrene-7,8-oxide (Belvedere and Tursi 1981; Norppa et al. 1980). The question now remains of what system in red blood cells is responsible for the oxidation of styrene. Belvedere and Tursi (1981) have reported that although this reaction requires oxygen, it is not catalysed by methemoglobin (without hydrogen peroxide) or erythrocyte membranes, and is independent of the cofactors that are required for metabolic reactions catalysed by microsomal enzymes. Since styrene oxidation is not inhibited by superoxide dismutase, catalase or scavengers of OH radicals, free oxygen radicals do not appear to be involved. Nevertheless, it has been shown that in deoxygenated erythrocytes and erythrocyte lysates the formation of styrene-7,8-oxide is related linearly to the molar fraction of oxyhemoglobin (Tursi et al. 1983). Thus, there are reasons to believe that the reaction is catalysed by partially activated oxygen in the oxyhemoglobin molecule.

References

Belvedere G, Tursi F (1981) Styrene oxidation to styrene oxide in human blood erythrocytes and lymphocytes. Res Commun Chem Pathol Pharmacol 33: 273–282

Linnainmaa K, Meretoja T, Sorsa M, Vainio H (1978) Cytogenetic effects of styrene and styrene oxide. Mutat Res 58: 277–286

Norppa H, Sorsa M, Pfäffli P, Vainio H (1980) Styrene and styrene oxide induce SCEs and are metabolised in human lymphocyte cultures. Carcinogenesis 1: 357–361

Norppa H, Hemminki K, Sorsa M, Vainio H (1981) Effect of monosubstituted epoxides on chromosome aberrations and SCE in cultured human lymphocytes. Mutat Res 91: 243–250

Norppa H, Vainio H, Sorsa M (1983) Metabolic activation of styrene by erythrocytes detected as increased sister chromatid exchanges in cultured human lymphocytes. Cancer Res 43: 3579–3582

Tursi F, Samai M, Salmona M, Belvedere G (1983) Styrene oxidation to styrene oxide in human erythrocytes is catalyzed by oxyhemoglobin. Experientia 39: 593–594

Vainio H, Norppa H, Hemminki K, Sorsa M (1982) Metabolism and genotoxicity of styrene. In: Snyder R, Parke DV, Kocsis J, Jollow DJ, Gibson GG, Witmer CM (eds) Biological reactive intermediates 2: Chemical mechanisms and biological effects, part A. Plenum, New York, pp 257–274

Waalkens DH, Joosten HFP, Taalman RDFM, Scheres JMJC, Yih TD, Hoekstra A (1981) Sister-chromatid exchanges induced in vitro by cyclophosphamide without exogenous metabolic activation in lymphocytes from three mammalian species. Toxicol Lett 7: 229–232

Disease, Metabolism and Reproduction in the Toxic Response to Drugs and Other Chemicals
Arch. Toxicol., Suppl. 7, 291–294 (1984)

Interaction of Acrylonitrile with the Liver Mixed Function Oxidases

D. Cova[1], E. Chiesara[2], and R. Rizzi[2]

[1] Department of Pharmacology, CNR Center of Cytopharmacology, Via Vanvitelli 32, 20129 Milan, Italy
[2] Department of Pharmacology, Chair of Toxicology, Via Vanvitelli 32, 20129 Milan, Italy

Abstract. The effect on the liver mixed function oxidases of acrylonitrile revealed an inhibition of the benzo(a)pyrene hydroxylase and of the epoxide hydrase whereas aniline hydroxylase is unaffected. These findings exclude the possibility that the inhibitory effect of certain hydroxylation activities of the liver microsomes can be secondary to a direct effect of acrylonitrile on cytochrome P-450 but suggest the hypothesis that the inhibition is mediated by the cyanide released during acrylonitrile metabolism.

Key words: Acrylonitrile – Metabolism – Reactive intermediates – Liver – Mixed function oxidases

The metabolism of acrylonitrile, a compound used on a large scale in the manufacture of acrylic polymers, has not been extensively studied but there is some evidence, during in vitro metabolism of acrylonitrile (Guengerich et al. 1981), of the formation of 2-cyanoethylene oxide, catalyzed by the liver microsomal mixed function oxidase (MFO).

It is important to confirm these findings, since there is increasing evidence that labile epoxide formed during metabolism of many chemicals may play an important role in carcinogenesis and in mutagenesis.

This communication summarizes recent findings concerning the effects of acrylonitrile on the activity of MFO and of epoxide hydrase, a key enzyme for the catabolism of epoxides, since it has been shown that some epoxides are able to decrease the activity of epoxide hydrase.

Microsomes were prepared according to the method of Mitoma et al. (1956) from the livers of Sprague-Dawley rats untreated or treated with phenobarbital (80 mg/kg i.p. for 5 days), methylcholanthrene (30 mg/kg i.p. for 2 days) and Aroclor 1254 (200 mg/kg i.p. once, 5 days before sacrifice). 3,4 Benzo(a)pyrene hydroxylase activity was determined by the fluorimetric method of Nebert et al. (1968). The activity of the epoxide hydrase was determined according to the method of Pachecka et al. (1977). Aniline hydroxylase activity was determined measuring the p-aminophenol formed, according to the method of Kato et al.

(1965). Acrylonitrile was added in the reaction mixture in order to obtain a final concentration of 5, 10 or 20 mM.

The results show that in the presence of microsomes obtained from the liver of normal rats, acrylonitrile is able to inhibit both benzo(a)pyrene hydroxylase (Table 1) and epoxide hydrase (Table 2) whereas it has no effect on aniline hydroxylase.

Considering this absence of effect on aniline hydroxylase and the fact that when acrylonitrile is incubated in vitro with the microsomes at even higher doses than those indicated in the tables, it is unable to diminish the content of

Table 1. Effect of acrylonitrile on benzo(a)pyrene (BP) hydroxylase in microsomes from control and differently treated rat livers

Acrylo-nitrile (mM)	Benzo(a)pyrene hydroxylase[a]			
	Control[b]	Phenobarbital[b]	3-Methyl-cholanthrene	Aroclor 1254
0	4.68 ± 0.51 (100)	4.62 ± 0.34 (100)	16.35 ± 1.11 (100)	15.96 ± 0.91 (100)
5	3.83 ± 0.45 (83)	4.28 ± 0.34 (93)	17.65 ± 1.42 (108)	15.89 ± 0.74 (99)
10	3.45 ± 0.72 (74)	3.94 ± 0.40 (85)	17.48 ± 1.38 (107)	16.28 ± 0.70 (102)
20	3.03 ± 0.18 (65)	3.60 ± 0.34 (78)	18.50 ± 2.64 (113)	15.89 ± 0.91 (99)

The BP hydroxylase reaction mixture contained 0.3 mg of microsomal protein, 0.1 M Tris-HCl (pH 7.5), 5 mM $MgCl_2$, 5 mM glucose-6-phosphate, 190 μM BP (added in 20 μl of acetone), 0.25 ml of the soluble fraction, and 1.2 mM NADP in a final volume of 1.0 ml. Reactions were carried out at 37° C for 10 min with mechanical shaking in the dark

[a] The values are expressed as nmoles × min^{-1} × mg $protein^{-1}$ ± SE (%) of 8-hydroxy-benzo(a)pyrene formed

[b] The inhibition is significant at 95% confidence level (Dixon plot slope significantly different from zero)

Table 2. Effect of acrylonitrile on epoxide hydrase (EH) in microsomes from control and differently treated rat livers

Acrylo-nitrile (mM)	Epoxide hydrase[a]			
	Control[b]	Phenobarbital[b]	3-Methyl-cholanthrene	Aroclor 1254
0	7.94 ± 0.23 (100)	10.05 ± 0.45 (100)	9.45 ± 0.51 (100)	11.07 ± 0.63 (100)
5	6.81 ± 0.31 (86)	9.15 ± 0.57 (92)	9.51 ± 0.77 (101)	11.23 ± 0.88 (101)
10	5.95 ± 0.28 (75)	8.43 ± 0.51 (85)	9.40 ± 0.85 (98)	10.95 ± 0.77 (98)
20	5.40 ± 0.33 (68)	8.05 ± 0.45 (80)	9.55 ± 0.69 (101)	11.31 ± 0.81 (102)

The EH reaction mixture contained 5 mg of microsomal protein, 0.05 M Tris-HCl (pH 7.4), 1.5 M NaCl, 5 mM $MgCl_2$, 5 mM glucose-6-phosphate, 0.5 mM styrene epoxide (added in 20 μl of acetone), 0.25 ml of the soluble fraction, and 1.2 mM NADP in a final volume of 1.0 ml. Reactions were carried out at 37° C for 10 min with mechanical shaking

[a] The values are expressed as nmoles × min^{-1} × mg $protein^{-1}$ ± SE (%) of phenylethylene glycol formed

[b] The inhibition is significant at 95% confidence level (Dixon plot slope significantly different from zero)

cytochrome P-450 [with or without a reduced nicotinamide adenine dinucleotide phosphate (NADPH) regenerating system] it is necessary to exclude the possibility that the inhibitory effect observed is due to the denaturation of microsomal cytochrome P-450 by the acrylonitrile itself or by its metabolites.

On the assumption that acrylonitrile undergoes metabolic oxidation similar to benzo(a)pyrene hydroxylase, competing for the same binding sites on the enzymes, the reciprocal of the rate of benzo(a)pyrene hydroxylase at the three substrate concentrations was plotted against acrylonitrile concentrations, the Dixon plot revealed that the mode of inhibition by acrylonitrile is not competitive (Fig. 1).

Taking into account the metabolic fate of acrylonitrile, as reported by Guengerich et al. (1981), it may be assumed that this inhibition is caused by the cyanide produced by the oxidation of the acrylonitrile which binds on cytochrome P-450 in its cyanide sensitive form.

Staundinger et al. (1965) described in fact two forms of terminal oxidase, one of which is inhibited by potassium cyanide (KCN), whereas the other is cyanide-resistant. To confirm this hypothesis the inhibitory effect of acrylonitrile was evaluated with microsomes obtained from livers pretreated with phenobarbital,3-methylcholanthrene or Aroclor 1254. Comai et al. (1973), who have separated chromatographically three spectrally distinguishable forms of cytochrome P-450 from rat liver microsomes which have differing activity with cyanide, reported that cytochrome P-450 with the lowest affinity for cyanide

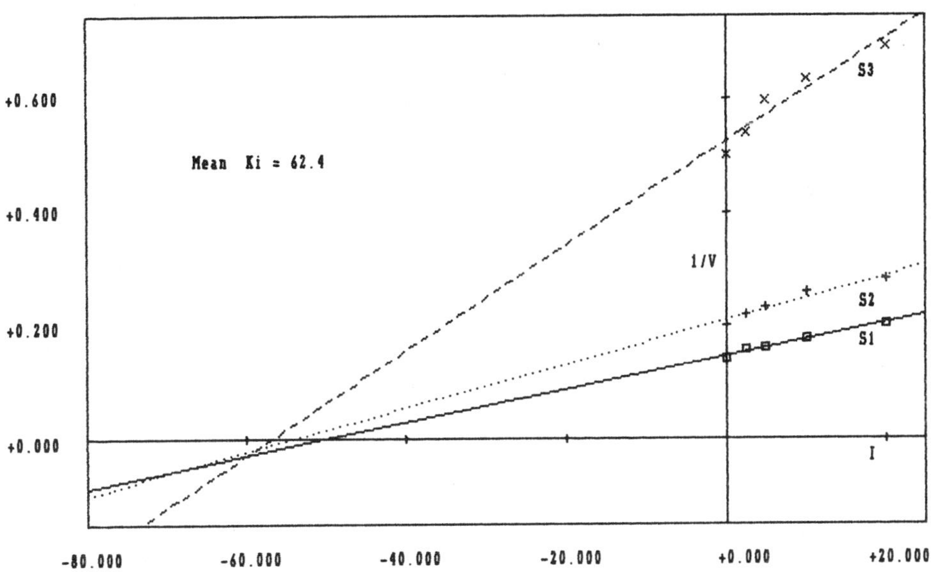

Fig. 1. Inhibition of benzo(a)pyrene hydroxylase by acrylonitrile. S_1, S_2, and S_3 represent respectively benzo(a)pyrene substrate concentrations of 0.1, 0.06, and 0.02 mM. Inhibition concentrations (I) are given in mM. Velocities (V) are given as nmoles of 8-hydroxy-benzo(a)pyrene formed per milligram of protein per minute. Each point shows the mean of at least three observations

(form III) is increased by pretreatment of animals with 3-methylcholanthrene, but not with phenobarbital.

From Tables 1 and 2 it can be seen that the inhibitory effect of acrylonitrile is evident in microsomes from control or in those from livers pretreated with phenobarbital, but the effect is absent in microsomes from livers pretreated with 3-methylcholanthrene or with Aroclor 1254.

In fact these inducers cause a significant increase in the content of cyanide-insensitive cytochrome P-450. This leads one to conclude that the inhibition of certain hydroxylation activities of liver microsomes by acrylonitrile is mediated by the cyanide released during acrylonitrile metabolism.

In the case of aniline hydroxylase, the absence of inhibitory effect could be linked with the different localization of the enzyme sites or to the fact that the enzyme proteins are too highly concentrated.

References

Comai K, Gaylor JL (1973) Existence and separation of three forms of Cytochrome P450 from rat liver microsomes. J Biol Chem 248: 4947–4955

Guengerich FP, Geiger LE, Hogy LL, Wright PL (1981) In vitro metabolism of Acrylonitrile to 2-cyanoethylene oxide reaction with glutathione and irreversible binding to proteins and nucleic acids. Cancer Res 41: 4925–4933

Kato R, Gillette J (1965) Effect of starvation on NADPH-dependent enzymes in liver microsomes of male and female rats. J Pharmacol Exp Ther 150: 279–284

Mitoma C, Posner HS, Reit HC, Udenfriend S (1956) Enzymatic hydroxylation of aromatic compounds. Arch Biochem Biophys 61: 431–441

Nebert DW, Gelboin HV (1968) Substrate-inducible microsomal aryl hydroxylase in mammalian cell culture. J Biol Chem 243: 6242–6249

Pachecka J, Salmona M, Cantoni L, Mussini E, Garattini S (1977) Inhibition of liver microsomal epoxide hydrase by ciproheptadine epoxide. Experientia 33: 484–485

Staudinger HJ, Kerekjàrtò B, Ullrich V, Zubrzyski Z (1965) In: King TE, Mason HS, Morrison M (eds) Oxidases and related redox systems. Wiley, New York, pp 815–837

Disease, Metabolism and Reproduction in the Toxic Response to Drugs and Other Chemicals
Arch. Toxicol., Suppl. 7, 295–297 (1984)

Induction of Microsomal Enzymes after Inhalation of Methanol

K. Aarstad, K. Zahlsen, and O. G. Nilsen

Department of Pharmacology and Toxicology, University of Trondheim,
7000 Trondheim, Norway

Abstract. Inhalation of 200, 2,000, and 10,000 ppm methanol increased several parameters in the microsomal cytochrome P-450 enzyme system in liver, lung, and kidney in a dose related manner. The most pronounced effect was observed in the kidney with an increase of 51% in the cytochrome P-450 concentration compared with the control. Cytochrome b_5 and NADPH cytochrome c reductase showed the same pattern of induction. The microsomal metabolism of n-hexane was enhanced in liver and kidney with the highest increase in the formation of the neurotoxic and preneurotoxic metabolite 2-hexanol with an increase of 41 and 17%, respectively, after inhalation of 10,000 ppm. A decreased formation of all n-hexane metabolites was observed in the lung. These results indicate an inter-organ difference in the induction pattern of methanol exposure.

Key words: Inhalation – Methanol – Cytochrome P-450 – Metabolic activation – n-Hexane

The acute toxicity of methanol after oral intake is well documented in man (Røe 1982). In industry, however, the main exposure will occur by inhalation. The purpose of the present investigation was to study the effects of methanol on the microsomal cytochrome P-450 enzyme system in different organs after inhalation.

Male Sprague-Dawley rats (200–250 g, five animals in each group) were exposed to 200, 2,000, and 10,000 ppm methanol for 5 days, 6 h a day, in inhalation chambers (volume 0.75 m^3) made of stainless steel and glass. The chambers were operated at six air changes per hour with a slight negative pressure. Animals were exposed at daytime in an atmosphere of 21–24° C and 40–60% humidity. The methanol was of 99.8% purity without any stabilizer added. Isolation of microsomes and enzyme assays of cytochrome P-450, cytochrome b_5, reduced nicotinamide adenine dinucleotide phosphate (NADPH) cytochrome c reductase, from liver, lung, and kidney were performed

Table 1. Concentration of microsomal cytochrome P-450 in liver, lung, and kidney after inhalation of methanol calculated in percent of control values ± SD (control = 100%)

Methanol concentration (ppm)	Liver	Lung	Kidney
200	104 ± 16	100 ± 7	111 ± 19
2,000	106 ± 6	120 ± 16	132 ± 51
10,000	126 ± 12[c]	111 ± 19	151 ± 26[c]
Control[a]	0.78 ± 0.04	0.052 ± 0.004	0.40 ± 0.07

Table 2. Formation of 2-hexanol catalyzed by liver, lung, and kidney microsomes after inhalation of methanol calculated in percent of contol ± SD (control = 100%)

Methanol concentration (ppm)	Liver	Lung	Kidney
2,000	119 ± 46	89 ± 23	103 ± 9
10,000	141 ± 26[b]	90 ± 21	117 ± 12[c]
Control[b]	2.43 ± 0.74	2.43 ± 0.34	0.57 ± 0.04

[a] Control absolute value ± SD given as nmol P-450/mg microsomal protein in liver or lung and nmol P-450/g kidney

[b] Control absolute value ± SD given as nmol 2-hexanol/min · mg microsomal protein in liver or lung and nmol 2-hexanol/min · g kidney

[c] Results significantly different from control, $p < 0.05$, $n = 5$ in a two-tailed Student's t-test

according to Dale et al. (1983). In vitro n-hexane metabolism was measured by a method described by Kraemer et al. (1974), and protein concentrations were determined according to Lowry et al. (1951).

Liver, lung, and kidney microsomes from rats exposed to methanol showed a dose related increase in the concentration of cytochrome P-450. The most pronounced effect was found in the kidney with a 51% increase of cytochrome P-450 after inhalation of 10,000 ppm (Table 1). A parallel increase was observed in the concentration of cytochrome b_5 and NADPH cytochrome c reductase activity in liver and kidney while the lung enzymes remained mainly unchanged.

The in vitro metabolism of n-hexane is shown in Table 2. Formation of the neurotoxic and preneurotoxic metabolite 2-hexanol increased in microsomes from kidney and liver after methanol exposure (17 and 41%, respectively, after 10,000 ppm). In the lung, however, a slight decrease was observed in the formation of 2-hexanol although the cytochrome P-450 enzyme level was elevated indicating a different pattern of induction of microsomal enzyme activities in different organs. Due to a high metabolizing capacity of n-hexane in the lung, this organ may still give a significant contribution to the total metabolic activation of this solvent in the organism.

The increased formation of 1- and 3-hexanol (16 and 36% in liver and 5 and 18% in kidney after 10,000 ppm) showed the same pattern as observed for

2-hexanol. It has been shown that inhalation of isopropanol increases the concentration of cytochrome P-450 in liver and kidney (Zahlsen et al., this volume) to about the same magnitude as after inhalation of methanol. The increase in the metabolism of n-hexane was, however, 5–10 times higher after inhalation of isopropanol. This is in accordance with observations made by Powis (1975) that methanol and isopropanol show different inducing properties on some cytochrome P-450 enzyme activities.

However, administration of methanol or isopropanol, prior to exposure to carbontetrachloride, potentiates liver damage to the same extent (Cantilena et al. 1979). It therefore seems likely that induction of the microsomal cytochrome P-450 enzyme system after inhalation of methanol share common properties but also show differences compared with the induction pattern obtained by isopropanol.

The present study has shown that inhalation exposure to methanol cause an induction of the cytochrome P-450 enzyme system which may alter the metabolic activation of xenobiotics significantly. Although an increase in the in vitro microsomal n-hexane metabolism has been observed, it seems likely that other cytochrome P-450 isoenzymes are induced to an equal and even higher extent.

Acknowledgement. The authors wish to thank Ms. Tenna Nørkov for skilful technical assistance.

References

Cantilena LR, Cagen SZ, Klaassen CD (1979) Methanol potentiation of carbontetrachloride-induced hepatotoxicity. Proc Soc Exp Biol Med 162: 90–95

Dale O, Nielsen K, Westgaard G, Nilsen OG (1983) Drug metabolizing enzymes in the rat after inhalation of halothane and enflurane: Different pattern of response in liver, kidney, and lung and possible implications for toxicity. Br J Anaesth 55: 1217–1224

Kraemer A, Staudinger H, Ullrich V (1974) Effect of n-hexane inhalation on the monooxygenase system in mice liver microsomes. Chem-Biol Interact 8: 11–18

Lowry OH, Rosebrough NJ, Farr AL, Randall RJ (1951) Protein measurement with the Folin phenol reagent. J Biol Chem 193: 265–275

Powis G (1975) Effect of a single oral dose of methanol, ethanol and propan-2-ol on the hepatic microsomal metabolism of foreign compounds in the rat. Biochem J 148: 269–277

Røe O (1982) Species differences in methanol poisoning. CRC Crit Rev Toxicol 10: 275–286

Disease, Metabolism and Reproduction in the Toxic Response to Drugs and Other Chemicals
Arch. Toxicol., Suppl. 7, 298–302 (1984)

Erythromycin Estolate Impairs the Mitochondrial and Microsomal Calcium Homeostasis: Correlation with Hepatotoxicity

P. Richelmi[1], C. Baldi[1], L. Manzo[2], F. Berte[1],
A. P. Martino[3], F. Mirabelli[3], and G. Bellomo[3]

[1] 2nd Institute of Pharmacology, [2] Chair of Toxicology, and [3] 2nd Medical Clinic,
University of Pavia, School of Medicine, Piazza Botta 10, 27100 Pavia, Italy

Abstract. The effects of erythromycin estolate, a well known hepatotoxic macrolide antibiotic, on isolated rat hepatocyte viability and on subcellular Ca^{2+} transport have been investigated. Erythromycin estolate (0.5 mM), but not erythromycin base and erythromycin ethylsuccinate, induced 100% cell death after 60 min incubation, and caused maximal inhibition of mitochondrial and microsomal Ca^{2+} sequestration activities at 0.1 mM concentration. Sodium lauryl sulphate, which is the surfactant moiety of the erythromycin estolate molecule, caused effects similar to those exhibited by erythromycin estolate. Disorders of the intracellular calcium homeostasis seem to play a role in the lauryl sulphate-mediated hepatotoxic action of erythromycin estolate.

Key words: Erythromycin – Macrolide antibiotics – Calcium pump – Hepatocytes – Lauryl sulphate – Hepatotoxicity

Disorders of liver cell function have been associated with the use of macrolide antibiotics and a special hepatotoxic potential has been attributed to erythromycin estolate (Keeffe et al. 1982). In accordance with the clinical observations, experimental studies have documented the in vitro hepatotoxicity of both erythromycin and lauryl sulphate in rat hepatoma cell cultures as well as in Chang cell cultures derived from human liver (Dujovne 1978).

The mechanism of the erythromycin-induced liver damage is still unclear. Recently, it has been proposed that alterations in subcellular calcium transport and intracellular calcium homeostasis play a major role in the hepatotoxicity associated with the exposure to a variety of chemicals (Schanne et al. 1979; Trump et al. 1981).

This work was aimed at studying the possible relationship between hepatotoxic action of erythromycin estolate and the effects of this drug on subcellular calcium transport systems. The role of the lauryl sulphate moiety in the mechanism of erythromycin estolate-induced liver damage has also been investigated.

Materials and Methods

Erythromycins were kindly supplied by Pierrel (Milan, Italy) and sodium lauryl sulphate was obtained from BDH Italia (Milan). Collagenase (grade IV) and arsenazo III were obtained from SIGMA (St. Louis, Missouri, USA). All other reagents and enzymes were obtained at the highest degree of purity.

Male Wistar rats (200 ± 20 g) fed ad libitum were employed. Isolated hepatocytes were prepared as described by Moldeus et al. (1978) and cell viability was monitored using the LDH leakage method. Mitochondria were isolated by differential centrifugation and intracellular Ca^{2+} movements were studied according to Bellomo et al. (1982). Microsomes (1 mg protein/ml) were

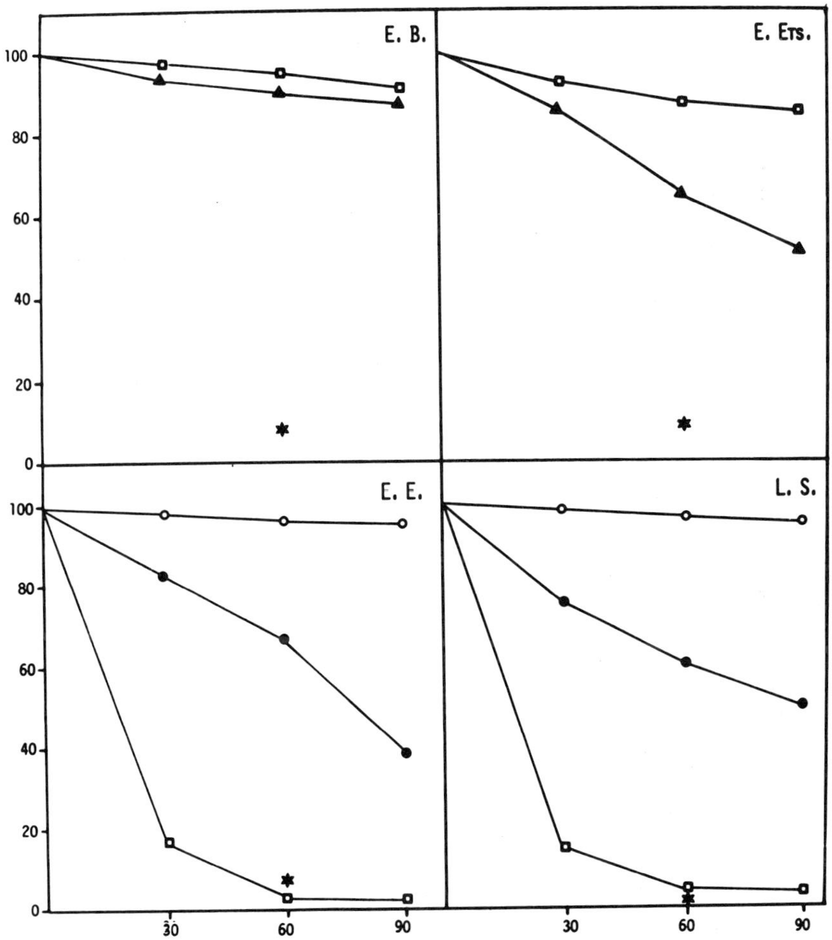

Fig. 1. Toxicity of various erythromycin derivatives and of sodium lauryl sulphate on isolated rat hepatocytes. *Ordinate:* Cell viability as per cent of control; *abscissa:* time (min) of incubation; *E.B.:* erythromycin base; *E.ETS.:* erythromycin ethylsuccinate; *E.E.:* erythromycin estolate; *L.S.:* sodium lauryl sulphate. Chlorpromazine 1 mM (*) was employed as internal control of hepatotoxicity. ○–○, 0.1 mM; ●–●, 0.25 mM; □–□, 0.5 mM; ▲–▲, 1.0 mM

preincubated for 10 min at 25° C in a medium containing 125 mM KCl, 2 mM K_2HPO_4, 4 mM $MgCl_2$, 25 mM Hepes pH 7.0 and 40 μM arsenazo III. After addition of ATP (3 mM final concentration) Ca^{2+} uptake was measured spectrophotometrically at the wavelenght pair 654–685 nm.

Results

Erythromycin estolate and sodium lauryl sulphate (0.5 mM) induced 100% cell death of the isolated hepatocytes after 60 min incubation. Erythromycin base and erythromycin ethylsuccinate were remarkably less toxic even when tested at higher concentrations (up to 1 mM) and for longer incubation periods (Fig. 1).

As depicted in Fig. 2, erythromycin estolate (0.1 mM) and sodium lauryl sulphate (0.1 mM) caused marked inhibition of the uptake (A) and retention (B) of Ca^{2+} by isolated mitochondria. This effect was not prevented by ATP (0.1 mM), dibucaine (0.2 mM), ruthenium red (1 μM), dithiotreitol (2 mM), isocitrate (0.5 mM) and β-OH-butyrate (0.5 mM). The microsomal ATPase-dependent Ca^{2+} translocase activities (C) were also inhibited by erythromycin estolate (0.1 mM) and sodium lauryl sulphate (0.1 mM), whereas erythromycin base and erythromycin ethylsuccinate had no effect at concentrations up to 1 mM.

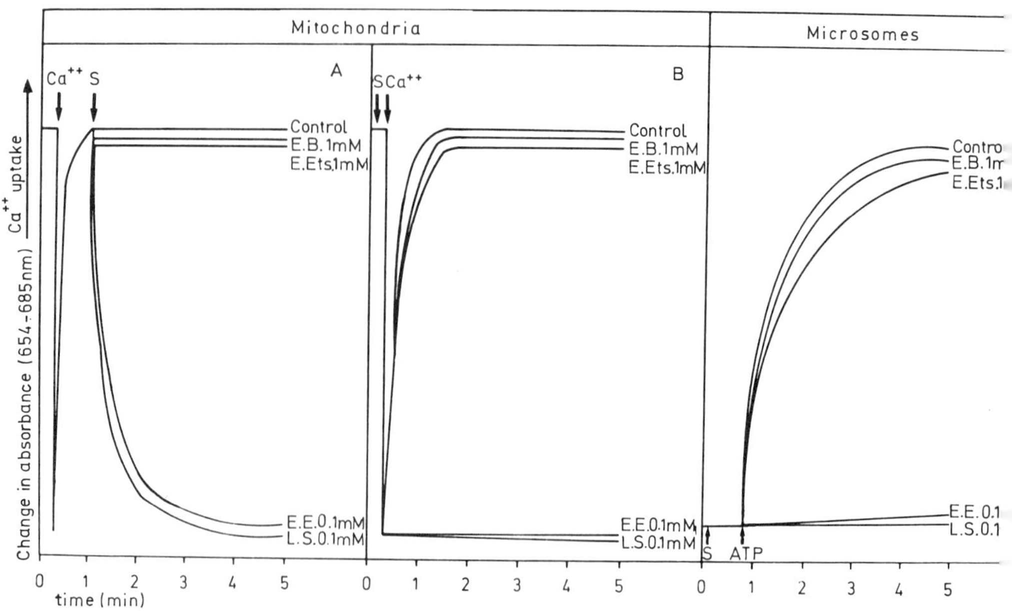

Fig. 2. Effects of various erythromycin derivatives and of sodium lauryl sulphate on intracellular calcium movements. **A** Mitochondrial calcium uptake; **B** mitochondrial calcium release; **C** microsomal calcium uptake. *S*, Substrates; Ca^{2+}, 50 nmoles/mg protein

Discussion

In the present investigation erythromycin estolate proved to be considerably more toxic than the parent compounds erythromycin base and erythromycin ethylsuccinate on isolated rat hepatocyte preparations. A cytotoxic potential was also exhibited by sodium lauryl sulphate, an agent with marked surface activity which is used to enhance the gastrointestinal absorption of erythromycin.

In previous studies on Chang cell cultures sodium lauryl sulphate was found to be at least equally or more toxic than the erythromycin moiety of the estolate derivative, and the hepatocellular toxicity of these compounds was markedly enhanced when they were placed together at the same concentration. This interaction was interpreted as the result of the increased cellular uptake of sodium lauryl sulphate promoted by the erythromycin derivative (Dujovne 1978). These experiments demonstrated intrinsic hepatotoxic effects of sodium lauryl sulphate that were of the same order of magnitude as those exerted by erythromycin estolate. The existence of a common intracellular target involved in the toxic action of erythromycin estolate and sodium lauryl sulphate was also observed. Thus, disorders of intracellular calcium homeostasis related to inhibition of mitochondrial and microsomal calcium pumps were produced by both erythromycin estolate and sodium lauryl sulphate. This effect was not secondary to an altered pyridine nucleotide and thiol redox status since the blockade of mitochondrial Ca^{2+} sequestration was not prevented by isocitrate, β-OH-butyrate and dithiotreitol. Moreover, the lack of protection by dibucaine, ATP and ruthenium red suggests that the hepatocellular toxicity of erythromycin estolate and sodium lauryl sulphate can not be accounted for by a direct membrane damage due to disturbed interaction of calcium with its uniporter (Bellomo et al. 1984a, b).

In conclusion the results of the present study indicate a non-specific membrane damage by the lauryl sulphate moiety as a causative factor leading to disorders of intracellular Ca^{2+} transport in the erythromycin estolate-induced hepatotoxicity.

References

Bellomo G, Jewell SA, Orrenius S (1982) The metabolism of menadione impairs the ability of rat liver mitochondria to take up and retain calcium. J Biol Chem 257: 11558–11562

Bellomo G, Martino AP, Mirabelli F, Fratino P, Baldi C, Manzo L, Richelmi P (1984a) Extramitochondrial calcium as a possible factor for mitochondria toxicity by xenobiotics. J Toxicol Med in press

Bellomo G, Martino AP, Mirabelli F, Richelmi P, Baldi C, Manzo L, Bertè F (1984b) The critical role of pyridine nucleotide redox level on the Ca^{2+}-mediated mitochondrial toxicity by xenobiotics. J Toxicol Med in press

Dujovne CA (1978) Hepatotoxic and cellular uptake interactions among surface active components of erythromycin preparations. Biochem Pharmacol 27: 1925–1930

Jewell SA, Bellomo G, Thor H, Orrenius S, Smith M (1982) Bleb formations in hepatocytes during drug metabolism is caused by disturbances in thiol and calcium homeostasis. Science 217: 1257–1259

Keeffe EB, Reis TC, Berland JE (1982) Hepatotoxicity to both erythromycin estolate and erythromycin ethylsuccinate. Dig Dis Sci 27: 701–704

Moldeus P, Högberg J, Orrenius S (1978) Isolation and use of liver cells. Methods Enzymol 51 : 60–71

Schanne FAX, Kane AB, Young EE, Farber JL (1979) Calcium dependence of toxic cell death: A final common pathway. Science 206 : 700–702

Trump BF, Berezesky IK, Osornio-Vargas AR (1981) Cell death and the disease process. The role of calcium. In: Bowen ID, Lockshin RA (eds) Cell death. Chapman and Hall, London, pp 209–242

Disease, Metabolism and Reproduction in the Toxic Response to Drugs and Other Chemicals
Arch. Toxicol., Suppl. 7, 303–306 (1984)

Relationships Between the Pharmacokinetics of Carbon Tetrachloride Conversion to Carbon Dioxide and Chloroform and Liver Injury

E. S. Reynolds †, R. J. Treinen, H. H. Farrish, and M. T. Moslen

Chemical Pathology Laboratory, The University of Texas Medical Branch, Galveston, Texas 77550, USA

Abstract. Rate and extent of CCl_4 metabolism by pathways leading to CO_2 and $CHCl_3$ were evaluated by measuring the amounts of these metabolites exhaled during discrete intervals following six different doses of CCl_4. Pulmonary pharmacokinetics of $^{14}CO_2$ and $CHCl_3$ exhalation after CCl_4 administration were compared with those after $Na_2{}^{14}CO_3$ and $^{14}CHCl_3$ administration. Exhalation of $^{14}CO_2$ metabolite declined more rapidly than expected after hepatotoxic doses of CCl_4. This decline could be due to injury associated changes in the metabolism of CCl_4.

Key words: Hepatotoxicity – Carbon tetrachloride – Chloroform – Carbon dioxide – Pharmacokinetics

Recently it was found that the magnitude of carbon tetrachloride (CCl_4) hepatotoxicity was strongly associated with the amounts of carbondioxide (CO_2) and chloroform ($CHCl_3$) metabolite exhaled when isopropanol pretreatment was the variable used to enhance liver injury (Reynolds et al. 1982). The purpose of this study was to further examine the relationship between $^{14}CCl_4$ hepatotoxicity and metabolism to $^{14}CO_2$ and $^{14}CHCl_3$ over a CCl_4 dose range causing minimal to severe acute liver injury. Since analysis of metabolite pharmacokinetics is frequently complex (Houston 1982), comparison time-course studies were carried out with sodium carbonate ($Na_2{}^{14}CO_3$) and $^{14}CHCl_3$.

$^{14}CCl_4$, $^{14}CHCl_3$, and $Na_2{}^{14}CO_3$ of 99% minimum purity were purchased from New England Nuclear Corp. (Boston, MA, USA). Male Sprague Dawley rats were obtained from Charles River Laboratories (Wilmington, MA, USA.). The rats were fasted overnight, and the next morning between 9.00 and 10.00 a.m. were given one of the following by gavage: CCl_4 (containing 10–80 μCi $^{14}CCl_4$) in 2.5 ml mineral oil/kg at doses of 0.1, 0.3, 2, 4, 10, and 26 mmoles/kg; $CHCl_3$ (containing 10–20 μCi $^{14}CHCl_3$) in 2.5 ml mineral oil/kg at doses of 0.1 and 0.3 mmoles/kg; or $Na_2{}^{14}CO_3$ (containing 10 μCi $^{14}CO_2$) in 2.5 ml 0.02 N

NaOH/kg at a dose of 0.005 mmole/kg. Each dose of CCl_4 and $CHCl_3$ was given to four rats, and $Na_2{}^{14}CO_3$ was given to three rats.

Immediately after compound administration each rat was placed in a one liter all glass and steel metabolism chamber. Amounts of parent compound and metabolites exhaled during discrete intervals (usually 15 min) were monitored for the next 8–12 h as previously described (Reynolds et al. 1982). Animals were killed at 24 h and liver injury assessed histologically and biochemically by measuring serum transaminases (SGPT and SGOT). Only the five larger CCl_4 doses (> 0.1 mmole/kg) were hepatotoxic with respective mean SGPT activities of 65, 77, 233, 821, and 1,333 IU increasing with CCl_4 dose as compared to control activities of 40 IU.

Exhalation data was plotted and pharmacokinetic parameters determined using NONLIN, a non-linear least squares program with initial estimates obtained by "graphic exponential curve stripping". The decay curve for $^{14}CO_2$ exhalation after $Na_2{}^{14}CO_3$ was biexponential and was well fit by a two compartment model. $CHCl_3$ exhalation data were at least biexponential and also best fit a two compartment model. CCl_4 exhalation data exhibited a monoexponential decay curve and was analyzed by a one compartment model.

The pulmonary pharmacokinetic parameters determined for the parent compounds and metabolites are summarized in Table 1. Comparison of the parent compounds shows that animals exhaled $^{14}CO_2$ more than twice as rapidly as $CHCl_3$ or CCl_4 which is consistent with more extensive uptake and slower release of the lipid soluble halocarbons from fatty tissues. Exhalation of CCl_4 was protracted, especially after the two largest doses with exhalation of peak amounts continuing for more than 4 h.

Animals, given the larger $^{14}CHCl_3$ dose, exhaled peak amounts of $^{14}CO_2$ metabolite later and for a longer period than animals given the smaller $CHCl_3$ dose. Apparent $t_{1/2}$ of $^{14}CO_2$ metabolite elimination after the larger $CHCl_3$ dose (5.5 h) was 2.5 times longer than after the smaller $CHCl_3$ dose (2.1 h). This slower apparent elimination rate of a metabolite is consistent with a dose-dependent increase in the oxidation of the parent compound by animals given a larger dose of the parent compound. Rose et al. (1981) similarly reported that the apparent elimination $t_{1/2}$ of prednisone's metabolite prednisolone increased with prednisone dose. In contrast to the findings with $^{14}CHCl_3$, animals given the larger $^{14}CCl_4$ doses exhaled peak amounts of $^{14}CO_2$ metabolite earlier than animals given the smaller $^{14}CCl_4$ doses. Also unlike $^{14}CHCl_3$, $^{14}CO_2$ exhalation by all animals given hepatotoxic doses of $^{14}CCl_4$ (i.e., > 0.1 mmoles/kg) declined abruptly from high initial rates, then stabilized for 3–4 h, and thereafter gradually decreased. Increases in $^{14}CCl_4$ dose were not consistently associated with slower apparent elimination half-times of $^{14}CO_2$ metabolite. It is possible that the extensive metabolism of CCl_4 to CO_2 at early times is relevant to the hepatotoxicity of CCl_4 since the rate of CO_2 exhalation by individual animals during the first hour correlated closely with injury (SGPT activities) at 24 h ($r = 0.88$, $n = 24$).

Peak values of $CHCl_3$ exhalation after $^{14}CCl_4$ were lower than expected and occurred several hours after the peak of $^{14}CO_2$ metabolite exhalation. Indeed as

Table 1. Exhalation pharmacokinetics of animals given $Na_2{}^{14}CO_3$, $^{14}CHCl_3$, or $^{14}CCl_4$

Compound given	Dose (mmoles/kg)	Total exhaled as (% dose/24 h)		
		CO_2	$CHCl_3$	CCl_4
$Na_2{}^{14}CO_3$	0.005	95	–	–
$^{14}CHCl_3$	0.1	67	5.0	–
$^{14}CHCl_3$	0.3	68	12	–
$^{14}CCl_4$	0.1	28	0.11	19
$^{14}CCl_4$	0.3	12	0.11	77
$^{14}CCl_4$	2	2.7	0.65	74
$^{14}CCl_4$	4	1.6	0.38	76
$^{14}CCl_4$	10	1.0	0.20	89
$^{14}CCl_4$	26	0.7	0.22	71

Compound given	Time peak exhaled (h)			Peak rate (μmoles/h · kg)		
	CO_2	$CHCl_3$	CCl_4	CO_2	$CHCl_3$	CCl_4
$Na_2{}^{14}CO_3$	0 –0.05	–	–	16	–	–
$^{14}CHCl_3$	0.5–0.75	0–0.25	–	37	6.0	–
$^{14}CHCl_3$	1.0–1.75	0–0.5	–	46	15.2	–
$^{14}CCl_4$	0.5–0.75	2–2.25	0 –2.25	11	0.02	2.6
$^{14}CCl_4$	0.5–0.75	4–7	0.5–2.25	15	0.06	102
$^{14}CCl_4$	0 –0.75	4–9	0.5–2.25	18	0.78	545
$^{14}CCl_4$	0 –0.25	4–9	0.5–1.5	37	0.90	845
$^{14}CCl_4$	0 –0.25	3–9	0.5–4	62	1.32	1,250
$^{14}CCl_4$	0 –0.25	2–9	0.5–6	88	3.40	1,550

the dose of CCl_4 and extent of injury increased, the duration of peak exhalation of $CHCl_3$ increased. After the most hepatotoxic dose of CCl_4, peak exhalation of $CHCl_3$ continued at peak rates for 7 h.

In order to confirm that the conversion of CCl_4 to CO_2 did decline abruptly after hepatotoxic doses although CCl_4 exhalation continued at peak rates, the fate of $^{14}CCl_4$ (0.3 mmole/kg) given 4 h before or 4 h after an equimolar dose of unlabelled CCl_4 was compared. Animals given unlabelled CCl_4 first exhaled one third as much $^{14}CO_2$ as animals given the labelled compound first. However, the order of administration did not affect the amount of ^{14}C-label recovered bound to liver macromolecules.

This working model for CCl_4 metabolism has at least two pathways. In the first pathway, the trichloromethyl radical ($\cdot CCl_3$) sequesters a molecule of oxygen forming a trichloromethyl radical ($\cdot OOCCl_3$) which is eventually converted to CO_2. In the second, $\cdot CCl_3$ sequesters a hydrogen atom forming $CHCl_3$ which is subsequently converted to CO_2 via the metabolic pathway postulated by Pohl (1979) to involve phosgene as an intermediate. Injury-associated alterations in components of one or more of these pathways of CCl_4 metabolism could account for the observed deviations in the pharmacokinetic patterns of CCl_4 metabolite exhalation from that anticipated based on these comparison studies with $Na_2{}^{14}CO_3$ and $^{14}CHCl_3$. The unexpected rapid decline in $^{14}CO_2$ exhalation following hepatotoxic doses of CCl_4 could be due to deactivation of the cytochrome P-450 isozyme that oxidizes CCl_4 via $^{\cdot}OOCCl_3$ to CO_2. This would be consistent with the recent reports on the specificity of cytochrome P-450 isozymes for the metabolism of CCl_4 (Noguchi 1982), and the disappearance of a specific cytochrome P-450 isozyme following CCl_4 poisoning, (Head et al. 1981). Furthermore the finding that nonhepatotoxic doses of $CHCl_3$ were more extensively metabolized to CO_2 than were hepatotoxic doses of CCl_4, strongly indicates that the $CHCl_3$ to phosgene to CO_2 pathway of CCl_4 metabolism is not relevant to the hepatotoxicity of CCl_4.

Acknowledgements. Supported by NIH grants AM-19814 and AM-27135.

References

Head B, Moody DE, Woo CH, Smuckler EA (1981) Alterations of specific forms of cytochrome P-450 in rat liver during acute carbon tetrachloride intoxication. Toxicol Appl Pharmacol 61 : 286–295

Houston JB (1982) Drug metabolite kinetics. Pharmacol Ther 15 : 521–552

Noguchi T, Fong KL, Lai EK, Alexander SS, King MM, Olson J, Poyer JL, McCay PB (1982) Specificity of a phenobarbital-induced cytochrome P-450 for metabolism of carbon tetrachloride to the trichloromethyl radical. Biochem Pharmacol 31 : 615–624

Pohl LR (1979) Biochemical toxicology of chloroform. Rev Biochem Toxicol 1 : 79–107

Reynolds ES, Moslen MT, Treinen RJ (1982) Isopropanol enhancement of carbon tetrachloride metabolism in vivo. Life Sci 31 : 661–669

Rose JQ, Yurchak AM, Jusko WJ (1981) Dose dependent pharmacokinetics of prednisone and prednisolone in man. J Pharmacokinet Biopharmacol 9 : 389–417

Disease, Metabolism and Reproduction in the Toxic Response to Drugs and Other Chemicals
Arch. Toxicol., Suppl. 7, 307–310 (1984)

Distribution and Metabolism of 2-*t*-Butyl-4-methoxyphenol in the Everted Rat Gut Preparation

L. Della Corte[1], M. G. Giovannini[1], and G. P. Sgaragli[2]

[1] Institute of Pharmacology and Toxicology, Viale G.B. Morgagni 65, 50134 Florence, Italy
[2] Institute of Pharmacological Sciences, Via Cassia Sud, Villa Betlem, 35100 Siena, Italy

Abstract. The distribution of BHA and its conversion to di-BHA in the everted rat gut preparation was monitored by GC/MS analysis of both compounds in the mucosal and serosal side solutions and in the ileum wall. Following 1 h incubation at 27° C, BHA concentration in the mucosal side solution was found to decay from an initial value of 0.1 mM down to 0.033 mM, while in the ileum it reached a 0.35 mM concentration. The amount of di-BHA found at this time in the ileum wall accounted for the transformation of 5% of the amount of BHA present in this compartment.

Key words: 2-*t*-Butyl-4-methoxyphenol – Distribution – Metabolism – 2,2′-Dihydroxy-3,3′-di-*t*-butyl-5,5-dimethoxydiphenyl – Everted gut preparation

Some aspects ot the toxicity of BHA, a widely used antioxidant food additive, are still unknown. It has been shown in this laboratory that the LD_{50} of BHA administered intraperitoneally to the rat is of two orders of magnitude lower than that reported for this agent given orally (Sgaragli et al. 1977). Subsequently, BHA has been shown to undergo peroxidative transformation catalysed by preparations of rat intestine peroxidase leading to the less toxic compound, di-BHA (Sgaragli et al. 1980). Furthermore in vivo, following the oral administration of BHA, di-BHA was found in rat intestine and plasma (Guarna et al. 1983).

BHA, recrystallised from light petroleum was obtained from Fluka A.G. (Buchs, S.G.); di-BHA was synthesized as previously described (Sgaragli et al. 1980). Sacs of everted rat [Sprague Dawley ♂ 150–200 g body weight (b.w.)]

Abbreviations: BHA, 2-*t*-butyl-4-methoxyphenol; BHA-d_3, 2-*t*-butyl-4-trideuteriomethoxyphenol; di-BHA, 2,2′-dihydroxy-3,3′-di-*t*-butyl-5,5′-dimethoxydiphenyl; di-BHA-d_6, 2,2′-dihydroxy-3,3′-di-*t*-butyl-5,5′-di(trideuteriomethoxy)diphenyl; GC/MS, gas chromatography/mass spectrometry

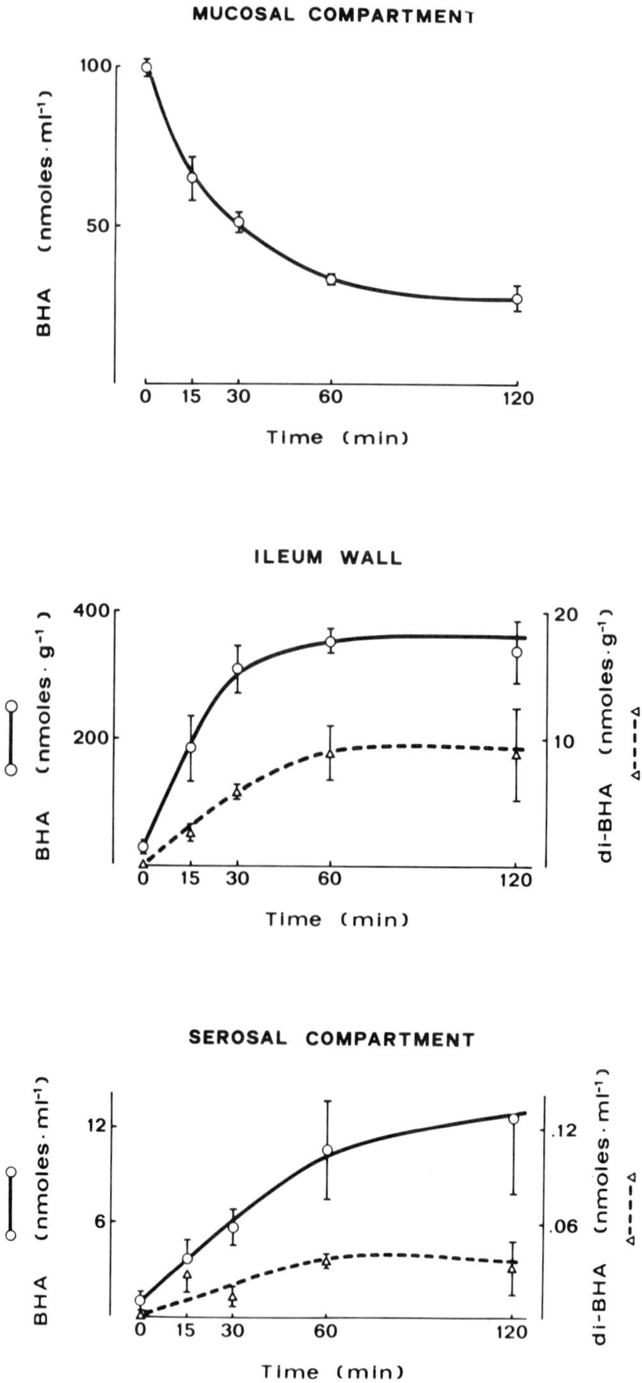

Fig. 1. Concentration vs. time profiles of BHA and di-BHA in different compartments of the everted gut preparation. *Data points* and *bars* represent mean values ± SE obtained from four different preparations

ileum, prepared according to Wilson and Wiseman (1954), filled with 0.5 ml of Krebs-Henseleit solution, were put into flasks containing 5 ml of Krebs-Henseleit solution gassed with 5% CO_2 in 95% O_2, incubated at 25° C and shaken at 90 oscillations · min^{-1}. BHA was present in the mucosal bathing medium at 0.1 mM concentrations. At the end of various experimental periods the sacs were emptied and, after gently blotting the surfaces with filter paper, were weighed and homogenised in 0.1 M buffer phosphate pH 7.2 (1 : 7, w : v). Aliquots of the mucosal and serosal side solutions and of ileum homogenates were analysed for BHA and di-BHA levels, using a gas chromatography/mass spectrometry (GC/MS) method with multiple ion detection as modified from Bailey et al. (1981). Deuterium labelled BHA-d_3 and di-BHA-d_6 were synthesized from *t*-butylhydroquinone (Bredereck et al. 1953) and added to the specimens as internal standards before methylene chloride extraction. The derivatives of the extracted compounds were produced with trifluoroacetic anhydride and analysed by mass fragmentography.

As shown in Fig. 1, the BHA concentration in the mucosal side solution showed a constant decay from an initial value of 0.1 mM down to 0.027 mM after 2 h incubation. The BHA concentration in the ileum increased with time reaching a maximum of about 0.35 mM after 1 h. BHA was also found to pass into the serosal side solution, where however the highest concentration reached after 2 h incubation was about 50% of that found on the mucosal side. di-BHA, while not detected on the mucosal side, was found to increase in the ileum wall, in a similar way to BHA, reaching a concentration of 0.009 mM and accounting for the conversion of 5% of the amount of BHA present in this compartment. The distribution of BHA and di-BHA among different compartments of the everted gut preparation is shown in Table 1. The initial amount of 90.7 µg of BHA present at the mucosal side progressively distributed into the ileum wall and, to a lesser extent, out at the serosal side. The entrance of BHA into the ileum wall was accompanied by the formation of di-BHA. However the amount of BHA which had left the mucosal solution was only partially recovered as BHA or di-BHA in the other compartments. It appears that in 1 h 35.5% of

Table 1. Distribution of BHA and di-BHA in the different compartments of the everted gut preparation

Incubation time (min)	Mucosal side (A)	Ileum wall (B)		Serosal side (C)		A + B + C	(%)[a]
	BHA	BHA	di-BHA	BHA	di-BHA		
15	58,860	14,202	387	232	1.2	73,682	(81)
30	46,170	23,868	834	380	1.7	71,254	(78)
60	29,790	28,332	1,352	635	4.3	60,113	(66)

Figures represent mean values of the total compartmental content (ng) calculated from data shown in Fig. 1. Volumes (ml) of compartments were (mean values ± SE), 5 (A), 0.443 ± 0.025 (B) and 0.353 ± 0.019 (C)

[a] Total (BHA + di-BHA) content expressed as percentage of the initial amount of BHA (90,720 ng) present at the mucosal side

BHA was metabolised, however its conversion into di-BHA only accounted for 1.5%. In previous experiments it was found that this conversion in vitro at 37° C, using a partially purified preparation of rat ileum peroxidase supplemented with H_2O_2, amounted to 6 μmoles · h^{-1}. $ileum^{-1}$ of di-BHA formed in the presence of 0.5 mM BHA. Furthermore, the actual capacity of the ileum to transform in vivo BHA into di-BHA in the first hour after BHA treatment was expressed by 2.8 μmoles of di-BHA formed at 5 mM average BHA concentration found in this tissue (manuscript in preparation). Thus in the everted gut preparation the efficiency of this pathway was almost 2 orders of magnitude lower. This discrepancy may be partially due to the lower temperature used in the present conditions. Furthermore, a role may also be played by a limited accessibility of the converting enzymes to BHA or by a poor availability of cosubstrates, such as hydrogen peroxide, in this preparation.

Acknowledgements. We are indebted to Prof. L. Zilletti and Dr. G. Moneti for the access and help in the use of the instruments of the "Centro di Spettrometria di Massa e Analisi Frammentografiche", Faculty of Medicine, University of Florence. This work was supported by Ministero Pubblica Istruzione and CNR grant no. 81-00187-04.

References

Bailey E, Della Corte L, Farmer PB, Gray AJ (1981) Determination of the antioxidant 3-tert-butyl-4-hydroxyanisole in rat plasma using high resolution gas chromatography-mass spectrometry. J Chromatogr 225: 83–89

Bredereck H, Hennig I, Ran W (1953) Alkilierungen mehrwertiger Phenole mit Dialkylsulfat. Chem Ber 86: 1085–1087

Guarna A, Della Corte L, Giovannini MG, De Sarlo F, Sgaragli GP (1983) 2,2′-dihydroxy-3,3′-di-*t*-butyl-5,5′-dimethoxydiphenyl (di-BHA) a new metabolite of 2-*t*-butyl-4-methoxyphenol (BHA) in the rat. Drug Metab Disposition 11: 581–584

Sgaragli GP, Rizzotti-Conti M, Garetti GL, Magi B, Puliti R, Megazzini I, Della Corte L (1977) Delayed toxicity exhibited by butylated hydroxyanisole (BHA) in the rat. Joint meeting of German and Italian pharmacologists, October 4–6, 1977, Isola di S. Giorgio, Venice, Italy. Abstracts: 213

Sgaragli GP, Della Corte L, Puliti R, De Sarlo F, Francalanci R, Guarna A, Dolara P, Komarynsky M (1980) Oxidation of 2-*t*-butyl-4-methoxyphenol (BHA) by horse-radish and mammalian peroxidase systems. Biochem Pharmacol 29: 763–769

Wilson TH, Wiseman G (1954) The use of sacs of everted small intestine for the study of the transference of substances from the mucosal to the serosal surface. J Physiol 123: 116–125

Disease, Metabolism and Reproduction in the Toxic Response to Drugs and Other Chemicals
Arch. Toxicol., Suppl. 7, 311 (1984)

Phenytoin Metabolites in Human Placental Tissue

M. Henneberg and E. Serowka

Medical Postgraduate Education Centre, Warsaw, Poland

Abstract. It had been suggested, by American epidemiological retrospective researchers, that phenytoin (DPH) is suspected of teratogenic effects in humans.

To study the mechanism of DPH biotransformation in the human placental tissue, its metabolites, in placental homogenates incubated in vitro, were investigated.

Thin layer chromatography and spectrophotometric methods (IR and UV) were used to detect the metabolites.

3–5 metabolites of DPH were isolated from placental tissue which had different physico-chemical characteristics from those of DPH metabolites in urine after oral administration.

Key words: Phenytoin – Biotransformation – Teratogenisis – Placenta

Disease, Metabolism and Reproduction in the Toxic Response to Drugs and Other Chemicals
Arch. Toxicol., Suppl. 7, 312 (1984)

The Placental Transfer and Detection of ^{14}C-Carmoisine Metabolites by HPLC Combined with a Radioactivity Monitor (RAM)

E. Tragni, M. Marinovich, and C. L. Galli

Institute of Pharmacology and Pharmacognosy, University of Milan, Milan, Italy

Abstract. Carmoisine (Azo Rubine; Ext. D&C Red No 10; C.I. (1956) No 14720; E 122) is the disodium salt of 2-(4′-sulpho-1′-naphthylazo)-1-naphthol-4-sulphonic acid, a water soluble sulphonated azodye currently permitted for food in the EEC member countries. Because of the lack of information on the metabolism and placental transfer of the red food color and its metabolites the absorption fate and excretion of ^{14}C-carmoisine has been determined in pregnant rats together with the presence of ^{14}C-metabolites in vivo and in vitro preparations. Pregnant rats received ^{14}C-carmoisine (200 mg/kg; 25 μCi) by gavage on days 16−19 of gestation. The animals were killed and the maternal tissues, amniotic fluid, placentae, foetal membranes and fetuses were analyzed for radioactivity. No evidence of the transplacental transfer of ^{14}C-carmoisine or its metabolites was obtained. More than 90% of the radioactivity was excreted in the faeces and urine within 64 h. The results suggested that there was no significant absorption of the azodye and no preferential concentration of the red food color or its metabolites in any particular tissue. The results are comparable to those obtained in a similar study in male rats. Analyses by high performance liquid chromatography (HPLC) combined with a radioactivity monitor of the urine and faeces of the animals and incubations of ^{14}C-carmoisine under anaerobic conditions with bacterial suspensions of human faeces show the same radioactivity profile. Five radioactive peaks were present in the radiochromatogram in addition to unmodified Carmoisine. The mean peak shows half of the specific activity of Carmoisine, at the retention time and with the UV spectrum of authentic naphthionic acid. The results demonstrate the value of transplacental studies because with chemicals that are poorly absorbed from the intestine and which do not cross the placenta, they will assist in the evaluation of adverse maternal effects which may result in foetal toxicity. Furthermore, with similar results obtained in vivo and in vitro one may use the in vitro preparations to prepare these compounds in amounts suitable for their identification by further chemical methods.

Key words: Carmoisine metabolism – Placental transfer – HPCL-RAM

Toxicity of Non-steroidal Antirheumatic Drugs: Molecular Mechanisms and Clinical Assessment

Disease, Metabolism and Reproduction in the Toxic Response to Drugs and Other Chemicals
Arch. Toxicol., Suppl. 7, 315–322 (1984)

A Biochemical Basis for the Gastrointestinal Toxicity of Non-steroid Antirheumatoid Drugs

B. J. R. Whittle and J. R. Vane

Wellcome Research Laboratories, Langley Court, Beckenham, Kent, Great Britain

Abstract. The non-steroid anti-inflammatory drugs inhibit cyclo-oxygenase and therefore the biosynthesis of prostaglandins, and it has been proposed that this biochemical intervention is the basis not only of their therapeutic activity but also contributes to their gastrointestinal side-effects. Since endogenous prostaglandins may exert mucosal protective actions, inhibition of cyclo-oxygenase by aspirin-like drugs would be expected to lead to gastric damage. The clinically-used anti-inflammatory compounds reduce prostaglandin levels in the experimental inflammatory exudate, but also inhibit prostacyclin formation in gastric tissue and induce gastric damage. In contrast, anti-inflammatory doses of sodium salicylate and an experimental drug BW755C (3-amino-1m-(trifluoromethyl)-phenyl-2-pyrazoline) fail to inhibit gastric mucosal prostacyclin formation (but do reduce prostaglandin levels in the inflammatory exudate) and causc only minimal gastric damage, supporting the relationship between production of gastric erosions and the inhibition of mucosal prostacyclin production. Anti-inflammatory doses of BW755C also fail to inhibit prostaglandin formation in the small intestine. Furthermore, studies on homogenates of gastric mucosa and ileum show that sodium salicylate, paracetamol and BW755C are only weak inhibitors of gastric mucosal cyclo-oxygenase in vitro. The development of nonsteroid anti-rheumatic drugs which have minimal action on prostaglandin production by the gastro-intestinal tract and exhibit reduced gastrointestinal toxicity, thus appears to be a feasible proposition.

Key words: Anti-inflammatory drugs – Gastrointestinal tract – Gastric ulcer – Prostaglandins – Cyclo-oxygenase

A major hypothesis concerning the gastric side-effects of aspirin, salicylates, non-steroid anti-inflammatory and similar compounds, was developed by Davenport (1964) and his colleagues in the mid 1960's. It was proposed that the normal resistance of the gastric mucosa to the back-diffusion of gastric acid from the lumen into the mucosal tissues could be disrupted by the topical administration of aspirin and other salicylates. Although an important mechanism, it is unlikely that such a topical action can be the only process leading to gastric toxicity since non-steroid anti-inflammatory compounds can cause gastric damage when administered parenterally in experimental animals as well as man (Grossman et al. 1961; Brodie and Hooke 1971; Main and Whittle 1975; Bugat et al. 1976).

In the early 1970's, Vane and his colleagues proposed that the biological actions of aspirin-like drugs were the result of inhibition of prostaglandin synthesis (Vane 1971; Flower 1974), a theory which has since had wide-based support from many biochemical and pharmacological experimental techniques. Of paramount importance was the observation that the doses required to inhibit cyclo-oxygenase, the prostaglandin synthesizing enzyme, were well within the range which would be achieved with therapeutic doses of these compounds.

Since prostaglandins exert potent protective actions on the gastric mucosa (Robert 1976; Robert et al. 1979; Whittle 1976) and may be involved in the local regulation of gastric function (see Whittle 1980), inhibition of prostaglandin biosynthesis by non-steroid anti-inflammatory agents could be expected to disrupt the functional integrity of the gastric mucosa. Such effects would occur whether the drugs were administered orally or parenterally. Furthermore, it has become clear that both hypotheses are of importance when considering the gastric toxicity of non-steroid anti-inflammatory agents, since both the topical irritancy (resulting presumably from their physico-chemical characteristics) and the biochemical actions on prostaglandin biosynthesis, may interact to produce more extensive gastric injury than either activity alone (Fig. 1). Such an interaction will occur in the clinical use of the aspirin-like drugs following oral administration.

Local Irritation

The ability of topically-applied aspirin to promote back-diffusion of acid into the mucosal tissue, increase luminal sodium ion concentrations and alter potential difference across the mucosa extends not only to other non-steroid anti-inflammatory drugs such as indomethacin, but also to other irritants such as ethanol and bile salts. These agents, which are not known to inhibit cyclo-oxygenase, appear to alter the structural organization of the mucosal membranes either by a local detergent-like action, or by some other mechanism following their uptake into the mucosal tissue. Thus, the "barrier-breaking" activity is unlikely to be directly related to the inhibition of prostaglandin biosynthesis. Furthermore, salicylate is equipotent with aspirin in causing such acid back-diffusion (Ligumsky et al. 1982), yet there are substantial differences in their ability to inhibit prostaglandin biosynthesis in the stomach. Biochemical changes, as indicated by a reduction in mucosal energy metabolism following local application of aspirin or salicylate, have been detected (Spenney and Bhown 1977; Ohe et al. 1980), which could reflect the effects of these

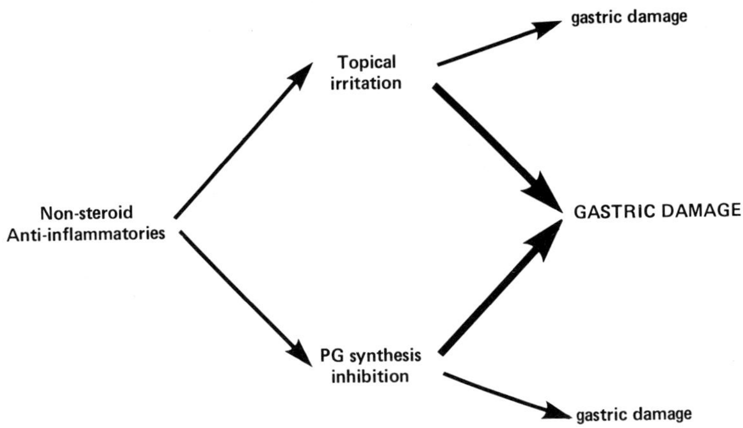

Fig. 1. Interactive process in gastric damage induced by non-steroid anti-inflammatory agents

compounds in very high concentrations used, in uncoupling oxidative phosphorylation. However, whether such changes are the cause or the result of tissue damage, or whether the newer anti-inflammatory agents have similar actions, remains to be fully investigated.

Inhibition of Gastrointestinal Prostaglandin Biosynthesis

In order to determine the actions of anti-inflammatory agents following oral or parenteral administration, on gastric mucosal and cyclo-oxygenase activity, a vortex-mixing procedure with mucosal tissue ex vivo has been utilized, which generates prostaglandins from endogenous substrate (Whittle 1981).

Segments of gastric mucosa, stripped from underlying muscle, and intestinal tissue (0.2 g) were freed from mesentery, washed in buffer (50 mM tris: pH 8.4, 0° C) chopped, rewashed (1 ml buffer) and incubated in buffer (0.5 ml) by vortex mixing for 1 min at 22° C. After centrifugation (15 s at 22° C) in a fixed-speed Eppendorf bench centrifuge (model 5412, maximum speed 9,000 *g*) the supernatant was removed for bioassay, using techniques involving platelet aggregometry as previously described (Whittle 1981). In further studies, the supernatant was transferred to plastic vials containing indomethacin (final concentration 10 $\mu g \cdot ml^{-1}$) and immediately frozen to prevent any further cyclo-oxygenase activity. Subsequently, the levels of both 6-oxo-$PGF_{1\alpha}$ (the chemical hydrolysis product of prostacyclin) and prostaglandin E_2 (PGE_2) in the supernatant were determined by radioimmunoassay (RIA) techniques (Whittle and Salmon 1983). As is shown in Table 1, parenteral administration of indomethacin in anti-inflammatory doses (10 $mg \cdot kg^{-1}$ s.c.) induced a significant inhibition ($p < 0.001$) of prostacyclin formation ex vivo as determined by bioassay techniques. The reliability of the bioassay for prostacyclin was confirmed by use of RIA for 6-oxo-$PGF_{1\alpha}$, which gave comparable data for the degree of inhibition of biosynthesis in both gastric mucosal and ileal extracts

Table 1. Inhibition of the formation of prostacyclin (determined by bioassay) and of 6-oxo-$PGF_{1\alpha}$ and PGE_2 (determined by radio-immunoassay) in the rat gastric mucosa and ileum, 3 h following indomethacin (10 mg · kg^{-1} s.c.) administration

	% Inhibition	
	Gastric mucosa	Ileum
PGI_2	88 ± 4	83 ± 3
PGE_2	75 ± 8	94 ± 2
6-oxo-$F_{1\alpha}$	77 ± 8	77 ± 3

Results shown as % inhibition of the control prostanoid formation following 1 min vortex incubation in vitro, are mean ± SE mean of three animals for each group. Data is taken from Whittle and Salmon (1983)

(Table 1). In addition, there was a comparable inhibition of PGE_2 formation ex vivo as determined by RIA.

Selective Inhibition of Tissue Cyclo-oxygenase

Prostaglandin E_2 and prostacyclin, which are the predominant cyclo-oxygenase products found in inflammatory exudates, have proinflammatory actions and are likely to be involved in the inflammatory process. These prostanoids can, however, exert protective actions on the gastro-intestinal tract and may have a physiological role in the gastric mucosa. Thus, to develop an anti-inflammatory agent with fewer gastric side-effects, it would be desirable to inhibit prostaglandin production only at the site of inflammation and not in the gastrointestinal tract. An investigation was, therefore, carried out on whether such differential inhibition of cyclo-oxygenase can be achieved in vivo and have correlated this with gastric damage (Whittle et al. 1980).

Inflammatory exudates were induced and collected by the subcutaneous implantation of carrageenin-impregnated polyester sponges in rats. After 24 h, the prostaglandin-like activity in the sponge was extracted and bioassayed on the rat superfused stomach strip (Vane 1957) in terms of PGE_2 equivalents (the major prostaglandin product in the exudate). The ex vivo generation of prostacyclin, the predominant prostaglandin in the gastric mucosa, was determined in strips of mucosal tissue by the vortex mixing procedure and bioassay techniques described above.

The anti-inflammatory compounds were administered orally three times during the 24 h period, after which time the incidence and severity of the gastric erosions was assessed. The doses of the compounds were all in the range causing 50–70% inhibition of inflammation, whereas BW755C, (3-amino-1 m-(trifluoromethyl)-phenyl-2-pyrazoline) a dual inhibitor of cyclo-oxygenase and lipoxygenase (Higgs et al. 1979) was administered in doses some tenfold greater than those required for such anti-inflammatory actions.

The clinically-used compounds, aspirin, indomethacin, ketoprofen, flurbiprofen and naproxen, all reduced cyclo-oxygenase products in both the inflammatory exudate and gastric mucosa in anti-inflammatory doses (Whittle et al. 1980). In contrast, sodium salicylate and BW755C, in doses causing a substantial reduction in prostaglandins in the inflammatory exudate, did not inhibit mucosal cyclo-oxygenase activity.

Indomethacin, ketoprofen, flurbiprofen and naproxen all induced a comparable degree of gastric erosions which paralleled their efficacy in inhibiting mucosal prostacyclin production. Aspirin, however, was more active in inducing gastric damage in doses causing a similar mucosal cyclo-oxygenase inhibition to the other compounds. This may reflect the synergistic interaction between the topical irritation with aspirin and the inhibition of mucosal cyclo-oxygenase (Fig. 1).

In contrast, sodium salicylate did not inhibit mucosal prostaglandin production in anti-inflammatory doses and caused little gastric damage. This is similar to findings in man showing that sodium salicylate produced far less gastrointestinal irritation than aspirin, measured by faecal blood loss (Grossman et al. 1961; Leonards and Levy 1973). Thus, although sodium salicylate may exert topical barrier-breaking activity, this action alone may not be sufficient to lead to pronounced gastric bleeding and erosion formation. However, in the clinical situation with the more chronic administration of sodium salicylate or under conditions of excess gastric acidity, the production of the more irritant salicylic acid may occur. Furthermore, the chronic ingestion of high levels of sodium salts may not be clinically desirable.

An overall association between the inhibition of gastric cyclooxygenase and the potential to induce gastric mucosal lesions has also been shown in the pig with seven of the eight anti-inflammatory drugs investigated. Four such compounds inhibited gastric prostaglandin synthesis and induced damage, whereas three further compounds failed to inhibit cyclo-oxygenase or cause gastric damage (Rainsford and Willis 1982).

BW755C, which also failed to inhibit mucosal cyclo-oxygenase activity, similarly caused little gastric damage, again giving support to a relationship between the production of gastric erosions and the inhibition of mucosal prostacyclin formation by anti-inflammatory drugs. Likewise, these doses of BW755C failed to inhibit prostaglandin formation in the rat small intestine (Whittle 1981), clearly demonstrating that this compound can selectively inhibit prostaglandin formation in the area of inflammation and not in the upper gastrointestinal tract. This experimental compound is of interest since it inhibits not only the cyclo-oxygenase pathway of arachidonic acid metabolism at the site of inflammation, but also inhibits the lipoxygenase pathway. The lipoxygenase enzyme gives rise to a series of hydroperoxy or hydroxy products and leukotrienes (Samuelsson et al. 1980). These latter products, especially leukotriene B_4, have potent chemotatic and chemokinetic activity and thus have a potential role in the control of leukocyte migration and inflammation. Inhibition of both pathways offers a novel approach in the development of more effective anti-inflammatory drugs (Higgs et al. 1979).

The tissue-selective action of BW755C has been confirmed by Peskar and co-workers (1982) who showed that this compound does not inhibit cyclo-oxygenase in vivo in the acid secreting corpus area of stomach, although it does

Table 2. Inhibition of prostacyciln formation from endogenous substrate in homogenates of rat gastric mucosa and ileum by anti-inflammatory agents

	ID_{50} (μM)	
	Mucosa	Ileum
Indomethacin	3.9	5.8
Flurbiprofen	0.5	0.4
Naproxen	3.9	6.3
Ketoprofen	5.5	7.3
Paracetamol*	1,325	>1,000
BW755C*	380	265

Results are shown as the ID_{50} values following 10 min preincubation in vitro with tissue homogenate, where * represents biphasic dose-response curves with stimulation of prostacyclin formation at lower concentrations. Data is taken from Boughton-Smith and Whittle (1983)

inhibit prostaglandin production in the antral mucosal region and muscular forestomach of rat. In further studies to investigate whether such in vivo selectivity was a result of pharmacokinetic distribution of the compound (Boughton-Smith and Whittle 1983), BW755C was found to inhibit prostacyclin production by homogenates of forestomach, but only at higher concentration in gastric mucosa and ileum in vitro (Table 2). Using whole-cell preparations, Peskar and co-workers (1982) likewise demonstrated a preferential inhibition of cyclo-oxygenase in the forestomach with BW755C. Such in vitro techniques should have minimized any differences in uptake or distribution between the compounds and tissues. Furthermore, in other in vitro systems, including horse platelets and rat leukocytes, BW755C exhibits comparable potency to indomethacin as a cyclo-oxygenase inhibitor (Randall et al. 1980).

In the absence of inhibition by low concentrations of BW755C in vitro, a substantial elevation of prostacyclin formation from endogenous substrate in the rat gastric mucosa was noted (Boughton-Smith and Whittle 1983). The mechanism underlying this enhancement of prostacyclin generation has yet to be characterized, but may involve a co-factor action or free-radical scavenging effect of BW755C. However, since BW755C is a potent inhibitor of the lipoxygenase pathway, the hydroperoxide products of which inhibit the prostacyclin-forming enzymes (Moncada et al. 1976), the actions of BW755C may also reflect the removal of a modulating influence of such lipoxygenase metabolites, or the diversion of available substrate to the cyclo-oxygenase pathway.

Interactive Mechanisms in Gastric Damage

Although inhibition of gastric mucosal cyclo-oxygenase appears to be an important biochemical mechanism underlying the gastric damage induced by non-steroid anti-inflammatory agents, reduction in prostaglandin biosynthesis may alone be insufficient to initiate extensive mucosal erosion. Likewise, direct topical irritancy following local application of these compounds also appears insufficient to produce substantial gastric damage. However, experimental studies in rat and dog have clearly demonstrated that there is a potentiating interaction between both effects, with cyclo-oxygenase inhibition reducing the ability of the gastric mucosa to withstand challenge (Whittle 1977; Whittle and Moncada 1983). Furthermore, inhibition of prostaglandin formation in the small intestine may act in concert with the damaging events which allow bacterial invasion and the subsequent development of intestinal lesions (Whittle 1981). An understanding of these interactive processes which are involved in gastrointestinal damage should be instrumental in directing research towards the development of novel anti-inflammatory drugs free of such side-effects.

References

Boughton-Smith NK, Whittle BJR (1983) Stimulation and inhibition of prostacyclin formation in the gastric mucosa and ileum in vitro by anti-inflammatory agents. Br J Pharmacol 78: 173–180

Brodie DA, Hooke KF (1971) Effects of route of administration on the production of gastric hemorrhage in the rat by aspirin and sodium salicylate. Am J Dig Dis 16: 985–989

Bugat R, Thompson MR, Aures D, Grossman MI (1976) Gastric mucosal lesions produced by intravenous infusion of aspirin in cats. Gastroenterology 71: 754–759

Davenport HW (1964) Gastric mucosal injury by fatty acid acetylsalicylic acids. Gastroenterology 46: 245–253

Flower RJ (1974) Drugs which inhibit prostaglandin biosynthesis. Pharmacol Rev 26: 33–67

Grossman MI, Matsumota KK, Lichter RJ (1961) Fecal blood loss by oral and intravenous administration of various salicylates. Gastroenterology 40: 383–388

Higgs GA, Flower RJ, Vane JR (1979) A new approach to antiinflammatory drugs. Biochem Pharmacol 28: 1959–1961

Leonards JR, Levy G (1973) Gastrointestinal blood loss from aspirin and sodium salicylate tablets in man. Clin Pharmacol Ther 14: 62–66

Ligumsky M, Grossman MI, Kauffman GL (1982) Endogenous gastric mucosal prostaglandins: their role in mucosal integrity. Am J Physiol 242: G337–341

Main IHM, Whittle BJR (1975) Investigation of the vasodilator and antisecretory role of prostaglandins in the rat gastric mucosa by use of non-steroidal anti-inflammatory drugs. Br J Pharmacol 53: 217–224

Moncada S, Gryglewski RJ, Bunting S, Vane JR (1976) A lipid peroxide inhibits the enzyme in blood vessel microsomes that generates from prostaglandin endoperoxides the substance (prostaglandin X) which prevents platelet aggregation. Prostaglandins 12: 715–737

Ohe K, Hayashi K, Shirakawa T, Yamada K, Kawasaki T, Miyoshi A (1980) Aspirin- and taurocholate-induced metabolic damage in mammalian gastric mucosa in vitro. Am J Physiol 239: G457–462

Peskar BM, Weiler H, Peskar BA (1982) Effect of BW755C on prostaglandin synthesis in the rat stomach. Biochem Pharmacol 31: 1652–1653

Rainsford KD, Willis C (1982) Relationship of gastric mucosal damage induced in pigs by anti-inflammatory drugs to their effects on prostaglandin production. Dig Dis Sci 27: 624–635

Randall RW, Eakins KE, Higgs GA, Salmon JA, Tateson JE (1980) Inhibition of arachidonic acid cyclo-oxygenase and lipoxygenase activities of leukocytes by indomethacin and BW755C. Agents Actions 10: 353–355

Robert A (1976) Antisecretory, antiulcer, cytoprotective and diarrhoegenic properties of prostaglandins. Adv Prostaglandin Thromboxane Res a: 507–520

Robert A, Nezamis JE, Lancaster C, Hanchar AJ (1979) Cytoprotection by prostaglandins in rats – prevention of gastric necrosis produced by alcohol, HCl, NaOH, hypertonic NaCl and thermal injury. Gastroenterology 77: 433–443

Samuelsson B, Hammarström S, Murphy RC, Borgeat P (1980) Leukotrienes and slow reacting substance of anaphylaxis (SRS-A). Allergy 35: 375–381

Spenney JG, Bhown M (1977) Effect of acetylsalicylic acid on gastric mucosa. II. Mucosal ATP and phosphocreatine content and salicylic effects on mitochondrial metabolism. Gastroenterology 73: 995–999

Vane JR (1975) A sensitive method for the assay of 5-hydroxytryptamine. Br J Pharmacol Chemother 12: 344–349

Vane JR (1971) Inhibition of prostaglandin synthesis as a mechanism of action of aspirin-like drugs. Nature (New Biol) 231: 232–235

Whittle BJR (1976) Relationship between the prevention of rat gastric erosions and the inhibition of acid secretion by prostaglandins. Eur J Pharmacol 40: 233–239

Whittle BJR (1977) Mechanisms underlying gastric mucosal damage induced by indomethacin and bile salts, and the actions of prostaglandins. Br J Pharmacol 60: 455–460

Whittle BJR (1980) Role of prostaglandins in the defense of the gastric mucosa. Brain Res Bull [Suppl 1] 5: 7–14

Whittle BJR (1981) Temporal relationship between cyclo-oxygenase inhibition, as measured by prostacyclin biosynthesis, and the gastrointestinal damage induced by indomethacin in the rat. Gastroenterology 80: 94–98

Whittle BJR, Moncada S (1983) Ulceration induced by an endoperoxide analogue and by indomethacin in the canine stomach. Prostaglandin Thromboxane Leukotriene Res 12: 373–378

Whittle BJR, Salmon JA (1983) Biosynthesis of prostacyclin and prostaglandin E_2 in gastro-intestinal tissue. In: Turnberg LA (ed) Proceedings of the third B.S.G./Smith Kline and French international workshop on intestinal secretion. Smith Kline & French, Welwyn Garden City, pp 69–73

Whittle BJR, Higgs GA, Eakins KE, Moncada S, Vane JR (1980) Selective inhibition of prostaglandin production in inflammatory exudates and gastric mucosa. Nature 284: 271–273

Disease, Metabolism and Reproduction in the Toxic Response to Drugs and Other Chemicals
Arch. Toxicol., Suppl. 7, 323–327 (1984)

Molecular Mechanisms of the Gastric Toxicity of Antirheumatic Drugs

U. Aehringhaus[1], H. Weiler[1], B. A. Peskar[1], and B. M. Peskar[2]

[1] Department of Pharmacology and Toxicology, Ruhr-Universität Bochum, 4630 Bochum, Federal Republic of Germany
[2] Department of Gastroenterology, University of Essen, 4300 Essen, Federal Republic of Germany

Abstract. Gastric toxicity of non-steroidal antiinflammatory drugs has been suggested to be due to inhibition of prostaglandin synthesis. Proquazone, which is less ulcerogenic than indomethacin, however, is a more potent inhibitor of gastric mucosal prostaglandin synthesis than indomethacin in vitro and equally effective in vivo. These results indicate that additional factors such as pharmacokinetic properties contribute to the gastric toxicity of non-steroidal antiinflammatory drugs. Furthermore, lipoxygenase products of arachidonic acid metabolism might modulate the effects of inhibition of prostaglandin synthesis by non-steroidal antiinflammatory drugs. Using a radioimmunoassay for leukotriene C_4 the capacity of ovalbumin-sensitized guinea pig gastric mucosa to release leukotriene C_4-like immunoreactivity after antigenic challenge has been demonstrated.

Key words: Non-steroidal antiinflammatory drugs – Prostaglandins – Cyclooxygenase – Lipoxygenase – Leukotrienes – Proquazone – Indomethacin

Introduction

Inhibition of prostaglandin (PG) synthesis in gastric mucosa has been suggested to be the biochemical mechanism underlying the damaging effect of non-steroidal antiinflammatory drugs (NSAID) like indomethacin or acetylsalicylic acid on gastric mucosal integrity (Vane 1971). It had, in fact, been observed that paracetamol, which is not ulcerogenic, has, contrary to indomethacin, no inhibitory effect on gastric mucosal PG synthesis in vitro (Peskar 1977). We have now further investigated the correlation between gastric mucosal damage and inhibition of gastric mucosal PG synthesis by NSAID using proquazone, which is less ulcerogenic than indomethacin in rat (Takesue et al. 1976; Gubler and Baggiolini 1978) and in man (Allan and Bleicher 1977). Furthermore, since NSAID, which inhibit fatty acid cyclooxygenase, could divert arachidonic acid metabolism to the lipoxygenase pathway, increased formation of lipoxygenase metabolites of arachidonic acid in gastric mucosa could contribute to the gastric toxicity of NSAID. Therefore, it was decided to investigate the capacity of guinea pig gastric mucosa to synthesize immunoreactive leukotriene (LT) C_4 using a radioimmunoassay developed recently (Aehringhaus et al. 1982).

Materials and Methods

Biopsy specimens of gastric mucosa obtained from healthy volunteers (age 22–41) were washed in ice-cold Krebs-Henseleit bicarbonate buffer, cut into small pieces and incubated as whole cell preparation (5–12 mg wet weight/incubate) at 37° C for 20 min as described previously (Peskar et al. 1980). Incubations were performed in the absence or presence of indomethacin (final concentrations 0.11–70 μmol/l) or proquazone (final concentrations 0.9–560 nmol/l). A stock solution of indomethacin pure compound (MSD, New Jersey) (2.8 mmol/l) was prepared in 0.1 mol/l sodium phosphate buffer, pH 7.4, and proquazone (5.8 mmol/l) was dissolved in ethanol. Further dilutions were made in Krebs-Henseleit bicarbonate buffer. Release of PGE_2 into the incubation media was determined by radioimmunoassay as described previously (Peskar et al. 1980).

Release of LTC_4-like immunoreactivity was investigated in fragments of gastric mucosa obtained from guinea pigs that had been sensitized with ovalbumin as described elsewhere (Liebig et al. 1974). The tissues (about 400 mg/incubate) were incubated in 3 ml oxygenated modified Tyrode solution [composition (g/l): NaCl 8.0, KCl 0.2, $MgCl_2 \cdot 6\ H_2O$ 0.21, $NaHCO_3$ 1.0,

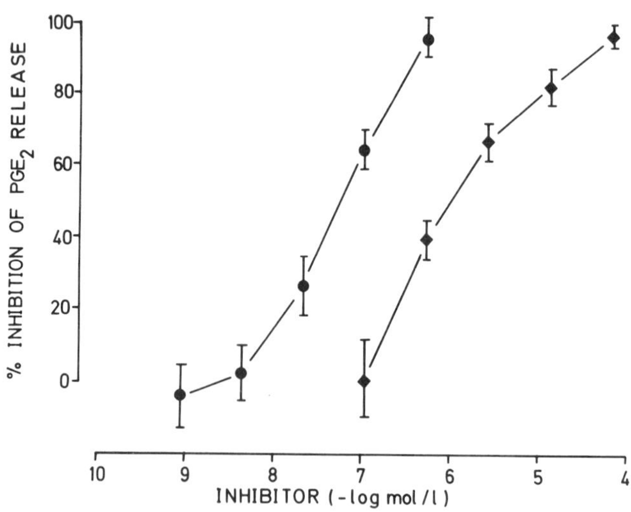

Fig. 1. Release of PGE_2 by whole cell preparations of human gastric mucosa is inhibited by proquazone (●) and indomethacin (⧫). Results represent the means ± SEM of six experiments

$NaH_2PO_4 \cdot H_2O$ 0.058, $CaCl_2 \cdot 2H_2O$ 0.13, glucose 1.1] at 37° C for 5 min. Then 1.5 ml of the incubation medium was removed and replaced by an equal volume of incubation medium containing 2 mg/ml ovalbumin. Incubation was continued for 20 min. Then the samples were boiled for 2 min and centrifuged (10,000 rpm, 20 min) to decrease non-specific interference, which may be due to protein binding or metabolism of LT, by the incubates in the radioimmunoassay for LTC_4. LTC_4-like immunoreactivity in the supernatants was determined using a radioimmunoassay described previously (Aehringhaus et al. 1982). In addition, biologically active slow-reacting substance of anaphylaxis (SRS-A) in the incubation media was measured using the isolated guinea pig ileum treated with mepyramine (1 μg/ml), atropine (0.2 μg/ml), methysergide (0.25 μg/ml) and phentolamine (1 μg/ml). Results were expressed in histamine equivalents (HE) (Liebig et al. 1974). The specificity of the bioassay was tested by the use of the SRS-A antagonist FPL 55712 (sodium 7-(3-(4-acetyl-3-hydroxy-2-propyl-phenoxy)-2-hydroxy propoxy)-4-oxo-8-propyl-4H-1-benzopyran-2-carboxylate, 200 ng/ml final bath concentration) (Augstein et al. 1973).

Results and Discussion

As shown in Fig. 1 proquazone is considerably more effective than indomethacin in inhibiting the release of PGE_2 from a whole cell preparation of human gastric mucosa incubated in vitro. This result indicates that proquazone, which is less ulcerogenic than indomethacin, is a potent inhibitor of human gastric mucosal cyclooxygenase. Similar results have been obtained with rat gastric tissues previously (Weiler et al., in press). Contrary to the in vitro results, proquazone and indomethacin administered orally, have been demonstrated to inhibit release of 6-keto-$PGF_{1\alpha}$ from fragments of rat gastric mucosa incubated ex vivo about equally effectively (Weiler et al., in press). These data indicate that pharmacokinetic properties of NSAID contribute considerably to the extent of inhibition of gastric cyclooxygenase in vivo. Similar conclusions have been drawn from autoradiographic studies with proquazone (Brune et al. 1979) and from experiments with another non-acidic NSAID, BW755C (3-amino-1-(3-tri-fluoromethylphenyl)-2-pyrazoline hydrochloride), which inhibits release of 6-keto-$PGF_{1\alpha}$ from rat gastric corpus mucosa in vitro (Peskar et al., 1982), but not when the tissue is incubated ex vivo after oral administration of the drug (Whittle et al. 1980; Peskar et al. 1982). However, contrary to BW755C, proquazone inhibits gastric mucosal PG synthesis ex vivo as effectively as indomethacin (Weiler et al., in press). Thus, the lower incidence of gastrointestinal side effects of proquazone as compared to indomethacin is not correlated to a less pronounced inhibition of PG synthesis in vivo and additional factors have to account for the differences in ulcerogenic potency.

It seems possible, that the effects of inhibition of PG synthesis in gastric mucosa by NSAID are modulated by products of the lipoxygenase pathway of arachidonic acid metabolism. Synthesis of the lipoxygenase product 12-hydro-xy-5,8,10,14-eicosatetraenoic acid by human gastric tissue has been observed (Bennett et al. 1981), while synthesis of leukotrienes by gastric tissue has so far not been described. Using radioimmunoassay as well as bioassay synthesis of LTC_4-like immunoreactivity and SRS-A by sensitized guinea pig gastric mucosa after antigenic challenge can be demonstrated. While before addition of antigen to the incubation media release of LTC_4-like immunoreactivity was close to or below the detection limit of the radioimmunoassay (0.6 ng/g wet weight), after antigenic challenge 33.0 ± 6.9 ng/g wet weight ($n = 23$, mean ± SEM) were released by the tissue. Similarly, significant release of biologically active SRS-A (0.29 ± 0.05 HE/g wet weight) after addition of antigen was found. The specific SRS-A antagonist FPL 55712 in the concentration used (200 ng/ml) inhibited the guinea pig ileum-contracting activity in the incubation media by 53 ± 7% ($n = 20$, $p < 0.005$). The effect of various NSAID on biosynthesis of lipoxygenase products of arachidonic acid metabolism in gastric mucosa remains to be investigated. However, increased formation of such metabolites in the presence of the NSAID indomethacin has been demonstrated in guinea pig lung tissue incubated in vitro (Morris et al. 1980). From these results, which demonstrate the capacity of guinea pig gastric mucosa to synthesize LTC_4-like immunoreactivity, it seems possible that increased formation of lipoxygenase products in the presence of NSAID could contribute to the gastric toxicity of these drugs.

Acknowledgement. This work was supported by the Deutsche Forschungsgemeinschaft.

References

Aehringhaus U, Wölbling RH, König W, Patrono C, Peskar BM, Peskar BA (1982) Release of leukotriene C_4 from human polymorphonuclear leucocytes as determined by radioimmunoassay. FEBS Lett 146: 111–114

Allen R, Bleicher M (1977) Die Behandlung degenerativer Gelenkerkrankungen mit Biarison. Schweiz Rundschau Med 46: 1481–1489

Augstein J, Farmer JB, Lee TB, Sheard P, Tattersall ML (1973) Selective inhibitor of slow-reacting substance of anaphylaxis. Nature (New Biol) 245: 215–217

Bennett A, Hensby CN, Sanger GJ, Stamford IF (1981) Metabolites of arachidonic acid formed by human gastrointestinal tissues and their actions on the muscle layers. Br J Pharmacol 74: 435–444

Brune K, Gubler H, Schweitzer A (1979) Autoradiographic methods for the evaluation of ulcerogenic effects of anti-inflammatory drugs. Pharmacol Ther 5: 199–207

Gubler HU, Baggiolini M (1978) Pharmacological properties of proquazone. Scand J Rheumatol 21: 8–11

Liebig R, Bernauer W, Peskar BA (1974) Release of prostaglandins, a prostaglandin metabolite, slow-reacting substance and histamine from anaphylactic lungs, and its modification by catecholamines. Naunyn-Schmiedebergs Arch Pharmacol 284: 279–293

Morris HR, Piper PJ, Taylor GW, Tippins JR (1980) The role of arachidonate lipoxygenase in the release of SRS-A from guinea-pig chopped lung. Prostaglandins 19: 371–383

Peskar BM (1977) On the synthesis of prostaglandins by human gastric mucosa and its modification by drugs. Biochim Biophys Acta 487: 307–314

Peskar BM, Seyberth HW, Peskar BA (1980) Synthesis and metabolism of endogenous prostaglandins by human gastric mucosa. Adv Prostaglandin Thromboxane Res 8: 1511

Peskar BM, Weiler H, Peskar BA (1982) Effect of BW 755C on prostaglandin synthesis in the rat stomach. Biochem Pharmacol 31: 1652–1653

Takesue EI, Perrine JW, Trapold JH (1976) The antiinflammatory profile of proquazone. Arch Int Pharmacodyn 221: 122–131

Vane JR (1971) Inhibition of prostaglandin synthesis as a mechanism of action for aspirin-like drugs. Nature (New Biol) 231: 232–235

Weiler H, Meier C, Fröhlich J, Peskar BM (1984) Effect of proquazone and indomethacin on gastric prostaglandin synthesis in vitro and in vivo. Agents Actions (in press)

Whittle BJR, Higgs GA, Eakins KE, Moncada S, Vane JR (1980) Selective inhibition of prostaglandin production in inflammatory exudates and gastric mucosa. Nature 284: 271–273

Disease, Metabolism and Reproduction in the Toxic Response to Drugs and Other Chemicals
Arch. Toxicol., Suppl. 7, 328–337 (1984)

Mechanisms of the Nephrotoxicity of Non-steroidal Anti-inflammatory Drugs

M. J. Dunn[1], L. Scharschmidt[1], and E. Zambraski[2]

[1] Department of Medicine, Case Western Reserve University, School of Medicine and Division of Nephrology, University Hospitals of Cleveland, 2065 Adelbert Road, Cleveland, Ohio 44106, USA
[2] Rutgers University, Department of Physiology, New Brunswick, New Jersey 08903, USA

Abstract. Renal cortical prostaglandin synthesis, particularly by arterioles and glomeruli, is important to preserve renal blood flow (RBF) and glomerular filtration rate (GFR). Glomeruli and arterioles synthesize not only the vasodilatory prostaglandins PGE_2 and PGI_2, but also the vasoconstrictor, thromboxane A_2. The primary renal cortical actions of these prostaglandins are renal vasodilatation and maintenance of GFR (PGE_2 and PGI_2) or renal vasoconstriction and reduction of GFR (thromboxane A_2). Vasodilatory renal prostaglandins are relatively unimportant under normal circumstances but play a modulatory role after ischemia or in the presence of increased concentrations of vasoconstrictor substances such as angiotensin II (ANG II), vasopressin or norepinephrine. ANG II and vasopressin stimulate the synthesis of PGE_2 in rat glomerular epithelial and mesangial cells maintained in cell culture. These stimulatory actions of constrictor peptides are dependent upon calcium entry into the cells since removal of extracellular calcium or co-incubation with verapamil or nifedipine block the prostaglandin stimulatory capacity of ANG II or vasopressin. In vivo indomethacin potentiates the actions of ANG II on the kidney, particularly the reduction of RBF and GFR. Isolated rat glomeruli contract in response to ANG II and this contractile effect, which reflects reduction in glomerular filtration surface area, can be potentiated by cyclooxygenase blockade. Conversely, arachidonic acid reduces the glomerular contractile effect of ANG II. The importance of renal prostaglandins in support of RBF and GFR has been studied in dogs after chronic bile duct ligation (CBDL). CBDL dogs have significant increase in renal PGE_2 and PGI_2 which maintain RBF and GFR since cyclo-oxygenase inhibition resulted in a 50% decrease in both RBF and GFR. Indomethacin, ibuprofen, naproxen, and sulindac sulfide had comparable effects. The pro-drug, sulindac sulfoxide, was tested

---

Abbreviations: PGE_2, PGI_2, etc., Prostaglandin E_2, I_2, etc.; ANG II, angiotensin II; TxA_2, thromboxane A_2; RBF, renal blood flow; GFR, glomerular filtration rate; CBDL, chronic bile duct ligation.

in normal volunteers and found to spare renal prostaglandin synthesis whereas indomethacin reduced renal synthesis of PGE_2 and $PGF_{2\alpha}$ by more than 50%. In vitro, sulindac sulfide is a potent inhibitor of renal prostaglandin synthesis by kidney cells in culture. It is, therefore, concluded that renal prostaglandins play an important vasoregulatory role. Furthermore, sulindac sulfoxide may spare renal cyclo-oxygenase and thereby preserve renal function.

Key words: Prostaglandin E_2 – Angiotensin II – Glomerular mesangium – Renal blood flow – Glomerular filtration rate – Indomethacin – Ibuprofen – Naproxen – Sulindac

Renal Synthesis of Prostaglandins

The kidney is a rich source of prostaglandin synthetic enzymes, particularly the medulla of the kidney. It has been known for some time that renal medullary synthesis of prostaglandins exceeds renal cortical synthesis; however, there has been growing emphasis on the importance of cortical sites of prostaglandin production in the kidney. Cortical synthesis of prostaglandins is primarily in glomeruli, arterioles and cortical collecting tubules (Hassid et al. 1979; Smith and Wilkin 1977; Smith and Bell 1978). Purified preparations of isolated rat glomeruli can be obtained with greater than 95% purity and these preparations, when incubated with arachidonic acid, synthesize substantial amounts of PGE_2 and $PGF_{2\alpha}$ with smaller amounts of PGI_2 and thromboxane A_2 (Hassid et al. 1979; Sraer et al. 1979; Folkert and Schlondorff 1979). Since prostaglandins are autacoids and, hence, exert their physiological and biochemical actions close to or at the site of synthesis, it seems quite likely that cortical synthesis of prostaglandins and thromboxane in arterioles and glomeruli affect arteriolar and glomerular function (see below). Medullary synthesis of prostaglandins has been documented using medullary microsomes, slices or homogenates of cells. The major medullary sites of prostaglandin synthesis seem to be renal medullary interstitial cells and the medullary collecting tubules (for a general review, see Dunn et al. 1983).

The Physiological Actions of Renal Prostaglandins

Most studies support the concept that renal medullary prostaglandins control medullary function and cortical prostaglandins regulate predominatly cortical function. The major medullary functions of the kidney are the reabsorption of salt and water, as well as the production of a concentrated or dilute urine. Prostaglandins, particularly PGE_2, inhibit sodium and chloride reabsorption by the tubule, particularly in the medullary portions of the tubule (Stokes 1981). There is good evidence supporting a role for PGE_2 in the control of water excretion since PGE_2 causes water diuresis and cyclo-oxygenase inhibition enhances water reabsorption and the production of a concentrated urine (Beck and Dunn 1981). Cortical prostaglandins appear important in the regulation of renin secretion by juxtaglomerular cells as well as in the control of renal blood flow (RBF) and glomerular filtration rate (GFR). PGE_2 and PGI_2 are potent renal vasodilators and hence, can alter renal cortical arteriolar resistance. PGE_2 and PGI_2 can increase GFR if it is depressed but will not increase GFR to supranormal levels. TxA_2 is a potent vasoconstrictor and can reduce both RBF and GFR through reductions in renal plasma flow and concomitant reductions of the glomerular ultrafiltration coefficient. Renal synthesis of PGE_2 and PGI_2, in glomeruli and cortical arterioles, will support or increase RBF only under circumstances of stress such as volume depletion, heart failure, kidney or liver disease. It has been previously theorized (Dunn and Zambraski 1980) that reductions of renal function after the use of cyclo-oxygenase inhibitors (nonsteroidal anti-inflammatory drugs) necessitated changes in the effective circulating plasma volume. The diseases which predispose to reduction in renal function, after prostaglandin inhibition, include congestive heart failure, severe hepatic disease, nephrotic syndrome and diuretic therapy. These conditions are characterized by an ineffective circulating plasma volume and, hence, are usually accompanied by increased plasma levels of ANG II, vasopressin and catecholamines. These compounds are potent stimuli of renal prostaglandin synthesis and the compensatory increase of renal cortical PGE_2 and PGI_2 modulates or regulates the amount of vasoconstriction mediated by ANG II, vasopressin or catecholamines (for review, see Dunn et al. 1983). In order to understand better the cellular mechanisms underlying the interactions of vasoconstrictor peptides and renal prostaglandins, in vitro studies have been conducted utilizing glomerular cell cultures and whole glomeruli.

Glomerular Epithelial and Mesangial Cell Culture

Purified preparations of isolated rat glomeruli were incubated in cell culture media for periods of 9–48 days (Petrulis et al. 1981; Dunn et al. 1982; Scharschmidt and Dunn 1983). Glomerular epithelial cells predominate during the first 7–14 days of outgrowth from explanted and incubated glomeruli. The epithelial cells progressively disappear after 7–14 days of culture and mesangial cells predominate thereafter. Fibroblast contamination is sparse, or nonexistent, and the morphology of both epithelial and mesangial cells was verified using transmission electron microscopy. The epithelial cells showed characteristic morphology including rudimentary microvilli and highly developed junctional complexes. The mesangial cells lacked intercellular junctional complexes and had characteristic intracellular myofibrils consistent with the contractile activity of the cells. The epithelial cell experiments were conducted 9 days after glomerular inoculation and the mesangial cell experiments were conducted after approximately 6 weeks. Samples of culture media were radio-immunoassayed for PGE_2, $PGF_{2\alpha}$, thromboxane B_2 (stable hydrolysis product of TxA_2) and 6-keto-$PGF_{1\alpha}$ (stable hydrolysis product of PGI_2) utilizing previously described antisera (Hassid and Dunn 1980). Table 1 summarizes the basal and stimulated prostaglandin synthesis in glomerular epithelial and mesangial cells in culture. It

Table 1. Prostaglandin synthesis by rat glomerular epithelial and mesangial cells in culture

	PGE_2	$PGF_{2\alpha}$	PGI_2[a]	TxA_2[b]
	ng/mg cell protein/30 min incubation			
Epithelial cells				
Basal	0.5 ± 0.2	ND[c]	ND	ND
Arachidonate (3 μM)	25 ± 3.0	3 ± 0.6	1.4 ± 0.35	11 ± 3.0
A 23187 (2 μM)	19 ± 4.0	1 ± 0.3	0.2 ± 0.07	3 ± 0.8
ANG II (1 μM)	8 ± 1.0	0.8 ± 0.4	0.07 ± 0.02	0.12 ± 0.03
Mesangial cells				
Basal	13 ± 2.0	4 ± 1.0	2 ± 1.0	ND
Arachidonate (3 μM)	373 ± 10.0	85 ± 3.0	13 ± 5.0	6 ± 2.0
A 23187 (2 μM)	176 ± 3.0	83 ± 2.0	20 ± 6.0	ND
ANG II (1 μM)	26 ± 2.0	5 ± 3.0	3 ± 1.0	ND

[a] PGI_2 measured as 6-keto-$PGF_{1\alpha}$
[b] TxA_2 measured as TxB_2
[c] Not detected

should be noted that intact glomeruli synthesize more $PGF_{2\alpha}$ than PGE_2, whereas glomerular epithelial and mesangial cells synthesize more PGE_2 than $PGF_{2\alpha}$. Since $PGF_{2\alpha}$ lacks any significant renal cortical action, it is believed that PGE_2 is the important glomerular prostanoid in the rat. Arachidonic acid, the substrate for the fatty acid cyclo-oxygenase which synthesizes prostaglandins, dramatically stimulates the glomerular synthesis of all prostanoids. Glomerular epithelial and mesangial cells are capable of synthesis of TxA_2 and PGI_2 as well as PGE_2 and $PGF_{2\alpha}$. This can be seen in the experimental data with both arachidonic acid or with the calcium ionophore, A 23187, which augments calcium entry into the cells and thereby activates phospholipase and the endogenous release of arachidonic acid to synthesize prostanoids. In order to evaluate the effect of pressor peptides on glomerular prostaglandin synthesis ANG II or vasopressin was incubated with glomerular epithelial and mesangial cells. The data for ANG II are summarized in Table 1 and the results with vasopressin were similar. ANG II increased cellular synthesis of PGE_2 with virtually no increment of the other prostanoids. Vasopressin also exclusively stimulated PGE_2. Calcium entry blockers such as verapamil or nifedipine eliminated the ANG II-stimulated PGE_2 synthesis of glomerular mesangial cells. It was concluded that glomerular epithelial and mesangial cells have specific receptors for ANG II and vasopressin and these receptors are tightly linked to intracellular pools of phospholipase and cyclo-oxygenase. The rat glomerular cells respond to the vasoconstrictor peptides with exclusive release of a vasodilatory prostanoid, namely PGE_2. This is not a function of cellular inability to synthesize the other prostanoids since arachidonic acid or calcium ionophore result in the release of the other prostaglandins and thromboxane. Glomerular release of PGE_2 may be important in modulating the effects of ANG II on the glomerulus.

Glomerular Contractility

Mesangial cells are modified smooth muscle cells which contain myofibrils and actomyosin. Mesangial cells can be shown to contract under phase contrast microscopy, after the addition of ANG II (Ausiello et al. 1980). Because it is difficult to quantitate mesangial contractility in cell culture, an assessment of glomerular contractility was substituted. Since the mesangial cell is the only contractile component of the glomerulus it is believed that measurements of glomerular contractility provide an accurate assessment of mesangial responsiveness to ANG II. Glomerular planar surface area was measured using a Millipore Particle Counter (Scharschmidt et al. 1983). All data have been normalized to the control glomerular planar surface area which is approximately 10,000 square micra in the rat. Reductions of glomerular planar surface area undoubtedly reflect reductions in the glomerular filtration surface area and, in vivo, would be accompanied by reductions in the glomerular ultrafiltration coefficient. Table 2 summarizes these experiments which were designed to evaluate the interactions between ANG II and glomerular prostaglandins. ANG II induced progressive reductions of glomerular planar surface area with the threshold being 1×10^{-13} M ANG II. Ang II-induced glomerular contraction did not reduce surface area more than 20% and maximum glomerular contraction was generally observed with ANG II concentrations of 1×10^{-10} M. If rat glomerular prostaglandin synthesis, especially PGE_2, served to regulate or antagonize ANG II-induced contraction, it is hypothesized that cyclooxygenase inhibitors such as indomethacin or meclofenamate, would potentiate ANG II-induced reductions in glomerular planar surface area. Table 2 shows that either indomethacin or meclofenamate, administered to the rat before sacrifice and also present in the incubation media, reduced the threshold concentrations of ANG II but did not maximize the extent of total glomerular contraction. In other words, when PGE_2 synthesis was blocked, isolated rat glomeruli were more sensitive to the contractile effects of ANG II to reduce glomerular filtration surface area. Conversely, incubation with arachidonic acid, which augmented glomerular synthesis of PGE_2, blunted the ANG II-induced glomerular contractility. The ANG II-induced contractility curve was shifted upward and to the right when glomeruli were co-incubated with arachidonic acid indicating that

Table 2. Rat glomerular contractility assessed by glomerular planar surface area[a]

	Angiotensin II (M)				
	10^{-14}	10^{-13}	10^{-12}	10^{-11}	10^{-10}
ANG II alone	98	95	88	83	80
Plus indomethacin (15 μM)	92	85	81	79	78
Plus meclofenamate (15 μM)	90	82	80	80	79
Plus arachidonate (3 μM)	104	104	98	95	90
Plus PGE_2 (1 nM)	98	96	96	97	95

[a] All data are shown as percent of control glomerular planar surface (approx. 10,000 square micra)

an arachidonic acid product antagonized the actions of ANG II. This was not a nonspecific fatty acid effect since linoleic acid had no actions in this system. Since PGE_2 is the most abundant vasorelaxant in rat glomeruli, PGE_2 and ANG II were incubated together with glomeruli. As shown in Table II, PGE_2 in concentrations of 1×10^{-9} M blocked ANG II-mediated reductions in glomerular planar surface area. Taken together, these data support the hypothesis that the actions of ANG II to reduce glomerular filtration surface area and GFR are modulated by PGE_2. Since ANG II stimulates PGE_2 synthesis in both glomerular epithelial and mesangial cells, it is believed that this is a physiologically important feedback system to regulate the actions of ANG II on GFR.

The Importance of Renal Prostaglandins in an Experimental Model of Liver Disease

Because the aforementioned work suggested important in vivo interrelationships between angiotensin, vasopressin, glomerular prostaglandins and renal function, a model of experimental renal disease was established in which renal prostaglandin production was important to maintain RBF and GFR. For this purpose chronic bile duct ligation (CBDL) was utilized in mongrel dogs. Twenty-four dogs had their common bile duct ligated and 10 animals served as sham-operated controls. After CBDL or sham operation, the animals were observed for periods ranging from 4 to 12 weeks with the mean duration of observation being 50 days. The CBDL dogs developed hyperbilirubinemia (serum total bilirubin 5.8 ± 0.9 mg/dl) and elevated serum alkaline phosphatase 3,211 ± 415 IU). Liver biopsies revealed cholestasis, biliary ductal proliferation and dilatation and early biliary cirrhosis (Zambraski and Dunn, 1984).

Approximately 50 days after initial ligation of the bile duct, the CBDL and sham-operated dogs were anesthetized and an electromagnetic flow probe was placed in the left renal artery to measure RBF. GFR was measured by inulin clearance. Urine was collected by bladder or ureteral catheter and was extracted and assayed for PGE_2, $PGF_{2\alpha}$, and 6-keto-$PGF_{1\alpha}$ as previously described (Dunn et al. 1978). The 23 CBDL dogs showed substantial increments of PGE_2 excretion from 1.5 ± 0.2 to 3.2 ± 0.4 ng/min and of 6-keto-$PGF_{1\alpha}$ excretion from 0.9 ± 0.1 to 4.8 ± 1.0 ng/min. The specific explanation for the stimulatory effect of CBDL on renal PGE_2 and PGI_2 synthesis is unknown, but it seems quite likely that circulating factors such as ANG II, vasopressin and catecholamines play a very important role since these animals have an ineffective circulating plasma volume and more than 50% of the dogs had ascites. In order to compare several cyclo-oxygenase inhibitors, the acute effects of intravenous treatment with indomethacin (2 mg/kg), sulindac sulfide (5 mg/kg), and naproxen (10 mg/kg) were studied. Table 3 summarizes the results. The renal synthesis of prostaglandins, as measured by urinary excretion from a single kidney, was decreased by more than 90% for PGE_2 and $PGF_{2\alpha}$ and by 50% or more for the prostacyclin metabolite, 6-keto-$PGF_{1\alpha}$. A similar percentage decrease was seen in the sham-operated animals. If the hypothesis was correct, namely that

Table 3. The effects of cyclo-oxygenase inhibitors on renal prostaglandin synthesis in CBDL dogs

	PGE_2	$PGF_{2\alpha}$	6-keto-$PGF_{1\alpha}$
	ng excreted/min[a]		
Indomethacin (n = 16, 2 mg/kg)			
Pre	3	3	15
Post	0.5	0.5	5
Sulindac sulfide (n = 4, 5 mg/kg)			
Pre	4	11	30
Post	0.2	1	8
Naproxen (n = 3, 10 mg/kg)			
Pre	2.5	5	4
Post	0.2	0.4	0.6

[a] Mean excretion from a single kidney; PG excretion was measured for 30 min before and after IV administration of the inhibitor

Table 4. The percent reduction of RBF and GFR in sham or CBDL dogs after prostaglandin inhibition[a]

	Sham		CBDL	
	RBF	GFR	RBF	GFR
Indomethacin (n = 23, 2 mg/kg)	14	8	32	33
Sulindac sulfide (n = 4, 5 mg/kg)	30	0	25	30
Naproxen (n = 3, 10 mg/kg)	–	20	39	20
Ibuprofen (n = 3, 20 mg/kg)	–	–	25	16

[a] Data are shown as the mean percentage decrease of RBF and GFR from the basal, control levels

augmented renal synthesis of vasodilatory prostaglandins modulate the vasoconstrictor effect of ANG II, vasopressin and catecholamines in the CBDL dogs, then cyclo-oxygenase inhibition should be accompanied by significant decrease in RBF and GFR in these animals. Table 4 summarizes the data for RBF and GFR in sham-operated and CBDL dogs after intravenous administration of four different inhibitors of cyclo-oxygenase. Since the dogs were anesthetized and had a retroperitoneal flank incision for the insertion of the electromagnetic flow probe and ureteral catheter, there were decreases ranging from 8–30% of RBF and GFR in the sham-operated animals after inhibition of prostaglandin synthesis. However, the reductions of RBF and GFR were always greater in the CBDL dogs ranging from 16 to 39% and renal vascular resistance doubled. These results reinforce the initial impression that some factor or factors in the CBDL dogs stimulated the renal synthesis and excretion of vasodilatory prostaglandins and these prostaglandins exhibit important vasoregulatory actions. The use of a nonsteroidal anti-inflammatory drug, such as indome-

Table 5. The effects of sulindac, indomethacin or placebo on renal prostaglandin excretion in normal female volunteers[a]

	Placebo (5)	Indomethacin (5)[b]	Sulindac (5)[b]
PGE_2			
Control (day 2)	190 ± 35	137 ± 20	170 ± 46
Exp (day 6)	224 ± 53	68 ± 24	187 ± 40
$PGF_{2\alpha}$			
Control (days 2 and 3)	832 ± 89	904 ± 193	977 ± 236
Exp (days 6 and 7)	912 ± 151	291 ± 49	566 ± 73
6-keto-$PGF_{1\alpha}$			
Control (days 2 and 3)	253 ± 27	257 ± 43	261 ± 55
Exp (days 6 and 7)	294 ± 27	193 ± 27	221 ± 48

[a] PG excretion in ng/24 h, mean ± SEM
[b] Indomethacin 25 mg four times daily over 4 days; sulindac sulfoxide 200 mg twice daily for 4 days

thacin, is not only accompanied by substantial inhibition of renal prostaglandin synthesis but also by 33% decreases in RBF and GFR (Zambraski et al. 1984).

The Effects of Sulindac on Renal Function and Renal Prostaglandin Synthesis in Normal Human Volunteers

Sulindac sulfoxide is a potent nonsteroidal anti-inflammatory drug which acts as a pro-drug since it must be reduced by the liver to sulindac sulfide in order to be activated. Sulindac sulfide is a potent inhibitor of cyclo-oxygenase activity and prostaglandin synthesis. An analysis of the urinary excretion of sulindac metabolites has shown that the active form of the drug, sulindac sulfide, does not appear in the urine after oral or intravenous administration of the sulfoxide pro-drug (Duggan et al. 1977). Based on these metabolic considerations, Ciabattoni and his coworkers (1980) evaluated the actions of sulindac sulfoxide, administered orally to female volunteers, on renal prostaglandin excretion. They observed no significant renal actions of sulindac sulfoxide based on measurements of urinary PGE_2, and 6-keto-$PGF_{1\alpha}$. In order to evaluate further the possibility that sulidac did not inhibit renal cyclo-oxygenase in vivo, 15 healthy female volunteers were used in a double-blind study comparing the effects of sulindac 200 mg twice daily, indomethacin 25 mg four times daily, or placebo. After a 3 day stabilization period, during which all subjects received placebo and a 60 mEq sodium, 60 mEq potassium diet, the treatment programs were then randomly assigned for the last 4 days of the study. The 24 h urinary excretion of PGE_2 was measured on days 2 and 6, whereas 24 h urinary excretion of $PGF_{2\alpha}$ and 6-keto-$PGF_{1\alpha}$ were measured on days 2 and 3 of the control period and days 6 and 7 of the experimental period. Table 5 summarizes the results. Whereas indomethacin significantly decreased mean PGE_2 excretion, sulindac did not alter the PGE_2 excretion rate as much as the placebo. Indomethacin significantly depressed 6-keto-$PGF_{1\alpha}$ on day 6 (compared to day 3) and day 7 (compared to placebo), whereas sulindac maintained excretion of 6-keto-$PGF_{1\alpha}$ as did the placebo. Although excretion of $PGF_{2\alpha}$ was decreased by both indomethacin and sulindac, the indomethacin effect was significantly greater. The mean 24 h urine values for sodium, potassium and chloride showed no changes of potassium excretion with any treatment and significant decrements of sodium and chloride excretion after indomethacin. There were no differences in 24 h urinary sodium and chloride between sulindac and the placebo control. RBF, measured by the clearance of para-aminohippurate and GFR, measured by inulin clearance, were unchanged by any of the treatment protocols.

In conclusion these data are consistent with the original report of Ciabattoni et al. (1980), showing minimal or negligible effects of sulindac on renal function and renal prostaglandin synthesis compared with a chemically similar cyclo-oxygenase inhibitor, indomethacin. The explanation for this phenomenon may be related to the capacity of the kidney to oxidize the reduced form of sulindac, sulindac sulfide, to the inactive pro-drug, sulindac sulfoxide. The kidney is rich in mixed-function oxidases and recent work by Miller et al. (1983) suggests that renal resistance to sulindac may depend upon continual inactivation, through oxidation, of the sulfide form of sulindac to sulfoxide and sulfone compounds. It has been demonstrated, in vitro with renal cell culture, that sulindac sulfide is an extremely potent inhibitor of renal prostaglandin synthesis and, consequently, one cannot conclude that the renal cyclo-oxygenase is intrinsically resistant to sulindac sulfide. It remains to be proved whether sulindac sulfoxide is safe in patients who are at risk of nephrotoxicity with the other nonsteroidal anti-inflammatory drugs. Patrono et al. (1982) have recently reported on their initial experience demonstrating the safety of sulindac in patients with mild renal insufficiency due to renal disease.

References

Ausiello DA, Kreisberg JI, Roy C, Karnovsky MJ (1980) Contraction of cultured rat glomerular cells of apparent mesangial origin after stimulation with angiotensin II and arginine vasopressin. J Clin Invest 65: 754–760

Beck TR, Dunn MJ (1981) The relationship of antidiuretic hormone and renal prostaglandins. Mineral Electrolyte Metab 6: 46–59

Ciabattoni G, Cinotti GA, Patrono C (1980) Renal effects of antiinflammatory drugs. Eur J Rheumatol Inflamm 3: 210–221

Duggan DE, Hare LE, Ditzler CA, Lei BW, Kwan KC (1977) The disposition of sulindac. Clin Pharmacol Ther 21: 326–335

Dunn MJ, Zambraski EJ (1980) Renal effects of drugs that inhibit prostaglandin synthesis. Kidney Int 18: 609–622

Dunn MJ, Liard JF, Dray F (1978) Basal and stimulated rates of renal secretion and excretion of prostaglandins E_1, $F_{1\alpha}$, and 13,14-dihydro-15-keto F_1 in the dog. Kidney Int 13: 136–143

Dunn MJ, Petrulis AS, Scharschmidt LS, Jim K, Hassid A (1982) The use of glomerular cell culture to evaluate cyclo-oxygenase and lipoxygenase products of arachidonic acid metabolism in the kidney. In: Morel F (ed) Biochemistry of kidney functions. Elsevier, Amsterdam

Dunn MJ, Patrono C, Cinotti G (1983) Prostaglandins and the kidney: biochemistry, physiology, pharmacology and clinical applications. Plenum, New York

Folkert VW, Schlondorff D (1979) Prostaglandin synthesis in isolated rat glomeruli. Prostaglandins 17: 76–86

Hassid A, Dunn MJ (1980) Microsomal prostaglandin biosynthesis of human kidney. J Biol Chem 255: 2472–2475

Hassid A, Konieczkowski M, Dunn MJ (1979) Prostaglandin synthesis in isolated rat kidney glomeruli. Proc Natl Acad Sci USA 76: 1155–1159

Miller M, Bednar M, McGiff J (1983) Renal vascular and urinary prostaglandin efflux is differentially affected by sulindac. Fed Proc 42: 499A

Patrono C (1983) Reduced prostacyclin production is associated with cyclo-oxygenase dependent renal function in chronic glomerulonephritis. Kidney Int 23: 282A

Petrulis AS, Aikawa M, Dunn MJ (1981) Prostaglandin and thromboxane synthesis by rat glomerular epithelial cells. Kidney Int 20: 469–474

Scharschmidt LA, Dunn MJ (1983) Prostaglandin synthesis by rat glomerular mesangial cells in culture: the effects of angiotensin II and vasopressin. J Clin Invest 71: 1756–1764.

Scharschmidt LA, Dunn MJ, Norris A (1983) Prostaglandins modulate angiotensin II stimulated glomerular contractility. Kidney Int 23: 283A

Smith WL, Bell TG (1978) Immunohistochemical localization of the prostaglandin-forming cyclo-oxygenase in renal cortex. Am J Physiol 235: F451–F457

Smith WL, Wilkin GP (1977) Immunochemistry of prostaglandin endoperoxide-forming cyclo-oxygenases: the detection of the cyclo-oxygenases in rat, rabbit and guinea pig kidneys by immunofluorescence. Prostaglandins 13: 873–892

Sraer J, Sraer JD, Chansel D, Russo-Marie F, Kouznetzova B, Ardaillou R (1979) Prostaglandin synthesis by isolated rat renal glomeruli. Mol Cell Endocrinol 16: 29–37

Stokes JB (1981) Integrated actions of renal medullary prostaglandins in the control of water excretion. Am J Physiol 240: F471–480

Zambraski E, Dunn MJ (1984) Importanca of renal prostaglandins in control of renal function after chronic ligation of the common bile duct in dogs. J Lab Clin Med 103: 549–559

Zambraski E, Chumos AN, Dunn MJ (1984) Comparison of the effect of sulindac with other cyclooxygenase inhibitors on prostaglandin excretion and renal function in normal and chronic bile duct – ligated dogs and swine. J Pharmacol Exp Ther 228: 560–566

Disease, Metabolism and Reproduction in the Toxic Response to Drugs and Other Chemicals
Arch. Toxicol., Suppl. 7, 338–349 (1984)

Clinical Assessment of the Renal Toxicity of Antirheumatic Drugs

G. A. Cinotti

Division of Nephrology, University of Rome "La Sapienza", Policlinico Umberto I°, 00100 Rome, Italy

Abstract. Antirheumatic drugs may cause a significant, although generally reversible, reduction of GFR, RPF, C_{Na} and hyperkalemia in a wide range of extrarenal and renal disease states (severe liver disease, congestive heart failure, SLE, nephrotic syndrome, etc.); chronic ingestion has been associated with analgesic nephropathy. Recently cases have been reported of reversible acute renal failure with massive proteinuria and interstitial nephritis. The acute effects of a renal PG-inhibiting (ibuprofen) or a renal PG-sparing (sulindac) cyclo-oxygenase inhibitor on renal functional parameters (GFR, RPF, C_{Na}, C_K, urine volume) and proteinuria have been studied in 24 patients with clinically and biopsy proven chronic glomerular disease; in all patients ibuprofen significantly reduced GFR, RPF, C_{Na}; these changes were fully reversible within a week of withdrawal of the drugs. A causal relationship exists between inhibited PG-synthesis and reduced renal function in these patients, since sulindac, which failed to reduce urinary PG excretion did not alter significanctly the renal function. Moreover proteinuria is not reduced by ibuprofen at doses comparable, as far as concerns inhibition of PG-synthesis, to those of indomethacin.

Key words: Kidney – Anti-inflammatory non-steroidal drugs – Sulindac – Ibuprofen – Prostaglandins – Proteinuria

Since the early 1900's transient proteinuria, increased tubular cell excretion, hematuria, fluid retention (salicylic edema), abnormal elevation of BUN have been reported following the administration of salicylates. In addition, acute tubular necrosis and renal failure are recognized complications of salicylate poisoning.

Abbreviations: AD, Antirheumatic drugs; BUN, blood urea nitrogen; CGD, chronic glomerular disease; GFR, glomerular filtration rate; GNF, glomerulonephritis; PG, prostaglandin; RPF, renal plasma flow; SLE, systemic lupus erythematosus; TxB_2, thromboxane B_2

In 1950 Spuhler and Zollinger observed an increasing incidence in Zurich of chronic interstitial nephritis at autopsy, possibly related to a history of chronic ingestion of large amounts of analgesic drugs.

Analgesic nephropathy is now recognized as a distinct form of chronic interstitial nephropathy different from pyelonephritis and clearly associated with the sustained consumption of high doses of certain analgesics over a period of several years.

Analgesic Nephropathy

The prevalence of analgesic nephropathy remains difficult to explain: not all patients consuming large quantities of analgesics develop renal papillary necrosis; many "abusers" present with a non obstructive chronic interstitial nephritis.

The importançe of bacterial infection was controversial for a long time; it is now evident that bacterial infection is a secondary phenomenon, which may be or may not be present. It has been demonstrated that dehydratation may be one of the predisposing factors (Core-Smith 1981). Furthermore two major issues remain unsolved. Firstly, which drug(s) should be considered as a prime offender and secondly the pathogenesis.

In a recent prospective longitudinal study (12 years) on a large number of Swiss women taking an analgesic drug with a matched control group, Dubach et al. (1983) reported a significant decrease in concentrating capacity and a rise in serum creatinine, with a relative risk of death from renal and urogenital causes of 5.9 times greater in the high-dose analgesic group compared with the controls.

The overall morbidity was relatively low but these authors concluded that "long standing analgesic abuse with drugs containing phenacetin is damaging for the urinary system, sometimes fatally".

Unfortunately, it was not possible to determine which drug(s) was responsible.

The Case of Phenacetin and Paracetamol

Phenacetin is the compound most commonly implicated as the causative agent; however, phenacetin was almost always taken in combination with other analgesics and nephropathy has only very rarely been described in patients abusing phenacetin alone. See Prescott (1982) for a review.

In experimental animals (rats, rabbits, mice, dogs, etc.) it was impossible to produce papillary necrosis with phenacetin alone, except with doses approaching the LD_{50} (3,000 mg/kg for 4 weeks) (Fordham et al. 1965; Axelsen 1976).

In man, phenacetin (3 g daily for 5 days) has no significant effect on the urinary excretion of red cells and leukocytes (Clausen and Harvald 1961).

Interestingly withdrawal of phenacetin from currently available analgesic mixture was not followed by the expected reduction in analgesic nephropathy (Burry and Hopkins 1977; Gault and Wilson 1978; Kincaid-Smith 1979).

Similarly, no properly documented cases of analgesic nephropathy with the use of paracetamol alone have been reported, and there is no experimental or clinical evidence of nephrotoxicity following administration of this agent (Prescott 1966).

The Case of Aspirin and Antirheumatic Drugs

Aspirin, amidopyrine and the other antirheumatic drugs (AD) usually present in analgesic mixtures can, in contrast to phenacetin and paracetamol, all produce renal papillary necrosis (Parsons 1963; Nanra 1980).

Even in therapeutic doses, aspirin produces acute tubular damage as indicated by the marked increase in urinary excretion of tubular cells and in enzymuria (Dubach and Josch 1967; Burry and Dieppe 1976).

Numerous cases of analgesic nephropathy with papillary necrosis have been reported in patients taking aspirin without phenacetin (Nanra 1980).

The question has recently been reexamined by Elizabeth Molland (1978) who demonstrated in rats that aspirin alone produces papillary necrosis and has a greater nephrotoxic effect than phenacetin and paracetamol and that the earlier changes occurred in interstitial medullary cells. This might be due either to direct toxicity or to ischemia, medullary blood flow being reduced possibly as a result of the inhibitory effect of aspirin upon prostaglandin (PG) synthesis (Molland 1978). Renal papillary necrosis may also be induced by other non steroidal anti-inflammatory drugs known to have an inhibitory effect upon PG synthesis, thus supporting a role for this mechanism in the development of papillary necrosis (Arnold et al. 1974; Wiseman and Reinert 1975).

To summarize, there is now overhelming evidence that chronic consumption of analgesics is causally associated with renal damage.

Until recently phenacetin was indicated as the major or exclusive culprit in the development of analgesic nephropathy however more recent reports suggest that other analgesics may have an even greater toxic effect upon the kidney.

The pathogenic role of a single drug is difficult to assess. Experimental evidence seems to indicate that the combination of different agents is more offensive than the intake of a single antirheumatic drug and would explain most of the observations to date (Goldberg 1982). Nanra (1976) considers analgesic nephropathy a reversible renal disease with a good prognosis if all analgesic drugs are withdrawn.

Some of the conflicting results are difficult to reconcile and are not without criticism. Experimentally, very high doses of drugs are required before anatomical lesions are observed in a consistent fashion. Sometimes the doses used in animals bear no relationship to those consumed by man, in fact many studies have employed doses which cannot be considered to be within the pharmacological range. All experimental animals have important anatomical dissimilarities or functional differences or both in comparison with man (i.e., the rat kidney has only a single papilla). Species differences in drug metabolism and pharmacokinetics may change the dose relationship from that in man. Some patient studies were retrospective and few data are available regarding the amount of drug consumed, the different combinations of analgesics and the baseline status of the renal function. Different methods have been used to evaluate renal function in man. Plasma creatinine enables only rough estimation of renal function to be made inasmuch as it does not rise above the normal range until after a consistent loss in renal function has taken place. Some drugs (salicylates) compete with tubular excretion and thus creatinine clearance cannot be considered a reliable index of GFR.

Renal Disease in Rheumatoid Arthritis

The New Zealand Rheumatism Association Study (1972) performed on over 1,000 patients concluded that there was no evidence that salicylates administered alone were significantly nephrotoxic.

In agreement with these findings Macklon et al. (1974) reported no clinically important impairment of renal function in 17 subjects with classical rheumatoid arthritis, with an intake of more than 5 kg of aspirin, and no significant changes in renal function in a group of patients who had continued taking aspirin during two years of observation. However, six out of 17 patients had a corrected GFR below 70 ml/min in the first test.

In contrast many studies demonstrate that renal disease is common in this condition. Vasculitis, amyloidosis and glomerular lesions may occur. Clinical evidence of interstitial nephritis and papillary necrosis has been reported in some patients (Whortmann et al. 1980) and a very high incidence (50%) has been demonstrated in most autopsy series (Nanra and Kincaid-Smith 1975).

Increased excretion of renal epithelial cells, increased enzymuria, significant correlation between reduction in GFR and urinary concentrating capacity and aspirin consumption has also been reported (Bulger et al. 1968; Fillastre et al. 1972; Burry 1972; Burry et al. 1976).

Here again, on account of the above-mentioned technical and methodological problems, evalutation may be difficult.

Taken together, the data available indicate that patients with rheumatoid arthritis seem to have a milder form of renal disease than those with analgesic nephropathy; probably these patients take analgesics intermittently and may not be considered analgesic abusers.

Recently many reports have appeared on the renal toxicity of analgesics administered acutely or for brief period of time. Here one is dealing with functional effects generally reversible with discontinuation of the drug.

Renal Toxicity in Healthy Subjects

Contradictory results have been reported in normal subjects. Robert et al. (1972) obtained a significant reduction in GFR and RPF with intravenous infusion of lysin-acetylsalicylate (0.9 g). Aspirin administration reduced GFR in two out of three subjects (Kimberly and Plotz 1977) and reversibly decreased urine volume and sodium excretion (Berg 1977a). However, other studies failed to demonstrate significant changes in GFR and RPF following aspirin, indomethacin and acetaminophen given for a period of up to 2 weeks in healthy adults receiving an unrestricted diet. In sodium depleted subjects treated with indomethacin, Donker et al. (1976) observed a constant reduction on GFR but no modification in RPF; similar results were obtained by Muther et al. (1981).

The preservation of RPF with a drop in GFR is difficult to explain, however, the inhibition of the PG-mediated renin-angiotensin system activity, may affect GFR regulation when renal perfusion is at a low level.

Renal Toxicity in Patients with Various Diseases

The growing awareness of the potential toxicity of AD and the interest in their effects on prostaglandin synthesis as a possible mechanism is reflected in the numerous clinical reports that have recently appeared, suggesting that AD may cause changes in renal function in a wide range of disease states and modify the expected response to therapy.

In hypertensive animals and man, indomethacin and related AD cause more severe hypertension. This effect is particularly apparent in experimental renovascular hypertension, showing some correlation with the severity of renal arterial stenosis and low sodium intake.

In Goldblatt hypertension Romero and Strong (1977) and Beirewaltes et al. (1979) also demonstrated that indomethacin induced a deterioration in renal function.

Renal clinical studies have focused on the interaction with diuretics and hypertensive drugs.

The natriuretic and antihypertensive effects of high ceiling diuretics (Frusemide, Bumetanide) and thiazides are blunted by indomethacin and aspirin (Tweeddale and Ogilvie 1973; Bartoli et al. 1980; Brater and Chennavasin 1980). Durao et al. (1977), Cangiano et al. (1978), Lopez-Ovejero et al. (1978) reported that indomethacin significantly reduces the antihypertensive efficacy of beta-blockers and hydralazine.

These results should induce caution in using these drugs in hypertensive patients.

The administration of AD resulted in a dramatic reduction of GFR and RPF in cirrhotic patients with ascites (Boyer et al. 1969; Zipser et al. 1979) and in patients with congestive heart failure (Walshe and Venuto 1979).

High doses of indomethacin (5 mg/day) used to effect closure of patent ductus arteriosus in premature infants resulted in: urine volume contraction, sodium retention and a rise in BUN and serum creatinine (Friedman et al. 1976; Haymann et al. 1976); these side-effects were not observed by Betkerur et al. (1981); with 0.3 mg/kg of indomethacin i.v.

In Bartter's syndrome, hyperreninemic hyperaldosteronism may be considered as secondary to an overproduction of PG in view of the demonstrated interrelationship between PG and the renin-angiotensin system. In these patients, the administration of a structurally different AD resulted in sodium retention and decreased GFR, a close correlation being observed between the magnitude of urinary PGE suppression and associated deterioration in renal function (Bowden et al. 1978).

It has been recently demonstrated that sulindac in contrast to indomethacin, does not reduce either elevated renal PG production or hyperreninemia in Bartter's syndrome. This observation extended to other experimental conditions, led to the conclusion that sulindac does not inhibit renal PG-synthesis even at the full therapeutic dosage of 200 mg b.i.d. which causes approximately 80% inhibition of platelet cyclo-oxygenase (Ciabattoni et al. 1980).

In very different conditions it is possible to demonstrate some common pathophysiological patterns. Many reports are concerned with disease states characterized by decreased effective blood volume. Increased urinary excretion rates of PG have been described in many patients prior to the treatment. Improvement in renal function follows discontinuation of drug administration.

Some cases of reversible acute renal failure, massive proteinuria and interstitial nephritis with eosinophil infiltration have recently been reported (Brezin et al. 1979; Curt et al. 1980; Finkelstein et al. 1982; Gary et al. 1980).

The pathogenesis of this disorder is unknown, but it may not be specifically related to AD since the syndrome has been observed after administration of other drugs and also described in a female patient receiving sulindac for arthritis (Lomvarias et al. 1981).

Antirheumatic Drugs in Patients with Renal Diseases

A similar phenomenon, i.e., a reversible drop in GRF and RPF, was observed in patients with renal parenchyma disease (Berg 1977b).

Kimberly et al. (1978) have clearly demonstrated that the renal function of patients with systemic lupus erythematosus (SLE) is particularly susceptible to the consequences of cyclo-oxygenase inhibition even in the absence of overt renal disease.

Nephrotic patients are particularly at risk of deterioration of renal function when submitted to AD therapy.

In a series of 19 patients, proteinuria showed a 55% decrease during indomethacin treatment, with a simultaneous reduction in GFR and RPF (35% and 23%, respectively) (Arisz et al. 1976).

Improvement in renal function generally occurs following discontinuation of indomethacin, but Kleinknecht et al. (1980) reported irreversible renal failure in six out of 25 children with steroid resistant nephrosis treated with indomethacin.

In common with the above mentioned pathological conditions, patients with a nephrotic syndrome have a variable degree of effective blood volume contraction.

In order to establish the PG dependance of renal function in chronic glomerular disease (CGD) and to determine whether a cause-effect relationship exists between the inhibition of PG synthesis and impaired renal function, the short term effects of ibuprofen (400 mg t.i.d.) have been randomly compared with those of sulindac (200 b.i.d.) on renal function as well as on renal PG synthesis in 24 female patients with clinically and biopsy proven CGD, maintained on a normal sodium and potassium intake (120 mEq/day and 80 mEq/day, respectively).

All drugs were withdrawn during the two weeks precedings the study. The age of the patients ranged between 18–70 years. Two patients presented the nephrotic syndrome and 6 patients had mild to moderate hypertension.

GFR, RPF, C_{Na}, urinary PGE_2 ($UPGE_2$) and platelet cyclo-oxygenase activity were performed on three consecutive occasions during the control, treatment and wash-out periods.

Endogenous creatinine and PAH clearances were used to measure GFR and RPF. In three patients C_{Cr} and inulin clearance were assayed simultaneously in order to evaluate GFR. A highly significant correlation was found between the two series of determination ($r = 0.984$, $p = 0.001$). $UPGE_2$ was measured by a previously described radioimmunoassay (Patrono 1982).

In order to monitor the extrarenal inhibitory effects of ibuprofen and sulindac, serum TxB_2 concentrations were measured as a reflection of platelets cyclooxygenase activity during whole blood clotting (Patrono 1980).

The results were submitted to parametric analysis of variance and Student's *t*-test for paired and umpaired data. All values are reported as mean ± on standard deviation (SD); a p value < 0.01 was considered statistically significant.

The two groups had similar baseline values of the parameters considered.

Ibuprofen for 7 days significantly reduced GFR, RPF, C_{Na} and $UPGE_2$, in all patients.

These changes were fully reversible within one week of withdrawal of the drug (Tables 1 and 2). However, both serum creatinine and GFR failed to return to normal by the fifth day of the recovery period.

Patients with SLE showed the same susceptibility as primary glomerular nephritis (Tables 2 and 3).

In contrast, sulindac for 7 days did not affect GFR, RPF, urinary sodium PGE_2 excretion (Table 1), but did lead to a significant reduction of serum TxB_2 (not shown).

It may thus be concluded that in CGD renal function is critically dependent upon the intact vasodilatatory PG synthesis irrespective of the actual status of renal function and that a causal relationship exists between inhibited PG synthesis and impaired renal function since sulindac, which does not affect urinary PG excretion, does not alter renal function.

It has not been consistently demonstrated that the changes in renal function are maintained or that an "escape" phenomenon could occur in long term treatment, possibly mediated by a resumption of the cyclooxygenase activity.

Kimberly et al. (1978) and Mitnick et al. (1980) have observed cases in which changes initially seen in renal function disappeared after a week of continuous treatment.

Table 1. Effect of 1 week randomly assigned ibuprofen or sulindac treatment on renal function in sodium replete patients with chronic glomerular disease

	C_{PAH}	C_{Cr}	C_{Na}
	ml/min · 1.73 m^2		
Control	514.9 ± 156.8	90.4 ± 19.8	0.38 ± 0.08
Ibuprofen 1.2 g/day	337.5 ± 95.6*	67.4 ± 16.2*	0.26 ± 0.06*
Wash-out	504.7 ± 171.8	86.1 ± 18.7	0.38 ± 0.06
Control	434.7 ± 159.3	91.1 ± 17.8	0.36 ± 0.07
Sulindac 0.4 g/day	443.2 ± 162.6 NS	89.5 ± 17.6 NS	0.37 ± 0.07 NS
Wash-out	433.3 ± 170.4	90.1 ± 17.1	0.37 ± 0.08

Mean ± SD
NS, not significant
* $p < 0.01$

Table 2. Percentage variation of renal parameters and urinary PGE_2 excretion during ibuprofen treatment in chronic glomerular diseases ($n = 12$)

GFR (ml/min)	RPF (ml/min)	C_{Na} (ml/min)	U-PGE_2 (ng/day)
−24.7 ± 5.5*	−33.8 ± 7.9*	−28.1 ± 7.6*	−75.8 ± 10.7*

Mean ± SD
* $p < 0.001$

Table 3. Percentage variation of renal parameters during ibuprofen treatment in lupus nephritis and primary glomerular diseases

	GFR	p	RPF	p
SLE ($n = 3$)	−26 ± 4.6	NS	−33 ± 10.6	NS
PGD ($n = 9$)	−25 ± 5.7	NS	−34 ± 6.7	NS

SLE, systemic lupus erythematosus; PGD, primary glomerular diseases; NS, not significant
Mean ± SD

The mechanism of this reversal to the pretreatment state is not understood. One sodium replete patient was rechallenged with the same agent (Ibuprofen) for one month. This promptly resulted in a deterioration of renal function similar to that previously observed and was maintained throughout treatment.

Figure 1 also demonstrates that there was no change in proteinuria during the month of continous treatment.

It is noteworthy that indomethacin has been employed in the treatment of a variety of forms of GNF and advocated as an effective drug for reducing proteinuria in patients with nephrotic syndrome (Michielsen and Lambert 1967). Decreased proteinuria following aminophenazone and phenylbutazone administration had previously been reported by Fieschi et al. (1964).

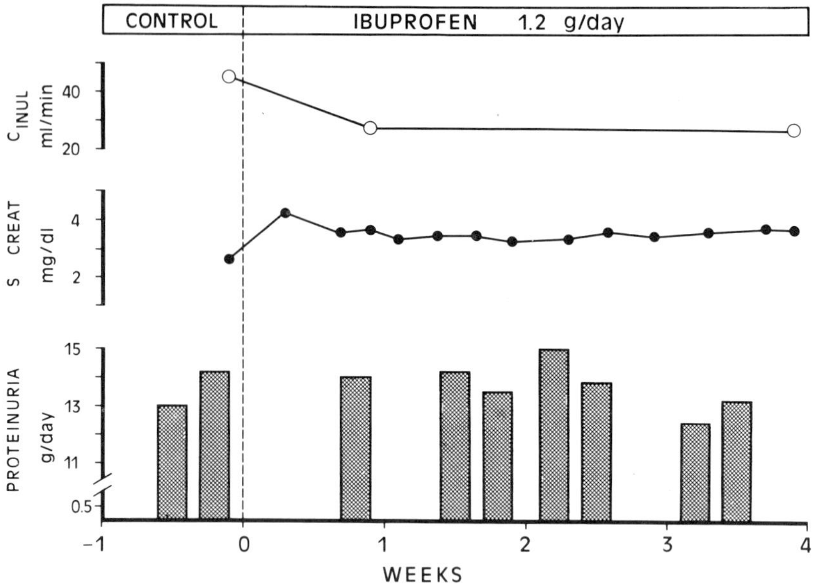

Fig. 1. B.V. (membranous glomerulonephritis) was rechallenged with ibuprofen (1.2 g/day) for 1 month on sodium unrestricted diet. The drug administration resulted in a drop in GFR and an increase in plasma creatinine maintained throughout treatment. No change in 24 h protein loss was observed

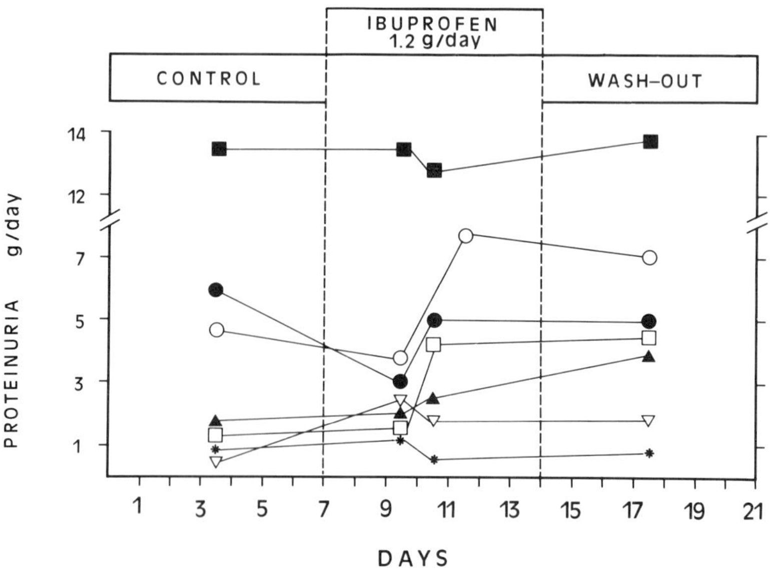

Fig. 2. The effect of ibuprofen (1.2 g/day) for 7 days on 24 h protein excretion in sodium replete patients with chronic glomerular disease

The mechanism of the effect still remains to be elucidated. The possibility that indomethacin interferes with the pathological process in the glomeruli, as advocated by Michielsen and Lambert (1967), has not been confirmed by others.

Interestingly, a reduction in proteinuria was not observed in the sodium replete patients treated with ibuprofen at doses comparable, as far as concerns inhibition of PG synthesis, to those of indomethacin (75.8%) (Fig. 2).

These results do not support the hypothesis that indomethacin reversibly affects proteinuria by influencing renal function or the permeability of the glomerular basement membrane, mediated by renal prostaglandins and the renin-angiotensin system (Tiggeler et al. 1979).

In conclusion, although further studies are required to identify which patients are at risk, the clinician must be aware that there is compelling evidence that AD may cause functional and structural renal damage and thus use these drugs with caution in a wide range of disease states.

References

Arisz L, Donker AJM, Brentjens JHR, Van de Hem GK (1976) The effect of indomethacin on proteinuria and kidney function in nephrotic syndrome. Acta Med Scand 199: 121–125

Arnold L, Collins C, Starmer GA (1974) Renal and gastric lesions after phenylbutazone and indomethacin in the rat. Pathology 6: 303–313

Axelsen RA (1976) Analgesic induced papillary necrosis in the Gunn rat: The comparative nephrotoxicity of aspirin and phenacetin. J Pathol 120: 145–149

Bartoli E, Arras S, Faedda R, Soggia G, Satta A, Olmeo NA (1980) Blunting of furosemide diuresis by aspirin in man. J Clin Pharmacol 10: 452–458

Beirewaltes WH, Britton SL, Romero JC (1979) Interrelationship between renin, prostaglandins and volume status in moderate and severe one two-kidney renovascular hypertension. Excerpta Medica Intern Congr Ser 496: 17–22

Berg JK (1977a) Acute effects of acetylsalicylic acid on renal function in normal man. Eur J Clinic Pharmacol 11: 117–123

Berg JK (1977b) Acute effect of acetylsalicylic acid in patients with chronic renal insufficiency. Eur J Clin Pathol 11: 111–116

Betkerur MV, Yeh TF, Miller K (1981) Indomethacin and its effect on renal function and urinary kallikrein excretion in premature infants with patent ductus arteriosus. Pediatrics 68: 99–102

Bowden RE, Gill JR Jr, Radfar N, Taylor AA, Keiser HR (1978) Prostaglandins synthetase inhibitors in Bartter's syndrome. Effect on immunoreactive prostaglandin excretion. JAMA 239: 117–121

Boyer TD, Zia P, Reynolds TB (1979) Effect of indomethacin and prostaglandin A_1 on renal function and plasma renin activity in alcoholic liver disease. Gastroenterology 77: 215–222

Brater DC, Chennavasin P (1980) Indomethacin and the response to bumetanide. Clin Pharmacol Ther 27: 421–425

Brezin JH, Katz SM, Schwartz AB, Chinitz JL (1979) Reversible renal failure and nephrotic syndrome associated with non-steroidal anti-inflammatory drugs. N Engl J Med 301: 1271–1273

Bulger RJ, Healey LA, Polinsky P (1968) Renal abnormalities in rheumatoid arthritis. Ann Rheum Dis 27: 339–344

Burry A, Hopkins J (1977) Phenacetin and analgesic nephropathy. Med J Aust 1: 879–882

Burry HC (1972) Reduced glomerular filtration rate in rheumatoid arthritis. Ann Rheum Dis 31: 65–68

Burry HC, Dieppe PA (1976) Apparent reduction of endogenous creatinine clearance by salicylate treatment. Br Med J 2: 16–17

Burry HC, Dieppe PA, Bresnihan FB, Brown C (1976) Salicylates and renal function in rheumatoid arthritis. Br Med J 1: 613–615

Cangiano JL, Rodriguez-Sargent C, Martinez-Maldonado M (1978) Modification of experimental renal hypertension in the rat by indomethacin and hydralazine. J Lab Clin Med 92: 516–520

Ciabattoni G, Pugliese F, Cinotti GA, Patrono C (1980) Renal effects of anti-inflammatory drugs. J Rheumatol Inflamm 3: 210–221

Clausen E, Harvald B (1961) Nephrotoxicity of different analgesics. Acta Med Scand 170: 469–474

Cove-Smith JR (1981) Analgesic nephropathy in the United Kingdom incidence, clinical features and pathogenesis. J Clin Pathol 34: 1255–1260

Curt GA, Kaldany A, Whitley LG, Crosson AW, Robla A, Merino MJ, Dielia JA (1980) Reversible rapidly progressive renal failure with nephrotic syndrome due to Fenoprofen Calcium. Ann Intern Med 92: 72–73

Donker AJM, Arisz L, Bretjens JRH, Van der Hem GK, Hollemans HJG (1976) The effect of indomethacin on kidney function and plasma renin activity in man. Nephron 17: 288–296

Dubach UC, Josch W (1967) Urinenzyme nach medikamentöser Nierenreizung durch Salicylat. Schweiz Med Wochenschr 97: 1314–1317

Dubach UC, Rosner B, Pfister E (1983) Epidemiologic study of abuse of analgesics containing phenacetin: renal morbidity and mortality (1968–1979). N Engl J Med 308: 357–362

Durao V, Prata MM, Goncalues LMP (1977) Modification of antihypertensive effect of beta adrenoreceptor blocking agents by inhibition of endogenous prostaglandin synthesis. Lancet 2: 1005–1007

Fieschi A, Bianchi V, Ghirardo G (1964) Results of treatment with phenylbutazone in albuminuric syndrome. In: Garattini S, Dukes NMG (eds) Non-steroidal anti-inflammatory drugs: proceedings of an international symposium, Milan. Excerpta Medica Intern Congr Series 82: 437; Excerpta Medica, Amsterdam

Fillastre RM, Berger H, Malandain H (1972) Effect of intravenous infusion of acetylsalicylate acid on renal function. Br Med J 2: 466–467

Finkelstein A, Fraley DS, Stachura I, Feldman HA, Gandy DR, Boucke E (1982) Fenoprofen nephropathy: lipoid nephrosis and interstitial nephritis. Am J Med 72: 82–87

Fordham C, Huffines WD, Welt LG (1965) Phenacetin-induced renin lesions in the rat. In: Kass EH (ed) Progress in pyelonephritis. Davis, Philadelphia 325–331

Friedman WF, Hirschklan MJ, Printz MP, Pitlich PT, Kirkpatrick SE (1976) Pharmacologic closure of patent ductus arteriosus in the premature infant. N Engl J Med 295: 526–529

Gary NE, Dodelsen R, Eisenger RP (1980) Indomethacin associated acute renal failure. Am J Med 69: 135–136

Gault MH, Wilson DR (1978) Analgesic nephropathy in Canada: Clinical syndromes, management and outcome. Kidney Int 13: 58–63

Goldberg M (1982) Analgesic nephropathy in 1981: Which drug is responsible? JAMA 247: 64–65

Heymann MA, Rudolph AM, Silverman NH (1976) Closure of the ductus arteriosus in premature infants by inhibition of prostaglandin synthesis. N Engl J Med 296: 418–424

Kimberly RP, Plotz PH (1977) Aspirin-induced depression of renal function. N Engl J Med 296: 418–424

Kimberly RP, Bowden RE, Keiser HR, Plotz PH (1978) Reduction of renal function by newer non-steroidal anti-inflammatory drugs. Am J Med 68: 804–807

Kincaid-Smith P (1978) Analgesic nephropathy in Australia. Contrib Nephrol 16: 57–64

Kleinknecht C, Broyer M, Gubler MC, Palcoux JB (1980) Irreversible renal failure after indomethacin in steroid-resistent nephrosis. N Engl J Med 302: 691

Lomvarias S, Pinn WV, Wadhwa ML, Koshy KM, Heller M (1981) Nephrotic syndrome associated with Sulindac. N Engl J Med 304: 424

Lopez-Ovejero JA, Weber MA, Drayer JIM, Sealey JE, Laragh JH (1978) Effects of indomethacin alone and during diuretic or beta-adrenoreceptor-blockade therapy on blood pressure and the renin system in essential hypertension. Clin Sci Mol Med 551: 2035–2056

Macklon AF, Craft AW, Thompson M, Kerr DNS (1974) Aspirin and analgesic nephropathy. Br Med J 1: 597–600
Michielsen P, Lambert PP (1967) Effets du traitment par les corticostéroids et l'indomethacine sur la protéinurie. Bull Mem Soc Med Hop Paris 118: 217
Mitnick PD, Greenberg A, De Oreo PB (1980) Effects of two non steroidal anti-inflammatory drugs: indomethacin and oxaprozin on the kidney. Clin Pharmacol Ther 28: 680–689
Molland EA (1978) Experimental renal papillary necrosis. Kidney Int 13: 5–14
Muther RS, Potter DM, Bennett WM (1981) Aspirin induced depression of glomerular filtration rate in normal humans: role of sodium balance. Ann Intern Med 94: 317–321
Nanra RS (1976) Analgesic nephropathy. Med J Aust 1: 745–748
Nanra RS (1980) Clinical and pathological aspects of analgesic nephropathy. A re-evaluation. Br J Clin Pharmacol [Suppl 2] 359S–368S
Nanra RS, Kincaid-Smith P (1975) Renal papillar necrosis in rheumatoid arthritis. Med J Aust 1: 194
New Zealand Rheumatism Association Study (1974) Aspirin and the kidney. Br Med J 1: 593–596
Parsons FM (1963) The use of the artificial kidney in salicylate poisoning. In: Dixon et al. (eds) Salicylates. An international symposium. Churchill, London, pp 281–285
Patrono C (1980) Radioimmunoassay of serum thromboxane B_2: a simple method to assess pharmacologic effects on platelet function. Adv Prostaglandin Thromboxane Res 6: 187–197
Patrono C, Pugliese F, Ciabattoni G, Maseri A, Chierchia S, Peskar BA, Cinotti Ga, Simonetti BM, Pierucci A (1982) Evidence for a direct stimulatory effect of prostacyclin on renin release in man. J Clin Invest 69: 231–239
Prescott LF (1966) The nephrotoxicity of analgesics. J Phar Pharmacol 18: 331–344
Prescott LF (1982) Analgesic nephropathy: a reassessment of the role of phenacetin and other analgesics. Drugs 23: 75–149
Robert M, Fillastre JP, Berger H, Malandain H (1972) Effect of intravenous infusion of acetylsalicylic acid on renal function. Br Med J 2: 466–467
Romero JC, Strong CG (1977) The effect of indomethacin blockade of prostaglandin synthesis on blood pressure of normal rabbits and rabbits with renovascular hypertension. Circ Res 40: 35–41
Tiggeler RGWL, Hulme B, Wijoleveld GAB (1979) Effect of indomethacin on glomerular permeability in the nephrotic syndrome. Kidney Int 16: 312–321
Tweeddale MG, Ogilvie RI (1973) Antagonism of spironolactone-induced natriuresis by aspirin in man. N Engl J Med 289: 198–200
Walshe JJ, Venuto RC (1979) Oliguric renal failure induced by indomethacin: possible mechanism. Ann Intern Med 91: 47–49
Whortmann DW, Kelsch RC, Kuhus L, Sullivan DB, Cassidy JT (1980) Renal papillar necrosis in juvenile rheumatoid arthritis. J Pediatr 97: 37–40
Wiseman EH, Reinert H (1975) Anti-inflammatory drugs and renal papillary necrosis. Agents Action 5: 322–325
Zipser RD, Hoefs JC, Speckart PF, Zia PK, Horton R (1979) Prostaglandins: modulators of renal function and pressor resistance in chronic liver disease. J Clin Endocrinol Metab 48: 895–900
Zollinger HU, Spuhler O (1950) Die nicht-eitrige chronische interstielle Nephritis. Schweiz Z Allg Pathol 13: 807

Disease, Metabolism and Reproduction in the Toxic Response to Drugs and Other Chemicals
Arch. Toxicol., Suppl. 7, 350–359 (1984)

Central and Peripheral Haemodynamic Effects of Non-steroidal Anti-inflammatory Drugs in Man

Å. Wennmalm, I. Carlsson, A. Edlund, S. Eriksson, L. Kaijser, and J. Nowak

Department of Clinical Physiology, Karolinska Institute, 104 01 Stockholm, Sweden

Abstract. The haemodynamic effects of non-steroidal anti-inflammatory (NSAI) drugs can be attributed either to their common property of inhibiting the formation of prostaglandins (PG) in the cardiovascular system, or to direct actions on the tone and sensitivity of the resistance vessels in various regions. Indomethacin (IND) is the most frequently studied NSAI drug, in animals and in man. Its cardiovascular effects differ somewhat from those of other NSAI, due to the fact that, besides inhibiting PG formation, IND acts as a direct vasoconstrictor. The stimulatory effect of IND in vascular smooth muscle results in an increased systemic vascular resistance which, although partially compensated by a decreased cardiac output, gives rise to a moderate increase in systemic blood pressure. The vasoconstrictor effect of IND is of particular interest in patients with ischemic heart disease, since it lowers their already decreased coronary flow, and may thereby accentuate the risk of myocardial infarction. Administration of IND also leads to a decreased blood flow in the splanchnic region, the kidneys, and the brain. The cerebral blood flow is lowered by 25–35%; in addition, IND almost entirely erases the hyperemic flow response to hypercapnia. Of other NSAI drugs, at least aspirin and naproxen are completely devoid of such actions on the cerebral circulation. A common vascular effect of all NSAI drugs is a diminution of reactive hyperemia, the local hyperemia that develops in a tissue subjected to a short period of arterial occlusion. Part of this hyperemic response is dependent on an intact vascular PG formation and consequently it is inhibited when PG formation is blocked. In contrast, NSAI drugs do not affect the functional increase in the blood flow in working skeletal muscle.

Key words: Cardiac output – Systemic vascular resistance – Regional blood flow – Non-steroidal anti-inflammatory drugs – Acetyl-salicylic acid – Naproxen – Ibuprofen – Indomethacin – Piroxicam

Introduction

The side effects of the non-steroidal anti-inflammatory (NSAI) drugs may be of two principal kinds: first, actions related to their property of inhibiting prostaglandin (PG) synthesis in organs or tissues in which this inhibition is undesirable and second, actions not related to this inhibitory effect. The wide spread use of such drugs, coupled with the fact that treatment often continues indefinitely, makes it important to obtain detailed information about these effects.

Patients given NSAI drugs are often elderly, and consequently it is likely that a number of them suffer from cardiovascular disease. This makes it particularly relevant to consider side effects of NSAI drugs in the cardiovascular system. Hitherto the actions of NSAI drugs in the cardiovascular system have been studied mainly with respect to their interference with platelet function, i.e., the balance between platelet thromboxane $A_2(TxA_2)$ and endothelial prostacyclin (PGI_2) production (see Ellis et al. 1980; Hanley et al. 1981; Patrignani et al. 1982). In the present study the direct cardiovascular actions of some NSAI drugs is reported, i.e., their central and peripheral haemodynamic effects.

Methods

Central Haemodynamic Effects of IND at Rest and During Exercise

Five healthy male volunteers, aged 22–35 years, were investigated. Short teflon catheters were inserted into a brachial artery and vein, respectively. A Swan-Ganz catheter (no 7) was inserted into a medial cubital vein and passed under fluoroscopic control to the pulmonary artery. Heart rate (HR) was measured via a continuous ECG recording. Cardiac output (CO) was measured using the direct Fick method. Arterial and right atrial blood pressures (BP) were recorded via the arterial catheter, and via a side hole in the Swan-Ganz catheter, respectively. All determinations were performed in supine position. Muscular work was performed as supine bicycle leg exercise at a work load of 150 W. Pure indomethacin (Merck, Sharp and Dohme) was dissolved in a small amount of ethanol and diluted in an appropriate volume of isotonic saline, before being infused via a sterile filter. The infusion rate was adjusted to result in a total drug amount of 25 mg infused during 10 min. Recordings of HR, CO, and BP were performed in the basal state and during leg exercise before and immediately after infusion of indomethacin.

Peripheral Haemodynamic Effects of NSAI Drugs

Effects on Basal and CO_2-Stimulated Cerebral Blood Flow (CBF)

Seventeen healthy male volunteers, aged 20–32 years, were investigated. A short teflon catheter was inserted into a brachial artery. A Cournand catheter (no. 7) was inserted into the right femoral vein and passed under fluoroscopic control to the right jugular venous bulb. CBF was measured according to Kety and Schmidt (1945) using inhalation of 2–4% N_2O in air. Arterial and jugular venous blood N_2O levels were analysed by gas chromatography. Stimulation of CBF was performed by inhalation of CO_2 (6–7%) in air. Either IND (Capsules Indomee, Merk, Sharp and Dome MSD, 0.8 mg/kg), naproxen (NAPR, Tablets Naprosyn, Astra-Syntex, 4 mg/kg), or acetyl-salicylic acid (ÁSP, Tablets Bamyl, Hässle, 45 mg/kg) was given orally. CBF was measured in the basal state and 10 min after the start of inhalation of CO_2 as indicated above, before and 60 min after administration of the drug.

Effect of IND on Coronary Blood Flow in Patients with Ischemic Heart Disease (IHD)

Twenty-one male patients with IHD, aged 34–62 years, were investigated. IHD was verified by typical chest pain and ECG changes during a previous bicycle exercise test. Most of the patients had an earlier history of myocardial infarction. A short teflon catheter was inserted in a brachial artery. Another teflon catheter was introduced into a medial cubital vein and passed under fluoroscopic control to the coronary sinus. Arterial and coronary sinus blood samples were drawn for analysis of O_2 content. Typical chest pain was elicited by atrial pacing, performed via an electrode in the coronary sinus catheter. Either ASP, IND, or NAPR was given orally as above. Arterial and coronary sinus blood samples for analysis of O_2 were drawn at supine rest and during pacing to moderately severe angina pectoris, before and 60 min after administration of the drug.

Effect on Skeletal Muscle Blood Flow in the Basal State, During Exercise, and After Arterial Occlusion

Six healthy males, aged 24–32 years, were studied. Short teflon catheters were introduced into both femoral veins, and into the femoral artery of the leg to be investigated. Leg blood flow was measured using the constant rate infusion technique (Jorfeldt and Wahren 1971) with indocyanine green dye. After repeated blood flow measurements at supine rest, exercise in upright body position was performed on a bicycle ergometer. The subjects performed a 6 min work at each of the loads 50, 100, and 150 W. Leg blood flow was measured four times at each work load. The procedure was repeated one week later, after 2 h pretreatment with IND (Suppository Indomee, Merk, Sharp and Dome, 1.25 mg/kg rectally).

In another ten healthy subjects, five males and five females, aged 18–48 years, basal forearm blood flow and the reactive hyperemia after a 5 min occlusion of forearm arterial flow were determined with venous occlusion plethysmography. For details of the flow determination technique, see Kilbom and Wennmalm (1976). The determinations were performed before and after one of the drugs ASP, IND, and NAPR in the doses indicated in the section on patients with ischaemic heart disease above, as well as after ibuprofen (Tablets Brufen, Boots, 10 mg/kg orally) or piroxicam (Tablets Voltaren, Ciba-Geigy, 0.9 mg/kg orally).

Effect of IND on Renal and Splanchnic Blood Flow

Ten healthy males, aged 23–41 years, were studied. Cournand catheters (no. 7) were inserted percutaneously and passed under fluoroscopic control to a right-sided hepatic vein and to either of the renal veins, respectively. Two short teflon catheters were inserted into a superficial forearm vein and a brachial artery, respectively. A mixture of indocyanine green dye and para-aminohippurate was infused into the short venous forearm catheter. Simultaneous arterial and renal and hepatic venous blood samples were drawn at regular intervals for determination of dye and para-aminohippurate concentrations. Splanchnic and renal blood flows were estimated using the constant infusion technique (Bradley 1948). IND was given i.v. as in the study on central haemodynamic effects above, but the total dose was 50 mg. Samples for splanchnic and renal blood flow determinations were drawn with the subjects in supine position, after a 25–35 min constant infusion of the indicator mixture. Subsequently IND was given and after another 25–35 min of constant rate indicator infusion, samples for determination of renal and splanchnic flows were drawn again.

Results

Central Haemodynamic Effects of IND at Rest and During Exercise

In the basal state, HR, CO, systemic BP and systemic vascular resistance of the subjects were within the normal range (Fig. 1a). Infusion of IND was followed by a significant ($p < 0.05$) decrease in CO. HR was unchanged, indicating that the lowered CO came from an impaired stroke volume. Systemic BP was significantly ($p < 0.01$) increased. Calculation of the systemic vascular resistance as the ratio between the blood pressure fall in the systemic circulation (mean systemic BP – mean right atrial BP) and the CO revealed a significant ($p < 0.01$) increase (Fig. 1a).

During supine leg exercise at a work load of 150 W, the CO rose to about 17 l/min. HR increased to about 135 beats/min and the systemic BP rose to about 120 mm Hg. The systemic vascular resistance fell to about 50% of the resting value (Fig. 1b). When the supine leg exercise was repeated after administration of IND, the haemodynamic response was almost the same as before drug. Thus, neither HR, CO, systemic BP nor systemic vascular resistance displayed significant differences from the corresponding values before IND.

Peripheral Haemodynamic Effects of NSAI Drugs

Effect on Basal and CO_2-Stimulated CBF

The basal CBF was about 45 ml/100 ml/min. After administration of ASP or NAPR, no significant change was found in CBF compared with before drug administration (Fig. 2). In contrast, administration of IND was followed by a

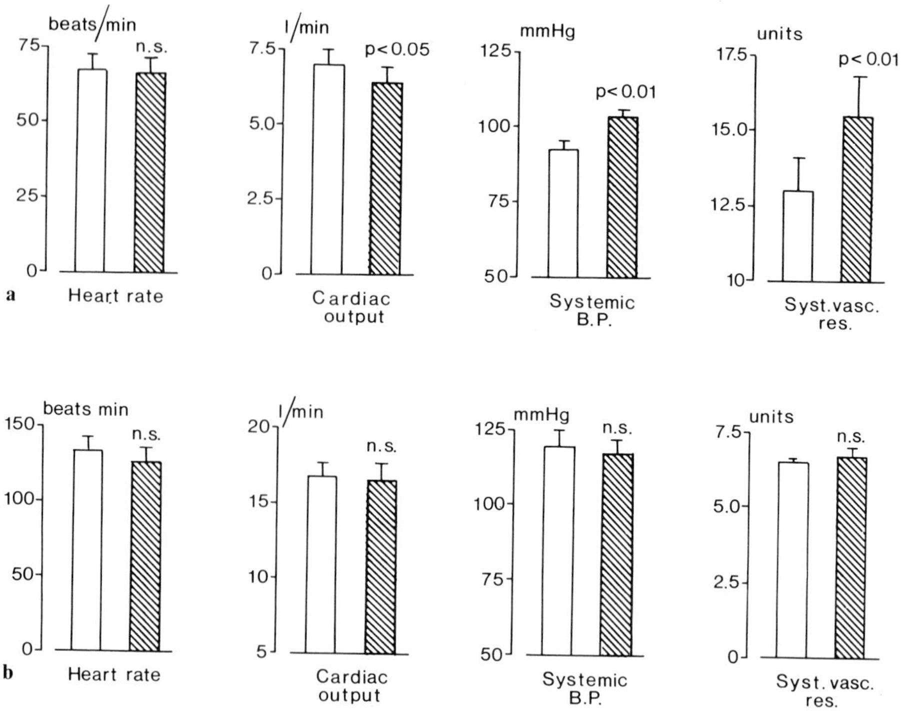

Fig. 1. **a** Heart rate, cardiac output, systemic blood pressure and systemic vascular resistance at supine rest before *(open columns)* and after *(striped columns)* an i.v. infusion of indomethacin. Values presented as mean ± SE. **b** As above, except that all data refer to recordings performed during leg exercise in the upright position on a bicycle ergometer at a work load of 150 W

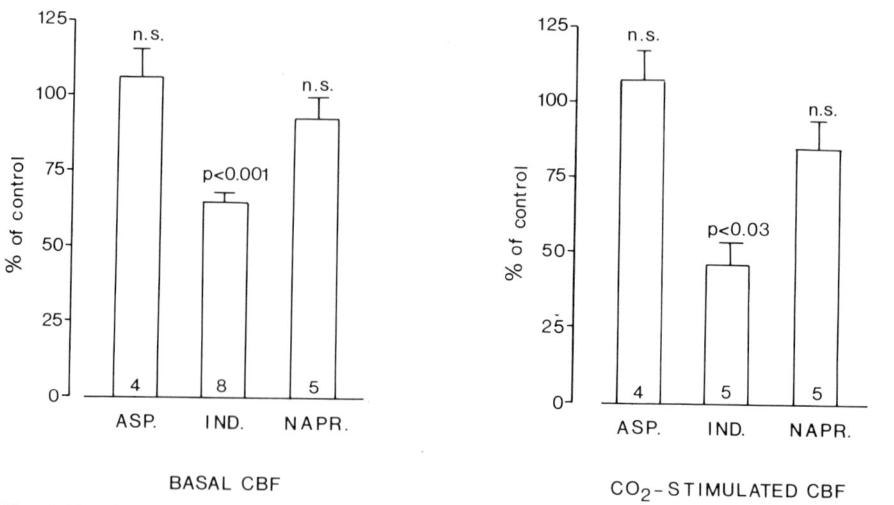

Fig. 2. Basal and CO_2-stimulated cerebral blood flow after administration of acetyl-salicylic acid *(ASP)*, indomethacin *(IND)*, or naproxen *(NAPR)*. Values presented as a percentage of the corresponding figures obtained before each drug. *Columns* and *bars* indicate means ± SE

considerable impairment of the basal CBF, down to about 65% of control (Fig. 2).

During inhalation of 6–7% CO_2 there was a considerable rise in CBF, to a level that ranged from 75 to 105 ml/100 ml/min. This CBF response to increased arterial CO_2 was not affected by ASP or NAPR, whereas IND abolished it almost completely (Fig. 2).

Effect of IND on Coronary Blood Flow in Patients with IHD

Before administration of IND, the basal coronary blood flow was 126 ± 14 ml/min. The difference in O_2 content between arterial and coronary sinus blood [d(A-CS)O_2] was 132 ± 3 ml/l. During atrial pacing to angina pectoris the coronary blood flow increased, to 270 ± 30 ml/ml. The cardiac oxygen extraction did not change significantly.

After administration of indomethacin the coronary blood flow was not changed, but the d(A-CS)O_2 was significantly increased (Fig. 3). During atrial pacing to angina pectoris the coronary blood flow rose less than before IND, to 237 ± 32 ml/min. The cardiac oxygen extraction during pacing was higher after IND than before. Since cardiac oxygen extraction after IND did not differ at rest and during atrial pacing, the d(A-CS)O_2 values at rest and during pacing before IND have been pooled, and compared to the corresponding values after administration of IND (Fig. 3). The increase in cardiac oxygen extraction was apparently sufficient to compensate for the decrease in coronary flow elicited by IND, since the calculated cardiac oxygen consumption was not significantly affected.

Effect on Skeletal Muscle Blood Flow in the Basal State, During Exercise, and After Arterial Occlusion

The resting leg blood flow was 0.4 ± 0.03 l/min. Exercise elicited a successive, marked increase in this flow (Table 1). Increasing work was paralleled by an augmented flow. The maximal figure for blood flow (4.3 ± 0.2 l/min) was reached at a work load of 150 W, implying more than a 10-fold rise above the

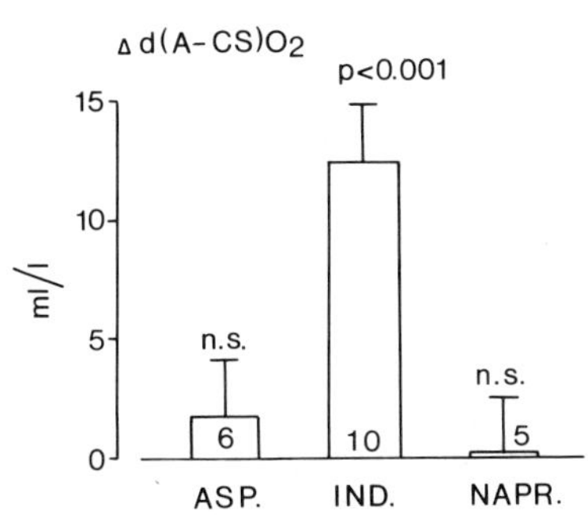

Fig. 3. Change in (arterial-coronary sinus) differences in oxygen content induced by acetyl-salicylic acid *(ASP)*, indomethacin *(IND)*, or naproxen *(NAPR)*. *Columns* and *bars* represent mean ± SE

Table 1. Leg blood flow at rest and during bicycle exercise at different work loads, before and after administration of indomethacin (1.25 mg/kg)

	Rest	50 W	100 W	150 W
Control	0.40 ± 0.03	2.09 ± 0.12	3.09 ± 0.10	4.30 ± 0.20
After indomethacin	0.45 ± 0.05	1.95 ± 0.06	3.10 ± 0.08	4.30 ± 1.10

Values presented in l/min as mean ± SE of 9–12 experiments

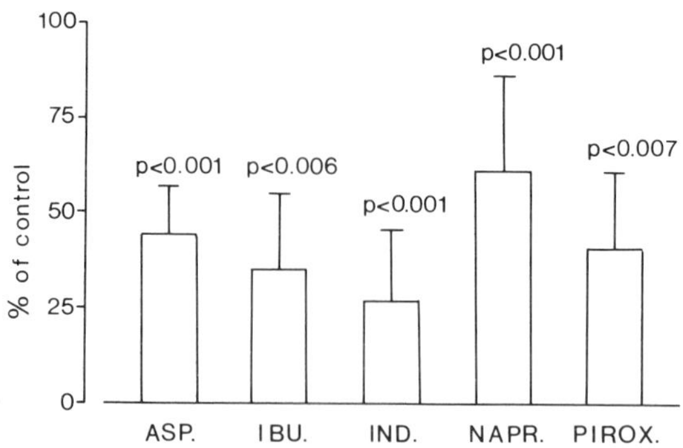

Fig. 4. Forearm reactive hyperemia after administration of acetyl-salicylic acid *(ASP)*, ibuprofen *(IBU)*, indomethacin *(IND)*, naproxen *(NAPR)*, or prioxicam *(PIROX)*. Values presented as a percentage of the corresponding figures obtained before each drug. *Columns* and *bars* indicate mean ± SE

Table 2. Effects of indomethacin on blood flow and vascular resistance in the kidneys and in the splanchnic region in 10 healthy humans

	Kidneys		Splanchnic region	
	Blood flow (l/min)	Vascular resistance (U)	Blood flow (l/min)	Vascular resistance (U)
Control	1.61 ± 0.07	58 ± 2.0	1.22 ± 0.17	78 ± 5.0
After indomethacin	1.41 ± 0.10**	75 ± 6.0**	1.17 ± 0.09 (NS)	91 ± 8.0*

Indomethacin (50 mg) was given as an i.v. infusion, and the flows were measured 25–35 min after drug administration. Values presented as mean ± SE
* and ** indicate that the value differs significantly ($p < 0.05$ and 0.01, respectively) from the corresponding value in the row above
NS, not significant

resting level. IND did not affect the resting leg blood flow, neither did it change the flow-enhancing effect of dynamic work; the leg blood flow following administration of IND was almost exactly the same as that obtained before drug (Table 1).

In the reactive hyperemia series the basal forearm blood flow was about 10 ml/100 ml tissue/min. Five min of occlusion of the brachial artery elicited a rapid but brief post-occlusive vasodilation, increasing the forearm flow to a peak value of about 25 ml/100 ml tissue/min. The duration of the reactive hyperemia only just exceeded 2 min. The amount of the reactive hyperemia, expressed as the total post-occlusive minus the preceding basal flow extrapolated to the 3 min during which the total post-occlusive flow was assessed, was about 13 ml/100 ml tissue/min.

As in the above-mentioned series on the effect of IND on basal leg blood flow the forearm basal flow was not affected by any of the NSAI drugs tested. The response to arterial occlusion was, however, changed. The peak post-occlusive flow was significantly decreased by ASP and ibuprofen, and the duration of the reactive hyperemia was shortened by piroxicam. All drugs significantly depressed the amount of reactive hyperemia (Fig. 4), although not to the same extent. Thus ibuprofen, most potent in this respect, impaired the reactive hyperemia by about 70%, while NAPR, which was least efficient, did so by about 35%.

Effect of IND on Renal and Splanchnic Blood Flow

The basal renal and splanchnic blood flows were well within the normal range, and are given in Table 2. After administration of IND, both the renal and the splanchnic flow values fell. This was accompanied by a moderate increase in systemic blood pressure, as in the series presented under the section on central haemodynamic effects above, indicating that the actual increase in vascular resistance was even greater than that indicated by the decrease in flow. Calculation of the local resistance values for the renal and splanchnic regions revealed that the renal vascular resistance in fact was increased by 30 ± 9% by IND, while the splanchnic vascular resistance was increased by 16 ± 6%.

Discussion

It was demonstrated a decade ago that IND lowers the basal CBF in anaesthetized baboons (Pickard and Mackenzie 1973). This observation was later extended to rats (Sakabe and Siesjö 1979). The present series, displaying a 35% decrease in CBF after administration of IND, confirms the drug effect in the conscious man. Unlike IND, neither ASP nor NAPR had any effect on the basal CBF, indicating that cerebral vasoconstriction is not a common property of NSAI drugs.

Recently it was reported that IND lowers coronary flow and elevates the cardiac oxygen extraction in patients with IHD (Friedman et al. 1981). The elevation of cardiac oxygenation was confirmed by the current experiments, displaying increased $d(A\text{-}CS)O_2$ both at rest and during atrial pacing. Furthermore, the coronary flow response to atrial pacing was lower after than before IND. However, neither ASP nor NAPR had any effect on the cardiac oxygen extraction, indicating that these NSAI drugs did not affect the coronary flow. Consequently it appears that IND, unlike ASP and NAPR, acts as a vasoconstrictor not only in the cerebral but also in the coronary circulation in humans. In the renal and splanchnic vascular beds IND also diminished the blood flow, by increasing the local vascular resistance. The only vascular bed investigated, in which IND did not impair the flow, was that of the forearm and leg skeletal muscle. Taken together, these observations on the actions of NSAI drugs in various vascular beds in the basal state indicate that IND has organ-specific vasoconstrictor properties that are not shared by ASP or NAPR.

Regional blood flow was stimulated by various means in the present study: by hypercapnia (cerebral flow), by atrial pacing (coronary flow), or by muscular work (leg flow). The vascular responses to these stimuli were affected differently by the NSAI drugs investigated. In the cerebral circulation IND almost completely abolished the hypercapnia induced hyperemia, while ASP and NAPR failed to induce a similar action. In the coronary circulation IND depressed the pacing induced increase in flow, as mentioned above; neither ASP nor NAPR affected the coronary flow, to judge from the unchanged differences in $(A\text{-}CS)O_2$. In the leg muscle circulation IND did not change the vasodilator response to muscle work at different loads. Neither did IND affect the total systemic resistance during heavy supine leg muscle work. During heavy exercise the total vascular resistance is largely dependent on the resistance in the working muscle; the latter results can therefore be regarded as support for the concept that functional hyperemia in working muscle is not affected by IND. The conclusion that can be drawn concerning the action of NSAI drugs on various types of hyperemia is consequently largely analoguous to that concerning basal flow: IND elicits organ- or stimulus-specific inhibition of these vasodilator responses.

Reactive hyperemia, the post-occlusive vasodilation following short-lasting arterial occlusion, represents a different type of vascular relaxation to that which develops during increased metabolic activity in the surrounding tissue. It is consequently not per se surprising that the NSAI drugs affected reactive hyperaemia in skeletal muscle in spite of their failure to change the muscle blood flow during exercise. More remarkable is the fact that all five NSAI drugs tested displayed mainly similar activities. This similarity strongly suggests that inhibition of muscle reactive hyperemia is a common property of NSAI drugs.

Effects shared by all NSAI drugs tested can most probably be ascibed to their known pharmacological action, i.e., inhibition of PG formation. By the same token, effects which are not common to all NSAI drugs can hardly be due to this action. On the basis of this assumption, some conclusions of a physiological character can be drawn concerning the role of locally formed PG in the cardiovascular system. Firstly, locally formed PG do not contribute to the basal blood flow in the human brain, heart and skeletal muscle, and possibly also not to the basal flow in the kidneys and the splanchnic region. Furthermore, locally formed PG do not participate in the development of hyperaemia induced by hypercapnia in the brain, by atrial pacing in the heart, or by muscular work in the legs. On the other hand, locally formed PG do contribute to the development of reactive hyperemia in skeletal muscle.

A conclusion of clinical importance can be drawn from the current data: IND impairs basal and stimulated blood flow in two regions that are susceptible to ischemia in the presence of atherosclerosis, i.e. the cerebral and coronary circuits. The consequence of this conclusion is that if ischemic disease in either of these regions is manifest or suspected, IND should not be the choice if treatment with an NSAI drug is deemed necessary.

Acknowledgements. This work presented here was supported financially by The Swedish Medical Research Council, project 04X-4341.

References

Bradley SE (1948) Measurements of hepatic blood flow. In: Potter VR (ed) Methods in medical research, Vol 1. Year Book Publishers, Chicago, p 99

Ellis EF, Wright KF, Jones PS, Richardson DW, Ellis CK (1980) Effect of oral aspirin dose on platelet aggregation and vascular prostacyclin (PGI_2) synthesis in humans and rabbits. J Cardiovasc Pharmacol 2: 387–397

Friedman PL, Brown EJ, Gunther S, Alexander RW, Barry WH, Mudge GH, Grossman W (1981) Coronary vasoconstrictor effect of indomethacin in patients with coronary-artery disease. N Engl J Med 305: 1171–1175

Hanley SP, Cockbill SR, Bevan J, Heptinstall S (1981) Differential inhibition by low-dose aspirin of human venous prostacyclin synthesis and platelet thromboxane synthesis. Lancet 2: 969–971

Jorfeldt L, Wahren J (1971) Leg blood flow during exercise in man. Clin Sci Mol Med 41: 459–473

Kety SS, Schmidt CF (1945) The determination of cerebral blood flow in man by the use of nitrous oxide in low concentrations. Am J Physiol 143: 53–66

Kilbom Å, Wennmalm Å (1976) Endogenous prostaglandins as local regulators of blood flow in man: Effect of indomethacin on reactive and functional hyperaemia. J Physiol (Lond) 257: 109–121

Patrignani P, Filabozzi P, Patrono C (1982) Selective cumulative inhibition of platelet thromboxane production by low-dose aspirin in healthy subjects. J Clin Invest 69: 1366–1372

Pickard JD, Mackenzie ET (1973) Inhibition of prostaglandin synthesis and the response of baboon cerebral circulation to carbon dioxide. Nature (New Biol) 245: 187–188

Sakabe T, Siesjo BK (1979) The effect of indomethacin on the blood flow-metabolism couple in the brain under normal, hypercapnic and hypoxic conditions. Acta Physiol Scand 107: 283–284

Disease, Metabolism and Reproduction in the Toxic Response to Drugs and Other Chemicals
Arch. Toxicol., Suppl. 7, 360–362 (1984)

Indomethacin Induced Intestinal Toxicity is Blocked by Sodium Salicylate at 24 and 48 Hours Post Treatment

E. Ezer

Pharmacological Research Centre, Chemical Works of Gedeon Richter, Ltd., Budapest, POB 27, 1475, Hungary

Abstract. Single 10 mg/kg oral dose of indomethacin induced so-called non-fatal intestinal ulceration. Tensile strength of the intestinal wall gradually decreased at 24, 48, and 72 h after treatment. In animals treated with sodium salicylate 24 and 48 h after administration of indomethacin the tensile strength of the intestinal wall was restored to normal value, the protective effect was related to dose.

Key words: Indomethacin – Intestinal ulcer – Cytoprotective effect – Sodium salicylate

One component of indomethacin toxicity is manifested as intestinal ulceration. A single 10 mg/kg oral dose of indomethacin induced so-called non-fatal intestinal ulceration in Rg : Han : Wistar rats (Fig. 1). Tensile strength (T.S.) of the small intestine has been determined by the inflatation technique (Ezer and Szporny 1975) to quantitate ulcerogenesis. The model is suitable for the study of potential protective effects against foci of intestinal ulcers induced 24 and 48 h after treatment with indomethacin. Three possibilities are taken into account: (1) ulcerogenesis might not be influenced; (2) ulcerogenesis might be promoted; (3) ulcerogenesis might be inhibited by the test compounds.

The results indicated (Table 1) that T.S. of the small intestinal wall was restored by sodium salicylate, the protective effect was related to dose, while further treatment with indomethacin increased ulcerogenesis. A protective effect of sodium salicylate, given as a combined preparation (Pelsonin, a combination of indomethacin : sodium salicylate 1 : 10), was observed. Different pharmacological studies (Ezer et al. 1976; Corell 1981; Whittle et al. 1980; Robert 1981; West 1982) demonstrated unambiguously that sodium salicylate or salicylic acid had a gastrointestinal cytoprotective effect. The relationship between gastrointestinal damage and inhibition of generation of prostaglandins by non-steroidal antiinflammatory compounds is well known.

There is a temporal relationship between cyclooxygenase inhibition and formation of gastric ulcer, 3 h after administration of 10 mg/kg indomethacin s.c.

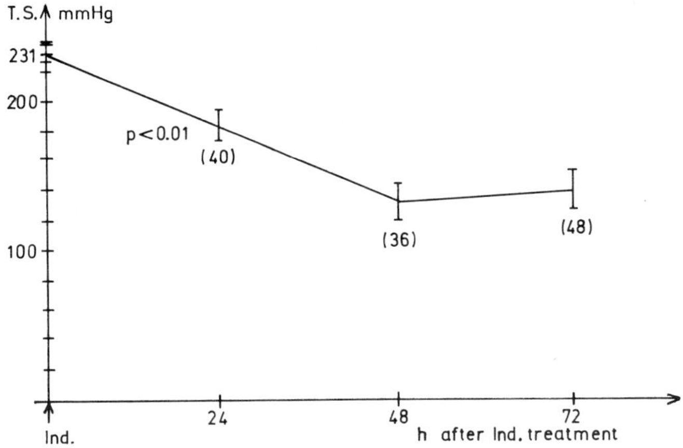

Fig. 1. Tensile strength *(T.S.)* of intestinal wall is gradually reduced due to intestinal ulceration induced by 10 mg/kg indomethacin p.o. (No. of animals in brackets)

Table 1. Modification of indomethacin induced intestinal ulcer by posttreatment with indomethacin, sodium salicylate and Pelsonin (group means ± SE)

Pretreatment p.o.	Posttreatment 24 and 48 h later p.o.	No. of animals	Tensile strength of small intestine, 24 h after last treatment (mm Hg)	Mortality (%)
None	None	30	231 ± 4	–
10 mg/kg indomethacin	Vehicle	31	140 ± 18[a]	0
	10 mg/kg indomethacin	10	20 ± 25	50
	25 mg/kg sodium salicylate	10	172 ± 25	0
	50 mg/kg sodium salicylate	10	109 ± 16[b]	0
	100 mg/kg sodium salicylate	10	223 ± 8[b]	0
	110 mg/kg Pelsonin	10	208 ± 12[b]	0

Pelsonin is a combined preparation of indomethacin : sodium salicylate 1 : 10
[a] = $p < 0.01$ compared with untreated group by Student's *t*-test
[b] = $p < 0.01$ compared with indomethacin-treated group by Student's *t*-test

(Whittle 1981). No such temporal relationship between cyclooxygenase inhibition and development of intestinal ulcers could be demonstrated. Development of intestinal ulcers can be inhibited by the simultaneous administration of several types of prostaglandins. Robert (1979) demonstrated that administration of prostaglandins 6 or 24 h after dosing with indomethacin had no protective effect against intestinal lesions. The results suggested that the later phase of the intestinal component of indomethacin toxicity was not dependent of prostaglandins.

References

Corell T (1981) Interaction of indomethacin and sodium-salicylate in rats as shown by gastro-ulcerogenicity and gastric prostacyclin release. Acta Pharmacol Toxicol (Suppl 1) 49 : 60–63

Ezer E, Szporny L (1975) A complementary method for the quantitative evaluation of rat stomach with shay-ulcer. J Pharm Pharmacol 27 : 867

Ezer E, Pálosi É, Hajós Gy, Szporny L (1976) Antagonism in gastrointestinal side effect experienced between sodium salicylate and some non-steroid anti-inflammatory agents. J Pharm Pharmacol 28 : 655–656

Robert A (1981) Gastric cytoprotection by sodium-salicylate. Prostaglandins [Suppl] 21 : 139–146

Robert A, Nezmais JE, Lancaster C, Hanchar AJ (1979) Cytoprotection by prostaglandins, Gastroenterology 77 : 433

West GB (1982) Testing for drugs inhibiting the formation of gastric ulcers. J Pharmacol Methods 8 : 33–37

Whittle BJR, Higgs GA, Eakins KE, Moncada S, Vane JR (1980) Selective inhibition of prostaglandin production in inflammatory exudates and gastric mucosa. Nature 284 : 271–273

Whittle BJR (1981) Temporal relationship between cyclooxygenase inhibition, as measured by prostacyclin biosynthesis, and the gastrointestinal damage induced by indomethacin in the rat. Gastroenterology 80 : 94–98

Disease, Metabolism and Reproduction in the Toxic Response to Drugs and Other Chemicals
Arch. Toxicol., Suppl. 7, 363–364 (1984)

The Preclinical Toxicity of Dazoxiben: A Specific Inhibitor of Thromboxane A_2 Synthetase

E. Irisarri, M. J. Kessedjian, C. Charuel, J. M. Faccini, P. Greaves, A. M. Monro, J. Nachbaur, and Y. Rabemampianina

Centre de Recherche-Pfizer, 37401 Amboise, France

Abstract. The recent discovery of highly selective inhibitors of thromboxane synthetase has opened exciting new therapeutic possibilities in cardiovascular disease, ranging from peripheral vascular disorders, angina and ischaemic heart disease to atherosclerosis. One such agent, dazoxiben (4-2-(1H-imidazol-l-yl)ethoxy benzoic acid) has been shown to be orally active in man. Clinical studies are currently in progress, the therapeutic dose being of the order of 2–3 mg/kg, three times per day (Tyler 1983).

The first animal toxicity studies with this compound are reported here. For reference, a long-lasting orally effective dose of dazoxiben in the dog is ca. 3 mg/kg. Beagle dogs and Sprague-Dawley rats which received dazoxiben orally for 6 months showed no evidence of toxicity at daily dose levels of 300 and 100 mg/kg respectively. Only in rats which received the highest dose level (400 mg/kg) were drug-related effects seen. Some changes in clinical chemistry and haematological parameters were seen and, in the females, some microscopically detected kidney changes. Reproductive studies in rats and rabbits revealed no adverse effects of dazoxiben on male or female fertility, embryogenesis, parturition or post-natal development up to the highest dose used, 400 mg/kg/day. The low toxicity found in these oral studies is not due to poor oral absorption of drug high and dose-related concentrations of drug were found in the plasma.

The generally favorable toxicological profile of dazoxiben, especially the absent or negligible effects on the g.i. tract, the kidney, coagulation and parturition (all prostaglandin sensitive organs or functions) augurs well for the safety of dazoxiben in clinical use.

Key words: Dazoxiben – Thromboxane – A_2 synthetase – Rats – Dogs – Preclinical toxicity

Acknowledgement. We wish to acknowledge the collaboration of Dr. M. Chvédoff who supervised the rabbit teratology study and Dr. C. Taradach who carried out all the ophthalmology.

Reference

Tyler HM (1983) Dazoxiben: A pharmacological tool or clinical candidate? Br J Clin Pharmacol 15: 13–16 and references cited therein

Disease, Metabolism and Reproduction in the Toxic Response to Drugs and Other Chemicals
Arch. Toxicol., Suppl. 7, 365–368 (1984)

Species Differences in the Acute Toxicity of Non-steroidal Anti-inflammatory Compounds

C. Pericin

Research Department, Pharma Division, Ciba-Geigy Limited, Basel, Switzerland

Abstract. The acute oral LD_{50} of 9 non-steroidal anti-inflammatory compounds were determined 24 hours and 14 days after administration in laboratory animals. The chinese hamsters exhibited greater median LD_{50s} than the other species.

Key words: Acute toxicity – LD_{50} – Species differences – Mice – Rats – Chinese hamsters – Syrian hamsters – Guinea pigs – Indomethacin – Piroxicam – Flufenamic acid – Pirprofen – Aspirin – Phenylbutazone – Oxyphenbutazone – Naproxen – Ibuprofen

Previous studies called attention to species differences in the acute toxicity of anti-inflammatory drugs (Wilhelmi 1974). Guinea pigs were markedly less susceptible to the lethal effects of indomethacin than rats (Mariani et al. 1978). This finding prompted the performance of additional studies concerning species differences between laboratory animals in relation to the acute toxicity of non-steroidal antiinflammatory compounds.

Indomethacin, piroxicam, flufenamic acid, pirprofen, aspirin, phenylbutazone, oxyphenbutazone, naproxen and ibuprofen were suspended in aqueous solutions of carboxymethylcellulose shortly before their use and administered between 7 and 10 a.m. as a single dose by oral intubation to animals which had been fasted overnight. Tif : MAGf (SPF) mice, Tif : RAIf (SPF) rats, Tif : chinese hamsters *(Cricetulus griseus)*, Tif: syrian hamsters *(Mesocricetus auratus)* and Tif : DHP guinea pigs were used. The LD_{50} values (with 95% confidence limits) were calculated on the basis of mortality after 24 h and 14 days after compound administration by the Probit Analysis Method (Goulden 1960).

Inter-species differences are considerable and no predictability of species susceptibility is evident (Figs. 1 and 2). In the majority of cases no autopsies were carried out on animals which died, due to advanced autolysis. A few autopsies which were performed revealed gastrointestinal lesions. The survivors

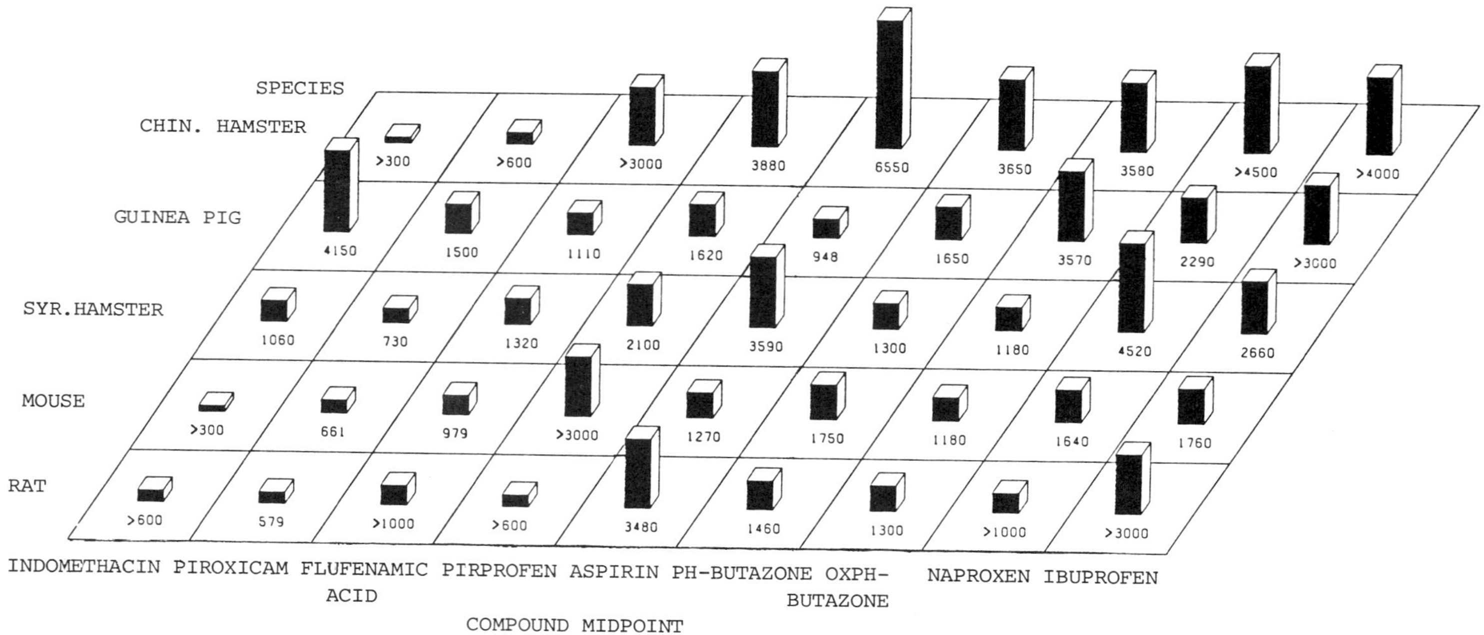

Fig. 1. 24 H LD_{50} (mg/kg) estimates for nine non-steroidal anti-inflammatory agents

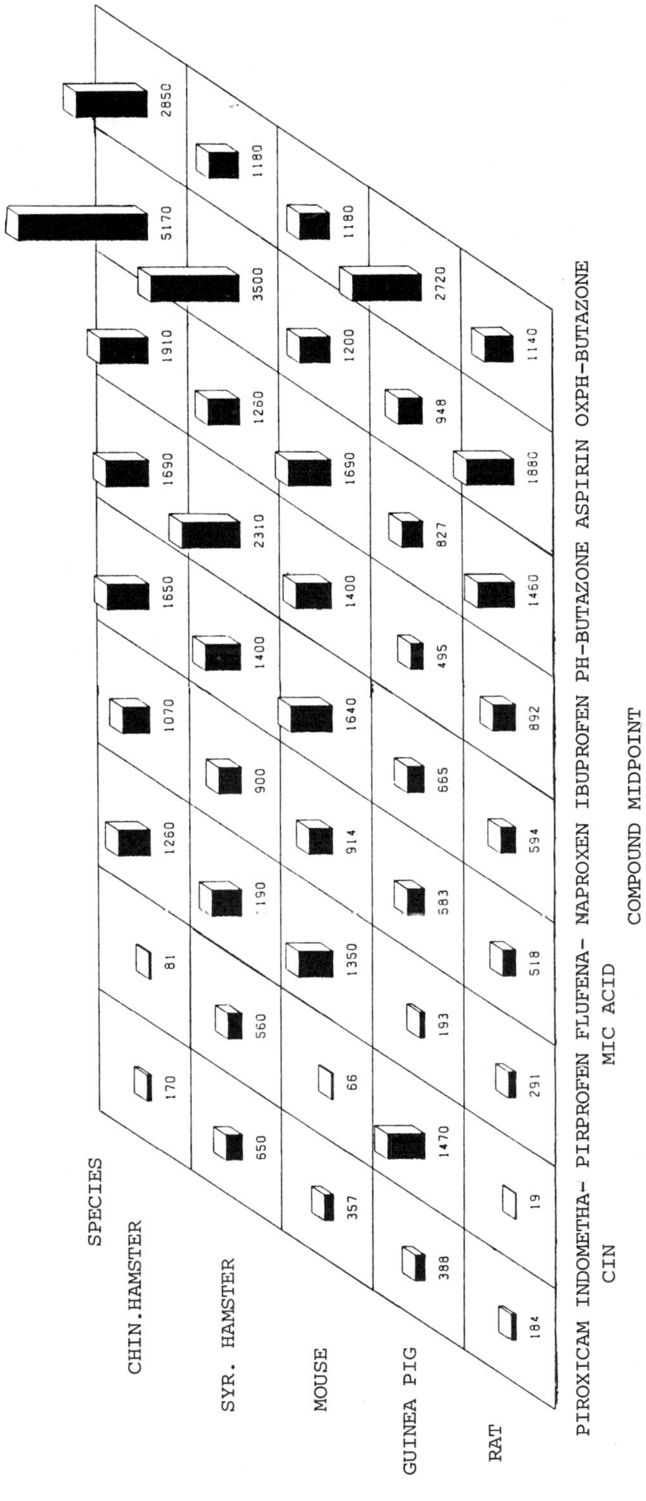

Fig. 2. 14 Day LD_{50} (mg/kg) estimates for nine non-steroidal anti-inflammatory agents

showed no pathological changes. The toxicological response of the chinese hamster might deserve further study.

Acknowledgement. I thank Mr. R. Gebus and Mr. G. Haby for skilful technical and Mr. A. P. Grieve for statistical assistance.

References

Goulden A (1960) Methods of statistical analysis. Wiley, New York London, p 404
Mariani L (1978) Resistance of the guinea pig to indomethacin ulcerogenesis. Toxicol Appl Pharmacol 45 : 637–639
Wilhelmi G (1974) Species differences in susceptibility to the gastro-ulcerogenic action of anti-inflammatory agents. Pharmacology 11 : 220–230

Heavy Metal Toxicity

Disease, Metabolism and Reproduction in the Toxic Response to Drugs and Other Chemicals
Arch. Toxicol., Suppl. 7, 371–373 (1984)

Renal Handling of Cadmium: A Study by Tubular Microinjections

E. Bosco, N. Porta, and J. Diezi

Institut de Pharmacologie de l'Université, Bugnon 21, 1011 Lausanne, Switzerland

Abstract. ^{109}Cadmium was microinjected, in different chemical forms, into the proximal or distal cortical tubules of adult rats and recovery in the pelvic urine from the ipsilateral kidney was measured. There was marked uptake of inorganic cadmium along the proximal tubules, and only negligible uptake in the distal nephron. The fractional uptake of the complex cadmium-cysteine in the proximal tubule was inversly related to the cysteine concentration. The chelate cadmium-pentetic acid was completely recovered in the pelvic urine.

Key words: Cadmium – Microinjection – Nephrotoxicity – Renal tubular transport – Pentetic acid (DTPA)

The kidney is one of the main target organs of cadmium (Cd) toxicity, particularly during chronic exposure. The renal lesions which have been reported included low molecular weight ("tubular") proteinuria (Piscator 1966), increased excretion of high molecular weight proteins (Lauwerys et al. 1974; Bernard et al. 1976) and various disorders of proximal tubule function in experimental conditions (Gonick et al. 1980). The mechanism of Cd uptake by tubular cells is poorly understood. It has been suggested (Friberg et al. 1974) that Cd reaches the kidney as Cd-metallothioneine complex, which would be taken up by tubular cells. Experiments indicate that the Cd-metallothioneine is ultrafilterable, and might be reabsorbed by specific processes (Foulkes 1978). However, direct investigation at the tubular level are lacking.

The tracer microinjection technique of Gottschalk et al. (1965) was used to characterize the pattern of Cd excretion after injection into defined nephron segments. The left kidney of anesthetized male Wistar rats was exposed, and samples (10 nl) containing ^{109}Cd (as $CdCl_2$, Cd-L-cysteine, Cd-DTPA) and ^{3}H-inulin were injected into the proximal or distal cortical tubules. The injection time was approximately 1 min. The pelvic urine was then collected serially (30–150 s samplings) from the left kidney over 10 min. The urine of the right

Table 1. ^{109}Cd recovery in pelvic urine after tubular microinjection

Microinjection site	*n*	[Cd] (mM)	[cys] (mM)	[DTPA] (mM)	Cd recovery (% ± SEM)
Prox. tubule	12	1	–	–	28.7 ± 4.6
Dist. tubule	6	1	–	–	91.9 ± 3.8
Prox. tubule	6	1	–	1	92.3 ± 2.8
Prox. tubule	6	0.8	0.8	–	17.7 ± 3.9
Dist. tubule	5	0.8	0.8	–	86.3 ± 2.9
Prox. tubule	11	1	5	–	46.4 ± 6.3
Prox. tubule	5	1	10	–	49.0 ± 10.8
Prox. tubule ($ZnCl_2$ infusion)	6	1	–	–	12.4 ± 4.2

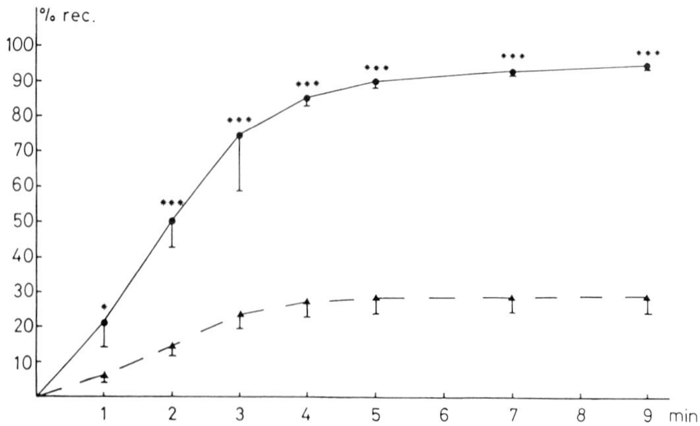

Fig. 1. Recovery of ^{3}H-inulin (●——●) and ^{109}Cd (▲ – – – ▲) in pelvic urine after microinjection in the proximal tubule (*n* = 12; mean ± SEM)

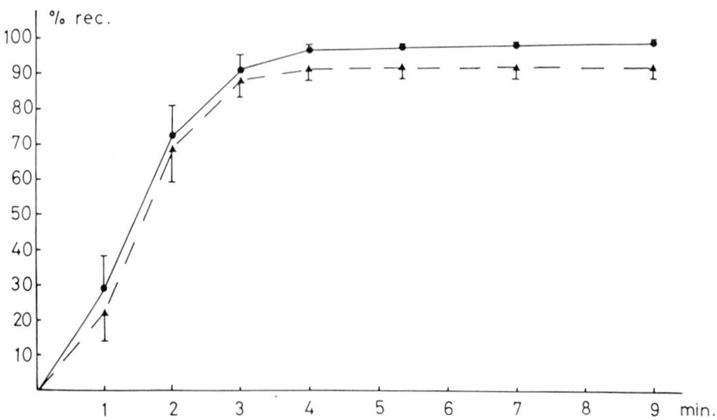

Fig. 2. Recovery of ^{3}H-inulin (●——●) and ^{109}Cd (▲ – – – ▲) in pelvic urine after microinjection in the distal tubule (*n* = 6; mean ± SEM)

kidney was also collected. The recovery of Cd and inulin is expressed as a fraction (%) of the amount microinjected (see Table 1; Figs. 1 and 2). The microinjections were considered as technically adequate if the recovery of inulin was equal to or greater than 95%. Uptake of inorganic Cd by the proximal tubules was approximately 70%. It might be explained by a reabsorptive transport, or by a binding to a brush border membrane protein, such as alkaline phosphatase, leucine-amino peptidase, carbonic anhydrase, or the formation of a reabsorbable complex with a constituant of the tubular urine.

The fractional uptake of the Cd-cysteine complex decreased when the molar ratio cys/Cd increased, possibly as a result of a saturation of the transport system of cysteine (Völkl and Silbernagl 1982). The chelate Cd-DTPA was quantitatively recovered in the pelvic urine after tubular microinjection. DTPA has been shown to be one of the most effective chelating agents allowing urinary excretion of Cd after acute exposure (Cantilena and Klaassen 1981, 1982). In another series of experiments, uptake of inorganic Cd was measured, by micro-injection technique, during an i.v. infusion of $ZnCl_2$ (4 μM/100 g × h in NaCl isotonic). Under these conditions, Cd recovery decreased to 12%. Interactions between these two ions have been described in the liver (Gunn et al. 1968). It was concluded from these experiments that luminal "uptake" of Cd in renal tubule is markedly influenced by the chemical form of the metal ion.

References

Bernard A, Roels H, Hubermont G, Buchet JP, Masson PL, Lauwerys R (1976) Characterisation of the proteinuria in Cd exposed workers. Int Arch Occup Environ Health 38: 19–30

Cantilena LR, Klaassen CD (1981) Comparison of the effectiveness of several chelators after single administration on the toxicity, excretion and distribution of Cd. Toxicol Appl Pharmacol 58: 452–460

Cantilena LR, Klaasen CD (1982) The effect of repeated administration of several chelators on the distribution and excretion of cadmium. Toxicol Appl Pharmacol 66: 361–367

Foulkes EC (1978) Renal tubular transport of Cd-metallotionein. Toxicol Appl Pharmacol 45: 505–512

Friberg L, Piscator M, Nordberg GF, Kjellström T (1974) Cadmium in the environment, 2nd edn. CRC Press, Cleveland

Gonick HC, Indraprasit S, Rosen VJ, Neustein H, Van de Velde R, Raghavan SRV (1980) Effect of cadmium on renal tubular function, the ATP-Na-K-ATPase transport system and renal tubular ultrastructure. Mineral Electrol Metab 3: 21–35

Gottschalk CW, Morel F, Mylle M (1965) Tracer microinjection studies of renal tubular permeability. Am J Physiol 209: 173–178

Gunn SA, Gould TC, Anderson WD (1968) Selectivity of organ response to cadmium injury and various protective measures. J Pathol 96: 89–96

Lauwerys R, Buchet JP, Roels H, Brouwers J, Stanescu D (1974) Epidemiological survey of workers exposed to cadmium: Effect on lung, kidney and several biological indices. Arch Environ Health 28: 145–148

Piscator M (1966) Proteinuria in chronic cadmium poisoning. Beckman's, Stockholm

Völkl H, Silbernägl S (1982) Mutual inhibition of L-cystine/L-cysteine and other neutral amino acids during tubular reabsorption. Pfluegers Arch 395: 190–195

Disease, Metabolism and Reproduction in the Toxic Response to Drugs and Other Chemicals
Arch. Toxicol., Suppl. 7, 374–377 (1984)

Cadmium Alters Arterial Baroreflex Control of Heart Rate in the Conscious Rat

D. Germanò[1], M. Pochiero[2], G. Romeo[1], A. Nunziata[3], G. Costa[2], and A. P. Caputi[2]

[1] Institute of Occupational Medicine, Faculty of Medicine, University of Messina, Viale Regina Elena, Villa Cappellani, 98100 Messina, Italy
[2] Institute of Pharmacology, Faculty of Medicine, University of Messina, Piazza XX Settembre, 4, 98100 Messina, Italy
[3] CRF, Via Tito Speri 14, 00040 Pomezia, Roma, Italy

Abstract. In conscious rats, a single oral dose of cadmium (Cd) chloride (up to 150 mg/kg) does not alter mean arterial pressure, heart rate and pressor response to phenylephrine 3, 7, and 14 days after loading. However, 150 mg/kg of Cd reduce reflex bradycardia and increase centrally mediated vagal decrease in heart rate. Therefore, it is suggested that Cd could modify baroreflex control of heart rate through an impairment of the afferent component of the reflex.

Key words: Cadmium – Arterial blood pressure – Heart rate – Baroreceptors – Rat

Since there is considerable controversy about the thesis that controlled cadmium (Cd) exposure can produce chronic hypertension in rat (Kotsonis and Klaessen 1977; Watkins 1980) the effect of a single oral administration of Cd chloride on arterial baroreflex control of heart rate was examined.

Methods

Female Sprague-Dawley rats, 165–195 g, were used throughout. Purina rat chow and water were supplied ad libitum. Under chloral hydrate anaesthesia, a permanent cannula was inserted into the left lateral cerebral ventricle (Caputi et al. 1980), at least one week before the animals received a single oral dose of 50 (n = 16) and 150 (n = 30) mg/kg of Cd chloride. Thirty rats given saline (2 mg/kg) orally were used as controls. Experiments were carried out 3, 7, and 14 days after dosing. One day before the experiments, the animals were anaesthetized with ether and catheters (PE 50) were chronically implanted into the left common carotid artery and into the right jugular vein, as previously described (Caputi et al. 1980). At the time of the experiment, the conscious rat was housed in a plexiglass chamber and mean arterial pressure (MAP), in mm

Hg, and heart rate (HR), as beats per minute, were measured continously, using a Statham pressure transducer and a Gemini polygraph with cardiotachometer. A pressor dose (2 μg/kg) of phenylephrine (Sigma) was injected intravenously (i.v.) in order to test peripheral vascular reactivity and reflex bradycardia. The rapid or vagal component of reflex bradycardia was calculated as the ratio of maximum decrease in HR (ΔHR) to maximum increase in MAP (ΔMAP), according to Coleman (1980). Pressor effect and ΔHR/ΔMAP were calculated in each animal as the average responses to triplicate injections of phenylephrine. In order to produce a centrally mediated increase in MAP and decrease in HR (Buccafusco and Brezenoff 1979) carbachol (Sigma) (250 ng) was given intracerebroventricularly (i.c.v.).

All drugs were diluted in 0.9% saline. All data are expressed as mean values ± SE. Statistical comparison of groups used the two-tailed Student *t*-test with significance reported at $p < 0.05$.

Results

The rats given 150 mg/kg Cd showed a decrease in body weight during the first 3 days (from 173.3 ± 10.7 to 143.7 ± 6.0 g); thereafter they had the same growth rate as the controls. They weighed significantly less than control rats from day 3 through to day 14. Rats receiving 50 mg/kg of Cd did not exhibit significant modifications in resting MAP and HR, or in the phenylephrine induced pressor response and ΔHR/ΔMAP. Basal MAP, HR and pressor response to phenylephrine also remained unchanged in the 150 mg treated animals, when compared with control (Table 1). ΔHR/ΔMAP showed, on the contrary, significant reduction 3 and 7 days after dosing by 40.4 and 52.3%, respectively, and returned towards the values observed in the controls within 14 days (Fig. 1).

Table 1. Effect of oral administration of cadmium (150 mg/kg) or saline (controls: 2 ml/kg) on mean arterial pressure (MAP), heart rate (HR), and phenylephrine induced pressor response (ΔMAP) and reflex bradycardia (ΔHR)

Parameter	Days after oral treatment		
	3	7	14
Controls	(*n* = 9)	(*n* = 10)	(*n* = 6)
MAP	105.0 ± 10.3	102.0 ± 7.9	108.0 ± 7.5
HR	457.0 ± 68.3	428.0 ± 45.3	466.0 ± 20.9
ΔMAP	20.1 ± 6.3	31.4 ± 10.2	18.6 ± 8.0
ΔHR	128.2 ± 43.4	185.8 ± 69.6	121.6 ± 33.4
Cadmium	(*n* = 9)	(*n* = 11)	(*n* = 8)
MAP	108.0 ± 13.0	100.0 ± 3.5	111.0 ± 8.2
HR	478.0 ± 34.5	435.0 ± 53.0	455.0 ± 49.6
ΔMAP	26.9 ± 8.4	24.3 ± 5.2	20.2 ± 9.4
ΔHR	102.2 ± 37.4	68.5* ± 15.6	155.3 ± 73.6

* $p < 0.05$ versus controls

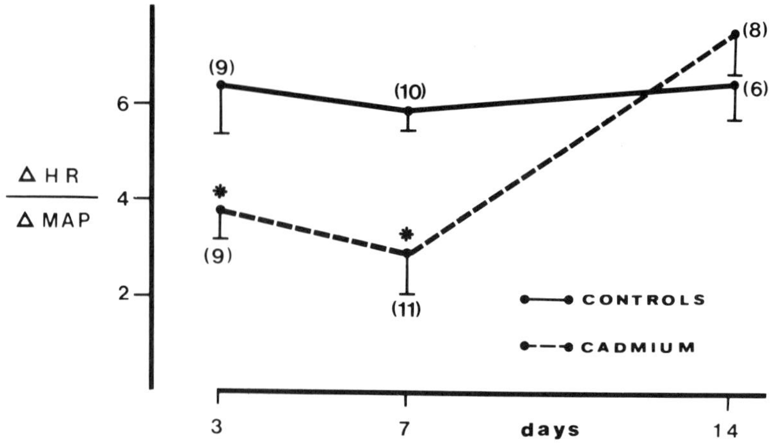

Fig. 1. Ratio of maximum decrease in heart rate (*ΔHR*) to maximum increase in MAP (*ΔMAP*) 3, 7, and 14 days after single oral cadmium (150 mg/kg) or saline (2 mg/kg) administration. Each point is the mean ± SE of the number of rats reported between parentheses. $^{*}p < 0.05$ versus the values obtained in saline treated rats

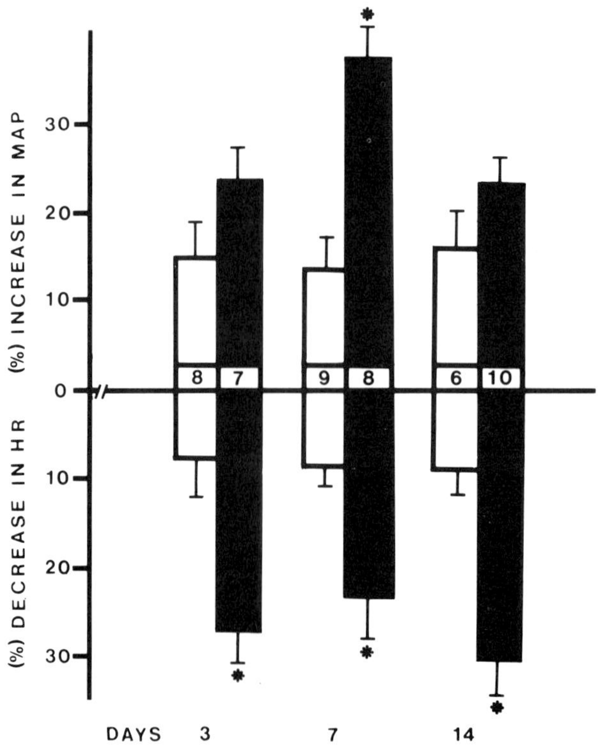

Fig. 2. Effects of intracerebroventricular injection of carbachol (250 ng/5 μl) on mean arterial pressure *(MAP)* and heart rate *(HR)* in cadmium *(closed bars)* or saline *(open bars)* treated animals. The value are reported as percentage increase in MAP or decrease in HR. Each column represents the mean ± SE of the number of rats reported into the column. $^{*}p < 0.05$ compared to the responses obtained in saline treated rats

The bradycardia induced by icv carbachol (250 ng) showed a significant increase 3, 7, and 14 days after cadmium ingestion (Fig. 2). The carbachol pressor response was also increased, but only 7 days after treatment (Fig. 2).

Discussion

A single oral dose of 150 mg/kg of Cd alters the arterial baroreflex control of heart rate, without changing basal MAP and HR.

Since the carbachol centrally mediated increase in MAP and decrease in HR (Buccafusco and Brezenoff 1979) are potentiated by Cd, a reduction of vagal and sympathetic activities, as a cause of the modification of the reflex, can be ruled out. Thus, it is tempting to speculate that arterial baroreflex control of heart rate is altered through an impairment of the afferent component of the reflex. Further experiments are obviously needed to investigate how central cholinergic control of arterial blood pressure and heart rate is modified.

References

Buccafusco JJ, Brezenoff HE (1979) Pharmacological study of a cholinergic mechanism within the rat posterior hypothalamic nucleus which mediates a hypertensive response. Brain Res 165: 295–310

Caputi AP, Rossi F, Carney K, Brezenoff HE (1980) Modulatory effect of brain acetylcholine on reflex-induced bradycardia and tachycardia in conscious rats. J Pharmacol Exp Ther 215: 309–316

Coleman TG (1980) Arterial baroreflex control of heart rate in the conscious rat. Am J Physiol 238: 515–520

Kotsonis FN, Klaessen CD (1977) Toxicity and distribution of cadmium administered to rats at sublethal doses. Toxicol Appl Pharmacol 41: 667–680

Watkins BE (1980) Effects of cadmium injections on arterial pressure regulation in the rat. Clin Exp Hypertens 2: 153–162

Disease, Metabolism and Reproduction in the Toxic Response to Drugs and Other Chemicals
Arch. Toxicol., Suppl. 7, 378–381 (1984)

Inhibition of Aortic Vessel Adenosine Diphosphate Degradation by Cadmium and Mercury

G. Togna[1], N. Dolci[1], and L. Caprino[2]

[1] Institute of Hygiene, [2] Institute of Pharmacology, Catholic University, Largo Francesco Vito 1, Rome, Italy

Abstract. The effects of cadmium and mercury on ADP breakdown by vessel walls were investigated. These metals reduce the ADP clearance promoted by arterial tissue. This effect could be attributed to the inhibition of vessel wall ADP-ase enzyme, which plays an important role in the genesis of thrombotic phenomena.

Key words: Mercury – Cadmium – Blood vessel – ADP degradation

Thrombosis of glomerular capillaries (Berry 1972), selective damage to vascular endothelium (Schlaepfer 1971), induction and progression of atherosclerosis and hypertension (Revis et al. 1981; Porter et al. 1975; Perry and Erlanger 1974; Shaper 1979), have been ascribed by many authors to several heavy metals. The non-thrombogenic properties of vascular endothelium are partially due to the production of prostacyclin by vessel wall and to the degradation of circulating adenonucleotides by adenosine diphosphatase (ADPase), a membrane-bound enzyme (Lieberman et al. 1977; Cooper et al. 1979). In previous studies it has been shown that cadmium chloride ($CdCl_2$), in vitro (Caprino and Togna 1979; Caprino et al. 1979) and in vivo (Caprino et al. 1982a), and mercuric chloride ($HgCl_2$), in vitro (Caprino et al. 1983) affect the vessel wall prostacyclin production and platelet responsiveness to the aggregating agents. In the present paper the in vitro activity of cadmium and mercury on the ADP breakdown induced by vascular tissue has been studied.

Methods

The ADP degradation by vascular tissue was evaluated by a biological assay previously described by Caprino et al. (1982b). Male Sprague Dawley rats were treated orally with aspirin (150 mg/kg) in order to inhibit the aortic prostacyclin production that could interfere with the biological assay. Two hours after the aspirin treatment the rats were sacrificed, the abdominal aorta was removed and cut into rings. About 10 mg wet weight of the tissue was incubated for 5 min at room temperature in saline (100 μl) or in saline containing cadmium (0.1; 0.5, and 1 μg/mg wet aortic tissue) or mercury (0.5, 1.25, and 2.5 μg/mg). Then platelet-poor plasma (PPP, 200 μl) and ADP (30 μg) were added to the mixture. Six, nine, and 15 min later, 50 μl of the incubation fluid were withdrawn, added to 1 ml of rabbit platelet-rich plasma (PRP) placed in the Born aggregometer and the platelet aggregation was recorded. The aggregation curves obtained were compared to the aggregating response induced by 5 μg of ADP. Additional control tests were performed evaluating the aggregating activity of a mixture consisting of saline (100 μl), ADP (30 μg), PPP (200 μl), devoid of aortic rings, both in the presence and in the absence of Cd or Hg.

Results and Discussion

The aggregating activity of the incubation liquid containing ADP and untreated aortic rings, decreases with the increase of the incubation time.

The rate of ADP disappearance induced by arterial tissue pretreated with cadmium or mercury remained unchanged after 6 min while it was significantly reduced after 9 and 15 min of incubation (Figs. 1 and 2). The aggregating activity

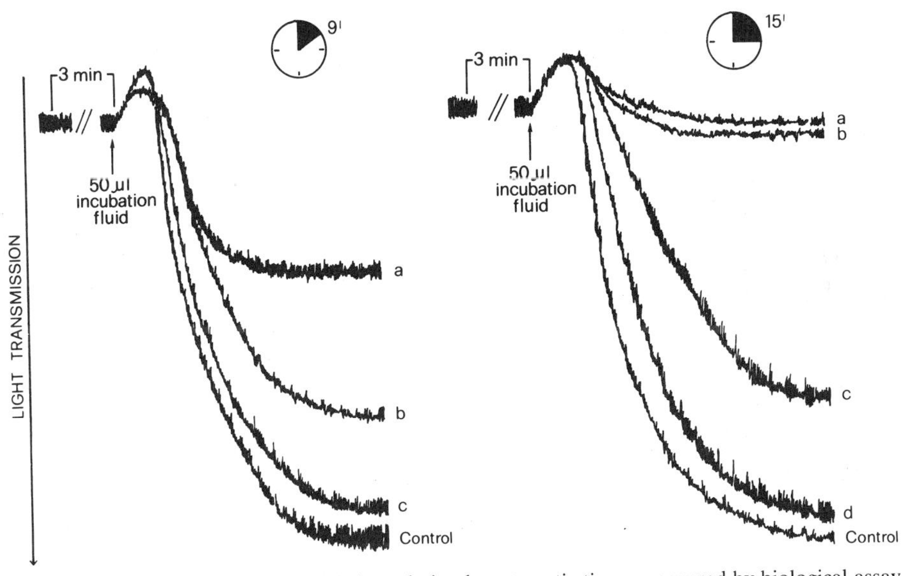

Fig. 1. Effects of $CdCl_2$ on the ADP degradation by rat aortic tissue measured by biological assay. The superimposed tracings were obtained by adding 50 μl supernatant of the incubation fluid, containing aortic rings, to rabbit PRP. The incubation fluid consisted of: saline (100 μl), PPP (200 μl), ADP (30 μg), and contained 10 mg of aortic rings previously pretreated with saline or the metal. Two different incubation times were assayed: 9 and 15 min. *(a)* Saline, *(b)* $CdCl_2$, 0.1 μg, *(c)* $CdCl_2$, 0.5 μg, *(d)* $CdCl_2$, 1 μg/mg wet aortic tissue. Control indicates platelet aggregation induced by 5 μg of ADP

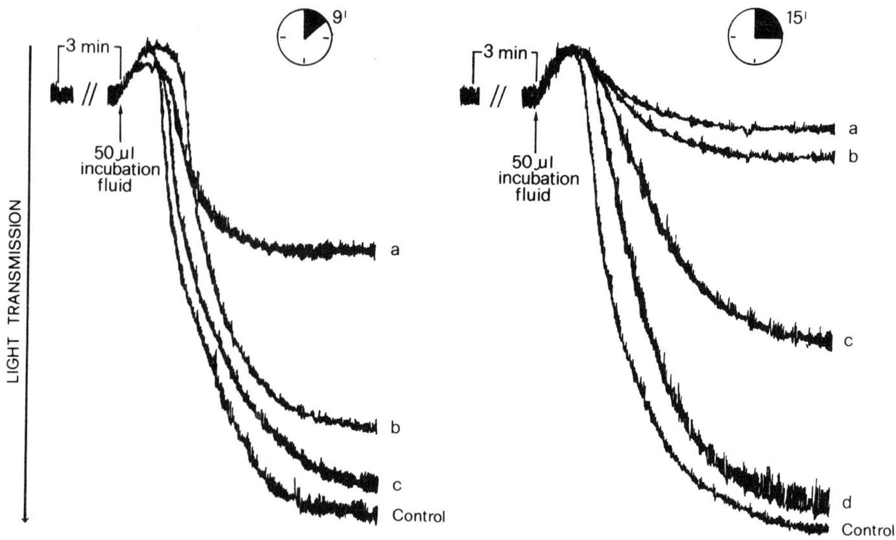

Fig. 2. Effects of $HgCl_2$ on the ADP degradation by rat aortic tissue measured by biological assay. Two different incubation times were assayed: 9 and 15 min. For details see Fig. 1. *(a)* Saline, *(b)* $HgCl_2$, 0.5 µg, *(c)* $HgCl_2$, 1.25 µg, *(d)* $HgCl_2$, 2.5 µg/mg wet aortic tissue. Control indicates platelet aggregation induced by 5 µg of ADP

of the incubation fluids, devoid of aortic rings, withdrawn at the three different times, was comparable with that induced by 5 µg/ml of ADP. The decreased rate of ADP disappearance observed in these experiments could be attributed to a vessel ADP-ase inhibition induced by Cd and Hg, which are known to affect several other enzymatic activities (Robinson et al. 1965; Vallee and Ulmer 1972; Singhal and Merali 1979).

The endothelium vessel ADP-ase plays an important role; it contributes to the non-thrombogenic properties of endothelium by degrading the circulating ADP (Lieberman et al. 1977) to products such as adenosine, which is an inhibitor of platelet aggregation and a modulator of local blood flow.

In conclusion, these data, in conjunction with the results previously obtained on the prostacyclin release by vessel walls (Caprino and Togna 1979; Caprino et al. 1982a; Caprino et al. 1983), provide useful information on the toxicological activity of Cd and Hg on vascular tissue; they could, at least partially, also clarify the mechanism of the genesis of vascular diseases, already ascribed to these metals.

Acknowledgment. This research was supported by a grant (83.02784.56) from the CNR.

References

Berry JP (1972) Les lésions rénales provoqueés par le cadmium. Etude au microscope électronique et au micro-analyseur a sonde électronique. Pathol Biol (Paris) 20: 401–412

Caprino L, Togna G (1979) Inhibition of prostacyclin-like material formation by cadmium. Toxicol Appl Pharmacol 48: 529–531

Caprino L, Togna G, Togna AR (1979) Cadmium-induced platelet hypersensitivity to aggregating agents. Pharmacol Res Commun 11: 731–737

Caprino L, Dolci N, Togna G, Villa P, Bucci R, Carunchio V (1982a) Effects of cadmium on platelet thromboxane and vascular prostacyclin production. Toxicol Appl Pharmacol 65: 185–188

Caprino L, Antonetti F, Borrelli F, Morelli L (1982b) In vitro activity of urokinase on platelet function and on ADP degradation by vascular tissue. Thromb Res 27: 447–456

Caprino L, Togna AR, Cebo B, Dolci N, Togna G (1983) In vitro effects of mercury on platelet aggregation and thromboxane and vascular prostacyclin production. Arch Toxicol Suppl 6: 48–51

Cooper DR, Lewis GP, Lieberman GE, Webb H, Westwich J (1979) ADP metabolism in vascular tissue. A possible-regulatory mechanism. Thromb Res 14: 901–914

Lieberman GE, Lewis GP, Peters TJ (1977) A membrane bound enzyme in rabbit aorta capable of inhibiting ADP-induced platelet aggregation. Lancet 2: 330–332

Perry HM Jr, Erlanger MW (1974) Metal-induced hypertension following chronic feeding of low doses of cadmium and mercury. J Lab Clin Med 83: 541–547

Porter MC, Miya TS, Bousquet WF (1975) Cadmium and vascular reactivity in the rat. Toxicol Appl Pharmacol 34: 143–150

Revis NW, Zinsmeister AR, Bull R (1981) Atherosclerosis and hypertension induction by lead and cadmium ions. Proc Natl Acad Sci USA 78: 6494–6498

Robinson CW, Kress SC, Wagner RH, Brinkhous KM (1965) Platelet agglutination and deagglutination with a sulphydryl inhibitor, methyl mercuric nitrate: Relationships to platelet ATPase. Exp Mol Pathol 4: 457–464

Schlaepfer WW (1971) Sequential study of endothelial changes in acute cadmium intoxication. Lab Invest 25: 556–564

Shaper AG (1979) Cardiovascular disease and trace metals. Proc R Soc Lond [Biol] 205: 135–143

Singhal RL, Merali Z (1979) Biochemical toxicity of cadmium. In: Mennear JH (ed) Cadmium toxicity. Dekker, New York, pp 61–112

Vallee BL, Ulmer DD (1972) Biochemical effects of mercury, cadmium and lead. Ann Rev Biochem 41: 91–128

Disease, Metabolism and Reproduction in the Toxic Response to Drugs and Other Chemicals
Arch. Toxicol., Suppl. 7, 382 (1984)

Embryotoxic Action Induced by Mercury Acetate in the Rat

A. Cerrati, P. A. Franco, G. Garrone, C. Puntrello, I. Raggi, and F. Viola

Chair of Toxicology, University of Milan, Milan, Italy

Abstract. In research into the toxic effect of mercury the teratogenicity of mercury acetate was investigated. In these experiments Sprague-Dawley female rats were used aged 90–100 days, average weight 242 ± 5 g. For coupling, male rats of the same strain and age were used, their average weight was 350 ± 3 g.

On the 10th day of pregnancy mercury acetate was administered intravenous to the treated group at a dosage of 3 mg/kg body weight, in distilled water (5 ml/kg). The control group was given only the vehicle. On the 17th day of pregnancy, the fetuses were surgically removed, weighed and examined. The average length, tail excluded, was 16 mm; that of the control group was 20.6 nm. The average body weight of the excised fetus was 512 mg and in the controls 785 mg. The results obtained in the mercury acetate-treated group showed delayed growth and hyposomatism in 100% of the rats. In 19%, a decrease in toe growth of the left hind paw was also found, although this change was not found in the controls.

Subcutaneous oedema was observed in 60% of the treated rats. Mercury probably alters the normal activity of mitochondria and the lysosomes. Mercury products seem also to cause chromosomes breakdown and to inhibit mitosis.

Key words: Embryotoxicity – Teratogenicity – Mercury

Disease, Metabolism and Reproduction in the Toxic Response to Drugs and Other Chemicals
Arch. Toxicol., Suppl. 7, 383–388 (1984)

Cardiovascular Homeostasis in Rats Chronically Exposed to Mercuric Chloride

M. Carmignani[1] and P. Boscolo[2]

[1] Institute of Pharmacology, and [2] Institute of Occupational Medicine, Faculty of Medicine and Surgery, Catholic University of the Sacred Heart, Via della Pineta Sacchetti 644, 00168 Rome, Italy

Abstract. Two groups of male Sprague-Dawley rats received from weaning 50 μg/ml of mercury as mercuric chloride ($HgCl_2$) in drinking water for 320 and 350 days. Hg exposure increased cardiac inotropism, without chronotropic changes, in both groups, and induced arterial hypertension in the rats exposed for 350 days. In the exposed rats, cardiovascular responses to the stimulation of peripheral alpha and beta adrenoceptors were decreased and increased, respectively, possibly through a reduced intracellular availability of calcium ions for contractile mechanisms. Hg exposure did not affect either vagal or sympathetic activity or cardiovascular reactivity to several physiological agonists. On the other hand, Hg exposure induced baroreflex hyposensitivity and produced a drastic alteration of the levels of copper and zinc in brain and kidney.

Key words: Mercury – Cardiovascular function – Blood pressure – Adrenoceptors – Vagotomy – Sympathetic nerves – Baroreflex pathways – Calcium – Copper – Zinc

Introduction and Experimental

Mercury (Hg) ions have been reported to increase the output of adrenal catecholamines (CA), to stimulate ganglionic neurotransmission, to induce contraction of aortic strips, to increase or decrease the arterial resistance, to induce hypertension without changes of cardiac output and to oppose the cardiovascular responses to norepinephrine (NE) and other pressor and depressor agonists (Perry and Erlanger 1974; Oka et al. 1979). There are also

---

Abbreviations: Mercury, Hg; catecholamines, CA; norepinephrine, NE; epinephrine, E; mercuric chloride, $HgCl_2$; maximum rate of rise of the left ventricular pressure, dP/dt_{max}; heart rate, HR; electrocardiogram, ECG; bilateral carotid occlusion, BCO; isoprenaline, ISO; blood pressure, BP; intravenous, i.v.; intraperitoneal, i.p.

sporadic clinical observations that $HgCl_2$ may increase both sympathetic activity and vascular response to epinephrine (E) in humans (Cheek et al. 1959). Two studies on rabbits exposed to Hg vapors showed some modifications in either chronotropism or the electrocardiogram (ECG), an altered response to vasopressin (Trachtenberg 1969) and early lesions in renal and extrarenal vessels (Zimmerman et al. 1977). In order to evaluate further the effects of chronic Hg exposure on cardiovascular function, some neurogenic and humoral mechanisms regulating cardiovascular function were investigated. Two groups of ten male Sprague-Dawley rats received 50 μg/ml of Hg (as $HgCl_2$) in deionized drinking water for 320 days (first group) and 350 days (second group). Two equal groups of rats received only deionized water for the same periods. The systolic and diastolic aortic blood pressure (BP) and the maximum rate of rise of the left ventricular pressure (dP/dt_{max}) were obtained by catheterization of the left carotid artery and by using a Biotronex BL 620 derivative computer. The heart rate (HR) and ECG were also monitored. Basal cardiovascular parameters were determined in both groups of rats under thiopental anaesthesia (40 mg/kg, i.p.). The cardiovascular responses to bilateral carotid occlusion (BCO), to i.v. administration of several physiological agonists, to vagotomy, carried out at the neck below the nodose ganglion, and to ganglionic blockade, under vagotomy, were evaluated. The levels of Hg in the kidney and of copper, zinc and iron in the brain and kidney of the rats of the first group were determined by flameless or flame atomic absorption spectrophotometry. The cardiovascular responses of the animals of the second group were assessed with i.v. NE (1 μg/kg) and isoprenaline (ISO; 0.50 μg/kg) during i.v. infusion with verapamil (1 μg/kg/min) or papaverine (1.5 mg/kg/min) in order to establish if the altered responses to CA, found in the first group, were dependent on a decrease of the intracellular availability of calcium ions for the contractile mechanisms.

Results

First Group

The basal BP levels, HR, and ECG pattern of the exposed rats were unchanged. On the other hand, these animals showed significantly higher values of dP/dt_{max}, demonstrating an increase of myocardial contractility. The rise of BP and dP/dt_{max}, observed during BCO, was greatly reduced in the exposed rats, while the slight reflex tachycardia was similar to that of the control rats. The cardiovascular responses to vagotomy and to graduated doses of i.v. hexamethonium were unchanged (Table 1). The pressor and inotropic responses to NE were significantly reduced in the exposed rats, without any chronotropic changes. Hg exposure was able to reverse and to potentiate, respectively, the systolic hypertensive and the diastolic hypotensive responses to a low dose (0.125 μg/kg) of E, with reduction of the inotropic response and no change in the chronotropic response. Pressor and inotropic responses to higher doses of E were significantly decreased by Hg exposure (Table 1). However, no difference was found in the cardiovascular responses to acetylcholine (1.25 μg/kg),

Table 1. Maximal cardiovascular changes[a] following bilateral carotid occlusion, vagotomy, hexamethonium (under vagotomy), norepinephrine, and epinephrine in control and mercury-exposed rats[b]

		Changes in							
		Systolic BP[c] (mm Hg)		Diastolic BP[c] (mm Hg)		Heart rate (beats/min)		dP/dt_{max}[d] (mm Hg/s)	
		Control	Exposed	Control	Exposed	Control	Exposed	Control	Exposed
Bilateral carotid occlusion		+37 ± 5	+19 ± 4*	+29 ± 4	+13 ± 2*	+13 ± 2	+15 ± 4	+3,011 ± 411	+1,850 ± 340*
Vagotomy		+ 8 ± 1	+12 ± 2	+ 6 ± 2	+12 ± 4	+ 8 ± 1	+12 ± 2	+ 854 ± 226	+1,298 ± 184
Hexamethonium (mg/kg, i.v.)	0.625	−23 ± 4	−29 ± 3	−22 ± 4	−27 ± 1	−15 ± 3	−19 ± 2	−2,067 ± 406	−2,293 ± 363
	1.25	−31 ± 3	−34 ± 3	−28 ± 3	−33 ± 3	−27 ± 7	−24 ± 4	−2,506 ± 585	−2,459 ± 326
	2.50	−44 ± 2	−50 ± 4	−34 ± 2	−42 ± 3	−48 ± 9	−49 ± 8	−4,040 ± 812	−3,304 ± 590
Norepinephrine (μg/kg, i.v.)	1	+44 ± 3	+26 ± 2*	+31 ± 2	+17 ± 1*	+14 ± 4	+12 ± 2	+4,314 ± 415	+3,097 ± 269*
Epinephrine (μg/kg. i.v.)	0.125	+10 ± 2	−17 ± 2*	−10 ± 0.5	−16 ± 1*	+ 9 ± 1	+11 ± 2	+1,562 ± 165	+ 562 ± 76*
	1	+28 ± 4	+17 ± 2*	+21 ± 2	+11 ± 2*	+12 ± 2	+12 ± 1	+3,186 ± 293	+1,264 ± 133*
	2	+49 ± 2	+36 ± 3*	+39 ± 3	+28 ± 3*	+14 ± 2	+17 ± 3	+3,568 ± 330	+1,624 ± 197*
Base line		124 ± 7	138 ± 7	97 ± 7	110 ± 5	333 ± 9	339 ± 14	5,527 ± 521	7,316 ± 428*

[a] Each value represents the mean ± SE (n = 10 in both groups)
[b] The exposed rats received 50 μg/ml of mercury (as $HgCl_2$) in deionized drinking water for 320 days
[c] BP, aortic blood pressure
[d] dP/dt_{max}, maximum rate of rise of the left ventricular pressure
* Indicates significant differences from the control (ANCVA, $p < 0.05$)

Table 2. Maximal changes[a] in aortic blood pressure induced by norepinephrine and isoprenaline in control ar mercury-exposed rats[b] before and during verapamil and papaverine i.v. infusion

Infusion	Agonist (μg/kg, i.v.)		Changes in aortic BP[c]			
			Systolic (mm Hg)		Diastolic (mm Hg)	
			Control	Exposed	Control	Exposed
None	Norepinephrine	1	+41 ± 3	+30 ± 3*	+30 ± 4	+22 ± 1*
	Isoprenaline	0.50	−19 ± 1	−30 ± 2*	−27 ± 2	−47 ± 3*
Verapamil (1 μg/kg/min)	Norepinephrine	1	+36 ± 3	+23 ± 3*	+27 ± 1	+19 ± 2*
	Isoprenaline	0.50	−16 ± 2	−32 ± 4*	−21 ± 3	−37 ± 4*
Papaverine (1.5 mg/kg/min)	Norepinephrine	1	+17 ± 4	+19 ± 4	+20 ± 1	+20 ± 4
	Isoprenaline	0.50	−10 ± 3	−19 ± 2*	−14 ± 1	−25 ± 3*
Base line			120 ± 6	162 ± 7	99 ± 4	131 ± 7

[a] Each value represents the mean ± SE (n = 10 in both groups)
[b] The exposed rats received 50 μg/ml of mercury (as $HgCl_2$) in deionized drinking water for 350 days
[c] BP, blood pressure
* Indicates significant differences from the control (ANOVA, $p < 0.05$)

Table 3. Copper, zinc, and iron levels[a] in kidney and brain of control and mercury-exposed rats[b]

	Kidney[c] (μg/g)			Brain[c] (μg/g)		
	Cu	Zn	Fe	Cu	Zn	Fe
Control	25.7 ± 2.4	81.0 ± 4.1	373.8 ± 27.4	11.8 ± 0.5	48.2 ± 1.7	133.2 ± 5.9
Mercury-exposed	162.9 ± 11.3*	168.4 ± 5.7*	412.5 ± 66.7	17.5 ± 0.8*	78.6 ± 6.5*	145.0 ± 4.3

[a] Each value represents the mean ± SE (n = 10 in both groups)
[b] The exposed rats received 50 μg/ml of mercury (as $HgCl_2$) in deionized drinking water for 320 days
[c] Values expressed on dry weight bases
* Indicates significant differences from the control (ANOVA, $p < 0.001$)

angiotensin I (0.50 μg/kg), angiotensin II (0.50 μg/kg), bradykinin (0.75 μg/kg), histamine (5 μg/kg) or serotonin (5 μg/kg). The kidney was the organ with the highest accumulation of Hg (371.7 ± 31.5 μg/g; mean ± SE; control: 1.6 ± 0.4 μg/g; values expressed as dry weight). Hg exposure caused an increase respectively of 48 and 63% in brain copper and zinc. These metals were also drastically increased in the kidney to levels of about 630% for copper and 210% for zinc, while the iron content of these organs was not significantly affected by Hg exposure (Table 3).

Second Group

Cardiac inotropism was significantly increased also in this group, without changes in HR or the ECG pattern. However, systolic and diastolic BP was higher than in the controls (Table 2). In these rats, systolic and diastolic BP responses to NE were reduced and to ISO were increased. The exposed rats showed, during verapamil infusion, pressor response to NE lower than those of controls. In the exposed rats, the depressor responses to ISO were greater, during infusion with either verapamil or papaverine, than those observed in the control rats (Table 2).

Discussion

Chronic exposure to inorganic Hg induces an increase of cardiac inotropism and may induce hypertension, without changes in HR. These effects cannot be explained either by an increased myocardial or vascular responsiveness to endogenous CA or by an effect of Hg on vagal or sympathetic activities. Hg was found to increase in vitro the output of NE from peripheral adrenergic neurons, without altering the nerve activity (Nakazato et al. 1979). If a similar mechanism occurs also in vivo, the increased cardiac inotropism and hypertension would be explained. Hg induces baroreflex hyposensitivity, possibly acting on the baro-afferent pathways and the central intermediary structures regulating cardiovascular responses to baroreflex stimulation or both. In this respect, polymercury sulfide complexes were found in the cervical part of the spinal cord and of the pontine region of rats chronically exposed to $HgCl_2$ (Danscher and Schrøder 1979). On the other hand, the reduced cardiovascular responses to BCO may depend also on the Hg-induced decrease of both vascular and cardiac responsiveness to the alpha adrenergic stimulation, since there was cardiovascular hyporeactivity to NE and higher doses of E. Hg seems to affect specifically the cardiovascular reactivity to CA. These results show that Hg decreases cardiovascular responsiveness to alpha adrenergic stimulation and potentiates vascular effects induced by stimulation of peripheral beta adrenoceptors. These actions of Hg may be explained by a reduced influx and intracellular availability of calcium ions for contractile mechanisms or both when the responses obtained in the second group of rats to NE and ISO during infusion with verapamil and papaverine are considered. The Hg-induced altered concentrations of copper and zinc may be related to the observed cardiovascular changes. This increase in essential metals may be explained by an augmented synthesis of metallothionein, a protein which may protect against the toxic effects of Hg (Cherian and Goyer 1978; Tandon et al. 1980). Increased brain copper following Hg exposure has not been previously reported. It remains to be established if the cardiovascular effects observed in the chronically exposed rats can be extrapolated to humans.

Acknowledgements. This study was supported by grants of the Commission of the European Communities (n. 71192) and of the Ministero Publica Istruzione (40%) 1981.

References

Cheek DB, Bondy RK, Johnson LR (1959) The effect of mercurous chloride (calomel) and epinephrine (sympathetic stimulation) on rats. The importance of the findings to mechanisms in infantile acrodynia. Pediatrics 23 : 302

Cherian MG, Goyer RA (1978) Metallothioneins and their role in the metabolism and toxicity of metals. Life Sci 23: 1–10

Danscher G, Schrøder HD (1979) Histochemical demonstration of mercury induced changes in rat neurons. Histochemistry 60: 1–7

Nakazato Y, Asano T, Ohga A (1979) The in vitro effect of mercury compounds on noradrenaline output from guinea-pig vas deferens. Toxicol Appl Pharmacol 48: 171–177

Oka M, Horrobin DF, Manku MS, Cunnane SC, Ally AI, Morgan RO (1979) Effect of mercuric chloride on the rat mesenteric vascular bed: relevance to the mechanism of mercury toxicity. Toxicol Appl Pharmacol 51: 427–438

Perry HM Jr, Erlanger MW (1974) Metal-induced hypertension following chronic feeding of low doses of cadmium and mercury. J Lab Clin Med 83: 541–547

Tandon SK, Magos L, Cabral JRP (1980) Protection against mercuric chloride by nephrotoxic agents which do not induce thionein. Toxicol Appl Pharmacol 52: 227–236

Trachtenberg IM (1969) The chronic action of mercury on the organism, current aspects of the problem of micromercurialism and its prophylaxis. Zdorov'ja, Kiev (Russian with German translation).

Zimmerman HD, Schmidt E, Weller E, Becker C, Dieker P (1977) Intra- and extrarenal vascular changes in the acute renal failure of the cat caused by mercuric chloride. Virchows Arch [Pathol Anat] 372: 259–285

Disease, Metabolism and Reproduction in the Toxic Response to Drugs and Other Chemicals
Arch. Toxicol., Suppl. 7, 389–390 (1984)

The Effects of a Dose of Mercuric Chloride, Below the Acute Toxic Dose, on Haemostasis in Rats

H.-P. Klöcking

Institute of Pharmacology and Toxicology, Medical Academy Erfurt,
Nordhäuser Strasse 74, 5010 Erfurt, German Democratic Republic

Abstract. Mercuric chloride ($HgCl_2$) intoxication in man may be associated with disturbances of haemostasis such as disseminated intravascular coagulation (DIC). The influence of subchronic effects of $HgCl_2$ on haemostasis in rats has been studied. The animals received a single dose of 20 mg $HgCl_2$/kg body weight intraperitoneally. After 2, 5, 24, 48, and 72 h of administration of $HgCl_2$ blood was taken for estimation of platelet counts, fibrinogen, fibrin monomer, antithrombin III, fibrinogen degreadation products, and plasminogen. Plasminogen activator activity was measured in the blood and kidney. The fibrinogen level rose from 2.5 g/l at 2 h to 6.3 g/l at 24 h. It returned to normal at 72 h. Fibrin monomer was observed at 24, 48, and 72 h after application of $HgCl_2$. Platelet counts and antithrombin III activity remained unchanged throughout the experiment. There was a progressive fall in plasminogen with minimum values occurring 72 h after $HgCl_2$ administration. After 2 h a 60% increase in plasminogen activator activity in blood was reached. It continued to fall to normal values after 72 h. Compared with the base-line data, plasminogen activator activity in the kidney was found to be significantly increased to 80–120% within 5–72 h after $HgCl_2$ application. Fibrin degradation products occurred to a very small extent only 72 h after the beginning of the experiment. These results show that during experimental $HgCl_2$ intoxication in rats, DIC did not develop. The alterations of plasminogen activator activity in blood and kidney may be explained as inhibition of transtubular secretion.

Key words: Mercuric chloride – Haemostasis – Disseminated intravascular coagulation

References

Hartert H (1948) Blutgerinnungen. Studien mit der Thrombelastographie, einem neuen Untersuchungsverfahren. Klin Wochenschr 26: 577–583

Kluft C, Brakman P (1975) Effect of flufenamate on euglobulin fibrinolysis: Involvement of C_1-inactivator. In: Davidson JF, Samama M, Desnoyers PC (eds) Progress in chemical fibrinolysis and thrombolysis, vol 1. Raven, New York, pp 375–381

Laurell CB (1966) Quantitative estimation of proteins by electrophoresis in agarose gel containing antibodies. Anal Biochem 15: 45–52

Mihara H, Fugii T, Okamoto S (1969) Fibrinolytic activity of cerebro-spinal fluid and the development of artificial cerebral haematomas in dogs. Thrombos Diathes Haemorrh 21: 294–303

Mussoni L, Raczka E, Chmielewska J, Donati MB, Latallo ZS (1979) Plasminogen assay in rabbit, rat and mouse plasma using the chromogenic substrate S-2251. Thromb Res 15: 341–349

Ødegård OR (1975) Evaluation of an amidolytic heparin cofactor assay method. Thromb Res 7: 351–360

Schönborn H, Prellwitz W, Schuster HP, Baum P, Poeplau W, Bordersen C (1970) Verbrauchskoagulopathien bei exogenen Vergiftungen. Dtsch Med Wochenschr 95: 2478–2481

Disease, Metabolism and Reproduction in the Toxic Response to Drugs and Other Chemicals
Arch. Toxicol., Suppl. 7, 391–393 (1984)

In Vitro Cytotoxicity of Nickel Chloride on a Human Pulmonary Epithelial Cell Line (A 549)

A. Dubreuil[1], G. Bouley[1], S. Duret[2], J.-C. Mestre[2], and C. Boudene[1]

U.122 INSERM, [1] Laboratoire de Toxicologie and [2] Laboratoire de Biologie Cellulaire, Centre Pharmaceutique de l'Université Paris-Sud, rue J.-B. Clément, 92290 Châtenay-Malabry, France

Abstract. The results of an in vitro study of the dose-effect response with nickel chloride on human epithelial cell line A 549 are reported. $NiCl_2$ in amounts ranging from 0 to 10^{-3} M, produced a decrease in cell growth rate, a diminished content of cell ATP, and a loss of viability at the highest concentration. No characteristic ultrastructural changes were seen on TEM preparations.

Key words: Cytotoxicity – Nickel – Lung – Cell line

Studies on the possible responsibility of nickel in some human respiratory diseases have given contradictory results (Sunderman 1976; Cox et al. 1981). Hence, this study on the cytotoxicity mechanisms of nickel, using $NiCl_2$ soluble salt.

The A 549 cell line (ATCC CCL 185) is of human lung origin, and probably derived from type II epithelial alveolar cells (Lieber et al. 1976) because it contains multilamellar inclusion bodies. The cells were cultured in 25 cm^2 Petri dishes, in Dulbecco's modified Eagle medium with 10% foetal calf serum and in monolayer conditions; each dish was seeded with 350,000 cells and $NiCl_2$ was added to the culture medium in concentrations ranging from 0 (controls) to 10^{-3} M. Cell growth rate was determined during the exponential phase of culture at 37° C in a CO_2 incubator (Dubreuil et al. 1979). For each point, cells of three Petri dishes were trypsinised and counted, using a Coulter counter (Coultronics).

At 48 h of culture, the adenosine triphosphate (ATP) content in control and exposed cells was measured (Jakubczak and Leclerc 1980). ATP was extracted with dimethylsulfoxide. ATPase was inhibited by ethylenediaminetetraacetic acid. Luciferine-luciferase reagent was added and bioluminescence measured using a LKB apparatus.

The cell viability was tested by the trypan-blue exclusion test (Phillips 1973). Preparations for transmission electron microscopy (TEM) were fixed with 2.5%

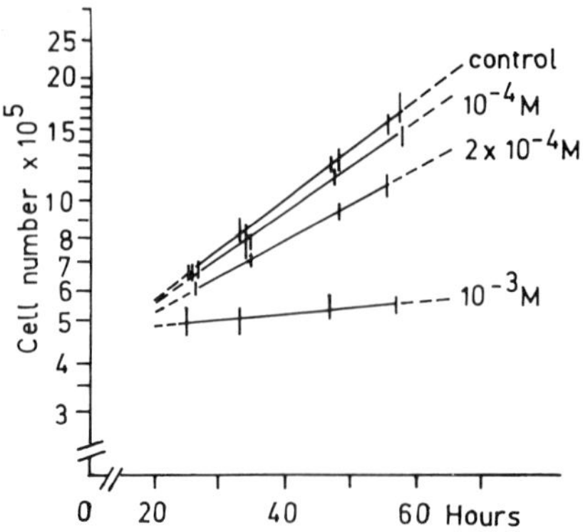

Fig. 1. Effect of $NiCl_2$ on the cell growth

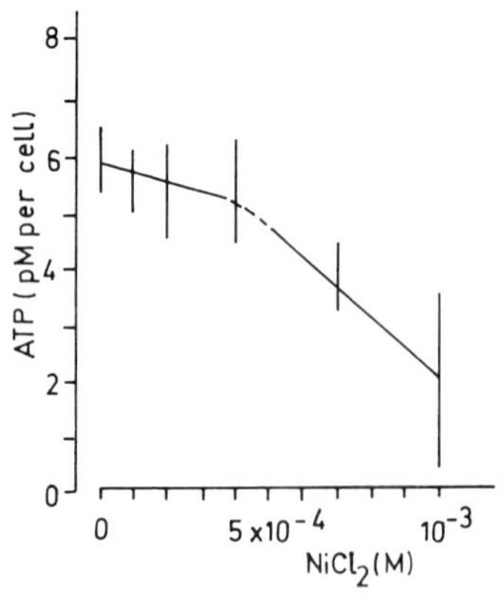

Fig. 2. Cell ATP content as a function of $NiCl_2$ amounts

glutaraldehyde in 0.1 M cacodylate buffer pH 7.2, post fixed with 2% OsO_4 in the same buffer, and embedded in Epon (Hayat 1981); TEM was performed in a Philips 301 apparatus.

The most sensitive method was found to be the study of cell growth rate, (Fig. 1) which indicated a 50% inhibiting dose (ID_{50}) of 3.5×10^{-4} M and a significant difference from the controls beginning at 2.0×10^{-4} M. The ATP concentration measurements were not so sensitive (Fig. 2); the ID_{50} was 8.0×10^{-4} M. The trypan-blue exclusion test, showed a significant difference with controls only at the highest dose of $NiCl_2$ used in these experiments (1.0×10^{-3} M). Finally, no characteristic ultrastructural changes were observed by TEM, even at 1.0×10^{-3} M and after 48 h.

Acknowledgement. This study was supported by a grant from INSERM and Ministère de l'Environnement (n° 996 122).

References

Cox JE, Doll R, Scott WA, Smith S (1981) Mortality of nickel workers: Experience of men working with metallic nickel. Br J Ind Med 38: 235–239

Dubreuil A, Hollande E, Bouley G, Boudene CL (1979) Effects of lead microparticles on the growth characteristics of the BHK^{21} fibroblast cell line. Toxicology 13 : 249–262

Hayat MA (1981) Fixation for electron microscopy. Academic Press, New York, pp 66–129

Jakubczak E, Leclerc H (1980) Mesure de l'ATP bactérien par bioluminescence: Étude critique des méthodes d'extraction. Ann Biol Clin 38 : 297–304

Lieber M, Smith B, Szakal B, Nelson-Rees W, Todaro G (1976) A continuous tumor-cell line from a human lung carcinoma with properties of type II alveolar epithelial cells. Int J Cancer 17 : 62–70

Phillips HJ (1973) Dye exclusion test for cell viability. In: Kruse PF, Patterson MK (eds) Tissue culture: Methods and applications. Academic Press, New York

Sunderman FW (1976) A review of the carcinogenicities of nickel, chromium and arsenic compounds in men and animals. Prev Med 5 : 279–294

Disease, Metabolism and Reproduction in the Toxic Response to Drugs and Other Chemicals
Arch. Toxicol., Suppl. 7, 394–397 (1984)

Changes in Endogenous Monoamine Levels of Rat Brain Induced by Tetraethyl Lead

H. Komulainen, R. Pietarinen, and J. Tuomisto

Department of Pharmacology and Toxicology, University of Kuopio, P.O.B. 6, 7021 Kuopio 21, Finland

Abstract. Tetraethyl lead (TEL) was given to adult rats at single doses of 30, 90, or 180 μmol/kg in soya bean oil by gavage. 24 h later the concentrations of three monoamines were measured in the hypothalamus, occipital cortex and corpus striatum. Cortical noradrenaline (NA) decreased by 17–31% with increasing TEL dose and hypothalamic NA by 32% at the highest TEL dose. After administration of the cumulative total doses of 3, 10, or 30 μmol/kg TEL over 3 weeks, the corpus striatum was most severely affected: levels of NA and dopamine (DA) decreased by 12–22% while that of 5-HT increased by 11% at the highest TEL dose. The changes of 5-HT levels were opposite to those of catecholamines in other brain regions as well suggesting a reciprocal interaction between serotonergic and catecholaminergic neurones.

Key words: Tetraethyl lead – Neurotoxicity – Dopamine – Serotonin – Noradrenaline – Rat

Organolead compounds are considered much more toxic than inorganic lead (Pb) and the brain is the organ most sensitive to the toxic effects (Grandjean and Nielsen 1979). In agreement with this, tetraethyl lead (TEL) increased net dopamine (DA) uptake into rat striatal synaptosomes ex vivo at one tenth the dose Pb (Komulainen et al. 1983). The toxic component of TEL in vivo is assumed to be triethyl lead (TriEL) (Grandjean and Nielsen 1979). Interestingly, TriEL appears to be somewhat selective in its toxicity affecting neurones rather than glia in brain tissue culture (Grundt et al. 1981). In ex vivo uptake studies, opposite effects of TEL on serotonergic and catecholaminergic neurones (Komulainen et al. 1983) were found. Hence, it is of interest to correlate monoamine uptake data to steady state levels of endogenous monoamines after a similar TEL schedule.

Abbreviations: TEL, tetraethyl lead; TriEL, triethyl lead; DA, dopamine; NA, noradrenaline; 5-HT, 5-hydroxytryptamine

Table 1. Concentrations of monoamines in rat striatum, occipital cortex, and hypothalamus 24 h after a single oral dose of tetraethyl lead. Figures are mean ± SEM (μg/g)

Monoamine	Tissue	Control	Tetraethyl lead (μmol/kg)		
			30	90	180
Noradrenaline	Cortex	0.29 ± 0.02 (6)[a]	0.28 ± 0.00 (5)	0.24 ± 0.01 (5)* −17%	0.20 ± 0.02 (6)** −31%
	Striatum	0.53 ± 0.02 (6)	0.53 ± 0.02 (6)	0.52 ± 0.02 (6)	0.56 ± 0.03 (6)
	Hypothalamus	1.29 ± 0.06 (6)	1.60 ± 0.08 (6)* +24%	1.24 ± 0.12 (6)	0.88 ± 0.08 (5)* −32%
Dopamine	Cortex	0.71 ± 0.06 (5)	0.84 ± 0.11 (6)	0.84 ± 0.12 (6)	0.84 ± 0.09 (6)
	Striatum	6.62 ± 0.19 (6)	6.85 ± 0.27 (5)	6.49 ± 0.14 (6)	6.57 ± 0.33 (6)
	Hypothalamus	1.27 ± 0.16 (6)	1.12 ± 0.10 (6)	1.25 ± 0.10 (6)	1.27 ± 0.09 (6)
5-Hydroxytryptamine	Cortex	0.85 ± 0.06 (6)	0.75 ± 0.03 (6)	0.75 ± 0.02 (6)	0.84 ± 0.02 (6)
	Striatum	1.19 ± 0.12 (6)	1.27 ± 0.10 (6)	1.14 ± 0.02 (6)	1.24 ± 0.05 (6)
	Hypothalamus	1.41 ± 0.11 (6)	1.41 ± 0.01 (6)	1.38 ± 0.10 (5)	1.36 ± 0.04 (5)

[a] Number of animals in each group are in parentheses; * $p < 0.05$; ** $p < 0.01$

Table 2. Regional concentrations of monoamines in rat brain after repeated administration of tetraethyl lead over 3 weeks. Values are expressed as μg/g (mean ± SEM)

Monoamine	Tissue	Control	Tetraethyl lead (μmol/kg, a cumulative dose)		
			3	10	30
Noradrenaline	Cortex	0.35 ± 0.02 (6)[a]	0.38 ± 0.02 (6)	0.32 ± 0.01 (6)	0.33 ± 0.02 (6)
	Striatum	0.58 ± 0.02 (6)	0.51 ± 0.02 (6)* −12%	0.45 ± 0.01 (5)** −22%	0.50 ± 0.01 (6)* −14%
	Hypothalamus	1.46 ± 0.02 (6)	1.46 ± 0.09 (6)	1.54 ± 0.09 (6)	1.42 ± 0.08 (6)
Dopamine	Cortex	0.75 ± 0.02 (6)	1.09 ± 0.14 (5)* +45%	0.77 ± 0.11 (6)	0.99 ± 0.10 (6)
	Striatum	6.76 ± 0.27 (6)	5.85 ± 0.14 (5)* −14%	5.66 ± 0.12 (5)** −16%	6.33 ± 0.20 (6)
	Hypothalamus	1.38 ± 0.12 (6)	1.63 ± 0.03 (6)	1.88 ± 0.14 (6)* +36%	1.50 ± 0.12 (6)
5-Hydroxytryptamine	Cortex	0.79 ± 0.02 (6)	0.68 ± 0.04 (5)* −14%	0.86 ± 0.05 (6)	0.87 ± 0.04 (6)
	Striatum	1.20 ± 0.02 (6)	1.19 ± 0.03 (5)	1.25 ± 0.06 (6)	1.33 ± 0.02 (6)** +11%
	Hypothalamus	1.54 ± 0.06 (6)	1.29 ± 0.04 (6)** −16%	1.35 ± 0.06 (6)* −12%	1.48 ± 0.02 (6)

[a] Number of animals are given in parentheses; * $p < 0.05$; ** $p < 0.01$

Materials and Methods

Adult male Wistar rats (Wis/Af/Han/Mol/Kuo strain) were housed in the animal room in the Animal Centre of the University of Kuopio in the following conditions: room temperature 20 ± 0.5° C, relative humidity 55–75%, and light cycle of 14 h light/10 h darkness. They were given TEL (TEL-CB, The Associated Octel Company Limited, England) by gavage in soya bean oil (1 ml/100 g) as a single dose of 30, 90, or 180 μmol/kg (10, 30, 60 mg/kg). 24 h later (9.00–11.00 a.m.) the rats were decapitated and the hypothalamus, corpus striatum and occipital cortex were dissected. The tissue pieces were quickly weighed and deep frozen (−70° C) for monoamine determination which was performed within a few days. In other experiments rats (60–90 g, 4 weeks old) were given TEL by gavage every other day (10 doses) over 3 weeks and decapitated 24 h after the last dose. The cumulative total doses of TEL were 3, 10, or 30 μmol/kg. Monoamines were assayed with spectrofluorometric methods: Noradrenaline and 5-HT according to Miller et al. (1970) and dopamine as described by MacDonald et al. (1975).

Results

After a single oral dose of TEL only NA levels changed significantly. There was a dose dependent decrease of NA in the occipital cortex while in the hypothalamus there was an increase with 30 μmol but a decrease with 180 μmol (Table 1).

After repeated administration of TEL, much lower doses than those given acutely induced slight changes in amine levels (Table 2). The corpus striatum was most severely affected. NA and DA concentrations decreased at low doses but 5-HT increased at the highest dose of TEL administered. By contrast, in the hypothalamus 5-HT decreased whereas DA tended to increase. In the occipital cortex the changes in amine levels were not dose dependent.

Discussion

Although the TEL-induced changes in monoamine levels were small and in the main not dose related, some interesting trends can be observed. After a single dose of TEL, the cortex appears to be particularly vulnerable. NA levels decreased at the doses at which TEL first increased NA uptake in cortical synaptosomes ex vivo (Komulainen et al. 1983). The vulnerability of cortex has also been detected histopathologically (Niklowitz 1974). The hypothalamus also appears to be affected after an acute administration of TEL. Changes in NA coincide with a decrease in 5-HT uptake by hypothalamic synaptosomes ex vivo (Komulainen et al. 1983).

After an extended TEL treatment the change in 5-HT concentration was usually opposite to those in catecholamines. The direction of this imbalance, however, varied between brain regions. In the striatum 5-HT concentration increased but in the hypothalamus and cortex it tended to be decreased. Hence, serotonergic and catecholaminergic neurons appear to be mutually interrelated during TEL administration. Similar observations have been made with neurotoxic agents such as chlordecone (Fujimori et al. 1982) and acrylamide (Ali et al. 1983).

Monoamine levels appear to be changed at lower doses of TEL than does monoamine uptake. This suggests that steps other than uptake are critical in the TEL-induced effects on monoaminergic neurotransmission.

Acknowledgements. The study was supported by the Research Council for Medical Sciences, Academy of Finland.

References

Ali SF, Hong JS, Wilson WE, Uphause LL, Bondy SC (1983) Effect of acrylamide on neurotransmitter metabolism and neuropeptide levels in several brain regions and upon circulating hormones. Arch Toxicol 52: 35–43

Fujimori K, Nabeshima T, Ho IK, Mehendale HM (1982) Effects of oral administration of chlordecone and mirex on brain biogenic amines in mice. Neurotoxicology (Park Forest Il) 3: 143–148

Grandjean P, Nielsen T (1979) Organolead compounds: Environmental health aspects. Residue Rev 72: 98–148

Grundt IK, Ammitzboll T, Clausen J (1981) Triethyl lead treatment of cultured brain cells. Effect on accumulation of radioactive precursors in galactolipids. Neurochem Res 6: 193–201

Komulainen H, Pietarinen R, Tuomisto J (1982) Increase in dopamine uptake in rat brain striatal synaptosomes after an acute in vivo administration of organic and inorganic lead. Acta Pharmacol Toxicol 52: 381–389

MacDonald E, Marselos M, Nousiainen U (1975) Central and peripheral catecholamine levels after pyrazole treatment. Acta Pharmacol Toxicol 37: 106–112

Miller FP, Cox RH, Snodgrass WR, Maickel RP (1970) Comparative effects of p-chlorophenylalanine, p-chloroamphetamine and p-chloro-N-methylamphetamine on rat brain norepinephrine, serotonin and 5-hydroxy-3-indole acetic acid. Biochem Pharmacol 19: 435–442

Niklowitz WJ (1974) Ultrastructural effects of acute tetraethyllead poisoning on nerve cells of the rabbit brain. Environ Res 8: 17–36

Disease, Metabolism and Reproduction in the Toxic Response to Drugs and Other Chemicals
Arch. Toxicol., Suppl. 7, 398–400 (1984)

Levels of Monoamines in Different Regions of the Rat Brain in Heavy Metal Intoxication

V. Anania[1], M. S. Desole[1], G. Esposito[1], F. Sanna Randaccio[2], and E. Miele[1]

[1] Institute of Pharmacology, University of Sassari, via Rolando 1, 07100 Sassari, Italy
[2] Chair of Occupational Health, University of Sassari, via Padre Manzella, 07100 Sassari, Italy

Abstract. In zinc intoxication, monoamines (5-HT, DA and NA) and 5-HIAA significantly increased in the rat hypothalamus; in cadmium intoxication, NA decreased in the hippocampus and amygdala; DA decreased in the hippocampus, however, 5-HIAA rose in the hypothalamus; in lead intoxication DA decreased in the hippocampus and amygdala. In the above brain regions, the levels of heavy metals did not differ from those of untreated rats.

Key words: Heavy metals – Brain monoamines – Brain heavy metal levels – Plasma corticosterone – Adrenal catecholamines

Chronic exposure to heavy metals induces behavioural changes both in humans and animals (Wender 1971). Attention has been focused on the changes in central monoaminergic functions which may cause behavioural disorders (Winder 1982). Levels of monoamines in the whole brain as well as in different brain regions have been investigated after chronic exposure to heavy metals but many of these studies do not report brain metal levels (for references, see Winder 1982). Heavy metals can affect uptake or release of monoamines (Komulainen and Tuomisto 1980) and dopaminergic and GABergic systems (Govoni et al. 1980). Levels of 5-hydroxytryptamine (5-HT), 5-hydroxyindoleacetic acid (5-HIAA), noradrenaline (NA) and dopamine (DA) were estimated (Welch and Welch 1969) in different regions [hippocampus (Hip), striatum (St), hypothalamus (Hyp) and amygdala (Amy)] of the rat brain, after daily treatment with 5 mg/kg orally for 15 consecutive days with zinc sulfate, cadmium sulfate or lead acetate. Plasma corticosterone (Givner and Rochefort 1965) and adrenal catecholamines (Anton and Sayre 1962) were also estimated. Male adult Wistar rats were used. The levels of brain monoamines and the 5-HIAA levels are reported in Table 1 and the plasma corticosterone levels in Table 2. Major changes were seen after zinc treatment; 5-HT, 5-HIAA, NA and DA levels rose significantly in the Hyp. After cadmium, NA decreased in the Hip and Amy; DA decreased in the Hip. 5-HIAA, however, rose in the Hyp. With lead, DA alone decreased in the Hip and Amy. In all the treated groups plasma

Table 1. Effects of heavy metal administration on the 5-HT, 5-HIAA, DA and NA levels (µg/g) in various brain regions of the rat. The heavy metals (5 mg/10 ml H_2O/kg) were administered daily by gastric intubation for 15 consecutive days. The controls received an equal volume of H_2O

	Controls	Pb-acetate	Cd-sulfate	Zn-sulfate
		5-HT		
Hippocampus	0.431 ± 0.049	0.378 ± 0.031 (−12.3%)	0.369 ± 0.032 (−14.4%)	0.456 ± 0.053 (+ 5.8%)
Striatum	0.468 ± 0.037	0.530 ± 0.041 (+13.2%)	0.543 ± 0.036 (+16.0%)	0.562 ± 0.033 (+20.1%)
Hypothalamus	0.577 ± 0.069	0.706 ± 0.031 (+22.3%)	0.729 ± 0.061 (+26.3%)	0.945* ± 0.039 (+63.8%)
Amygdala	0.702 ± 0.065	0.736 ± 0.058 (+4.8%)	0.663 ± 0.075 (−5.6%)	0.773 ± 0.068 (+10.1%)
		5-HIAA		
Hippocampus	0.300 ± 0.016	0.259 ± 0.012 (−13.8%)	0.268 ± 0.046 (−10.8%)	0.292 ± 0.034 (− 2.8%)
Striatum	0.430 ± 0.033	0.487 ± 0.028 (+13.2%)	0.450 ± 0.026 (+ 4.6%)	0.448 ± 0.052 (+ 4.2%)
Hypothalamus	0.427 ± 0.025	0.435 ± 0.019 (+ 1.9%)	0.680* ± 0.041 (+59.2%)	0.658* ± 0.144 (+54.1%)
Amygdala	0.374 ± 0.023	0.269 ± 0.065 (−28.1%)	0.278 ± 0.046 (−25.7%)	0.344 ± 0.041 (− 8.1%)
		DA		
Hippocampus	0.394 ± 0.002	0.273* ± 0.039 (−30.8%)	0.348* ± 0.009 (−11.7%)	0.409 ± 0.013 (+ 3.8%)
Striatum	6.534 ± 0.538	5.912 ± 0.443 (− 9.6%)	7.100 ± 1.336 (+ 8.6%)	7.162 ± 1.960 (+ 9.6%)
Hypothalamus	0.795 ± 0.030	0.755 ± 0.037 (− 5.1%)	0.986 ± 0.131 (+24.0%)	1.159** ± 0.057 (+45.8%)
Amygdala	0.856 ± 0.043	0.589* ± 0.043 (−31.2%)	0.694 ± 0.164 (−19.0%)	0.869 ± 0.112 (+ 1.5%)
		NA		
Hippocampus	0.315 ± 0.032	0.274 ± 0.017 (−13.1%)	0.236* ± 0.013 (−25.1%)	0.271 ± 0.028 (−14.0%)
Striatum	1.150 ± 0.055	1.007 ± 0.172 (−12.5%)	0.998 ± 0.164 (−13.3%)	1.056 ± 0.225 (− 8.2%)
Hypothalamus	0.884 ± 0.091	0.801 ± 0.053 (− 9.4%)	1.063 ± 0.071 (+20.2%)	1.155* ± 0.049 (+30.6%)
Amygdala	0.419 ± 0.019	0.385 ± 0.0078 (−8.2%)	0.336* ± 0.028 (−19.9%)	0.408 ± 0.049 (− 2.7%)

Values are expressed as mean ± SE. Five animals were used for each group.
In parentheses are given as percentages taking the values of controls as 100%
$^{*}P < 0.05$; $^{**}P < 0.001$ if compared to control values

Table 2. Effects of heavy metal administration on the plasma corticosterone levels (μg/100 ml) of the rat. The heavy metals (5 mg/10 ml H_2O/kg) were administered daily by gastric intubation for 15 consecutive days. Controls received an equal volume of H_2O

Controls	Pb-acetate	Cd-acetate	Zn-sulfate
18.40 ± 2.106	54.25* ± 2.322 (+ 194.83%)	44.37* ± 2.110 (+ 141.14%)	57.25* ± 4.732 (+ 211.14%)

Values are expressed as mean ± SE. Five animals were used for each group
In parentheses are given as percentages taking the values of controls as 100%
* $P < 0.001$ if compared to control values

corticosterone (Table 2) significantly increased as compared with the controls. Adrenal NA content was also affected, while adrenaline remained unchanged. In Zn-treated rats NA was significantly reduced by 45%. In brain regions reported above the levels of Zn, Cd and Pb did not differ from the controls.

Acknowledgment. This work was supported by Ministero Publica Istruzione, quota 60% (1982).

References

Anton AH, Sayre DF (1962) A study of the factors affecting the aluminum oxide trihydroxyindole procedure for analysis of catecholamines. J Pharmacol Exp Ther 138 : 360–375
Givner M, Rochefort J (1965) An improved assay of corticosterone in rat serum and adrenal tissue. Steroids 6 : 486
Govoni S, Memo M, Lucchi L, Spano PF, Trabucchi M (1980) Brain neurotransmitter systems and chronic lead intoxication. Pharmacol Res Commun 12 : 447–460
Komulainen H, Tuomisto J (1981) Effect of heavy metals on dopamine, noradrenaline and serotonin uptake and release in rat brain synaptosomes. Acta Pharmacol Toxicol 48 : 199–204
Welch AS, Welch BL (1969) Solvent extraction method for simultaneous determination of norepinephrine, dopamine, serotonin and 5-hydroxyindoleacetic acid in a single mouse brain. Anal Biochem 30 : 164–179
Wender PH (1971) Minimal brain dysfunction in children. Wiley, New York
Winder C (1982) The interaction between lead and catecholaminergic function. Biochem Pharmacol 31 : 3717–3721

Xenobiotic Toxicology

Disease, Metabolism and Reproduction in the Toxic Response to Drugs and Other Chemicals
Arch. Toxicol., Suppl. 7, 403–404 (1984)

Experimental Evidence on the Pulmonary Carcinogenicity of Arsenic Trioxide

G. Pershagen[1], G. Nordberg[2], and N.-E. Björklund[3]

[1] Department of Environmental Hygiene, Karolinska Institute,
and the National Institute of Environmental Medicine, 104 01 Stockholm, Sweden
[2] Department of Environmental Medicine, Umeå University, 901 87 Umeå, Sweden
[3] National Veterinary Institute, 750 07 Uppsala, Sweden

Abstract. Pulmonary carcinomas were obtained in male hamsters given intratracheal instillations of arsenic trioxide together with a carrier dust (charcoal carbon) and sulfuric acid. No malignant lung tumours appeared in sham treated control animals.

Key words: Arsenic trioxide – Lung cancer – Intratracheal instillation – Hamster

In spite of strong epidemiological evidence of the carcinogenicity of inorganic arsenic compounds, conclusive support from experimental studies is lacking (Pershagen 1981). In this study, arsenic trioxide has, for the first time, been tested in an experimental carcinogenicity system which often has been employed successfully, i.e. intratracheal instillations in hamsters together with a carrier dust (Saffiotti et al. 1968). Arsenic trioxide is the most common arsenic compound in many occupational exposure situations, e.g., in copper smelters.

Male syrian golden hamsters, 7–9 weeks of age at the start of the experiment, were given 15 intratracheal instillations according to the method described by Saffiotti et al. (1968). At each instillation one group of animals received 0.15 ml 0.9% saline solution containing arsenic trioxide, charcoal carbon and sulfuric acid in doses of about 3, 40, and 0.4 mg/kg body weight, respectively. Arsenic trioxide (As_2O_3) and sulfuric acid were obtained from Merck Chemikalien, (Darmstadt, Federal Republic of Germany) and had a certified purity of 99.5 and 96%, respectively. The charcoal carbon dust (Sigma Chemicals, Saint Louis, Missouri, USA) contained less than 40 mg/kg of antimony, chromium and nickel and less than 1 mg/kg of polyaromatic hydrocarbons. The control animals received instillations with charcoal carbon and sulfuric acid at the same doses as the arsenic treated animals. Detailed histopathological examinations were performed on coded samples of the larynx, trachea, bronchi, and lungs and on other tissues showing macroscopic

Table 1. Respiratory tract lesions in male hamsters given 15 weekly intratracheal instillations of arsenic trioxide (As) and in control animals[a]

Exposure[a]	Number of animals	Lesions in the larynx, trachea, bronchus, or lung			
		Carcinomas	Adenomas	Papillomas	Adenomatoid lesions
As	47	3	2	6	16
–	53	0	1	4	2

[a] Both groups received charcoal carbon and sulfuric acid (see text)

abnormalities in all animals dying after the 15 week exposure period. The average age at death was somewhat greater for the animals given arsenic trioxide than for the control animals, 77 and 63 weeks, respectively. However, differences in longevity between the treatment groups are controlled by the methods used for statistical testing (Peto et al. 1980).

Table 1 shows the number of animals examined in the two treatment groups as well as the number of respiratory tract lesions, e.g., benign and malignant tumours. Among the 47 arsenic treated animals, three pulmonary carcinomas werer found, i.e., one laryngeal squamous cell carcinoma, one bronchiolar adenocarcinoma and one bronchiolar small cell anaplastic carcinoma. No malignant lung tumours appeared in 53 control animals. The three carcinomas in the arsenic treated group do not constitute a statistically significant increase ($p \approx 0.07$). However, there was a significantly higher incidence of non-malignant lung lesions (adenomas, adenomatoid lesions and papillomas) in the arsenic exposed animals ($p < 0.01$). As a rule the number of these lesions is increased in groups of hamsters exposed to carcinogens giving rise to an increased frequency of malignant lung tumours (Saffiotti et al. 1968; Pershagen 1982). This indicates that the pulmonary carcinomas in the arsenic treated group were not a chance finding.

Taken together the data provide strong evidence that arsenic trioxide can induce carcinomas of the respiratory tract. The use of the carrier dust increased the lung retention of arsenic (Pershagen 1982), which may have had an influence, as well as the concomitant administration of sulfuric acid.

References

Pershagen G (1981) The carcinogenicity of arsenic. Environ Health Perspect 40: 93–100

Pershagen G (1982) Arsenic and lung cancer, with special reference to interacting factors – Epidemiological and experimental evidence. Thesis at the dept. of environmental hygiene. Karolinska Institute, Stockholm

Peto R, Pike M, Day N et al. (1980) Guidelines for simple, sensitive significance tests for carcinogenic effects in long-term animal experiments. In: Long-term and short-term screening assays for carcinogens: A critical appraisal. IARC Monographs on the evaluation of the carcinogenic risk of chemicals to humans; Supplement 2. Int. Agency for Research on Cancer, Lyon, pp 311–426

Saffiotti U, Cefis F, Kolb N (1968) A method for the experimental induction of bronchogenic carcinoma. Cancer Res 28: 104–124

Disease, Metabolism and Reproduction in the Toxic Response to Drugs and Other Chemicals
Arch. Toxicol., Suppl. 7, 405–406 (1984)

Molecular Interaction of Acrylonitrile at Target Sites of Carcinogenicity in Rats

A. E. Ahmed and M. Y. H. Farooqui

Departments of Pathology, Pharmacology and Toxicology, University of Texas Medical Branch, Keiler Building, Rm 230, Galveston, Texas 77550, USA

Abstract. Acrylonitrile ($CH_2 = CH-CN$), a plastic monomer, is known to produce microglioma of the central nervous system, cell papillomas of the stomach and squamous cell carcinoma. The molecular interaction of [2,3^{14}C]-acrylonitrile (VCN), its metabolites or both with proteins, RNA and DNA of various rat tissues after a single oral dose of 46.5 mg/kg has been studied. RNA and DNA molecules were separated by hydroxyapatite chromatography, and the DNA nucleosides were separated after enzymic hydrolysis by high performance liquid chromatography (HPLC). Binding of VCN to proteins of various tissues was extensive and time dependent. Radioactivity incorporated in the nucleic acids was highest in liver and the target organs stomach and brain. DNA alkylation, which increased by time, was significantly higher in the target organs, brain and stomach (119 and 81 pmol/mg respectively) than that in the liver (25 pmol/mg). The covalent binding indices for liver, stomach and brain were 6, 52, and 65 respectively. HPLC analysis of DNA hydrolysate revealed that by 24 h most of the applied radioactivity appeared in peaks corresponding to standard deoxyguanosine and deoxyadenosine. These results are consistent with the ability of VCN to act as a multipotent carcinogen by preferential alkylation of DNA in the extrahepatic target tissues, stomach and brain.

Key words: Carcinogenicity – Molecular interaction – DNA binding – Covalent binding – Environmental toxicology

References

Abreu M, Ahmed AE (1980) Metabolism of acrylonitrile to cyanide in in vitro studies. Drug Metab Dispos 8: 376–379

Beland FA, Dooley KL, Casciano DA (1979) Rapid isolation of carcinogen-bound DNA and RNA by hydroxyapatite chromatography. J Chromatogr 174: 177–186

Abbreviations: VCN, acrylonitrile; HPLC, high pressure liquid chromatography; CBI, covalent binding index

Bergman K (1982) Reaction of vinyl chloride with RNA and DNA of various mouse tissues in vivo. Arch Toxicol 49: 117–129

Bradford MM (1976) A rapid and sensitive method for the quantitation of microgram quantities of protein, utilizing the principle of protein-dye binding. Anal Biochem 72: 248–254

Burton K (1968) Determination of DNA concentration with diphenylamine. In: Grossman L, Moldave K (eds) Methods in enzymology, vol 12B. Academic Press, New York, pp 163–165

Ghanayem BI, Boor PJ, Ahmed AE (1982) Gastric gluthatione depletion mediates acrylo-nitrile-induced gastric ulceration (Abstract). Pharmacologist 24: 110

Guengerich FP, Geiger LE, Hogy LL, Wright PL (1981) In vitro metabolism of acrylonitrile to 2-cyanoethylene oxide: Reaction with glutathione and irreversible binding to proteins and nucleic acids. Cancer Res 41: 4925–4933

Lutz WK (1979) In vivo covalent binding of organic chemicals to DNA as a quantitative indicator in the process of chemical carcinogenesis. Mutat Res 65: 289–356

Maltoni C, Ciliberti A, Dimaio V (1977) Carcinogenicity bioassays of rats of acrylonitrile administered by inhalation and by ingestion. Med Lav 68: 401–411

O'Berg MT (1980) Epidemiological studies on workers exposed to acrylonitrile. J Occup Med 22: 245–252

Ottenwalder H, Laib RJ, Bolt HW (1979) Alkylation of RNA by vinyl bromide metabolites in vitro and in vivo. Arch Toxicol 41: 279–286

Quast JF, Enriques RM, Wade CM, Humiston CG, Schwetz BA (1977) Toxicity of drinking water containing acrylonitrile (AN) in rats. Fed Red 43: 2589

Schneider WC (1957) Determination of nucleic acids in tissue by pentose analysis. In: Grossmann L, Moldave K (eds) Methods in enzymology, vol 3. Academic Press, New York, pp 680–684

Secrist JA, Barrio JR, Leonard NJ, Weber G (1972) Fluorescent modification of adenosine-containing co-enzymes. Biological activities and spetroscopic properties. Biochemistry 11: 3499–3506

Szabo S, Reynolds ES, Komanicky P, Moslen MT, Melby JC (1976) Effect of chronic acrylonitrile ingestion on rat adrenal (Abstract). Toxicol Appl Pharmacol 37: 133

Disease, Metabolism and Reproduction in the Toxic Response to Drugs and Other Chemicals
Arch. Toxicol., Suppl. 7, 407 (1984)

Mutagenic Activity of Nitriloacetic Acid

A. Nunziata[1], M. Monaco[1], N. Loprieno[2], G. Boncristiani[2], P. Venier[3], and A. Montaldi[3]

[1] L.S.R. Roma Toxicology Centre, 00040 Pomezia, Rome, Italy
[2] Institute of Genetics, University of Pisa, Pisa, Italy
[3] Institute of Animal Biology, University of Padua, Padua, Italy

Abstract. Nitriloacetic acid (NTA) has been demonstrated to be unable to produce gene mutations in prokariotic and eukaryotic cells or chromosomal aberrations in cells grown in vitro, as well as in living animals. However a very slight mutagenic activity has been found when *Drosophila* and higher plants were used.

NIDA, a N-nitroso derivative of NTA, has been found negative on bacterial cells.

It is known from the literature that NTA solubilize some insoluble metal salts.

This study attempted to further investigate the mutagenicity of NTA and NIDA and on the potential genotoxic effect of insoluble Cr^{VI} salt when NTA was present.

For this study the Ames test (5 strains), the tests on yeast for the induction of gene-mutations and mitotic gene-conversions, and the test for the induction of SCE in CHO cells have been employed. Preliminary results indicate that NTA and NIDA are not mutagenic in *Salmonella* and yeasts. When, however an hexavalent Cr salt (insoluble) was assayed in the presence of NTA, the mixture was found positive on TA 98 and TA 100 Salmonella's strains: this activity correlates positively with the amount of soluble Cr in the mixture. NTA moreover increases the induction of SCE on CHO cells induced normally by an insoluble Cr^{VI} salt.

Key words: Mutagenesis – Nitriloacetic acid – Ames test

Disease, Metabolism and Reproduction in the Toxic Response to Drugs and Other Chemicals
Arch. Toxicol., Suppl. 7, 408–409 (1984)

Neurotoxicity in Rats Dosed with Peppermint Oil and Pulegone

P. Olsen and I. Thorup

Institute of Toxicology, National Food Institute, 2860 Søborg, Copenhagen, Denmark

Abstract. Rats dosed with peppermint oil and pulegone up to 100 or 160 mg/kg body weight/day, respectively, in 28 days developed encephalopathy. Microscopically dose-related cyst-like spaces were found in the white matter of the cerebellum.

Key words: Peppermint oil – Pulegone – Food flavouring – Encephalopathy – Rats

Peppermint oil and pulegone isolated from Mentha species are used as flavourings, particularly in the manufacture of chewing gum, flavoured candies, beverages, toothpastes and pharmaceutical products. Peppermint oil is composed of different substances of which pulegone constitutes 2–4% (Morison Smith and Levi 1961).

Very little is known about the toxicity of these oils although the consumption as food additives is several thousand metric tons per year (Greenhalgh 1979).

The histopathological findings presented here are from two 28-days studies in rats dosed with peppermint oil and pulegone. The experiments included clinical, biochemical, haematological and pathological parameters (Thorup et al. 1983).

Groups of 10 male and 10 female rats were given by gavage 0, 10, 40, or 100 mg/kg/day of peppermint oil and 0, 20, 80, or 160 mg/kg/day of pulegone, respectively. The peppermint oil and pulegone were obtained from Dandy Ltd. and Fluka (82569), respectively.

Microscopical examination revealed similar dose-related lesions in the white matter of the brain for both substances (Table 1). Cyst-like spaces were seen scattered in the white matter, especially in the cerebellum, without any cellular reaction in the surrounding tissue. Demyelination could not be demonstrated using staining procedures appropriate for myelin sheets. This resembles the neuropathy in rats induced by hexachlorophene (Kennedy et al. 1976).

Table 1. Number of rats with microscopic changes after dosing with peppermint oil or pulegone. 10 males and 10 females per group

	Peppermint oil (mg/kg bw/day)				Pulegone (mg/kg bw/day)			
	0	10	40	100	0	20	80	160[a]
Cyst-like spaces in cerebellum	0	0	4	11	0	0	4	13

[a] 17 animals

References

Greenhalgh P (1979) The markets for mint oils. Tropical Products Institute, London, pp 1–44

Kennedy GL Jr, Dressler IA, Richter WR, Keplinger ML, Calandra JA (1976) Effects of hexachlorophene in the rat and their reversibility. Toxicol Appl Pharmacol 35: 137–145

Morison Smith D, Levi L (1961) Essential oils treatment of compositional data for the characterization of essential oils. Determination of geographical origins of peppermint oils by gas chromatographic analysis. Agric Food Chem 9: 230–244

Thorup I, Würtzen G, Carstensen J (1983) Short term toxicity study in rats dosed with peppermint oil. Toxicology Letters 19: 211–215

Thorup J, Würtzen G, Carstensen J, Olsen P (1983) Short term toxicity study in rats dosed with pulegone and menthol. Toxicology Letters 19: 207–210

Disease, Metabolism and Reproduction in the Toxic Response to Drugs and Other Chemicals
Arch. Toxicol., Suppl. 7, 410–411 (1984)

Neurotoxicological Profile of Carbon Disulphide After Intraventricular Administration in Rats

D. Rotiroti, F. Naccari, S. Gratteri, R. Anfosso, and G. Nisticò

Institute of Pharmacology, Faculty of Medicine, University of Messina, Piazza XX. Settembre, 4, 98100 Messina, Italy

Abstract. The effects of different concentrations of CS_2 given into the III cerebral ventricle in rats on behaviour, on GABA content and on glutamate-decarboxylase activity (GAD), the rate limiting step for GABA synthesis, were assessed. A stereotyped behaviour (licking, sniffing) was elicited by CS_2 in a dose-dependent manner; in addition tonic-clonic convulsions were produced after the highest doses used (5 and 10 μl of a 99% solution). At the same time 10 μl of this solution produced a significant decrease in GAD activity and GABA content in the rat diencephalon.

Key words: Carbon disulphide – Behaviour – Glutamate decarboxylase – Amino butyric acid

Exposure to carbon disulphide (CS_2) can lead to widely different pathological conditions such as mental aberrations, extrapyramidal symptoms, hypertension, atherosclerosis and an increased frequency of coronary death (Szobor 1962). In addition, carbon disulphide decreases noradrenaline synthesis in rat brain as a consequence of dopamine-β-hydroxylase inhibition (Magos and Jarvis, 1970; McKenna and Di Stefano, 1977) and it potentiates amphetamine and apomorphine-induced stereotyped behaviour (Magos 1971, 1976).

The aim of the present work was to investigate whether CS_2 given directly into the III cerebral ventricle of rats was able to produce behavioural changes and to assess, since strict interrelationships exist between catecholaminergic and GABA-ergic mechanisms (see Nisticò 1980), whether CS_2 was able to affect GABA metabolism in the diencephalon.

Wistar Morini rats (200–220 g) were used. The cannula was chronically implanted into the III cerebral ventricle according to the DeGroot's atlas coordinates (1959). GAD activity was assayed by measurement of $^{14}CO_2$ formed from L-(1-^{14}C)-glutamic acid in a liquid scintillator according to Nisticò et al. (1979). The GABA content was determined by the enzymatic fluorimetric procedure of Graham & Aprison (1966) as modified by Balcom et al. (1975).

Table 1. Effects of an intraventricular injection of CS_2 on GAD activity and GABA content in the rat diencephalon 30 min after the administration

Experimental group	n	GAD activity (µmol CO_2/100 mg/protein/h)	GABA content (µmol/100 mg/protein)
Controls (vehicle)	6	30.4 ± 0.40	5.26 ± 0.24
CS_2 10 µl	6	18.3 ± 0.32*	3.53 ± 0.15*

n = Number of experiments, each from triplicate assay; * $p < 0.01$ in comparison to controls

Behavioural changes after intraventricular CS_2 were dose-related. Ten animals were used at each dose level. In fact after the administration of 2.5 µl of a 99% solution only a slight pattern of stereotyped movements (licking, sniffing) was observed, whereas a higher dose (5 µl) produced an intense pattern of stereotyped behaviour accompanied by ataxia and in 20% of the rats short-lasting episodes of tonic-clonic convulsions occurred; these were present in 80% of rats after 10 µl. In addition after the latter dose a significant ($p < 0.01$) decrease in glutamate-decarboxylase activity and in GABA content (Table 1) was observed in the rat diencephalon 30 min after the administration.

In conclusion, the present experiments show that CS_2 after intraventricular injection produces extrapyramidal effects and at high doses possess marked neurotoxicity culminating into tonic-clonic convulsions associated with a decrease in GABAergic mechanisms in the diencephalon.

References

Balcom GJ, Lenox RH, Meyerhoff JL (1975) Regional γ-aminobutyric acid levels in rat brain determined after microwave fixation. J Neurochem 24: 509–513

De Groot J (1959) The rat forebrain in stereotaxic coordinates. Noord-Hollandsche Uitgevers Maatschappij, Amsterdam

Graham GJ, Aprison MH (1966) Fluorimetric determination of aspartate, glutamate and GABA in nerve tissue using enzymatic methods. Anal Biochem 15: 487–497

Magos L (1971) Amphetamine induced stereotypy in carbon disulphide exposed and diethyldithiocarbamate-treated male rats. Proc Eur Soc Study Drug Toxicity 12: 24–27

Magos L (1976) The effect of carbon disulphide on the stereotypic effect of dopamine agonists. Eur J Pharmacol 36: 257–258

Magos L, Jarvis JAE (1970) The effects of carbon disulphide exposure on brain catecholamines in rats. Br J Pharmacol 39: 26–33

McKenna MJ, Di Stefano V (1977) A proposed mechanism of the action of carbon disulphide on dopamine-β-hydroxylase. J Pharmacol Exp Ther 202: 253–266

Nisticò G (1980) Relations between dopaminergic and GABAergic mechanism in avian brain. Pharmacol Res Commun 12: 507–514

Nisticò G, Di Giorgio RM, Rotiroti D, Macaione S (1979) GABA depletion and GABA transaminase increase after intraventricular 6-hydroxydopamine. Biochem Pharmacol 28: 3030–3032

Szobor A (1962) Contribution à la question de sulfocarbonisme. Psychiatria Neurol 143: 178–196

Disease, Metabolism and Reproduction in the Toxic Response to Drugs and Other Chemicals
Arch. Toxicol., Suppl. 7, 412–417 (1984)

Immediate Effects of m-Xylene on the Human Central Nervous System

K. Savolainen[1], J. Kekoni[2], V. Riihimäki[2], and A. Laine[2]

[1] National Public Health Institute, P.O.B. 138, 70101 Kuopio 10, Finland
[2] Institute of Occupational Health, 00290 Helsinki 29, Finland

Abstract. Male volunteers were exposed to m-xylene vapour for 4 h a day either sedentary or with a period of 10 min exercise twice a day with stable (8.2 μmol/l) m-xylene concentrations or fluctuating concentrations with peaks (16.4 μmol/l). The TWA concentration was always the same (8.2 μmol/l). The body balance of the subjects was clearly impaired in the anteroposterior (a−p) direction, especially with their eyes closed during the peaks at rest, whereas it was improved when exercise was included in spite of the higher blood m-xylene concentrations. When on the contrary, the situation was reversed in the lateral direction. Complex audiomotor reactions were impaired after the peaks combined with exercise, whereas changes in simple reaction times were similar in pattern to those found for body balance in the a−p direction. The results suggest a complex interaction between physiological factors and m-xylene and development of adaptation or tolerance during the exposure.

Key words: m-Xylene – Inhalation exposure – Central nervous system – Kinetics – Human

Several industrial solvents are narcotic in higher atmospheric concentrations, and mixtures of xylene isomers, being widely used in paints and lacquers as well as printing links, can induce inebriation of the human CNS even at rather low concentrations, such as 4.1−16.4 μmol/l (Riihimäki and Savolainen 1980). Due to practical and theoretical reasons, adaptation of the human CNS to different exposure situations, such as rapid fluctuations of the concentration of the solvent, e.g., xylene, in the workroom air, merits more attention (Savolainen et al. 1979). In addition, interactions of physical exercise with these processes carry important consequences in a real working situation (Savolainen et al. 1980).

Abbreviations: CNS, central nervous system; TWA, time-weighted average

Materials and Methods

Nine healthy male volunteers were exposed to m-xylene (Laboratory grade, Merck, F.R.G.) in a dynamically controlled exposure chamber 4 h a day, 3 h in the morning and 1 h in the afternoon with a 40 min break between. The subjects were sedentary or had a period of exercise at 100 W for 10 min at the beginning

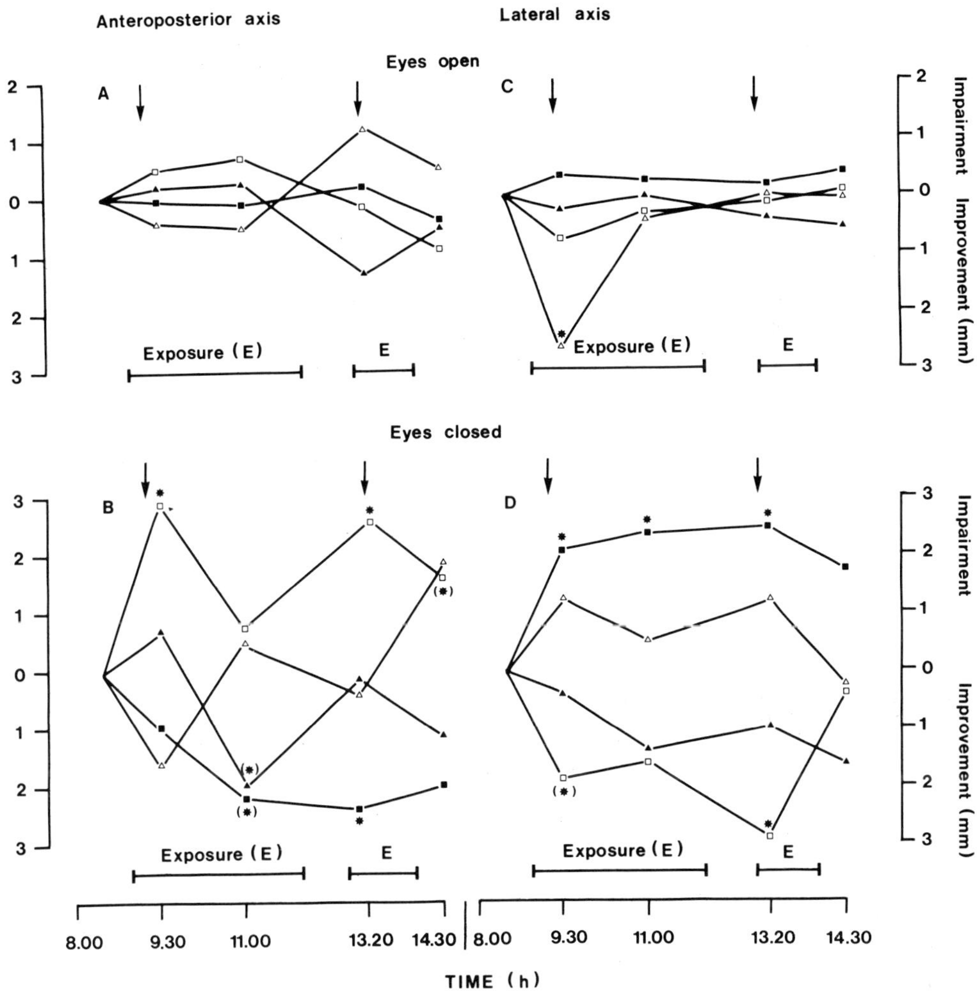

Fig. 1. Body balance along the anteroposterior (a–p) and lateral axes. Changes in the body balance are shown along the a–p axis with the subjects' eyes open **(A)** and closed **(B),** as well as along the lateral axis with open **(C)** and closed **(D)** eyes. Changes between control and exposure situations are given for exposure to stable concentration (8.2 μmol/l) of m-xylene at rest (△) and with exercise (▲), as well as for fluctuating concentrations (5.3–16.4 μmol/l) of m-xylene at rest (□) and with exercise (■). The morning values have been used as a reference. Periods of exposure have been indicated with *straight lines* and those of exercise with *arrows*. * $0.1 > p > 0.05$; *$p < 0.05$, Student's paired *t*-test, two-tailed

of each session. The exposures were presented as either stable m-xylene concentrations (8.2 μmol/l) or fluctuating concentrations with peaks (16.4 μmol/l) the TWA concentration being always 8.2 μmol/l (Table 1). The subjects were divided into three groups and exposed in a balanced order to avoid the effect of learning. The measurements were done before the subjects entered the chamber, in the chamber always at the time of the peak and exercise, and after the exposure. Body balance was measured with a straingauge transducer platform and reaction times were recorded with a device in which subjects responded manually to visual stimuli in a simple reaction time task, and to auditory stimuli in a choice reaction time task. Blood samples were also drawn and analysed with gas chromatography (Savolainen et al. 1979).

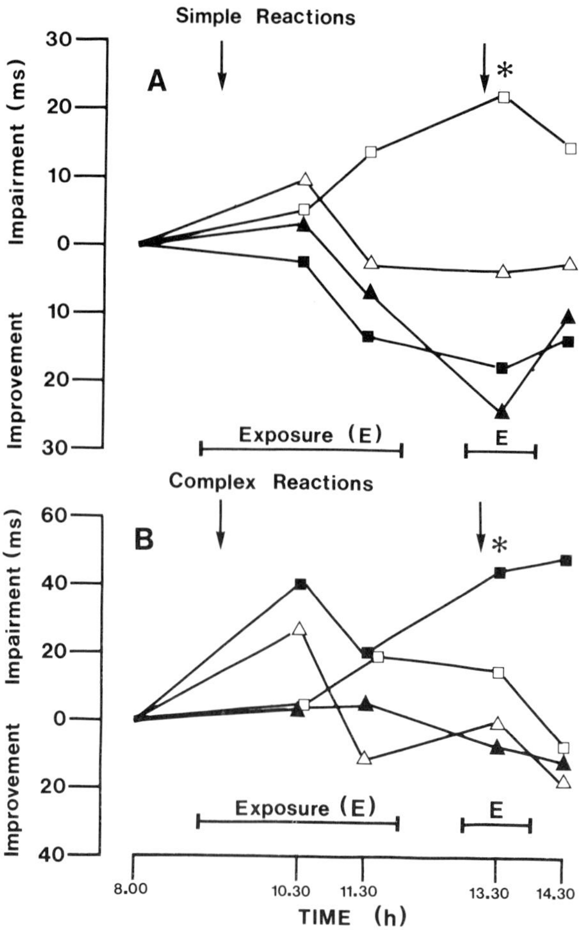

Fig. 2. Simple visuo-motor and complex audio-motor reaction times. The changes in simple **(A)** and complex **(B)** reaction times between control and exposure situations are shown. The morning values have been used as a reference. Periods of exposure are indicated with *straight lines* and those of exercise with *arrows*. Symbols indicating the different exposure situations are as in Fig. 1. * $p < 0.05$, Student's paired t-test, two-tailed

Table 1. Atmospheric (μmol/l) and venous blood (μmol/l) m-xylene concentrations during different experimental situations. The atmospheric exposure and venous blood m-xylene levels each day are given at the time of different measurements because the atmospheric concentrations of m-xylene occasionally fluctuated (5.3–16.4 μmol/l; 130–400 ppm), the TWA concentrations being always the same (8.2 μmol/l; 200 ppm). The periods of physical exercise at 100 W for 10 min a time are indicated (+). The experiment also included two control days, one at rest and the other in which periods of physical exercise were included

Time of day	Exposures to m-xylene							
	Stable 8.2 μmol/l		Stable 8.2 μmol/l (+)		5.3–16.4 μmol/l		5.3–16.4 μmol/l (+)	
	In air	In blood	In air	In blood	In air	In blood	In air	In blood
09.30	8.2	17.5	8.2 (+)	38.0 (+)	16.4	25.0	16.4 (+)	50.0 (+)
10.30	8.2	26.0	8.2	32.5	5.3	26.0	5.3	31.0
11.00	8.2	29.0	8.2	33.0	5.3	26.0	5.3	28.0
11.30	8.2	30.0	8.2	31.0	5.3	22.5	5.3	26.5
13.10	8.2	25.0	8.2 (+)	35.0 (+)	16.4	31.0	16.4 (+)	58.0 (+)
13.30	8.2	19.0	8.2	23.0	5.3	23.0	5.3	37.5
14.30	–	10.0	–	11.0	–	15.0	–	20.0

The subjects entered the chamber at 09.00, and during the days on which fluctuations of m-xylene concentrations took place the peaks at rest or with exercise occurred 09.10–09.30 and 13.00–13.10. The subjects always left the chamber at 14.00

Results

m-Xylene peaks significantly impaired body balance along the antero-posterior (a–p) axis in the morning and in the afternoon at rest whereas exercise in the same situation counteracted this effect inducing an improvement in body balance, especially with the eyes closed. Along the lateral axis, however, the fluctuating m-xylene concentrations combined with exercise significantly impaired the body balance, whereas at rest in an otherwise identical situation the body balance was improved, especially with the eyes closed (Fig. 1).

Complex audiomotor reaction times were somewhat impaired after the peaks combined with exercise. Changes in simple visual reaction times had a pattern rather similar to that found for body balance along the a–p axis (Fig. 2).

Venous blood m-xylene concentrations increased rather rapidly during the peaks, especially during the exercise, and they tended to reach a steady state at the end of the morning exposure (Table 1).

Discussion

Impairment of body balance during the m-xylene peaks in the morning and in the afternoon was an expected finding based on earlier results (Savolainen and Linnavuo 1979). Development of a rapid tolerance of adaptation during a day might partly explain these findings for body balance and simple reaction time recordings when the venous blood m-xylene concentrations are taken into consideration. A strong counteraction to the xylene effect on body balance along the a–p axis by simultaneous physical exercise was a surprising finding which can probably be explained by an increased arousal level induced by the exercise (Seppäläinen et al. 1981; Seppäläinen et al. 1983). This finding was supported by the changes in simple reaction times whereas the changes in body balance along the lateral axis and the auditory reactions were logically impaired related to the xylene dose at the same situation, the latter possibly due to the complexity of the task. The reason for the clearly opposite changes in body balance along the a–p and lateral axes might indicate in addition to the impairment of body balance, a more specific effect of m-xylene on the pattern of body sway, and thus also to the central vestibular system. These findings emphasize the importance of studying interactions not only between different chemicals, but also between them and physiological factors such as physical exercise on the human CNS in a working situation.

References

Riihimäki V, Savolainen K (1980) Human exposure to m-xylene: Kinetics and acute effects on the central nervous system. Ann Occup Hyg 23: 411–422

Savolainen K, Linnavuo M (1979) Effects of m-xylene on human equilibrium measured with a quantitative method. Acta Pharmacol Toxicol 44: 315–318

Savolainen K, Riihimäki V, Linnoila M (1979) Effects of short-term xylene exposure on psychophysiological functions in man. Int Arch Occup Environ Health 44: 201–211

Savolainen K, Riihimäki V, Seppäläinen AM, Linnoila M (1980) Effects of short-term m-xylene exposure and physical exercise on the central nervous system. Int Arch Occup Environ Health 45: 105–121

Seppäläinen AM, Savolainen K, Kovala T (1981) Changes induced by xylene and alcohol in human evoked potentials. Electroencephalogr Clin Neurophysiol 51: 148–155

Seppäläinen AM, Salmi T, Savolainen K, Riihimäki V (1983) Visual evoked potentials in short-term exposure of human subjects to m-xylene and 1,1,1-trichloroethane. In: Zbinden G, Cuomo V, Racagni G, Weiss B (eds) Application of behavioral pharmacology in toxicology. Raven, New York, 349–352

Disease, Metabolism and Reproduction in the Toxic Response to Drugs and Other Chemicals
Arch. Toxicol., Suppl. 7, 418–419 (1984)

Potentiation of Hexane and Organophosphate Neurotoxicities

E. Vilanova, J. L. Vicedo, M. D. Zafra and M. C. Pellín

Department of Physiology and Biochemistry, Faculty of Medicine, University of Alicante, Alicante, Spain

Abstract. Long-term exposure to hexane and acute or accumulative chronic ingestion of many organophosphates induce peripheral neuropathies (Spencer et al. 1980; Johnson 1982). Many cases of similar peripheral neuropathies have been reported in workers handling solvents or adhesives in leather factories in Italy, Spain, Japan and other countries (Vilanova 1981). Many of them have been attributed either to hexane or organophosphates (mainly TOCP). This laboratory has observed a possible potentiation of the hexane and organophosphate neurotoxicities. Hens were exposed to hexane at doses producing slight weakness, but not ataxia. They devolped a severe ataxia (3–4 points in a 4-points scale) after a single TOCP dose which induced only a slight ataxia in the hexane non-exposed hens (1–2 points). The possibility that the impurities in the industrial solvents could play a significant role is shown by the observation that the non-hydrocarbon impurities in many samples of commercial hexane inhibited S-ChE "in vitro" but not AChE. An inhibition without preincubation is observed and also a time progressive inhibition with kinetic properties in accord with organophosphate inhibitors. Organic elemental phosphorus has been measured. Several fractions have been isolated by preparative chromatography. In one of them dibutyl, hexyl and dioctyl phthalates, adipates and triphenylphosphate have been identified by GC-mass spectrometry. The presence of dibutylphthalate could explain the non-progressive inhibition. The progressive inhibition is not explained by the triphenylphosphate. Another unidentified organophosphate has to be in the hexane impurities to explain the non-progressive inhibition. The potentiation effect of organophosphates and hexane, besides the presence of organophosphates and inhibitors of sterases are facts to take into consideration in understanding a multifactor explanation of occupational toxic neuropathies.

Key words: Hexane – Tri-o-cresylphosphate (TOCP) – Neurotoxicity – Potentiation

Acknowledgements. To Dr. Bailey from MRC-Toxicology Unit (Carshalton, Surrey, U.K.) and Dr. J. Font from the "Universidad Autónoma de Barcelona" (Bellaterra, Barcelona, Spain) for their help in the GC-mass studies. To the students Mr F. Pascual and V. Prieto for technical assistance.

References

Bermejillo M (1971) Intoxicación laboral por el triortoxcresilfosfato. Rev Med Segur Trabajo 74: 49–58

Capellini A, Chiappino S, Zurlo N (1968) Osservazioni cliniche e sperimentali sulle polineuriti considerate da tricresilfosfato. Med Lav 59: 721–759

Perbellini L, Brugnone F, Gaffuri E (1981) Neurotoxic metabolites of "commercial hexane" in the urine of shoe factory workers. Clin Toxicol 18: 1377–1385

Vicedo JL, Vilanova E (1982) Anticolinesterasas en impurezas de hexano comercial. X Congreso de la Sociedad Española de Bioquímica. Com No 347. Santander, Spain

Vilanova E, Vicedo JL (1983) Serum cholinesterase inhibitors in the commercial hexane impurities. Arch Toxicol 53: 59–69

Xintaras C, Burg JR, Tanaka S, Lee ST, Johnson BL, Cottrill CA, Bender J (1978) NIOSH health survey of Velsicol pesticide workers. Occupational exposure to leptophos and other chemicals. DHEW (NIOSH) publication No 78–136. US Govern Printing Office, Washington

Yamamura Y (1969) n-Hexane polineuropathy. Folia Psychiatr Neurol Jpn 23: 45–57

Disease, Metabolism and Reproduction in the Toxic Response to Drugs and Other Chemicals
Arch. Toxicol., Suppl. 7, 420–424 (1984)

Behavioural and Electrocortical Spectrum Power Changes After Intraventricular Injection of Patulin in Rats

G. B. De Sarro, A. Donato, G. Bagetta, A. Pujia and G. Nisticò

Institute of Pharmacology, Faculty of Medicine, University of Messina
Piazza XX Settembre, 4, 98100 Messina, Italy

Abstract. The effects of patulin when given into the third cerebral ventricle of rats, on behaviour and electrocortical spectrum power have been investigated. Patulin (10 μg i.v.t.) produced behavioural sedation, hypoalgesia, tail rigidity, piloerection and postural changes. This symptomatology lasted approx. 3 h and was accompanied by slower frequency and larger amplitude potentials in the electrocorticogram (ECoG) and by an increase in total voltage power. A larger dose (50 μg) produced a more dramatic picture characterized by catatonic posture with kyphosis, loss of the righting reflex, tail rigidity and on a few occasions short-duration episodes of tonic-clonic convulsions. Such a symptomatology was accompanied by a flattening of ECoG activity with a significant fall in total voltage power, as well as in preselected bands (0–3, 3–6, 6–9, 9–12, and 12–16 Hz). A lower dose (1 μg) of patulin, on the other hand, produced behavioural sedation without significant changes in ECoG spectrum power.

Key words: Patulin – Mycotoxins – Neurotoxicity – Electrocortical spectrum power – Behaviour

Patulin (4-hydroxy-4-H-furo [3,2c]-pyran-2(6H)-one), a mycotoxin produced by *Penicillum patulum* and other species of *Penicillum* and *Aspergillus* was originally isolated and studied as an antibiotic, but, because of its toxicity both for animals and plants, it has not been accepted as a practical antimicrobial agent (see Chu 1977). However, many reports indicate that patulin occurs as a contaminant in foods especially in agricultural products such as apples and apple juices. This suggests that this mycotoxin is a potential hazard for humans and animals (see Chu 1977). It is also very stable during processing (Stoloff 1975; Pohland and Allen 1970). Patulin is toxic in several biological systems and produces, in various animal species, hemorrhage and capillary damage in the liver, spleen, and kidney together with oedema of the brain and nervous symptoms (Abraham and Florey 1949; Katzman et al. 1944; Yamamoto 1954).

Patulin inhibits aerobic respiration in fungi and in liver homogenates in several animal species (Gottlieb and Singh 1964; Hayes 1977).

In addition several experiments have shown that patulin is a potent inhibitor both in vivo and in vitro of Na^+ and K^+-ATPase (Phillips and Hayes 1977, 1978) suggesting that inhibition of this enzymatic activity may be responsible for the neurotoxicity produced by patulin.

The aim of the present work was to characterize better the neurotoxicological profile of patulin, after its infusion into the third cerebral ventricle of rats, by following changes in behaviour and in electrocortical activity which was continously analyzed as total voltage power and the voltage power of preselected bands of frequency (Nisticò et al. 1980).

Patulin (10 µg, $n = 6$) given into the third cerebral ventricle produced behavioural sedation, decreased responsiveness to external stimuli, hypoalgesia, tail rigidity, hunched back and piloerection. The rats kept the same posture and the same position in the box. This symptomatology lasted 3 h and was

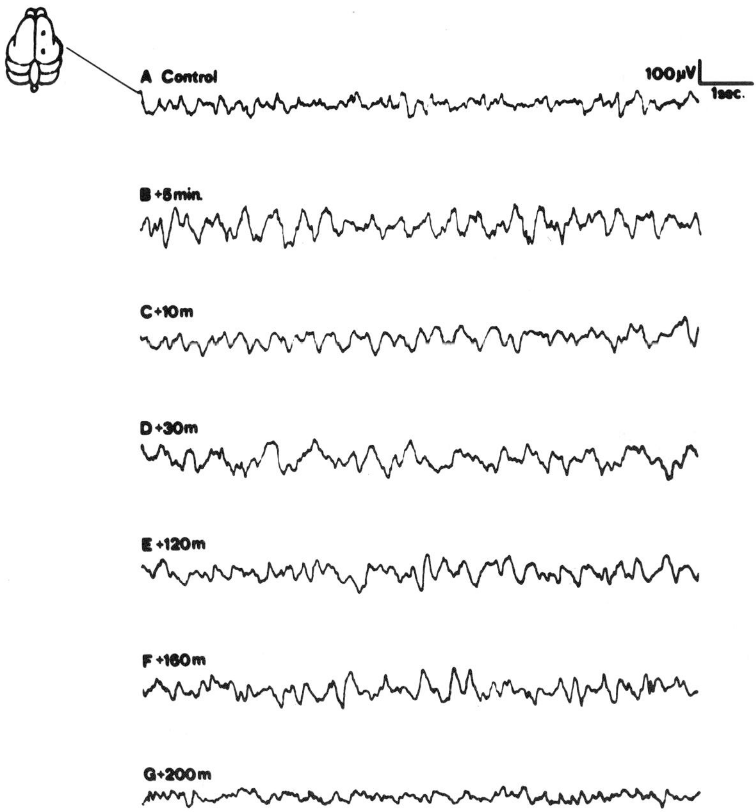

Fig. 1. Electrocortical effects of patulin (10 µg) after intraventricular administration. *A.* Control ECoG pattern. *B, C, D, E, F* Slow wave, higher amplitude potentials 5, 10, 30, 120, and 160 min after patulin administration. *G.* Return to control ECoG activity 200 min after patulin administration

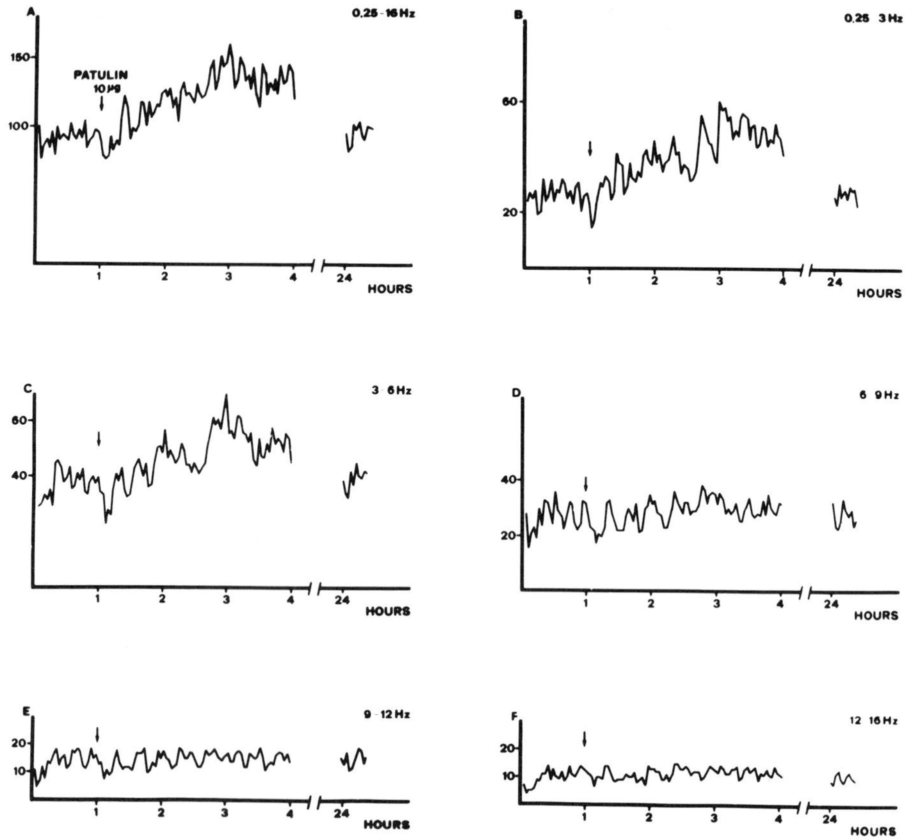

Fig. 2. Spectrum power effects of patulin (10 µg) after intraventricular administration. In comparison with the same period of control activity, patulin produced a significant ($p < 0.01$) increase in total voltage power *(A)* lasting 3 h and at the same time a significant increase of power in 0.25–3 *(B)* and 3–6 *(C)* Hz bands. No significant changes occurred in 6–9 *(D)*, 9–12 *(E)*, and 12–16 *(F)* bands

accompanied by slower frequency ECoG potentials of increased amplitude (Fig. 1) and by a significant increase in ECoG total voltage power and in the voltage power of 0.25–3 and 3–6 Hz bands (Fig. 2). A more dramatic picture culminating åfter 12–18 h in death was observed after a larger dose (50 µg, $n = 8$). This was characterized by catatonic posture with kyphosis, loss of the righting reflex, tail rigidity and on a few occasions, short-duration episodes of tonic-clonic convulsions. In addition, flattening of ECoG activity and a decrease in total voltage power and in the voltage power of the preselected bands (0.25–3, 3–6, 6–9, 9–12 Hz) (Fig. 3) was evident during this time. A lower dose (1 µg, $n = 4$) produced only behavioural sedation for approx. 3 h without significant changes in the ECoG spectrum power.

In conclusion, the present experiments provide neurophysiological evidence suggesting the high neurotoxicological profile of patulin in animals and presumably in man.

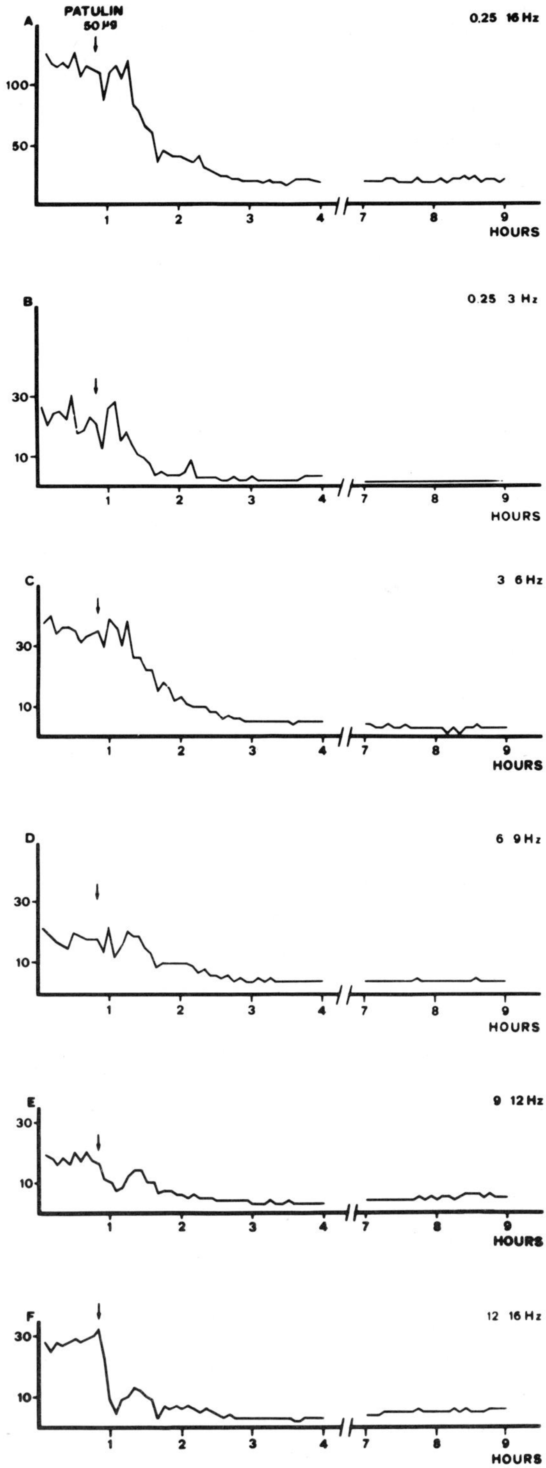

Fig. 3. Spectrum power effects of patulin (50 μg) after intraventricular administration. In comparison with the same period of control activity, patulin produced a significant decrease in total voltage power *(A)* as well as in all the preselected frequency bands *(B, C, D, E, F)*

References

Abraham EP, Florey HW (1949) Substances produced by imperfecti and ascomycetes. In: Florey H, Chain E, Heatley NG, Jenning MA, Sanders A, Abraham E, Florey ME (eds) Antibiotics, vol I. Oxford University Press, London, p 273

Chu FS (1977) Mode of action of mycotoxins and related compounds. Adv Appl Microbiol 22: 83–143

Gottlieb D, Singh J (1964) The mechanism of patulin inhibition of fungi. Riv Patol Veg Ser III 4: 455–479

Hayes AW (1977) Action of patulin on mouse liver mitochondria. Toxicol Appl Pharmacol 41: 165

Katzman PA, Hays EE, Cain CK et al. (1944) Clavacin, an antibiotic substance from aspergillus clavatus. J Biol Chem 154: 475–486

Nisticò G, De Sarro GB, Rotiroti D, Silvestri R, Marmo E (1980) Antagonism by classical antiepileptics and sodium valproate of cefazolin induced experimental epilepsy in rats. Res Commun Chem Pathol Pharmacol 29: 429–444

Phillips TD, Hayes AW (1977) Effects of patulin on adenosine triphosphatase activities in the mouse. Toxicol Appl Pharmacol 42: 175–187

Phillips TD, Hayes AW (1978) Effects of patulin on the kinetics of substrate and cationic ligand activation of adenosine triphosphatase in mouse brain. J Pharmcol Exp Ther 205: 606–616

Pohland AE, Allen R (1970) Stability studies with patulin. J Assoc Off Anal Chem 53: 688–691

Stoloff L (1975) Patulin, a contaminant of apple juice. In: Downing DL, Labelle RL (eds) N.Y. State agricultural experimental station special report 19. pp 51–53

Yamamoto T (1954) Studies on the poison-producing molds isolated from dry malt. I. Distribution, isolation, cultivation and formation of the toxic substances. J Pharmacol Soc Jpn 74: 797–804

Disease, Metabolism and Reproduction in the Toxic Response to Drugs and Other Chemicals
Arch. Toxicol., Suppl. 7, 425–426 (1984)

The Effects of Radiological Contrast Media on the Reproduction System of the Rat

P. Tirone and E. Boldrini

Bracco Industria Chimica, S.p.A., Via E. Folli 50, Milan, Italy

Abstract. During preclinical studies on new radiological contrast media the potential effect on reproductive performance and fertility must be evaluated. Two conventional oral cholecystographic agents, iopanoic acid and iopronic acid, were administered to rats through the periods of gametogenesis, mating, gestation, parturition and lactation. They produced a dose related weight loss in both males and females. All males proved fertile; in the females a selective maternally orientated effect of the two compounds on the process of gestation was assessed (Tables 1 and 2).

Table 1. Reproductive performance and litter parameters of female rats given iopanoic acid

Observations	Control	Iopanoic acid (g/kg)		
		0.1	0.2	0.4
Fertility index[a]	92	100	100	100
Litter size at birth				
Total	13.5	13.0	13.8	11.7
Live	13.4	12.8	13.8	11.2*
Mean pup weight (g) at birth[b]	6.0	5.6**	5.3**	5.6**

[a] Percentage of pregnant females after mating
[b] Including liveborn and stillborn
* Value differing significantly from control ($p < 0.05$)
** Value differing significantly from control ($p < 0.01$)

Iopamidol, a new low osmolality compound was also studied and it did not show any adverse effects on fertility and reproductive performance (Table 3).

Key words: Reproduction – Rats – Iopanoic acid – Iopronic acid – Iopamidol

Table 2. Reproductive performance and litter parameters of female rats given iopronic acid

Observations	Control	Iopronic acid (g/kg)		
		0.15	0.3	0.6
Fertility index[a]	92	100	100	100
Litter size at birth				
Total	13.5	13.8	10.8	10.2
Live	13.4	12.5	10.0	4.6**
Mean pup weight (g) at birth[b]	6.0	5.6**	5.5**	4.3**

[a] Percentage of pregnant females after mating
[b] Including liveborn and stillborn
** Value differing significantly from control ($p < 0.01$)

Table 3. Reproductive performance and litter parameters of female rats given iopamidol

Observations	Control	Iopamidol (g/kg)		
		1.2	3.1	8.2
Fertility index[a]	100	100	96	100
Litter size at birth				
Total	13.0	12.3	11.8	11.6
Live	13.0	11.8	11.5	10.9
Mean pup weight (g) at birth[b]	5.7	5.8	6.1*	5.5

[a] Percentage of pregnant females after mating
[b] Including liveborn and stillborn
* Value differing significantly from control ($p < 0.05$)

Disease, Metabolism and Reproduction in the Toxic Response to Drugs and Other Chemicals
Arch. Toxicol., Suppl. 7, 427–429 (1984)

Short-term Studies with the Cryptating Agent Hexaoxa-diaza-bicyclo-hexacosane in Rats

M. Baumann, E. Schäffer, and H. Greim

Gesellschaft für Strahlen- und Umweltforschung, Department of Toxicology, 8042 Neuherberg, Federal Republic of Germany

Abstract. In short-term experiments rats received single doses of 50, 100, and 500 µmoles/kg of the cryptating agent A 222. A dose-related increase in the activities of GOT and GPT in the serum was observed 6 h after treatment, reaching values up to eleven and three times that of the controls, respectively. However, the enzyme activities returned to the control levels within 3 days. The activity of alkaline phosphatase and the levels of protein and cholesterol in serum were not altered during the observation period of 7 days. Histopathological examinations did not show any changes in the liver, kidney, heart, lung, thymus, spleen, or intestine. The elevations of GOT and GPT seem to be due to a transient liver lesion, since no histopathological alterations of the liver became apparent. These results show, that after single applications of A 222 at all doses used, no severe lesions occur in the observed organs.

Key words: Cryptating agent – Hexaoxa-diaza-bicyclo-hexacosane – Serum analysis – Histopathology – Rat

Introduction

The hexaoxa-diamine macrobicycle A 222 is a new type of complexing agents, which forms cryptate complexes with alkaline earths. This cryptating agent is effective to selectively eliminate the bone-seeking radionuclides Sr-85, Ba-133 and Ra-224 from the body (Müller et al. 1977) and its use for evacuation of these radionuclides has been suggested. It has been shown (Müller and Beaumatin 1976) that after a single administration of A 222 to rats up to 90% of the substance is excreted in the urine and feces of the rats after 3 days. However, no information on the toxicological potential of this chemical is available. The dose proposed for the therapeutic use in man is 50–100 µmoles A 222/kg.

Abbreviations: A 222, hexaoxa-diaza-bicyclo-hexacosane; GOT, glutamic oxalacetic transaminase; GPT, glutamic pyruvic transaminase,

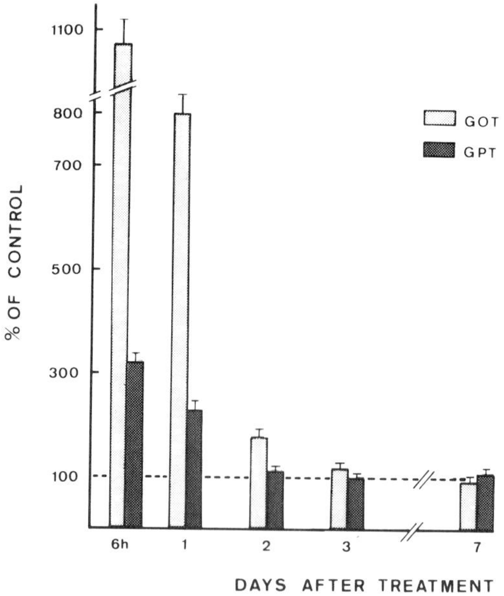

Fig. 1. Effect of a single dose of 500 µmoles A222/kg on the activities of GOT and GPT in rat serum

Methods

In short-term experiments, 6 weeks old male Wistar rats were treated with single doses of 50, 100, and 500 µmoles A 222/kg. Six hours and 1, 2, 3, and 7 days after application groups of six rats each were sacrificed and blood was collected for the subsequent investigations. GOT, GPT, and alkaline phosphatase activities were measured and the levels of cholesterol, protein and creatinine were determined in the rat serum. Histopathological examinations were carried out in all groups of animals, treated with the highest dose of 500 µmoles A 222/kg at 1–7 days after application. Immediately after sacrifice, tissues of the animals were excised and fixed in 4% formalin. They were embedded in paraffin and sections of 5 µm were stained with haematoxylin-eosin.

Results and Discussion

Even at 6 h after treatment with A 222, a marked dose-related increase in the activities of the transaminases GOT and GPT in rat serum was observed. At the same time the activity of GOT was elevated up to two, three and eleven times over that of the controls after the doses of 50, 100, and 500 µmoles A 222/kg, respectively. An increase of GPT levels up to 1.2-times and up to 3-times that of the control was found within 6 h after the application of 50 and 500 µmoles A 222/kg, respectively. This initial increase of GOT and GPT was followed by a rapid decrease during the first days after treatment. Within 3 days the activities of the enzymes returned to the control levels and remained unchanged up to 7

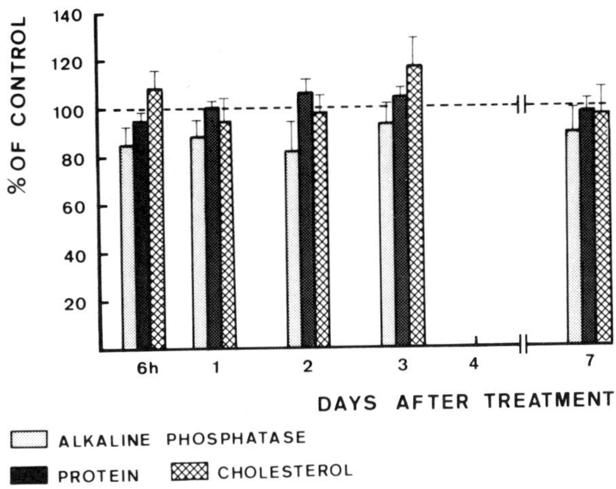

Fig. 2. Activity of alkaline phosphatase and levels of protein and cholesterol in rat serum after treatment with a single dose of 500 μmoles A222/kg

days after application. For clarity, in Fig. 1, only the data obtained with 500 μmoles A 222/kg are presented. The activity of alkaline phosphatase, the levels of protein and cholesterol as well as the concentration of creatinine in the serum were not altered throughout the experiment at any dose level. Again for the purpose of clarity the absence of any significant changes of these parameters is presented in Fig. 2 for the highest dose of 500 μmoles A 222/kg. The body weight gain, the liver and kidney weight did not show any changes when compared with the controls. The histopathological examinations of the liver, kidney, heart, lung, thymus, spleen, and large and small intestine did not show any substance related effects during the observation period of 1–7 days after treatment with the highest dose of 500 μmoles A 222/kg. The initial elevations of GOT and GPT, observed at the dose levels of 50–500 μmoles A 222/kg seem to be due to a degenerative change of the liver in an early stage of development. However, since no histopathological alterations of the liver became apparent during the 7 day observation period it is concluded, that these initial liver lesions are transient and of a low degree. These results suggest, that after single applications of low doses of A 222 no severe lesions occur in the observed organs.

References

Müller WH, Beaumatin J (1976) Distribution of a cryptating agent in excreta and its influence on urinary elimination of Na, K, Mg, Ca, and Zn in the rat. Life Sci 17: 1815–1820

Müller WH, Müller WA, Linzner U (1977) Enhanced $^{140}Ba/^{140}La$ excretion provoked by a cryptating agent in the rat. Naturwissenschaften 64: 96–97

Disease, Metabolism and Reproduction in the Toxic Response to Drugs and Other Chemicals
Arch. Toxicol., Suppl. 7, 430 (1984)

Evaluation of the Toxicological Risk in Animals Following the Ingestion of Cheese Obtained from Milk with Added Formaldehyde

M. Marinovich, P. Campagner, P. Restani, E. Tragni, and C. L. Galli

Institute of Pharmacology and Pharmacognosy, University of Milan, Via A. del Sartro, 21, 20129 Milan, Italy

Abstract. The epidemiological evidence concerning the carcinogenicity of formaldehyde (FA) to man, provides no proof of causal relationship between previous exposure and the occurrence of malignant neoplasma. The use of FA as an antimircobiol agent in food has caused concern mainly because of the lack of toxicological data about oral FA toxicity and because of the potential hazard caused by the stable reaction compounds between FA and food proteins. The aim of the present work was to study the absorption fate and excretion of the complex $H^{14}CHO$-milk protein in mice and rats. Unlabelled FA and C^{14}-FA were added to milk to obtain a final concentration of 35–40 ppm. Groups of rats and mice were given the ^{14}C-cheese obtained; 2.2 g (18 μCi) and 0.5 g (4.0 μCi) respectively and were killed at different times. Blood, liver, gastrointestinal tract, kidney, lungs, spleen, testes, muscle, and adipose tissue were removed; urine and faeces were collected from the metabolic chambers. Within 16–32 h after the administration, when radioactivity was almost completely excreted in the faeces and urine (65–70%), 25–30% of radioactivity was exhaled as CO_2 in both species. The radioactivity profile of blood indicated a maximum content corresponding to 0.08% and 0.3% of the dose per milliliter of blood for rats and mice respectively. No concentration of the ^{14}C-activity occurred in any of the tissues of either species. Although a study is in progress on the identification of radioactivity associated with the catabolites of ^{14}C-cheese, very likely represented by methylated aminoacids, the present opinion is that no hazard would result from the ingestion of cheese produced with such concentrations of formaldehyde.

Key words: Milk proteins – Formaldehyde – Cheese – Rats – Mice

Disease, Metabolism and Reproduction in the Toxic Response to Drugs and Other Chemicals
Arch. Toxicol., Suppl. 7, 431–434 (1984)

The Influence of Soil Particle Adsorption on 2,3,7,8-Tetrachlorodibenzo-p-dioxin Biological Uptake in the Rabbit

A. Bonaccorsi[1], A. di Domenico[2], R. Fanelli[1], F. Merli[2], R. Motta[1], R. Vanzati[2], and G. A. Zapponi[2]

[1] Istituto di Ricerche Farmacologiche "Mario Negri", Via Eritrea, 62, 20157 Milan, Italy
[2] Laboratorio di Tossicologia Comparata ed Ecotossicologia, Istituto Superiore di Sanità, Viale Regina Elena, 299, 00161 Rome, Italy

Abstract. A comparative study on the biological uptake in the rabbit of 2,3,7,8-tetrachloridibenzo-p-dioxin (TCDD) in different formulations, including accident-contaminated Seveso soil, was attempted. On the whole, these results indicated that soil-borne TCDD had a bioavailability lower than that of free (solvent-borne) TCDD.

Key words: 2,3,7,8-TCDD Uptake – Bioavailability – Seveso soil – ICMESA accident – Environmental TCDD

Introduction

TCDD (2,3,7,8-tetrachlorodibenzo-p-dioxin) is the most toxic of the polychlorodibenzodioxins and is generally an unwanted trace contaminant of the widely-produced 2,4,5-trichlorophenol. TCDD has also been formed in relatively high amounts in a number of industrial accidents of which the one that occurred at the ICMESA chemical plant at Seveso (Milan), in July 1976, is an example. This event yielded a widespread TCDD contamination of the environment and its extreme seriousness could still be appreciated over 5 years later as was shown by Pocchiari et al. (1983).

The literature offers many instances of toxicological studies on isolated TCDD normally aimed at evaluating its toxicity rather than its absorption (Poiger and Schlatter 1980). However, contact with TCDD in the environment most often involves the compound in a form bound to environmental substrata rather than as a pure chemical. Therefore, it was thought of interest to assess the effects of using different formulations of TCDD on its absorption in the rabbit. As the liver was known to be the main target organ for TCDD in such species (Fanelli et al. 1980a), the TCDD concentration in the liver was taken as a measure of uptake. TCDD was administered via gavage with different solvents and soils. Maximum uptake was assumed to be associated with solvent-administered TCDD and was taken as a reference to evaluate the relative bioavailability of soil-borne TCDD. Bioavailability may have a bearing on the assessment of the toxicological risk.

Analytical Methods

Determination of TCDD levels in soil was carried out by adapting a previously described gas chromatography-mass spectrometry GC-MS method (di Domenico et al. 1980) to small samples (~ 2 g) and using the following steps: Soxhlet extraction, and multilayer and alumina column chromatography. Determination of TCDD levels in the liver was carried out by applying a GC-MS method reported in the literature (Fanelli et al. 1980b) and using the following steps: alkaline digestion, extraction, and Kieselguhr and alumina column chromatography. Recoveries of analytical procedures are summarized in Table 1. The identity of TCDD in some pooled soil or pooled liver samples was ascertained by hrGC-MS (Buser and Rappe 1978). Purity of chemicals used was as per referenced papers.

Treatments and Results

(a) Soil was taken from a highly TCDD-contaminated area at Seveso. It was allowed to dry and then sieved to obtain a powder (200–400 mesh) which exhibited a mean TCDD content of 81 ± 8 ppb. (b) TCDD-free soil (200–400 mesh) was contaminated at 10 and 40 ppb TCDD levels by adding the toxicant in acetone which was allowed to evaporate prior to use. In some cases, contaminated soil samples were allowed to age for 30 days before use. (c) Solutions of TCDD in acetone-vegetable oil (1 : 6) and alcohol-water (1 : 1) had a titre of 20 and 40 ppb.

Albino male rabbits (2.6 ± 0.3 kg at sacrifice) were kept in individual cages for the entire period of the experiment. TCDD was administered by gavage every day for 7 days in any one of the formulations mentioned above. Soil (1–2 g) was given suspended with 10 ml water. The rabbits were sacrificed on the eight day and their livers assayed. Treatment results are shown in Table 2 (all figures rounded to two digits). It can be pointed out that at 40 and 80 ng/day, data from administration-homogeneous groups (i.e., alcohol or acetone-oil, soil, and again soil) were pooled to evaluate the final statistical figures shown in the table.

Conclusions

Table 3 summarizes the statistical appraisal (ANOVA and Duncan test) of TCDD bioavailability as estimated from Table 2 data, as follows:

a) No difference was observed between uptakes at the lowest administration level (20 ng/day) with either solvent or soil vehicles.

Table 1. Recoveries of analytical procedures

Item	No. of date	Recovery (%)
Multilayer column	67	96 ± 10
Alumina column	22	94 ± 5
TCDD-added soil	19	94 ± 14
TCDD-added soil (aged)	16	92 ± 8
TCDD(Cl^{37}), added to soil	28	94 ± 6
TCDD(Cl^{37}), added to liver	57	80 ± 10

Table 2. TCDD levels in rabbit liver after 7-day treatment

TCDD (ng/day)	Vehicle	No. of rabbits	TCDD (ppb) in the liver	
			$\bar{x} \pm \sigma$	Conf. int. (99%)
20	Acetone-oil	5	0.26 ± 0.07	0.12 ± 0.40
	Lab-contaminated soil	7	0.26 ± 0.08	0.15 ± 0.37
40	Alcohol or acetone-oil	16	1.1 ± 0.3	0.94 ± 1.3
	Lab-contaminated soil	13	0.81 ± 0.31	0.54 ± 1.1
80	Alcohol	5	2.7 ± 0.5	1.7 ± 3.8
	Lab-contaminated soil	10	1.5 ± 0.2	1.3 ± 1.8
	Seveso soil	7	0.88 ± 0.28	0.48 ± 1.3
160	Seveso soil	7	2.2 ± 1.0	0.84 ± 3.5

Table 3. Statistical evaluation of the bioavailability of soil-borne TCDD versus TCDD in solution (bioavailability: 100%)

TCDD (ng/day)	Item	Group difference meaningfulness	Relative decrease (%) $\bar{x}$	Conf. int. (99%)
20	Lab-contaminated soil	Not significant		
40	Lab-contaminated soil	$p < 0.01$	29	5.0–53
80	Lab-contaminated soil	$p < 0.01$	44	19 –68
80	Seveso soil	$p < 0.01$	68	40 –95

b) Uptake of soil-borne TCDD appeared to be an average of 29 and 44% lower than that of solvent-borne TCDD at 40 and 80 ng/day respectively. However, the lower confidence limits ($p < 0.01$) of such means appear at 5 and 19% only.

c) Uptake of Seveso soil-borne TCDD may be seen to be on average 68% lower than solvent-borne TCDD. Here again however, the lower confidence limit ($p < 0.01$) of the mean is only at 40%.

d) Statistical analysis of individual groups at the 40-ng/day administration level (unreported in this text) shows that no significant difference exists between data obtained with non-aged lab-contaminated soil and TCDD given in two solvent media out of three.

e) Two highly significant linear regressions can be determined on solvent-borne TCDD and lab-contaminated soil treatment data sets, respectively. These regressions allow extrapolated TCDD levels in liver to be estimated at 160 ng/day doses. Unlike the case for laboratory-contaminated soil, the value obtained, for the solvent-borne TCDD set, appears to be significantly higher than the Seveso soil value.

In summarizing, it may be said that, in the rabbit, uptake of soil-borne TCDD appears to be lower than that of solvent-borne TCDD. Differences in uptake are more evident at higher doses of TCDD.

Acknowledgements. The authors wish to express their appreciation to the Regione Lombardia, Ufficio Speciale di Seveso, for providing financial support for this research project.

References

Buser HR, Rappe C (1978) Identification of substitution patterns in polychlorinated dibenzo-p-dioxins (PCDDs) by mass spectrometry. Chemosphere 7: 199–211

di Domenico A, Silano V, Viviano G, Zapponi G (1980) Accidental release of 2,3,7,8-tetrachlorodibenzo-p-dioxin (TCDD) at Seveso, Italy: I. Sensitivity and specificity of analytical procedures adopted for TCDD assay. Ecotoxicol Environ Safety 4: 283–297

Fanelli R, Bertoni MP, Castelli MG et al. (1980a) 2,3,7,8-tetrachlorodibenzo-p-dioxin toxic effects and tissue levels in animals from the contaminated area of Seveso, Italy. Arch Environ Contam Toxicol 9: 569–577

Fanelli R, Bertoni MP, Bonfanti M et al. (1980b) Routine analysis of 2,3,7,8-tetrachlorodibenzo-p-dioxin in biological samples from the contaminated area of Seveso, Italy. Bull Environ Contam Toxicol 24: 818–823

Pocchiari F, di Domenico A, Silano V, Zapponi G (1983) Environmental impact of the accidental release of tetrachlorodibenzo-p-dioxin (TCDD) at Seveso (Italy). In: Human health aspects. Coulston F, Pocchiari F (eds) Accidental exposure to dioxins. Academic Press, New York, pp 5–35

Poiger H, Schlatter C (1980) Influence of solvents and adsorbents on dermal and intestinal absorption of TCDD. Food Cosmet Toxicol 18: 477–481

Disease, Metabolism and Reproduction in the Toxic Response to Drugs and Other Chemicals
Arch. Toxicol., Suppl. 7, 435–436 (1984)

The Subchronic Toxicity of 3,5-Dinitro-4-chloro-α,α,α-trifluorotoluene in the Rat

A. Macrì, A. R. Bucchi, C. Guastadisegni, F. Gramenzi, C. Ricciardi, and G. Salvatore

Laboratorio di Tossicologia Comparata ed Ecotossicologia, Istituto Superiore di Sanità, Viale Regina Elena, 299, 00161 Rome, Italy

Abstract. Since 1978 this department has been engaged in carrying out investigations on the acute and subchronic toxicity of 3,5-dinitro-4-chloro-α,α,α-trifluorotoluene (DNCTT) and 3-nitro-4-chloro-α,α,α-trifluorotoluene (NCTT) which in 1977 were detected as surface water contaminants in northern Italy. This paper is a progress report of an on-going study of the subchronic toxicity of DNCTT. Diets containing different levels of DNCTT (20; 200; 2,000 ppm) were administered to different groups of young male and female rats for 28 days. No animal deaths were observed at any dose levels. A slight reduction of body weight increase, and of food and water intake was observed in both male and female rats, particularly at the highest dose level tested (Fig. 1). A dose-related increase was observed in liver and spleen relative weights in both sexes, but it was significant ($p < 0.005$) only at the highest dose level (liver: m 6.6%, f 22.3%; spleen:

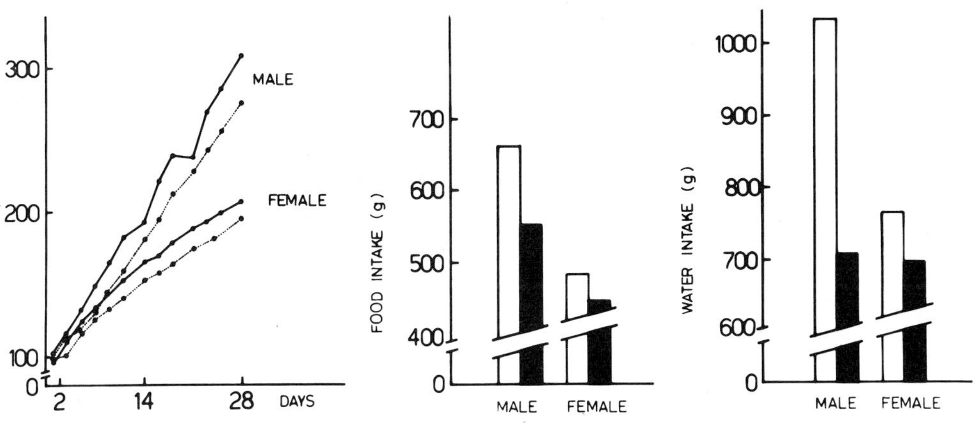

Fig. 1. Male ($p < 0.01$) and female ($p < 0.05$) body weight decrease at 2,000 ppm of DNCTT. Food and water intakes decrease (20% and 25%, respectively) at 2,000 ppm of DNCTT. ●——●, control; ●- - -●, DNCTT 2,000 ppm

m 41%, f 27%). Significant alterations were also seen in blood parameters. Glycemia was increased dose-dependently in both sexes (2,000 ppm: m 43%, f 66%) as were triglycerides in the treated females. Cholesterol and triglycerides were significantly higher (40.7% and 31.3% respectively) only in male animals treated with 2,000 ppm of DNCTT. Animals treated with this dose level also showed a significant decrease in haemoglobin (m 9.3%, f 12%) and erythrocyte count (m 5%, f 18%). Cage-side observations, carried out on a daily basis, did not show any major change in the treated animals with the exception of the finding a yellow coloration of urine and fur seen only at 2,000 ppm of DNCTT. The available findings on the toxicity of DNCTT are closely related to those observed in a previous similar investigation on the oral toxicity of NCTT and are consistant with a possible role of DNCTT as an inhibitor of the mitochondrial respiratory chain.

Key words: 3,5-Dinitro-n-chloro-α,α,α-trifluorotoluene benzotrifluorides – Rat – Subchronic toxicity

References

Benigni R, Bignami M, Conti L, Crebelli R, Dogliotti E, Falconi E, Carere A (1982) In vitro mutational studies with trifluralin and trifluorotoluene derivatives. Ann Ist Super Sanità 18: 123–126

Bucchi AR, Macrì A, Pellegrini N, Pisani A, Ricciardi C (to be published) Acute oral toxicity of 3-nitro-4-chloro-α,α,α-trifluorotoluene (NCTT) and of 3,5-dinitro-4-chloro-α,α,α-trifluorotoluene (DNCTT) on rat. Ann Ist Super Sanità

Pasquinelli F (1980) Diagnostica e tecniche di laboratorio, 2nd edn. Rosini, Firenze, pp 841–982

Schiller CM (1980) In vitro effects of substituted toluenes on mitochondria isolated from rat liver. Biochem Pharmacol 29: 2485–2489

Working group on criteria and guidelines for halogenated aromatic compounds. WHO, Venice 3–7 sept. 1979

Disease, Metabolism and Reproduction in the Toxic Response to Drugs and Other Chemicals
Arch. Toxicol., Suppl. 7, 437–439 (1984)

Trihalomethane in Drinking Waters: A Statistical Study

C. Cremisini, S. De Fulvio, L. Giannico, A. Piccioni, and G. A. Zapponi

Laboratorio Igiene del Territorio, Laboratorio Tossicologia Comparata ed Ecotossicologia, Istituto Superiore di Sanità, Viale Regina Elena, 299, 00161 Rome, Italy

Abstract. The formation of trihalomethane compounds (T.H.M.C.) in drinking water after chlorination is a cause of considerable health concern. This paper deals with a mathematical-statistical analysis of data obtained from a collaborative T.H.M.C. monitoring programme on several water distribution systems in Italy, carried out jointly by a number of Italian Public Institutions. Levels of T.H.M.C. were determined at different intervals after chlorination treatment. As far as levels of T.H.M.C. determined 1–3 hours after chlorination are concerned, a statistically-significant increase of chloroform ($CHCl_3$), dichlorobromomethane ($CHCl_2Br$), and dibromochloromethane ($CHClBr_2$) levels (as an average, respectively $\simeq$ 300%, $\simeq$200%, $\simeq$ 30%), was detected. Levels of $CHCl_3$, $CHCl_2Br$ and $CHClBr_2$ in chlorinated waters appeared correlated with those of Total Organic Carbon (T.O.C) in water before chlorination as well as with those of water residual

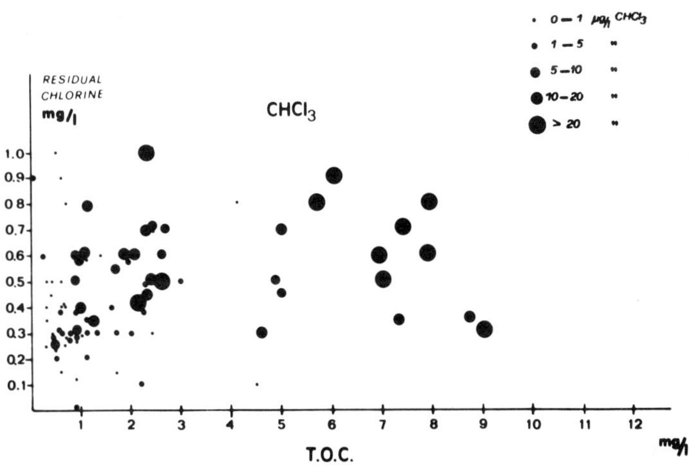

Fig. 1. Increase of $CHCl_3$ with the increase of T.O.C. and residual chlorine values

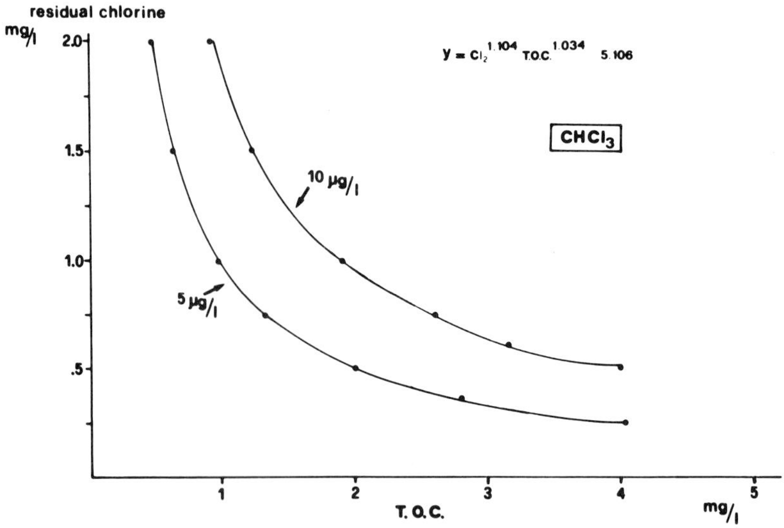

Fig. 2. $CHCl_3$ functions derived from regression analysis with fixed T.H.M. levels

chlorine (Fig. 1). Water temperature was positively related to formation of $CHCl_3$ and $CHCl_2Br$. Finally, an increase of water pH also resulted in an increase of $CHCl_3$. The formation of the three above organochlorinated compounds appeared to follow a substantially identically pattern. As far as the levels of T.H.M.C. determined 24 and 72 hours after the chlorination treatment, they were, as an average, 1.5–2.3 and 1.6–2.8 times higher, thus showing that formation of organohalogens takes place to a large extent within a short interval of the water treatment. A mathematical model of the T.H.M.C. formation was carried out (Fig. 2).

Key words: Trihalomethane – Drinking waters – Mathematical model – T.O.C. – Chlorination – Statistical analysis

References

Bellar TA, Lichtenberg JJ, Kroner RC (1974) The occurrence of organohalides in chlorinated drinking waters. J AWWA December: 703–706

Carns KE, Stinson B (1978) Controlling organics: The East Bay Municipal utility District experience. J AWWA November: 637–644

Cohen RS, Hwang CJ, Krasner SW (1978) Controlling organics: The Metropolitan water District of Southern California experience. J AWWA November: 647–652

Cooley W, Lohnes PR (1971) Multivariate analysis. Wiley & Sons, New York

Cotruvo JA (1981) T.H.M.s in drinking waters. ES & T 15: 268–274

EPA (1979) National interim primary drinking water regulations control of trihalomethane in drinking water; final rule. Federal Register 44/231: 68624–68705

Jekel MR, Roberts PV (1980) Total organichalogen as a parameter for the characterization of reclaimed waters: Measurement, occurrence, formation and removal. ES & T 14/8: 970–975

Lison L (1961) Statistica applicata alla biologia sperimentale. Ambrosiana, Milano

McBride DG (1978) Controlling organics: The Los Angeles Department of water and power experience. J AWWA November: 644–646

Nelson SJ, Khalifa S (1980) Trihalomethane levels in public suppliers drawn from Sacramento river system. J AWWA July: 423–426

Quaghebeur D, De Wulf E (1980) Volatile halogenated hydrocarbons in Belgian drinking waters. Sci Total Environ 14: 43–52

Rook JJ (1977) Chlorination reactions of fulvic acids in natural waters. ES & T 11/5: 478–482

Senter RJ (1969) Analysis of data. Scott, Foresman, Glenview

Symons JM, Bellar TA et al. (1975) National organic reconnaissance survey for halogenated organics. J AWWA November: 634–647

Trussel RR, Umphres MD (1978) The formation of trihalomethanes. J AWWA November: 604–612

Veenstra JM, Schnoor JL (1980) Seasonal variations in trihalomethane levels in Iowa river water supply. J AWWA October: 583–590

Disease, Metabolism and Reproduction in the Toxic Response to Drugs and Other Chemicals
Arch. Toxicol., Suppl. 7, 440 (1984)

Inhalation Toxicology: Correlation Between the Concentration of the Test Compound and the Exposure Time Using Carbon Tetrachloride

T. W. McSheehy, A. Nunziata, P. Mercatelli, A. Argentino, and R. O. Salerno

L.S.R. Roma Toxicology Centre, 00040 Pomezia, Rome, Italy

Abstract. In order to determine the toxic effects of a compound administered by the inhalation route it is frequently necessary to employ exposure periods of long duration. It is of interest, therefore, to establish whether or not an inverse relationship exists between exposure time and the concentration of the test compound. Here some preliminary data on the toxicity of carbon tetrachloride when administered to rats via the inhalation route is presented. Exposure of the rats was performed with whole body equipment and the concentration of carbon tetrachloride (CCl_4) in the air stream was routinely monitored. The rats were exposed once on each of 5 consecutive days. Blood samples were taken at the end of this period and the haematological and blood chemistry parameters were analysed. Samples of lung, trachea, stomach, liver, and kidney were processed for histopathological evaluation. The results of the biochemical analyses (see Table) indicated that the toxicity was a function of the total concentration of CCl_4 absorbed. These data suggest that a threshold exists at the highest doses administered during the shortest exposure time, resulting in a decrease in toxicity.

Table

CCl_4 (ppm)	h exp.	Enzymatic activities			
		SGOT	SGPT	Alk. phos.	LDH
0	4	52 ± 2.7	31 ± 1.7	80 ± 7.2	195 ± 22.3
2.5	4	496* ± 78.7	227* ± 39.3	72 ± 4.9	2 093* ± 325.7
5.0	4	602* ± 63.0	302* ± 33.6	86 ± 4.4	2 626* ± 200.3
10.0	1	275* ± 21.2	198* ± 75.0	66 ± 4.7	673 ± 122.5

Means ± SE; * p 0.05

Key words: Inhalation – Carbon tetrachloride – Rats

Reference

Phalen RF (1976) Inhalation exposure of animal. Environ Health Perspect 16: 17–26

Disease, Metabolism and Reproduction in the Toxic Response to Drugs and Other Chemicals
Arch. Toxicol., Suppl. 7, 441–443 (1984)

Circulating Concentrations of Testosterone, Luteinizing Hormone and Follicle Stimulating Hormone in Male Rats After Inhalation of Methanol

A. M. Cameron[1], O. G. Nilsen[2], E. Haug[3], and K. B. Eik-Nes[1]

[1] Division of Biophysics, The Norwegian Institute of Technology, Trondheim, Norway
[2] Department of Pharmacology and Toxicology, University of Trondheim, Trondheim, Norway
[3] Aker Hospital, Oslo, Norway

Abstract. Male mature rats were examined for alterations in circulating free testosterone, luteinizing hormone (LH) and follicle-stimulating hormone (FSH) after inhalation of methanol vapour in a dynamic system for up to 6 weeks at doses ranging 200 ppm to 10,000 ppm. The most extensive effects were observed after exposure to 200 ppm of methanol for 6 weeks with serum testosterone concentrations being 32% of the controls. A significant change in LH concentration after exposure to 10,000 ppm of methanol for 6 weeks was also demonstrated. FSH remained unchanged throughout these experiments. Such exposure did not change the elimination rate of testosterone from blood which indicated effects on the testicular synthesis of testosterone.

Key words: Methanol inhalation – Reproductive function – Testosterone – Follicle stimulating hormone – Luteinizing hormone

Due to the many uses of methanol in industry and its employment as a potential substitute in petrol, effects of inhaled methanol on the male reproductive system are of significance. The changes in testicular function have been explored following the inhalation of methanol in male, mature rats.

Groups of five male, mature Sprague-Dawley rats were exposed in inhalation chambers to methanol vapours in concentrations of 200, 2,000 and 10,000 ppm for 1, 2, 4, and 6 weeks. Control animals were subjected to air only. The animals were exposed 8 h a day, 5 days a week and the chamber temperature varied between 20° and 22° C with a relative humidity of 40–60%. No food or water were allowed during the 8 h exposure. The steady state levels of methanol during the exposure were 10,000 ppm ± 400, 2,000 ppm ± 100 and 200 ppm ± 10. Sixteen hours after the last exposure, the animals were sacrified using CO_2. Blood for the measurement of the serum values of testosterone, LH and FSH was taken from the heart immediately after sacrifice. Measurements of the circulating hormones were performed by standard radioimmunoassay procedures. Student's *t*-test was used and *p*-values less than 0.05 were considered significant. Methanol p.a. was purchased from Merck and was 99.5% pure.

Significant effect on levels of circulating free testosterone was demonstrated after 2 and 6 weeks at a concentration of 200 ppm (260 mg/m^3 ≡ TLV) and after 6 weeks at a concentration of 2,000 ppm methanol (Table 1). Significant augmentation in circulating LH was demonstrated only after 6 weeks exposure to 10,000 ppm. No significant change was found with respect to concentrations of circulating FSH in any group of animals.

Male mature rats were exposed to methanol at a dosage level of 200 ppm for 6 weeks and then injected intravenously (i.v.) with ^{14}C-testosterone (58 mCi/mmol C^{14}-testosterone) 3 μCi per animal 16 h after the last exposure. The radioactive steroid was purchased from Amersham and purified by chromatography before use. Groups of five animals were sacrified by decapitation 1, 2, 4, and 6 h after i.v. injection, and the plasma concentrations of ^{14}C-testosterone determined. The testosterone metabolism of the methanol exposed animals was the same as that of the controls.

No change in circulating LH and FSH was seen at exposure levels of 200 and 2,000 ppm methanol for 6 weeks which makes an effect at the hypothalamic-hypophyseal axis unlikely. Thus exposure to 200 ppm methanol for 6 weeks will lower testicular production of testosterone. Rats subjected to 10,000 ppm methanol for 6 weeks showed a significant increase in circulating LH, pointing to a possible decrease, at this dose of methanol, of LH metabolism, and a decreased testicular use of LH or both. It has been reported that ingestion of ethanol in rats will result in a reduced amount of testicular enzymes involved in testosterone production (Chiao et al. 1981). Elevated blood concentrations of either endogenous or exogenous adrenal steroids will decrease testicular

Table 1. Effects of inhaled methanol on the serum concentration of testosterone, LH, and FSH in male mature rats

Methanol (ppm)	Length of exposure			
	1 week	2 weeks	4 weeks	6 weeks
Testosterone				
0	100 ± 25	100 ± 22.3	100 ± 16	100 ± 23
200	98 ± 33	55 ± 17*	79.2 ± 22	32 ± 31*
2,000	115 ± 38	74 ± 8.8	73 ± 16	59 ± 18*
10,000	152 ± 43	111 ± 32	83 ± 20	119 ± 45
LH				
0	100 ± 25	Not done	Not done	100 ± 20
200	70 ± 14	Not done	Not done	83 ± 60
2,000	Not done	Not done	Not done	120 ± 110
10,000	80.3 ± 14	Not done	Not done	311 ± 107*
FSH				
0	100 ± 17	Not done	Not done	100 ± 26
200	91 ± 7.4	Not done	Not done	106 ± 15.5
2,000	Not done	Not done	Not done	125 ± 24
10,000	84.3 ± 8.3	Not done	Not done	105 ± 17

Mean concentration of hormones ± SD are given in % of respective controls (n = 5); * $p < 0.05$

testosterone production (Gabrilove et al. 1979; McKenna et al. 1979; Welsh and Johnson 1981). A direct inhibitory effect of glucocorticoids on testicular function has also been shown (Bambino and Hsueh 1981). It is, however, not known whether inhalation of methanol results in increased adrenal function in rats or not. These data demonstrate that inhalation of methanol at a dosage equal to the 200 ppm threshold limit value in industry causes a depression of free circulating testosterone in male rats. This effect seems due to decreased testicular formation of testosterone. A possible effect of methanol inhalation on increased adrenocortical function (Bambino and Hsueh 1981) should, however, not be overlooked.

References

Bambino TH, Hsueh AJW (1981) Direct inhibitory effect of glucocorticoids upon testicular luteinizing hormone receptor and steroidogenesis in vivo and in vitro. Endocrinology 108 : 2142–2148

Chiao Y, Johnston DE, Gavaler JS, Van Thiel DH (1981) Effect of chronic ethanol feeding on testicular content of enzymes required for testosteronogenesis. Alcoholism 5 : 230–236

Gabrilove JL, Nicolis GL, Sohval AR (1979) The testis in Cushing's syndrome. J Urol 112 : 95–99

Mckenna TJ, Lorber D, Lacroix A, Rabin D (1979) Testicular activity in Cushing's disease. Acta Endocrinol (Kbh) 91 : 501–509

Welsh TH, Johnson BH (1981) Stress induced alterations in secretion of corticosteroids, progesterone, luteinizing hormone and testosterone in bulls. Endocrinology 109 : 185–190

Disease, Metabolism and Reproduction in the Toxic Response to Drugs and Other Chemicals
Arch. Toxicol., Suppl. 7, 444–445 (1984)

The Effect of Sodium Selenite on Respiratory Function in Mitochondria Isolated from Guinea Pig Heart

G. Ignesti[1], G. Antonini[1], F. Bennardini[1], R. Matucci[1], G. Dini[2], and F. Franconi[1]

[1] Istituto Interfacoltà di Farmacologia e Tossicologia, Universitá degli Studi di Firenze, Florence, Italy
[2] Istituto di Patologia Generale, Università degli Studi di Firenze, Florence, Italy

Abstract. It is known that sodium selenite produces cardiac mitochondrial alterations in vivo and in vitro (Franconi et al. 1980; Dini et al. 1981, 1982). The effect of sodium selenite are reversed by pyruvate administration in vitro and pyruvate treatment also prevented the mitochondrial lesions produced by sodium selenite in vivo. The oxygen consumption of guinea-pig heart isolated mitochondria was studied with glutamate (10 mM) or malate-pyruvate (5 and 10 mM, respectively) as substrates. Sodium selenite (0.1–00.1 mM) significantly reduced (47%–14%) the respiratory control index (RCI) in a dose-dependent manner with glutamate as substrate; on the other hand in the presence of malate-pyruvate no significant difference was observed between the controls and the selenite-treated mitochondria. Moreover, the transaminase and cytochrome-oxidase activities were not changed either in the sodium selenite-treated or the control mitochondria. The above findings suggest that the effects of sodium selenite on mitochondrial oxygen uptake are exerted in a step in which glutamate but not pyruvate-malate are involved.

Key words: Sodium selenite – Respiratory function – Mitochondria – Guinea pig – Heart

Acknowledgments. This research was supported by CNR grant 82.002247.56 PF. MP.

References

Dini G, Franconi F, Martini F (1981) Mitochondrial alterations induced by selenium in guinea-pig myocardium. Exp Mol Pathol 34: 226–235

Dini G, Martini F, Standardi I, Bennardini F, Franconi F (1982) Time course of sodium selenite-induced ultrastructural alterations in guinea-pig hearts. Exp Mol Pathol 36: 326–332

Franconi F, Manghi N, Giotti A, Martini F, Dini G (1980) Effect of selenium on the contractile force of isolated and perfused guinea-pig heart. Acta Pharmacol Toxicol 46: 98–104

Khan MY, Gilani SH (1980) Selenium poisoning and embryogenesis: Light and electron microscopic studies of heart. Environ Res 23: 98–109

Lowry OH, Rosebrough NJ, Farr AL, Randall RJ (1951) Protein measurement with the folin phenol reagent. J Biol Chem 193: 265–275

Sobel B, Jequier E, Sjoerdsma A, Lovemberg W (1966) Effect of catecholamines and adrenergic blocking agents on oxidative phosphorilation in rat heart mitochondria. Circ Res 29: 1050–1061

Disease, Metabolism and Reproduction in the Toxic Response to Drugs and Other Chemicals
Arch. Toxicol., Suppl. 7, 446–450 (1984)

Intestinal Absorption and Excretion of Thallium (^{201}Tl) in the Rat

E. Sabbioni[1], A. Di Nucci[2], J. Edel[1], C. Gregotti[2], E. Marafante[1], and L. Manzo[3]

[1] Radiochemistry and Nuclear Chemistry Division,
Commission of the European Communities Joint Research Centre, Ispra, Italy
[2] 2nd Institute of Pharmacology and
[3] Chair of Toxicology, University of Pavia Medical School, Piazza Botta 10, 27100 Pavia, Italy

Abstract. The gastrointestinal transport of ^{201}Tl-labelled monovalent thallium has been studied in normal and rats with cannulated bile ducts using an in vivo ligated loop technique. A marked difference in the Tl absorptive capacity among the various sections of the gut was observed. ^{201}Tl was taken up more quickly from the colon than from any other segment and the uptake from the ileum and jejunum was higher than from the stomach. In addition, considerable amounts of the intravenously administered thallium were excreted into the intestinal lumen. The biliary excretion was very low compared with the direct transfer of ^{201}Tl across the gastrointestinal wall that occurred against a tissue-to-plasma concentration gradient. In the rat, the large intestine seems to be the major area for the enteral reabsorption and recycling of thallium (I) ions.

Key words: Thallium – Gastrointestinal tract – Enteral recycling – Biliary excretion – Absorption

Thallium is a cumulative toxic element which is rapidly absorbed after ingestion and is eliminated in remarkable quantities with the feces after parenteral administration to rats (Sabbioni and Manzo 1980). Thallium is very slowly excreted from the body. It has been detected for weeks or months in excreta (urine and feces) of both laboratory animals and humans after a single-dose exposure (Smith and Carson 1977; Van der Stock and De Schepper 1978). A mechanism of enteral recycling contributing to the prolonged body retention of this element has been suggested (Rauws 1974). Accordingly, the repeated oral administration of Prussian Blue, an agent forming with thallium a non-absorbable complex in the gut, accelerated the fecal elimination of the intravenously injected thallium and increased the survival of thallium-intoxicated rats (Heydlauf 1969; Manninen et al. 1976).

Correspondence should be addressed to Dr. L Manzo

The present study was conducted to determine and compare the sites of thallium (I) absorption and excretion in the rat gastro-intestinal tract.

Materials and Methods

Female rats of the COBS strain (Charles River, Calco, Italy) weighing 240–260 g were used in these experiments. ^{201}Tl was prepared carrier-free by proton activation of an Hg target in the cyclotron of Milan University. The preparative procedures and methods for the assessment of Tl radiochemical purity have been reported elsewhere (Edel-Rade et al. 1981).

The animals were deprived of food, but not water, for 16 h prior to the beginning of the experiment. Under sodium pentobarbital anesthesia, the peritoneal cavity was opened and ligated segments of the proximal jejunum, distal ileum and colon were prepared as described by Sasser et al. (1978). The stomach was also ligated at the pylorus and the esophagus. The intestines were cleared of contents by repeated washing with saline (38° C). Body temperature was maintained at 36–38° C by a heating lamp regulated by continuous rectal temperature measurements. Thallium was injected intravenously or directly instilled into the individual gastrointestinal segments in doses ranging from 2 μg to 2,000 μg Tl/rat as ^{201}Tl-labelled thallium sulphate. 0.25 ml and 1.0 ml volumes of a saline solution with pH adjusted to 7.2 were used for the intravenous injection and intestinal instillation of thallium, respectively. At various time intervals after dosing (5–240 min) the animals were killed by exsanguination. The loops were dissected free of mesenteric tissue, weighed and then measured by direct gamma-counting. Blood, liver, kidney, and lung were also taken for ^{201}Tl analysis.

In a separate group of rats, the bile duct was exposed and cannulated with PE 10 tubing. Thallium was injected intraperitoneally in doses ranging from 2 μg Tl/rat to 10.5 mg Tl/rat as ^{201}Tl thallium sulphate. Bile was collected during timed intervals and the biliary excretion of the radiotracer was measured during the initial 240-min period after dosing.

Results

Figure 1 illustrates the absorption of thallium from ligated segments of the rat gut over a 60 min period after instillation of 20 μg of ^{201}Tl-labelled thallium. Marked regional differences in the absorptive capacity of the individual gastrointestinal sites were observed. ^{201}Tl was taken up more quickly from the colonic segment than from any other segment, and the uptake from the jejunum and ileum was higher than from the stomach. The accumulation of ^{201}Tl-derived radioactivity was measured in tissues and carcasses 60 min after dosing as an index of the isotope absorption. As the dose was increased from 2 μg Tl to 2,000 μg Tl a proportional increase of thallium concentrations in the tissues was noted.

Direct secretion of thallium into the gut was indicated by the appearance of ^{201}Tl radioactivity in the lumen of ligated gastrointestinal segments of the

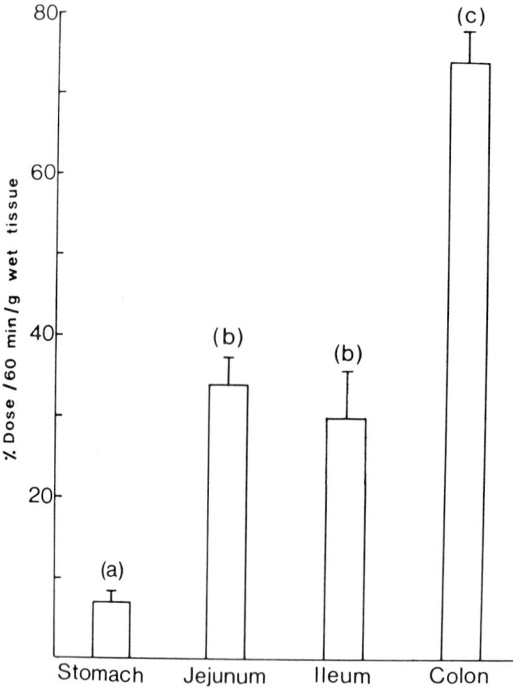

Fig. 1. ^{201}Tl absorption from ligated gastrointestinal segments 60 min after instillation of 20 μg of ^{201}Tl thallium. Each value represents the mean ± SE of four to five rats. Bars not marked by the same letter indicate significantly different values ($p < 0.05$)

Table 1. Secretion of thallium in in vivo isolated segments of the gastrointestinal tract. Percentage of dose appeared in the gut lumen 60 min after the administration of 20μg Tl/rat i. v. (n = 4 to 5 experiments ± SE)

Segment	^{201}Tl Secretion	
	dose/g wet tissue (%)	Dose/cm (%)
Stomach	0.83 ± 0.09	
Jejunum	2.05 ± 0.25	0.272 ± 0.032
Ileum	1.53 ± 0.19	0.301 ± 0.017
Colon	1.20 ± 0.23	0.448 ± 0.034

animals injected with the radiotracer intravenously (Table 1). The transfer of thallium into the loops occurred against a tissue-to-plasma concentration gradient at all of the thallium doses tested.

Figure 2 depicts representative data of the biliary excretion of thallium in rats given 20 μg Tl/rat intraperitoneally. Less than 0.12% and 0.3% of the thallium dose was excreted in bile within 1 h and 4 h, respectively. During the initial 4-h post injection period, the bile-to-plasma ^{201}Tl concentration ratios were approximately at unity and the ^{201}Tl biliary excretion rate exhibited a rapid decay. An identical pattern of thallium excretion into the bile was seen at all of the dosage levels tested. No changes in the biliary flow were found in animals injected with thallium at doses as high as 10.5 mg Tl/rat.

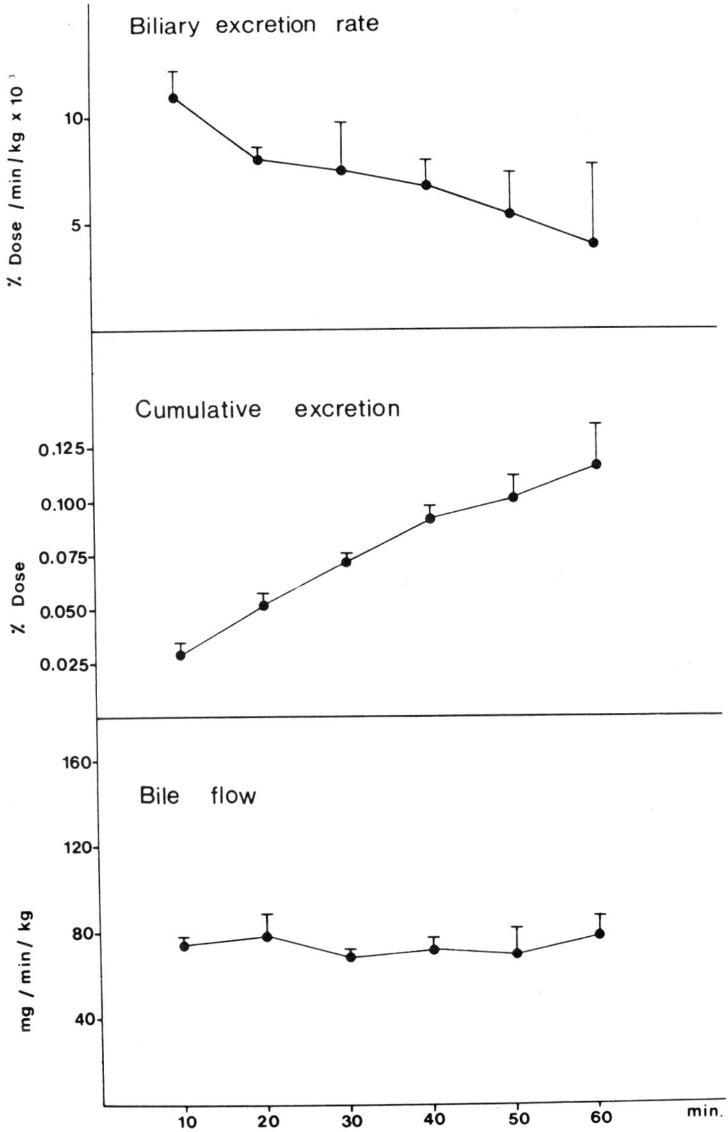

Fig. 2. ^{201}Tl biliary excretion after the i.p. administration of 20 µg Tl/rats as ^{201}Tl-labelled thallium sulphate. Mean ± SE of four experiments

Discussion

Recent studies (Schäfer et al. 1981) on unidirectional movements of thallium (I) ions across the mucosal epithelium of descending rat colon have demonstrated a thallium transfer by diffusion from the mucosal to the serosal side as well as active thallium transport from serosa to mucosa occurring against an electrochemical gradient. In the present work, all sections of the rat gastrointestinal tract were functional with respect to the absorption of monovalent thallium and marked regional differences were noted. The colon proved to be a major absorptive segment and the trend for ^{201}Tl uptake from the various sites was as follows: colon > jejunum and ileum > stomach. Moreover, appreciable levels of ^{201}Tl-derived radioactivity were detected in the gut after i.v. injection of the radiotracer. The biliary excretion of thallium was very low. 4 h after the administration, the cumulative recovery of ^{201}Tl in the bile was less than 0.3% of the dose. At this time up to 8% of the injected thallium was found in the gut segments (stomach and intestine plus their contents) of the bile duct cannulated rats. This suggests a direct transport of thallium across the gastrointestinal wall as a major pathway for the passage of thallium from the plasma to the digestive tract.

In mammals, almost all thallium ions are concentrated into the cells and only a small fraction of the body load is retained in plasma and extracellular fluid (Sabbioni et al. 1980). It may be assumed that the thallium concentration gradient between the intestine and plasma promotes the reabsorption of the element from the various sections of the gut so that only a limited proportion of the intestinal thallium becomes available for elimination in feces. Due to the intensive thallium uptake from the colon, the large intestine probably represents the most important section for the reabsorption and enteral recycling of thallium in the rat.

Acknowledgment. This work was in part supported by the National Research Council (CNR), Roma. Res. Project "Controllo del Rischio Tossicologico".

References

Edel-Rade J, Sabbioni E, Manzo L (1981) Environmental toxicology research on thallium. Metabolic and toxicological studies in the rat. Commission of the European Communities Official Report, Rep EUR 7604 EN

Heydlauf H (1969) Ferric-cyanoferrate (II): An effective antidote in thallium poisoning. Eur J Pharmacol 6: 340–344

Manninen V, Mäikönen M, Skulskii IA (1976) Elimination of thallium in rats as influenced by Prussian Blue and sodium chloride. Arch Toxicol 39: 256–261

Rauws AG (1974) Thallium pharmacokinetics and its modification by Prussian Blue. Naunyn-Schmiedebergs Arch Pharmacol 284: 295–306

Sabbioni E, Manzo L (1980) Metabolism and toxicity of thallium. In: Manzo L (ed) Advances in neurotoxicology. Pergamon, Oxford New York, pp 249–270

Sabbioni E, Goetz L, Marafante E, Gregotti C, Manzo L (1980) Metabolic fate of different inorganic and organic species of thallium in the rat. Sci Total Environ 15: 123–128

Sasser LB, Jarboe GE, Walter BK, Kelman BJ (1978) Absorption of mercury from ligated segments of the rat gastrointestinal tract. Proc Soc Exp Biol Med 157: 57–60

Schäfer SG, Nell G, Henning CH (1981) Movement of thallium (I) ions in vitro. Arch Toxicol 48: 271–279

Smith IC, Carson BL (1977) Trace elements in the environment. I. Thallium. Ann Arbor Sci Publ, Ann Arbor, Michigan, pp 309–325

Van der Stock J, De Schepper J (1978) The effect of Prussian Blue and sodium ethylendiaminetetraacetic acid on the faecal and urinary elimination of thallium by the dog. Res Vet Sci 25: 337–342

Disease, Metabolism and Reproduction in the Toxic Response to Drugs and Other Chemicals
Arch. Toxicol., Suppl. 7, 451–452 (1984)

Evaluation of Pollution Levels by Analysis of the Pesticide Residues in Algerian Sheep

B. Alamir[1], A. Venant[2], and L. Richou Bac[2]

[1] Laboratory of Toxicology, Institute of Pharmacy, University of Algiers, Algeria
[2] Department of Physico-Chemistry II, Central Laboratory of Alimentary Hygien, Paris, France

Abstract. In Algeria, some organochlorine pesticides such as hexachlorocyclohexane, lindane and dichlorodiphenyltrichloroethane are still in use. The present study was designed as a first evaluation of the pollution level by the chlorinated residues in the Algerian sheep. For this evaluation, the kidney fat was chosen.

Key words: Pesticides residues – Hexachlorocyclohexane – Dichlorodiphenyltrichloroethane – Sheep fat

130 samples of sheep fat were collected from five regions (Table 1). All kidney fat, once sampled, was packed in aluminium foil; contact with container or wrapping material made of plastic was avoided to prevent any contamination by polychlorinated biphenyls or phtalates (Mestres et al. 1966). The samples were stored at −20° C until assay.

To proceed to the quantitative analysis of the samples, the low temperature method developed by Venant et al. (1982) was used. Its principle rests on extraction of fat and residues (using a mix of acetonitrile and dichloromethane: 3/1 and centrifuging at −15° C) followed by purification on florisil. The determination of residues was made by gas chromatography; two columns were used, the first packed with 5% DOW-Chromosorb W AW-DMCS, the second, with 5% QF_1-Chromosorb W AW-DMCS. The working conditions were as follows: column temperature: 190° C; injection temperature: 220° C; E.C. detector temperature: 300° C; carrier gas: nitrogen at a flow rate of 30 ml/min; sample volume: 5 µl.

The results are presented in Table 1. No residue of heptachlor epoxide was found; dieldrin has not been detected. Only residues of HCH isomers (α, β, γ)

Abbreviations: HCH, Hexachlorocyclohexane; γ-HCH, lindane; DDT, dichlorodiphenyltrichloroethane; DDE, dichlorodiphenyldichloroethane; AW-DMCS, acid-washed dimethyldichlorosilane, treated

Table 1. Chlorinated pesticides content in ovine fat tissues (ppb)

Regions	Samples (*n*)	Average			Total HCH		DDT + Metabolites	
		α HCH	β HCH	γ HCH	X	R	X	R
Biskra (South)	26	17	100	25	142	20–240	60	20–125
Chellala (Center)	29	15	15	13	43	ND–90	50	20–200
El-Eulma (Center-East)	18	8	12	9	29	ND–30	40	25– 70
Souk-Ahras (East)	29	10	12	10	32	ND–30	60	30–130
Tebessa (East)	30	6	8	6	20	ND–50	16	ND–50

X = average R = range ND = not detectable (< 5 ppb)

have been found, as well as residues of DDT (essentially DDE, the main DDT metabolite in the ovine species). To make the interpretation of results easier, only total HCH isomers are given. For the same reason, only the amount calculated for DDT and its metabolites is given.

Among the five regions studied it will be noted that the Tebessa region is the least polluted and the Biskra region the most contaminated. The different levels seem perfectly related to the anti-insect campaigns undertaken in Algeria. In the Tebessa region anti-insect campaigns are not systematic whereas they are undertaken every year elsewhere. All the figures are well below the internationally accepted norms set by FAO/OMS and Codex Alimentarius: DDT+metabolites-5ppm,HCH-2ppm (Codex Alimentarius Commission 1978).

Finally, it cannot be claimed that the results are representative of the pollution level of the Algerian ovine stock because the samples are coming from only five regions; however they can be taken as a preliminary estimation which may show the worth of extending the study.

References

Codex Alimentarius Commission (1978) Guide concernant les limites maximales Codex pour les residus de pesticides, 1. ed. FAO/OMS, Rome, pp 1–233

Mestres R, Barthes F, Priu M (1966) Résidus de pesticides, sur une cause d'erreur dans la recherche des insecticides organochlorés. Trav Soc Pharm Montpellier 26: 93–98

Venant A, Borrel S, Richou Bac L (1982) Méthode rapide pour la détermination des résidus de composés organo-chlorés dans les produits laitiers et les graisses animales. Analusis 10: 333–335

Miscellaneous Toxic Effects

Disease, Metabolism and Reproduction in the Toxic Response to Drugs and Other Chemicals
Arch. Toxicol., Suppl. 7, 455–458 (1984)

A 2′Guanidyl Derivative of Gentamicin (S86451) with Reduced Nephrotoxicity: Studies at Low and Medium Dose Levels in the Rat

P. Maldague[1], G. Laurent[2], M. B. Carlier[2], and P. Tulkens[2]

[1] Laboratoire de Pathologie et Cytologie expérimentales, Université Catholique de Louvain, Avenue Mounier, 52, 1200 Brussels, Belgium
[2] Laboratoire de Chimie physiologique and International Institute of Cellular and Molecular Pathology, Université Catholique de Louvain, Avenue Hippocrate, 75, 1200 Brussels, Belgium

Abstract. The nephrotoxic potential of S86451 (2′guanidyl, 2′deamino gentamicin C_1) has been investigated in Sprague-Dawley rats at 10 and 25 mg/kg, in comparison with gentamicin at 4 and 10 mg/kg. The criteria were (i) the severity of the lysosomal phospholipidosis, as assessed by both biochemical and morphological investigations; (ii) the degree of tubular regeneration, a consequence of the aminoglycoside-induced focal necrosis measured by ^{3}H-thymidine incorporation into kidney cortex DNA. S86451 was found at least 2–5 times less toxic than gentamicin. Thus, this compound should be a safer antibiotic than gentamicin in combating organisms with a similar sensitivity to either drug.

Key words: Aminoglycoside – Nephrotoxicity – Phospholipidosis – Regeneration – Gentamicin – S86451

A severe limitation in the use of aminoglycosides is their nephrotoxicity. Animal studies have demonstrated that aminoglycosides are accumulated by the kidney cortex and localize in the lysosomes of the proximal tubular cells, after pinocytic uptake from the luminal fluid (Just et al. 1977). The first conspicuous alteration concerns the lysosomes of proximal tubular cells, which show morphological evidence of phospholipidosis (Kosek et al. 1974). Gentamicin inhibits lysosomal phospholipases, both in vivo and in vitro; in vivo, a loss of activity of sphingomyelinase has also been demonstrated (Laurent et al. 1982). Lysosomal phospholipidosis is associated with early focal necrosis of proximal tubular cells, and concomitant tissue regeneration (Laurent et al. 1984). These alterations can be quantified in animals treated with low doses of gentamicin (4–10 mg/kg) for 10 days or less, i.e., under conditions close to the clinical use of this drug. The importance of toxicological evaluation at low doses has been stressed by Hottendorf et al. (1981) and Laurent et al. (1984).

A report is presented here on toxicological studies with a new derivative of gentamicin (S86451 [2′guanidyl, 2′deamino gentamicin C_1] from Sandoz

Table 1. Biochemical evaluation of the lysosomal alterations (phospholipidosis) induced by S86451 and gentamicin. All values are expressed in % ± SD of matched controls

	Drug			
	S86451		Gentamicin	
	Dose (mg/kg daily)			
	10	25	4	10
4 Days treatment				
Sphingomyelinase	88.1 ± 3.6**	76.3 ± 5.0**	84.4 ± 6.8**	74.8 ± 7.6*
Phospholipase A_1	99.6 ± 9.2	91.8 ± 11.5	93.1 ± 5.1	89.6 ± 8.9
Phospholipids	96.5 ± 3.8	96.2 ± 6.3	103.4 ± 2.6	104.9 ± 6.6
10 Days treatment				
Sphingomyelinase	96.2 ± 2.8	81.4 ± 6.6**	79.4 ± 10.1*	79.8 ± 6.2**
Phospholipase A_1	87.0 ± 12.3	67.8 ± 10.4	79.1 ± 15.6	69.5 ± 11.7**
Phospholipids	100.1 ± 3.3	104.5 ± 4.6	103.8 ± 5.2	109.5 ± 4.6**

*$p < 0.05$; **$p < 0.01$ (statistical analysis by Students t-test for comparison between each treated group and matched controls (degree of freedom = 10)

Forschungsinstitut, Vienna). S86451 and gentamicin are equally potent against most sensitive organisms, except *Ps. aeruginosa.*

Earlier studies have shown that S86451 is significantly less toxic than gentamicin at equal doses (Wilmotte et al. 1983). In the present study, S86451 has been administered at doses 2.5 times greater than gentamicin to investigate the safety margin of this new compound.

Sprague-Dawley rats were treated intraperitoneally (i.p.) with S86451 or gentamicin for 4 and 10 days and compared with animals receiving only 0.9% NaCl. Biochemical assays [phospholipids; phospholipase A_1 (E.C. 3.1.1.31); sphingomyelinase (E.C. 3.1.4.12) and morphological studies (electron microscopy and "plastic sections") were performed according to published techniques] (Kosek et al. 1974; Aubert-Tulkens et al. 1979; Laurent et al. 1982). Tubular regeneration was measured by the incorporation of radioactivity into cortex DNA and by autohistoradiography after ^{3}H-thymidine injection (Laurent et al. 1984).

Biochemical evaluation (Table 1) indicates a 2.5 times reduction in the effect of S86451 upon lysosomal enzymes, and little effect on total phospholipids. The latter data are somewhat surprising since significant inhibition of phospholipases was found with S86451 at the highest dose. The mild increase of phospholipids was, however, confirmed by the morphological investigations (Fig. 1). Little or no myeloid bodies were seen in animals treated with 10 mg/kg of S86451. At 25 mg/kg, typical myeloid bodies were detected but not to the extent seen with gentamicin at 10 mg/kg. Examination of the plastic sections confirmed the milder alterations induced by S86451 in comparison with gentamicin.

Regeneration studies (Table 2) showed also a clear difference between S86451 and gentamicin. Considerably less ^{3}H-thymidine was incorporated into

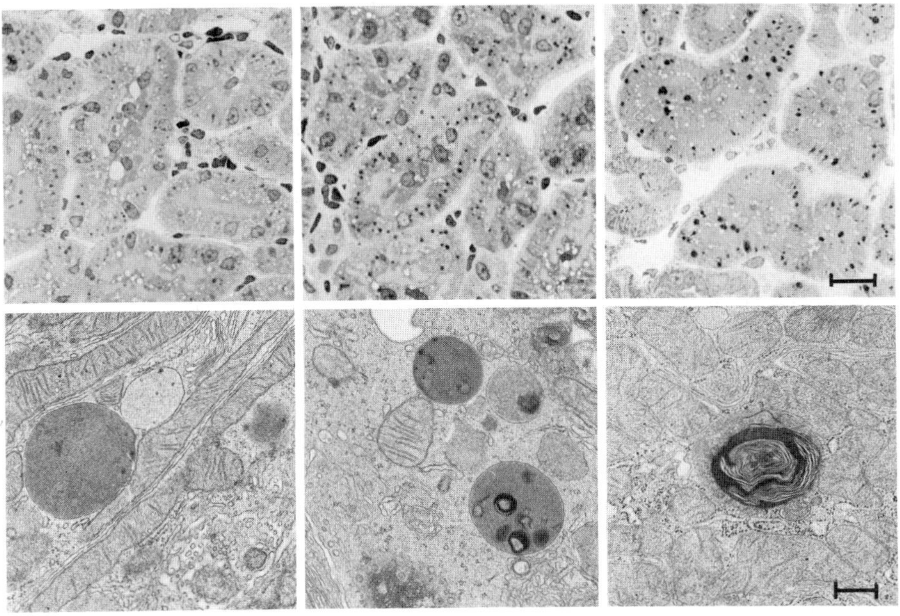

Fig. 1. Morphological appearance of proximal tubular cells in a control animal and in animals treated 10 days with S86451 (10 mg/kg) or gentamicin (4 mg/kg) treated animals (10 days). *Upper row:* "plastic sections" (1 μm-thick sections of material fixed and processed as for electronmicroscopy, toluidine blue staining; bar = 20 μm). Lysosomes appear swollen in gentamicin-treated animals. Upon higher magnification, the lysosome content is highly heterogenous (not shown). S86451 induces only a modest change of lysosome size, with no heterogenous content. The apparently larger number of lysosomes seen in this photograph of S86451-treated animal was not confirmed in the examination of a large series of slides. *Lower row:* electron micrographs (bar = 0.5 μm). Lysosomes in gentamicin-treated animals are overloaded with osmiophilic material made of closely apposed layers at 5 nm distance (not visible at this magnification; see Kosek et al. 1974 and Wilmotte et al. 1983). By contrast to gentamicin, S86451-treated animals show little alteration of lysosomes

Table 2. Influence of a 10 days treatment with S86451 and gentamicin on the incorporation of ^{3}H-thymidine in cortex DNA

	Controls (saline)	S86451 (25 mg/kg)[a]	Gentamicin (10 mg/kg)[a]
dpm/mg DNA (± SD)	19,709 ± 4,292 (n = 8)	33,713 ± 13,294 (n =3)	85,748 ± 35,661* (n = 11)

Animals were injected with 200 μCi of ^{3}H-thymidine 1 h before sacrifice (Laurent et al. 1983). The n value refers to the number of animals. For each animal, both kidneys were processed separately; data were pooled, since variations between kidneys observed from the same animal were consistently lower than that between kidneys from different animals

* Significantly different from control ($p < 0.05$); Students t-test

[a] Daily dose (in mg of base)

DNA after 10 days of treatment with S86451 (25 mg/kg daily) than with gentamicin (10 mg/kg). In both cases, autohistoradiography showed that the label was predominantly associated with nuclei in regenerating tubules.

This study demonstrates that S86451, at doses 2.5 times greater than those of gentamicin, induces similar, or less marked alterations in the kidney cortex. If these data are transposable to humans, S86451 should be a safer antibiotic than gentamicin in combating organisms with similar sensitivity to either drug.

References

Hottendorf GH, Bartnett D, Gordon LL, Christensen EF, Madison H (1981) Non parallel nephrotoxicity dose-response curves of aminoglycosides. Antimicrob Agents Chemother 19: 1024–1028

Just M, Erdmann G, Haberman E (1977) The renal handling of polybasic drugs. 1. Gentamicin and aprotinin in intact animals. Naunyn-Schmiedebergs Arch Pharmacol 300: 57–66

Kosek JD, Mazze RI, Cousins MJ (1974) Nephrotoxicity of gentamicin. Lab Invest 30: 48–57

Laurent G, Carlier MB, Rollman B, Van Hoof F, Tulkens P (1982) Mechanism of aminoglycoside-induced lysosomal phospholipidosis: In vitro and in vivo studies with gentamicin and amikacin. Biochem Pharmacol 31: 3861–3870

Laurent G, Toubeau G, Maldague P, Carlier MB, Stienon-Heuson JA, Tulkens P (1984) Tubular regeneration in rat kidney cortex during treatment with gentamicin at a low dose (10 mg/kg). Arch Toxicol Suppl 7: 459–463

Wilmotte E, Maldague P, Tulkens P, Baumgartner R, Schmook F, Walzl H, Obenaus H (1983) S86451, a new derivative of gentamicin with reduced nephrotoxicity: Biochemical, morphological and functional studies. Drug Exp Clin Res 9: 467–477

Disease, Metabolism and Reproduction in the Toxic Response to Drugs and Other Chemicals
Arch. Toxicol., Suppl. 7, 459–463 (1984)

Tubular Regeneration in Rat Kidney Cortex During Treatment with Gentamicin at a Low Dose

G. Laurent[1], G. Toubeau[2], P. Maldague[3], M. B. Carlier[1], J. A. Heuson-Stiennon[2], and P. Tulkens[1]

[1] Laboratoire de Chimie physiologique and International Institute of Cellular and Molecular Pathology, Université Catholique de Louvain, Avenue Hippocrate, 75, 1200 Brussels, Belgium
[2] Service d'Histologie, Université de l'Etat à Mons, Avenue du Champ de Mars, 24, 7000 Mons, Belgium
[3] Laboratoire de Pathologie et Cytologie expérimentales, Université Catholique de Louvain, Avenue Mounier, 52, 1200 Brussels, Belgium

Abstract. Tissue injury induced in rat kidney cortex by gentamicin at a low dose (10 mg/kg) has been studied by measuring subsequent regeneration after treatment for 4, 7, and 14 days. Cell proliferation was demonstrated by the incorporation of [^{3}H]-thymidine into kidney cortex DNA. In treated animals, the specific radioactivity of DNA increased up to 4.6 times the mean value found in the controls. Autoradiography showed labelling of nuclei in proximal tubular cells. Electron microscopy showed that a subpopulation of tubular cells, devoid of myeloid bodies, which are characteristic of gentamicin intoxication, is also poorer in peroxisomes, and therefore may belong to less differentiated, regenerating cells. It is concluded that a low dose of gentamicin induces measurable tissue regeneration.

Key words: Gentamicin – Aminoglycosides – Nephrotoxicity – Kidney – Regeneration – [^{3}H]-thymidine – Peroxisomes – Screening

Patients treated with aminoglycosides show a significant incidence of nephrotoxic reaction, especially if aged or critically-ill (Appel and Neu 1978). Toxicological or screening studies in animals are, however, complicated by the fact that conventional histopathology or kidney function studies fail to reveal constant and significant alterations, unless doses several times higher than human therapeutic doses are used. The validity of a "high dose" model has been questioned because the uptake of aminoglycosides by kidney shows dose-dependent saturation (Josepovitz et al. 1982). Moreover, non-parallel response curves have been reported when comparing various aminoglycosides (Luft et al. 1978).

Ultrastructural and biochemical investigations have demonstrated that low doses of aminoglycosides induce a lysosomal phospholipidosis in proximal tubular cells (Laurent et al. 1982). Focal necroses and various indirect signs of tubular injury have also been reported. Damaged tubular cells are, however, quickly eliminated in urine, and evaluations based on direct tissue examination tend therefore to underestimate the toxicity. The present study describes a method based on the early measurement of tissue regeneration, subsequent to the gentamicin-induced necrosis of proximal tubules.

Rats were treated with gentamicin (10 mg/kg per day) in two daily intraperitoneal (i.p.) injections for 4, 7, and 14 days, and killed 12 h after the last injection. One hour before sacrifice, the animals were injected (i.p.) with 200 μCi of [^{3}H]-thymidine. The kidney cortex was dissected and a large fragment was fixed in Bouin's fluid and processed for autohistoradiography. Small blocks (± 1 mm^3) were fixed with glutaraldehyde and processed for cytochemical demonstration of catalase (H_2O_2-diaminobenzidine reaction, Novikoff et al. 1972), with morphometrical evaluation (Baudhuin 1974). The specific radioactivity of DNA was measured on the remaining material after extraction, purification and assay (Munro and Fleck 1966). Both the cortices from each animal were processed separately. Variation between corresponding cortices was usually less than 10% and the data were pooled. The levels of radioactivity in serum and the amounts of acid-soluble radioactivity in the tissue did not significantly differ in the treated and control animals. The amount of extracted DNA was consistently approx. 3.75 mg DNA/g tissue.

Table 1 shows that gentamicin treatment induced a significant increase of [^{3}H]-thymidine incorporation into the cortex DNA. The localization of the radioactivity was investigated by autohistoradiography (Fig. 1). Labelled nuclei were scattered throughout the cortex. About two-third of them were seen in the proximal tubular cells. The remaining labelled nuclei were mostly found in endothelial cells. Distal tubular and glomerular cells occasionally showed a labelled nucleus. The control animals displayed less labelled nuclei, but their distribution between proximal and endothelial cells was roughly similar.

The presence of regenerating tissue in proximal tubules was assessed by morphometry of the peroxisomes. Regenerating, less differentiated parts of proximal tubules are indeed poorer in peroxisomes than fully differentiated segments (Böti et al. 1979). In control animals, peroxisomes occupy a surface area of 3.3% of the surface of the cytoplasm (total area of proximal tubular sections scanned: 3,500 μm^2). This percentage was very constant from one zone of the cortex to another and between individual animals. In contrast, two cell populations were recognized in animals treated 7 days with gentamicin (n = 4; total area scanned: 24,000 μm^2). The former (about 73% of surface section) contained prominent myeloid bodies, characteristic of gentamicin intoxication (Fig. 2a) and peroxisomes occupied 3.5% of their surface area. The latter showed either no lysosome or normal lysosomes in the section (Fig. 2b); this subclass may belong to regenerative tissue, not yet intoxicated or refractive to gentamicin. In these sections, the surface of peroxisomes was reduced to 1.6% of the cytoplasmic area.

It is concluded that low doses of gentamicin are associated with early signs of cell proliferation in kidneys, concomitant with the development of a population of less differentiated cells. In the absence of a malignant process, tubular proliferation occurs only to compensate for previous tissue damage (necrosis) or a partial loss of active tissue (compensatory hyperplasia) (Robbins and Cotran

Table 1. Increase of the specific radioactivity of cortex DNA after treatment of the animals with gentamicin (10 mg/kg daily, in two injections)

Duration of treatment		Difference from controls	
		Student's t-test[a]	Kolmogorov-Smirnov test[b]
Controls[c)]	14,700 ± 4,600 ($n = 11$)[d)]		
4 days	17,557 ± 6,389 ($n = 3$)	NS	
7 days	63,706 ± 20,110 ($n = 3$)	$p < 0.025$	$p < 0.01$
14 days	68,310 ± 31,297 ($n = 4$)	$p < 0.025$	

NS = Not significant
[a]) Each group compared to controls
[b]) All treated animals compared to controls
[c]) Mean of all controls injected with saline; no influence of the number of injection was noticed
[d]) Number of animals; both cortices were processed separately. Variation between corresponding cortex was minimal and data were pooled

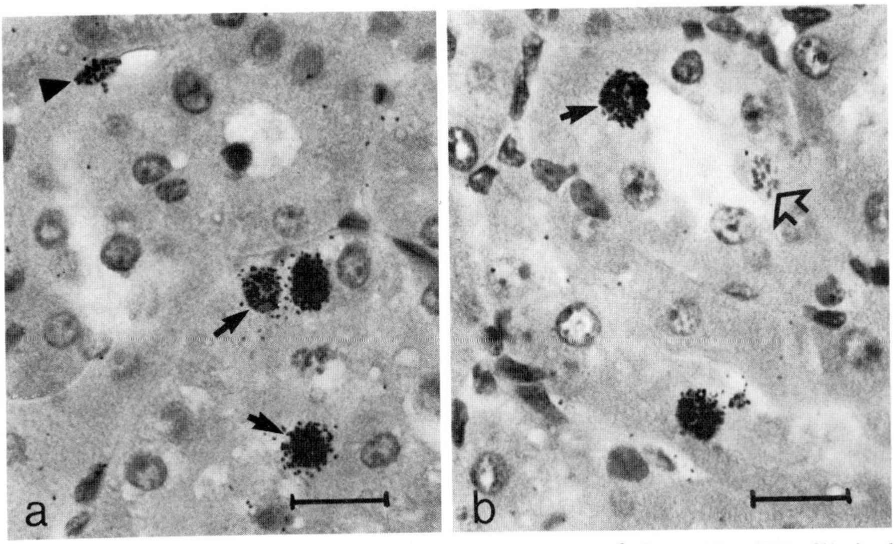

Fig. 1 a, b. Autohistoradiography of kidney cortex after injection of [^{3}H]-thymidine (200 μCi/animal) to gentamicin-treated rats. Scale bar is 15 μm. **a.** 4 Days treatment. Labelled nuclei are seen in proximal tubular cells *(filled arrows)* and in one endothelial cell *(arrow-head)*. **b.** 14 Days treatment. A labelled nucleus *(filled arrow)* and a mitosis *(open arrow)* are present in the same proximal tubule section

1979). In the present case, the kidney function is not altered, and the proliferation is therefore likely to be the consequence of focal, undetected necroses, induced by gentamicin at low dose.

These observations may have both clinical and toxicological implications. First, humans may regenerate less easily than rats, and factors such as age, debilitating diseases or co-administration of anticancer agents are likely to

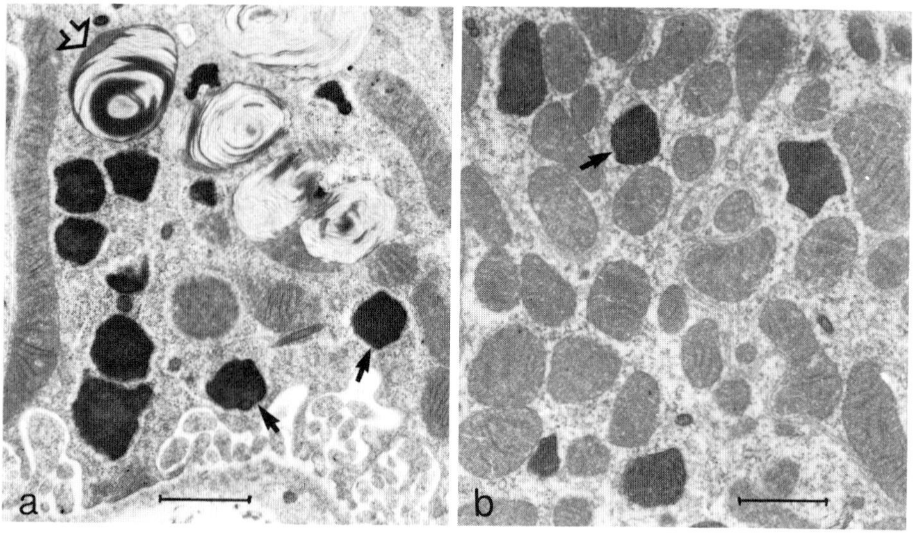

Fig. 2 a, b. Proximal tubular cells of gentamicin treated rats. Peroxisomes are stained with diaminobenzidine/H_2O_2. Scale bar is 1 μm. **a.** Field with typical myeloid bodies (concentric lamellar material in lysosomes, an early sign of gentamicin intoxication; Kosek et al. 1974) *(open arrow)*. **b.** Field devoid of myeloid bodies. Three peroxisomes are indicated by the *filled arrows*

decrease this regenerative capacity. This may explain how some subpopulations of patients, identified by the above criteria, go on more easily to develop acute renal dysfunction, although the doses and the duration of treatment are appropriate on pharmacokinetic criteria. Second, this approach may be useful to compare or to screen the nephrotoxic potential of aminoglycosides at low doses and after short term administration, i.e., under conditions that are directly relevant to the clinical use of these drugs.

Acknowledgement. This work was supported in part by the Belgian Ministère de la Santé Publique.

References

Appel GB, Neu HC (1978) Gentamicin in 1978. Ann Intern Med 89: 528–538

Baudhuin P (1974) Morphometry of subcellular fractions. Methods Enzymol 32B: 3–20

Böti ZS, Ivanyi B, Kobor J, Ormos J (1979) Histochemical studies on peroxisomes in regenerating proximal tubules of the kidney. Br J Exp Pathol 60: 620–626

Josepovitz C, Pastoriza-Munoz E, Timmerman D, Scott M, Feldman S, Kaloyanides G (1982) Inhibition of gentamicin uptake in rat renal cortex in vivo by aminoglycosides and other organic polycations. J Pharmacol Exp Ther 223: 314–321

Kosek JD, Mazze RI, Cousins MJ (1974) Nephrotoxicity of gentamicin. Lab Invest 30: 48–57

Laurent G, Carlier MB, Rollman B, Van Hoof F, Tulkens P (1982) Mechanism of gentamicin-induced lysosomal phospholipidosis: In vitro and in vivo studies. Biochem Pharmacol 31: 3861–3870

Luft FC, Bloch R, Sloam RS, Yun MN, Costello R, Merwell DR (1978) Comparative nephrotoxicity of aminoglycoside antibiotics in rats. J Infect Dis 138: 541–545

Munro HN, Fleck A (1966) The determination of nucleic acids. Methods Biochem Anal 14: 113–176

Novikoff AB, Novikoff PM, Davis C, Quintana N (1972) Studies on microperoxisomes. II. A cytochemical method for light and electron microscopy. J Histochem Cytochem 20: 1006–1023

Robbins SL, Cotran RS (1979) Pathologic basis of disease, 2nd edn. Saunders, Philadelphia

Disease, Metabolism and Reproduction in the Toxic Response to Drugs and Other Chemicals
Arch. Toxicol., Suppl. 7, 464–466 (1984)

Aminoglycoside Antibiotics: A Study of Their Neurotoxic Effects at Peripheral Nerve Fibres

D. Mitolo-Chieppa and M. R. Carratù

Institute of Pharmacology, Faculty of Medicine, University of Bari, Piazza Giulio Cesare, 70124 Bari, Italy

Abstract. Some antibiotics with aminoglycoside structure (streptomycin, neomycin, gentamicin, kanamycin, sisomicin, amikacin) are endowed with a marked neurotropism. They have been investigated on myelinated nerve fibres isolated from the frog sciatic nerve. The drugs affect the electric activity of both sensory and motor fibres; their action has been evaluated comparatively.

Key words: Neurotoxicity – Node of Ranvier – Aminoglycoside antibiotics

The availability of several aminoglycosides has raised questions regarding their comparative efficacy and toxicity. Most of these drugs are endowed with strong neurotropism, and ototoxicity is a recognized side effect. It is reported to be due to degenerative changes in the vestibular sensory epithelia and in the organ of Corti. Although various kinds of new aminoglycoside antibiotics have been developed, these drugs still have some degree of ototoxicity (Akiyoshi 1977; Federspil 1981). Streptomycin, which seems endowed with more marked neurotropism, has been reported to display a neuromuscular blocking action probably by reducing the release of acetylcholine (Brazil and Pinto Corrado 1957). The effects of streptomycin have also been investigated on the tibial nerve in toto of the frog (Sokoll and Diecke 1969); this drug was found to affect the amplitude of the action potential, the maximum rate of the action potential conduction and the upstroke of the action potential. All these effects could account for the peripheral neuropathy observed during chronic treatment with streptomycin.

The present study was carried out to evaluate the effects of some aminoglycoside antibiotics on the electrical activity of peripheral nerve fibres.

Single myelinated nerve fibres were isolated from the frog sciatic nerve and transferred to a special chamber where one node of Ranvier was continuously superfused. The perfusion liquid was a balanced salt solution for amphibia

(110.5 NaCl, 2.5 KCl, 1.8 $CaCl_2$, and 2.4 $NaHCO_3$, in mM) to which the following drugs could be added: neomycin, streptomycin, gentamicin, kanamycin, sisomicin, amikacin. One of the neighbouring nodes was stimulated by a short rectangular current pulse (of 0.2 ms) and the electrical activity was recorded using the airgap technique (Staempfli 1959).

Table 1 shows the main effects induced by the drugs tested. They all slightly increase the threshold for electrical excitability without altering substantially the amplitude of the action potential; thus, the main effect is the increase of the action potential duration. The effect is dose-dependent (e.g., streptomycin, Fig. 1). From some experiments using the voltage-clamp technique, it appears that the increase of the action potential duration is to be attributed to a reduced potassium conductance. The increase of the action potential duration and the prolongation of the refractory period could account for a reduction of the maximum number of transmissible impulses, per unit of time, along the nerve fibre and could contribute to the neurotoxic effect of the drugs under investigation. The order of the ability of these drugs to modify the electrical

Table 1. The concentration (mg/ml) ± SE which increased by 20% the duration of the action potential (AP) and the refractory period (RP) (five experiments)

Drugs	AP Duration	RP Duration
Neomicin	0.07 ± 0.002	0.23 ± 0.006
Streptomycin	0.10 ± 0.008	0.43 ± 0.034
Gentamicin	0.30 ± 0.011	0.61 ± 0.023
Kanamycin	0.34 ± 0.010	0.68 ± 0.020
Sisomicin	0.47 ± 0.023	0.93 ± 0.057
Amikacin	0.51 ± 0.042	0.98 ± 0.095

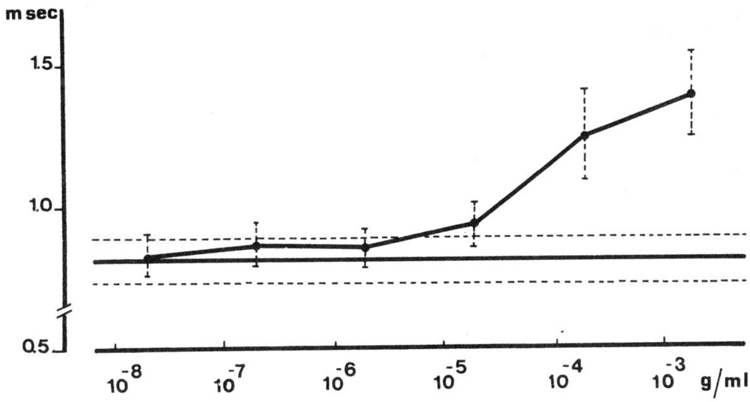

Fig. 1. Relationship between the concentration of streptomycin *(abscissa)* and the duration of the action potential *(ordinate)*. Mean ± SE is calculated from five experiments. The duration of the action potential in Ringer is indicated by the *horizontal full line* and the corresponding SE is indicated by the *horizontal dashed lines*

parameters examined is as follows: neomycin > streptomycin > gentamicin > kanamycin > sisomicin > amikacin; with ratios of relative potency approximately 1, 0.7, 0.23, 0.20, 0.15, 0.13. The ratio between the blood concentration for therapeutic doses and the concentration active in vitro is calculated to be 1/3–1/2 for the old aminoglycosides (neomycin, streptomycin) and 1/100–1/50 for the new aminoglycosides (sisomycin, amikacin). It is noteworthy that the relative potency of the aminoglycosides tested on the electrical activity of nerve fibres is consistent with their neurotoxic potential in vivo.

Note added in proof. This work was supported by a grant from the Italian National Research Council (C.N.R. No. CT83.434).

References

Akiyoshi M (1977) Evaluation of ototoxicity and safety of aminoglycoside antibiotics in the guinea pig. Adv. Clin Pharmacol 13: 374–386

Brazil OV, Pinto Corrado A (1957) The curariform action of streptomycin. J Pharmacol 120: 452–459

Federspil P (1981) Drug- induced sudden hearing loss and vestibular disturbances. Adv Otorhinolaryngol 27: 144–158

Sokoll MD, Diecke FPJ (1969) Some effects of streptomycin on frog nerve. Arch Int Pharmacodyn Ther 177: 332–339

Staempfli R (1959) Is the resting potential of Ranvier nodes a potassium potential? Ann NY Acad Sci 81: 265–284

Disease, Metabolism and Reproduction in the Toxic Response to Drugs and Other Chemicals
Arch. Toxicol., Suppl. 7, 467 (1984)

The Use of Physostigmine in Heroin Overdose

J. Rupreht[1], B. Dworacek[1], M. Valkenburg[2], and H. Oosthoek[1]

[1] Department of Anaesthesiology, Erasmus University Rotterdam,
P.O. Box 1738, 3000 DR Rotterdam, The Netherlands
[2] Department of Anaesthesiology, Zuider Ziekenhuis, Rotterdam, The Netherlands

Abstract. Two groups of 10 patients who were brought into the emergeny room for a heroin-overdose respiratory depression were treated aselectively with 0.003 mg/kg naloxone intravenously (i.v.) or 0.04 mg/kg physostigmine salicylate i.v. Blood gases, consciousness, heart rate, blood pressure, pupil diameter and subjective well-being were recorded. Patients treated either with naloxone or physostigmine awoke from coma within 10 min.

The important difference between the two groups was in the subjective feeling of well-being: naloxone caused opiate withdrawal and the patients felt "rotten" while patients after physostigmine felt "fine". The effect of physostigmine, however, wore off within 40 min.

Key words: Heroin overdose – Respiratory depression – Naloxone hydrochloride – Physostigmine salicylate – Blood gases – Subjective well-being – Opiate withdrawal syndrome

References

Jhamandas K, Phillis JW, Pinsky C (1971) Effects of narcotic analgesics and antagonists on the in vivo release of acetyl-choline from the cerebral cortex of the cat. Br J Pharmacol 43 : 53–66

Rupreht J (1980) Clinical aspects of the central cholinergic blockade. In: Kovatsis A (ed) Toxicological aspects. Technica Studio, Thessaloniki, pp 520–524

Rupreht J, Dworacek B (1976) Central anticholinergic syndrome in anaesthetic practice. Acta Anaesthesiol Belg 27 : 45–60

Weinstock M, Erez E, Roll D (1981) Antagonism of the cardiovascular and respiratory depressant effects of morphine in the conscious rabbit by physostigmine. J Pharmacol Exp Ther 218 : 504–508

Weinstock M, Davidson JT, Rosin AJ, Schnieder H (1982) Effect of physostigmine on morphine-induced postoperative pain and somnolence. Br J Anaesth 54 : 429–434

Disease, Metabolism and Reproduction in the Toxic Response to Drugs and Other Chemicals
Arch. Toxicol., Suppl. 7, 468 (1984)

4-Aminopyridine: An Anticurare and Reawakening Drug

E. Malizia, P. Nicolai, R. Romano, and G. Pinto

Institute of Anaesthesiology and Resuscitation, Rome University "La Sapienza" Medical School, Policlinico Umberto I°, 00161 Rome, Italy

Abstract. 4-Aminopyridine has been used experimentally in the reawakening phase of general anaesthesia induced by two different procedures: neuroleptoanalgesia type II, using fentanyl and droperidol and midazolan-ketamine ataranalgesia. Both groups were curarized with a nondepolarizing drug: pancuronium bromide. A rapid decurarization and in the subjects of the second group a remarkable shortening of the time to awakening has been observed after 4-aminopyridine administration.

Key words: 4-Aminopyridine – Anticurare and reawakening effect

References

Agoston S, Salt PJ, Erdmann W, Hilkemejer J, Bencini A, Langrehr D (1980) Antagonism of ketamine-diazepam anaesthesia by 4-Aminopyridine in human volunteers. Br J Anaesth 52 : 367–370

Folgering H, Rutten J, Agoston S (1979) Stimulation of phrenic nerve activity by an acetylcholine releasing drug: 4-Aminopyridine. Pfluegers Arch 379 : 181–189

Langrehr D, Agoston S, Erdmann W, Newton D (1981) Pharmaco dynamics and reversal of benzodiazepine-ketamine ataranalgesia. S Afr Med J 59 : 425–428

See WR, Folgering H, Schlafke ME (1978) Central respiratory and cardiovascular effect on the acetylcholine releaser: 4-Aminopyridine. Pfluegers Arch 377 : R20

Sia RL, Salt PJ, Langrehr D, Agoston S, Erdmann W (1979) Effect of the analeptic drug, 4-Aminopyridine upon post-operative respiratory depression in patients. Acta Anaesth Belg [Suppl] 30 : 195–199

Uges DRA (1982) 4-Aminopyridine, clinical pharmaceutical, pharmacological and toxicological aspects. State Univ., Groningen/Netherlands, p 230

Thesleff S (1980) Aminopyridine and synaptic transmission. Neuroscience 5 : 1413–1419

Disease, Metabolism and Reproduction in the Toxic Response to Drugs and Other Chemicals
Arch. Toxicol., Suppl. 7, 469–471 (1984)

The Influence of Dose Schedules and Administration Routes on the Toxicity of Potential Antiviral Drugs

R. Amlacher and H. Hoffmann

Academy of Sciences of the GDR, Central Institute of Microbiology and Experimental Therapy, Beutenbergstrasse 11, 6900 Jena, German Democratic Republic

Abstract. The influence of two differently constructed dose schedules and of two dissimilar administration routes on the subacute toxicity of the potential antiviral drug benzoxazolyl-2-formyl-S-ethyl-isothiosemicarbazone was investigated in mice. Administration of identical aliquots of the, route dependent, maximally tolerated, dose was found to cause no significant differences in weight gain in any of the schedules used, but marked changes in lethality after oral or subcutaneous administration could be demonstrated.

Key words: Subacute toxicity – Mouse – Antiviral drug – Benzoxazolyl-2-formyl-S-ethyl-isothiosemicarbazone – Dose schedules – Administration routes

In the course of in vivo screening of potential antiviral drugs therapeutic trials are performed in virus infected animals. The basis of an effective therapy for these animals is to reach and to maintain antiviral, but nontoxic, drug levels for a period long enough for optimal treatment. However, as many of the frequently used dose schedules do not take into consideration the special pharmacokinetic and toxicological properties of the drugs tested. Moreover, the pharmacokinetics of a drug and its toxicological effects are considerably dependent on the route of administration. Therefore, it was the first aim of the present study to investigate the influence of two alternatively constructed dose schedules on the degree of the toxic effect of a drug to be tested. Additionally, the influence of different administration routes on the degree and the kinetics of the toxic effect of the drug was to be described.

For these investigations the potential antiviral drug ZIMET 111/74 (benzoxazolyl-2-formyl-S-ethyl-isothiosemicarbazone; Heinisch et al. 1977) was used. As a result of the calculation of its acute toxicity, the maximally tolerated single dose (MTD) was found to be 1240 mg/kg after subcutaneous administration, and 410 mg/kg after oral administration. The lower toxicity after s.c.

Table 1. Effect of different aliquots of the acute maximally tolerated dose (MTD) on lethality to mice after subcutaneous or oral administration of ZIMET 111/74 according to scheme A

Dose in aliquots of MTD on day 1–5		No. of animals surviving: treated	
Single	Total	s.c.	p.o.
1	5	Not done	3:5
6/10	3	Not done	5:5
1/2	2.5	0:5	5:5
3/10	1.5	Not done	5:5
1/4	1.25	5:5	5:5
1/8	0.625	5:5	Not done

Table 2. Effect of different maintenance doses (D'') on lethality to mice after subcutaneous or oral administration of ZIMET 111/74 according to scheme B

Dose in aliquots of MTD			No. of animals surviving: treated	
Day 1 (D')	Day 2–5 (D'')	Total	s.c.	p.o.
1	1	5	Not done	3:5
1	1/2	3	0:5	5:5
1	1/16	1.25	5:5	5:5
1/2	1/2	2.5	0:5	5:5
1/2	1/4	1.5	4:5	5:5
1/2	1/8	1.0	Not done	5:5
1/2	1/32	0.625	5:5	Not done

administration may be explained by the very slow absorption of the drug from the injection site.

All dosages used in the experiments were related to the respective MTD. For both routes, the subacute toxicity of the drug was studied using the following dose schedules: Scheme A: Administration of identical single doses (D) on 5 consecutive days; Scheme B: Administration of an inital dose (D') on day 1 and 4 identical maintenance doses (D'') on the next 4 consecutive days.

According to these schemes total dosages of ZIMET 111/74 in a range between 0.625 and 5 MTD were administered. Treatment with identical aliquots of the route dependent MTD caused marked differences in lethality dependent on the administration route. For instance, a total dose of 2.5 MTD according to scheme A resulted in the death of all treated animals after subcutaneous (s.c.) administration, while after oral treatment no deaths were observed (Table 1). Similiar results were obtained after subcutaneous or oral administration of the drug at a total dose of 3 MTD according to scheme B (Table 2). Using D' = 1 MTD, the maximally tolerated non-lethal maintenance dose D'' was found to be $^1/_2$ for oral and $^1/_{16}$ for subcutaneous administration. On the other hand, administration of identical total doses of the drug (5 D = D' + 4 D'') caused no significant differences in weight gain in any of the schedules used (Fig. 1). This

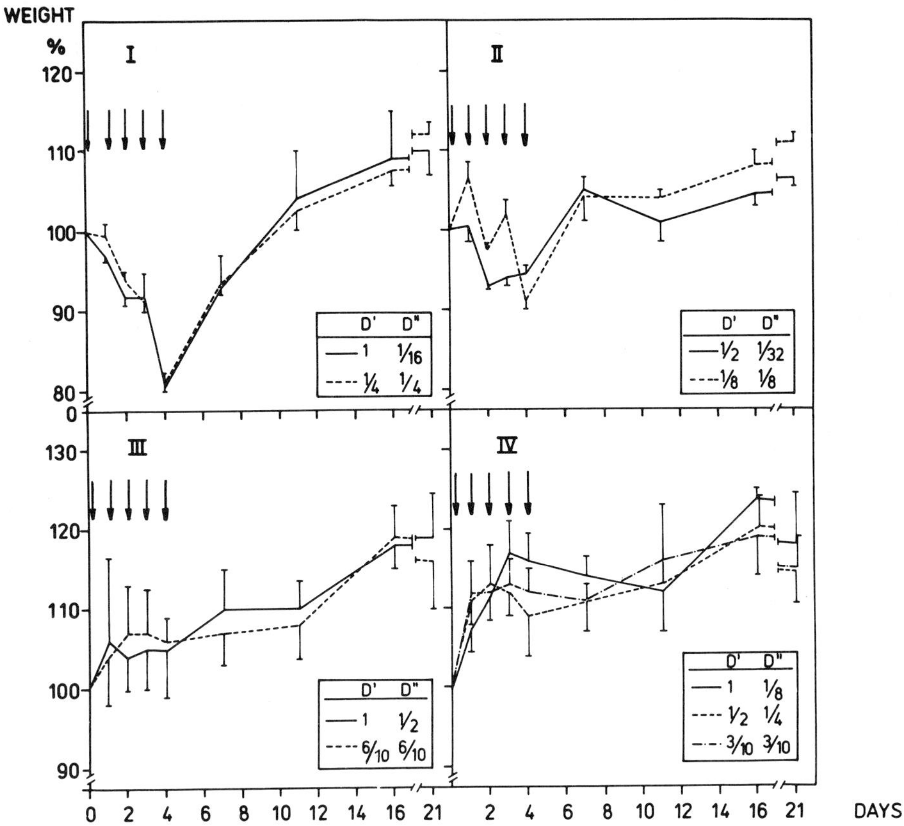

Fig. 1. Weight gain of mice following subcutaneous (*I, II*) or oral (*III, IV*) administration of ZIMET 111/74 on two differently constructed dose schedules. Dose on day 1 (*D'*) and doses on days 2–5 (*D''*) are aliquots of the respective MTD. ↓ Drug administration

could be stated for the varying levels of the total doses administered and for both administration routes.

From these results the following conclusions can be drawn for the in vivo screening of potential antiviral drugs: Drug administration according to scheme B has the advantage of producing higher initial antiviral drug levels without higher toxicological risks in comparison with scheme A treatment. Moreover, using the treatment according to scheme B, route dependent peculiarities of the toxicological and pharmacokinetic properties of drugs can be taken into consideration using route dependent initial and maintenance doses. In general, for evaluation of the antiviral in vivo activity of a drug, dose schedules which neglect its pharmacokinetic and toxicological data should be avoided.

References

Heinisch L, Tonew M, Tonew E (1977) Synthese und antivirale Wirkung N-heterocyclischer Formylisothiosemicarbazone. Pharmazie 32: 752–756

Disease, Metabolism and Reproduction in the Toxic Response to Drugs and Other Chemicals
Arch. Toxicol., Suppl. 7, 472–475 (1984)

Intramuscular Injections and Muscle Damage: Effects of Concentration, Volume, Injection Speed and Vehicle

O. Svendsen and L. Blom

Research Laboratories, H. Lundbeck A/S, Ottiliavej 7–9, 2500 Copenhagen-Valby, Denmark

Abstract. An intramuscular injection was given to rabbits with the needle inserted in the longissimus dorsi muscle. The muscle tissue at the injection site was examined post-mortem 3 days after the injection and areas of necrotic muscle tissue were dissected for weighing. With a fixed dose of the neuroleptic drug cis(Z)-clopenthixol it was shown that a small volume of a concentrated solution caused less muscle damage than a larger volume of a relatively less concentrated solution. Injection speed, on the other hand, was not an important factor. Aqueous solutions of neuroleptic drugs caused local muscle damage which was diminished or prevented by oily vehicles.

Key words: Injection – Intramuscular – Local damage – Neuroleptics – Rabbits

From studies in animals it is known that various therapeutic agents for intramuscular use cause local muscle tissue damage at the injection site (Steiness et al. 1978). Studies in patients, on the serum creatine phosphokinase levels after intramuscular injection, have provided indirect evidence that some of these drugs also cause local muscle tissue damage in humans (Steiness et al. 1978). Such damage may contribute to the experience of pain and discomfort. Local tissue damage caused by the therapeutic agent may also be an important factor in intramuscular injection-site complications.

The present studies in rabbits were undertaken in order to investigate the influence of the concentration, volume, vehicle, and injection speed on the local damaging effect.

New Zealand White rabbits of both sexes were used. Each animal received one single intramuscular injection. Four rabbits were used for each preparation. The injections were given by a needle inserted centrally into the right longissimus dorsi muscle. The fix point for introduction of the needle was a transversal plane through the lumbar region halfway between the last rib and the crest of ilium bone and a sagittal plane in the middle of the muscle. This corresponds to about 4 cm ahead of the crest of ilium and 2 cm laterally from the spinous process of lumbar vertebrae. The needle was inserted about halfway (1.5 cm) into the vertical plane of the muscle. The thickness of the muscle at the injection site was evaluated from immediately preceding palpation.

Three days after the injection the rabbits were anaesthetized (50 mg/kg of pentobarbital intravenously) and killed by exsanguination. The muscle tissue at the injection sites was examined for macroscopic changes by serial sectioning. The areas of necrotic muscle tissue were isolated by careful trimming from the surrounding tissue and weighed. This procedure for demonstrating muscle damaging effect of injectable formulations has been described before (Svendsen et al. 1979).

A dose of 10 mg cis(Z)-clopenthixol (Lundbeck, Copenhagen), a neuroleptic drug, was administered in concentrations of 0.1, 0.3, 1.0, 3.0, and 10% in saline. The weight of necrotic muscle tissue was 5.7, 4.7, 4.6, 2.3, and 1.4 g, respectively. These results indicate that a small volume of a concentrated solution causes less muscle damage than a large volume of a relatively less concentrated solution.

In another study the same volume (2 ml) of different concentrations (1.0, 0.5, and 0.1% in saline) of cis(Z)-clopenthixol was administered. The weight of necrotic muscle tissue was 7.7, 5.6, and 0.6 g. This demonstrates that a 10 times dilution reduced the local toxic effect to a large extent although it was inadequate in totally avoiding the local toxicity.

The effect of injection speed was investigated after injection of saline or cis(Z)-clopenthixol (1%) in saline (Svendsen 1983a). Saline was administered as a constant volume (2 or 6 ml) or at constant injection speed (1.0 or 0.1 ml/s). Cis(Z)-clopenthixol was administered in a constant volume (2 ml) at injection speeds of 0.03, 0.1, 0.3, or 1.0 ml/s. Very fast injection of saline caused slight bleeding in the muscle tissue (autopsy 30 min after injection) indicating modest disruption. Slight bleeding in the needle track was the only finding after slow injection. In the rabbits given cis(Z)-clopenthixol there was no difference in the weight of necrotic muscle tissue after injection speeds of 0.03, 0.1, or 1.0 ml/s. The weight obtained at an injection speed of 0.3 ml/s was slightly but significantly higher than those obtained at injection speeds of 0.03 and 0.1 ml/s. Form these data it is concluded that injection speed is not an important factor for the muscle damaging effect of intramuscular drug preparations.

Vegetable oils have been used for decades as vehicles for intramuscular drug preparations. Vegetable oils are tolerated well at the injection site (Svendsen and Aaes-Jørgensen 1979). The muscle damaging effect of a series of neuroleptic drugs formulated in water or in oily vehicles [Viscoleo, sesame oil (EP), methyl oleate (EP), or squalane (EP)] was investigated by the same procedure as in the above studies (Svendsen 1983b). All aqueous preparations caused damage at the injection site as shown by the presence of a large and well-defined necrotic area in all rabbits (Table 1). The mean weight of the necrotic muscle tissue varied from 3.8 g (Buronil) to 8.8 g (cis(Z)-clopenthixol). The individual necrotic area varied considerably after injection of cis(Z)-clopenthixol (4.4–15.9 g), Klorpromazin (3.2–11.1 g), and fluphenazine (EP) (1.3–8.3 g).

Little or no necrotic muscle tissue was found at the injection site after injection of the same drugs dissolved in Viscoleo (Table 1). The most consistent

Table 1. Post mortem findings at the injection site 3 days after intramuscular injection of 2 ml of different neuroleptic drug preparations into rabbits

Preparation	Aqueous solution		Viscoleo solution	
	Weight (g) of isolated necrotic muscle tissue (Mean and range)	Macroscopic findings	Weight (g) of isolated necrotic muscle tissue (Mean and range)	Macroscopic findings
Cis(Z)-clopenthixol, 10 mg/ml	8.8 (4.4–15.9)	Well-defined necrosis	0.3 (0–0.7)	Focal hemorrhages and grey stripes
Cis(Z)-flupentixol, 10 mg/ml	4.0 (3.2– 4.8)	Well-defined necrosis	0	No chances
Clorpromazine, 25 mg/ml (Klorpromazin)	7.9 (3.2–11.1)	Well-defined necrosis	0.3 (0–0.7)	Focal hemorrhages and grey stripes
Chlorprothixene, 5 mg/ml (Truxal)	4.5 (3.6– 5.3)	Well-defined necrosis	0	Focal hemorrhage
Fluphenazine, 10 mg/ml	4.9 (1.3– 8.3)	Well-defined necrosis	0	Focal hemorrhages and grey stripes
Haloperidol, 5 mg/ml (Serenase)	5.2 (3.5– 7.6)	Well-defined necrosis	0.2 (0–0.8)	Focal hemorrhages and grey stripes
Levomepromazine, 25 mg/ml (Nozinan)	4.9 (4.7– 5.2)	Well-defined necrosis	0	Focal hemorrhages and grey stripes
Melperone, 25 mg/ml (Buronil)	3.8 (3.2– 4.4)	Well-defined necrosis	0	Focal hemorrhages and grey stripes
Perphenazine, 5 mg/ml W (Trilafon)	4.3 (3.3– 5.4)	Well-defined necrosis	0	Focal hemorrhages and grey stripes
Thiethylperazine maleate, 6.5 mg/ml (Torecan)	5.8 (4.6– 7.0)	Well-defined necrosis	0	Focal hemorrhages and grey stripes

findings were focal haemorrhages, stripes of grey muscle fibres between normal muscle fibres and occasionally very small areas of necrotic muscle tissue. Sesame oil, methyl oleate and squalane also reduced the local damaging effect of chlorpromazine and cis(Z)-clopenthixol but not to the same extent as with Viscoleo. Methyl oleate was less effective than sesame oil and squalane was less effective than methyl oleate. No necrotic muscle tissue was found at the injection site after injection of haloperidol (Serenase) in sesame oil, methyl oleate or squalane.

From the present studies it is concluded that the local damaging effect to muscle tissue of injectable formulations is related to the injected volume and concentration of the preparation. The injection speed is not an important factor. The muscle damaging effect of aqueous preparations of neuroleptic drugs can be diminished or even prevented by oily vehicles.

References

Steiness E, Rasmussen F, Svendsen O, Nielsen P (1978) A comparative study of serum creatine phosphokinase (CPK) activity in rabbits, pigs and humans after intramuscular injection of local damaging drugs. Acta Pharmacol Toxicol (Kbh) 42: 357–364

Svendsen O (1983a) Intramuscular injections and local muscle damage. An experimental study of the effect of injection speed. Acta Pharmacol Toxicol (Kbh) 52: 305–309

Svendsen O (1983b) Local muscle damage and oily vehicles. A study on local reactions in rabbits after intramuscular injection of neuroleptic drugs in aqueous or oily vehicles. Acta Pharmacol Toxicol (Kbh) 52: 298–304

Svendsen O, Aaes-Jørgensen T (1979) Studies on the fate of vegetable oil after intramuscular injection into experimental animals. Acta Pharmacol Toxicol (Kbh) 45: 352–378

Svendsen O, Rasmussen F, Nielsen P, Steiness E (1979) The loss of creatine phosphokinase (CK) from intramuscular injection sites in rabbits. A predictive tool for local toxicity. Acta Pharmacol Toxicol (Kbh) 44: 324–328

Disease, Metabolism and Reproduction in the Toxic Response to Drugs and Other Chemicals
Arch. Toxicol., Suppl. 7, 476–477 (1984)

Evidence of an Interaction Between Opioids and Histaminergic Systems on Cannabis Sativa-Induced Catalepsy

R. Arrigo-Reina[1], C. Cosentino[1], M. Reina[1], and S. Ferri[2]

[1] Chair of Pharmacology and Pharmacognosy, Faculty of Pharmacy, University of Catania, Viale A. Doria 6, 95125 Catania, Italy
[2] Institute of Pharmacology, University of Bologna, Bologna, Italy

Abstract. Behavioral responses of rat to an extract of Cannabis Sativa L., consisting of stereotyped behavior, hyperreactivity to touch with characteristic vocalisation, followed by a state of general depression, lack of responsiveness to noxious stimuli and atonic muscular prostration alternating with muscle rigidity were observed. Analgesic effects and modification of the rectal temperature were also noted. Pretreatment with an opiate receptor blocker naloxone (3 mg/kg) significantly modified these parameters and also induced a cataleptic state with muscle rigidity. Pretreatment with anti-H_1 antazoline (20 mg/kg) or anti-H_2 cimetidine (25 mg/kg) receptor drugs modified the behavioral syndrome elicited by cannabis extract but failed to induce catalepsy, which was enhanced by pretreatment with compound 48/80. These results suggest that cannabis or its active constituents may interact with central histaminergic systems through specific opiate sites.

Key words: Cannabis – Stereotypy – Hyperreactivity – Catalepsy – Body temperature – Analgesia – Opioid receptor blocker – Anti-H_1-H_2 receptor drugs – Rat

References

Arrigo-Reina R, Scoto GM, Spadaro C, Mazzone G (1978) Behavioral effects of an extract of Cannabis in rats: Role of catecholamines. Boll Soc Ital Biol Sper 23: 2348–2354

Bhargava H (1976) Inhibition of naloxone-induced withdrawal in morphine dependent mice by L-trans-delta-9-tetrahydrocannabinol. Eur J Pharmacol 36: 259–262

Bloom A, Dewey L (1978) A comparison of some pharmacological action of morphine and delta-9-tetrahydrocannabinol in the mouse. Psychopharmacology (Berlin) 57: 243–248

D'Amour FE, Smith D (1941) Method for determining loss of pain sensation. J Pharmacol Exp Ther 72: 74–79

Ferri S, Costa G, Murari G, Panico AM, Rapisarda E, Speroni E, Arrigo-Reina R (1981) Investigations on behavioral effects of an extract of Cannabis Sativa L. in the rat. Psychopharmacology (Berlin) 75: 144–147

Gough AL, Olley JE (1977) Delta-9-tetrahydrocannabinol and the extrapyramidal system. Psychopharmacology (Berlin) 54: 87–99

Hirschorn ID, Rosecrans JA (1974) Morphine and delta-9-tetrahydrocannabinol: Tolerance to the stimulus effects. Psychopharmacology (Berlin) 36: 243–253

Kaakkola S, Ahtee L (1977) Effects of muscarinic cholinergic drugs on morphine-induced catalepsy, antinociception and changes in brain dopamine metabolism. Psychopharmacology (Berlin) 52: 7–15

Kamikawa Y, Shimo Y (1978) Antagonistic effect of compound 48/80 on the inhibitory actions of morphine and methionine-enkephalin on electrically-induced contractions of the guinea-pig ileum. Br J Pharmacol 64: 511–518

Koffer KB, Berney S, Hornykiewicz O (1978) The role of the corpus striatum in neuroleptic- and narcotic-induced catalepsy. Eur J Pharmacol 47: 81–86

Lomax P (1971) Animal pharmacology of marijuana. Proc West Pharmacol Soc 14: 10

Muley MP, Balsara JJ, Jadhav JH, Chandorkan AG (1982) Involvement of histaminergic mechanisms in the cataleptogenic effect of morphine in mice. J Pharm Pharmacol 34: 34–37

Nakamura K, Kuntzman R, Maggio A, Conney AH (1973) Decrease in morphine's analgesic action and increase in its cataleptic action by 6-OHDA injected bilaterally into caudate and putamen areas: Partial restoration by 1-DOPA plus decarboxylase inhibition. Neuropharmacology 12: 1153–1158

Sofia RD Nalepa SD, Harakal JJ, Vassar HB (1973) Anti-edema and analgesic properties of delta-9-tetrahydrocannabinol (THC). J Pharmacol Exp Ther 186: 646–655

Taylor DA, Fennessy MR (1977) Biphasic nature of the effects of delta-9-tetrahydrocannabinol on body temperature and brain amines of the rat. Eur J Pharmacol 46: 93–99

Turker RK, Kaymakçalan S, Ercan ZS (1975) Antihistaminic action of (−)trans-delta-9-tetrahydrocannabinol. Arch Int Pharmacodyn Ther 214: 254–257

Disease, Metabolism and Reproduction in the Toxic Response to Drugs and Other Chemicals
Arch. Toxicol., Suppl. 7, 478 (1984)

Fever Reaction of Rabbits After Repeated Intravenous Injections of Antigens

H. Ronneberger

Research Laboratories of Behringwerke AG, POB 1140, 3550 Marburg/Lahn, Federal Republic of Germany

Abstract. In some pharmacopoeial pyrogen tests the re-use of rabbits which have received an antigenic drug is not prohibited for the same substance. Human albumin (HA), aprotinin (Ap), or streptokinase (Sk) were injected week-by-week over 5 weeks or with different latent periods between 1 and 5 weeks. The clinical reaction and the fever response after the applications were divided into three types:

Repeated injection of HA caused an increase of body temperature in most rabbits from the 2nd application or after a latent period of at least 2 weeks (> 0.6° C).

After repeated Ap injection only one animal showed an increase of temperature after a period of 2 weeks, all other rabbits had normal values for this parameter.

Repeated Sk application caused extreme falls or increases of body temperatures in most rabbits from the 2nd injection in both test series. Some animals died between 1 and 4 h after the second injection due to anaphylactic shock.

The re-use of rabbits, which have already received antigenic drugs, in the pyrogen assay cannot be recommended, because they may show immunological reactions not caused by pyrogens, such as anaphylactic fever or a fall of body temperature due to shock reactions.

Key words: Pyrogen test – Antigens – Fever – Rabbits – Human albumin – Aprotinin – Streptokinase

References

Test on pyrogens (1975). In: Europäisches Arzneibuch II. pp 56–60, Deutscher Apotheker-Verlag, Stuttgart

Farr RS (1959) Fever as a manifestation of an experimental allergy. J Allergy 30: 268–269

Ronneberger H (1975) On eventual temperature rises following streptokinase infusion, results of animal experiments. Arzneim Forsch 25: 641–644

Disease, Metabolism and Reproduction in the Toxic Response to Drugs and Other Chemicals
Arch. Toxicol., Suppl. 7, 479 (1984)

Cardiovascular Effects of Tetanus Toxin After Systemic and Intraventricular Administration in Rats

G. Nisticò[2], S. Gratteri[2], G. Vairo[1], F. Rossi[1], and E. Marmo[1]

[1] Institute of Pharmacology, Faculty of Medicine, University of Naples, Naples, Italy
[2] Institute of Pharmacology, Faculty of Medicine, University of Reggio Calabria, Italy

Abstract. Evidence exists that GABAergic mechanisms in the brain may play an important role in the control of cardiovascular activity; thus GABA and GABA receptor agonists given intracerebroventricularly reduce blood pressure and heart rate in rats and cats (De Feudis 1982). In addition, bicuculline, a GABA receptor antagonist, microinjected into the nucleus ambiguous of the brain-stem in cats produces hypotensive and bradycardiac effects which are apparently vagally mediated (Di Micco 1979). Tetanus toxin has been used for a long time as a valid tool to decrease GABA release in the brain (Collingridge and Davies 1982). Thus the purpose of the present experiments was to assess changes in blood pressure and heart rate after systemic and intraventricular administration of tetanus toxin in rats.

In comparison with a control group (n = 15) receiving the same volume of vehicle (0.1 ml/100 g body weight), a single intraperitoneal injection of tetanus toxin [200 minimal lethal dose (MLD), n = 30] in unanaesthetized rats produced, 3 days later, a significant increase in systolic blood pressure (185 ± 15 min mm Hg against control values of 132 ± 6) and in heart rate. On the other hand, in anaesthetized rats the intraventricular administration of tetanus toxin (20 and 40 MLD, n = 6 for each dose) produced a gradual decrease in blood pressure accompanied by bradycardia.

In conclusion, the present findings show that tetanus toxin is able to affect cardiovascular activity very likely through an interference with central GABAergic mechanism.

Key words: Tetanus toxin – Cardiovascular

References

Collingridge GL, Davies J (1982) The in vitro inhibition of GABA release by tetanus toxin. Neuropharmacology 21: 851–855
De Feudis F (1982) GABA an inhibitory neurotransmitter that is involved in cardiovascular control. Pharmacol Res Commun 14: 567–575
Di Micco JA, Gale K, Hamilton B, Gillis RA (1979) GABA receptor control of parasympathetic antiflow to heart: Characterization and brainstem localization. Science 204: 1106

Disease, Metabolism and Reproduction in the Toxic Response to Drugs and Other Chemicals
Arch. Toxicol., Suppl. 7, 480–481 (1984)

The Incidence of Drug Overdosage in Patients Admitted to General Hospitals in the Canary Islands

E. Sanz and J. Boada

Department of Pharmacology, Faculty of Medicine, University of La Laguna, Tenerife, Canary Islands, Spain

Abstract. The incidence of adverse reactions caused by drug treatment was explored in patients admitted to General Hospitals in Canary Islands. Partial results of this study have been reported elsewhere (Sanz and Boada 1982). The present communication deals with new data about unwanted effects produced by drug overdosage. A randomized sample of 864 in-patients was studied. Forms used by the Boston Collaborative Drug Surveillance Program (Miller 1974) were simplified and conveniently adapted to be used by 20 instructed pregraduate medical students who were going to continue their clinical training in six General Hospitals during a period of 6 months. At the end of this period, all data, suitably coded, were submitted to analysis using a Digital VAX-VMS-11/780 computer. Drug overdosage was found in 30 patients and the drugs involved were: digitalis (10 patients), anticonvulsants (3 patients), anxiolytics (3 patients), combinations of barbiturates plus analgesics (6 Patients), antibiotics (2 patients) and miscelaneous (6 patients). Children (10 patients) and the eldery (10 patients) were more frequently affected. The average of drugs administrated to each patient was 3 · 4. Eighteen patients were admitted as a consequence of drug toxicity. Drug overdosage gave rise to a severe clinical picture in 23 patients. The symptomatology was variable and depended on the type of drug employed. Thus, arrythmia and vomiting were seen in digitalis overdosage, and drowsiness and ataxia were common symptom in the patients exposed to central nervous system depressants. Two cases of slight and temporary renal failure, without definitive confirmation, were observed after gentamycin therapy. Atypical reactions were not detected. After drug withdrawal and suitable treatment, the symptoms disappeared in 3–4 days, except for four patients who exhibited sustained alterations. Two cases of ataxia with benzodiazepins and phenytoin lasted about 1 week; a dermatological mercurial preparation produced a marked skin reaction which persisted for 2 weeks; one of the two probable cases of renal failure by gentamycin lasted about 4 weeks. 208 patients in the sample suffered from undesirable reactions to drugs, 80 of them corresponded to hypersensitivity reactions and

76 to expected side-effects. The results presented confirm the high incidence of drug overdosage reactions. It seems to be clear that special attention must be given to the pharmacokinetic and pharmacodynamic interchange in children and the elderly.

Key words: Drug surveillance – Overdosage – Adverse reactions

References

Miller R (1974) Pharmacol Weekblad 109: 461

Sanz E, Boada J (1982) Communication to the VII Reunión Asoc Esp Farm, Salamanca, p 28, 180

Disease, Metabolism and Reproduction in the Toxic Response to Drugs and Other Chemicals
Arch. Toxicol., Suppl. 7, 482–484 (1984)

The Toxic Effects of Clofibrate and Its Metabolite on Mammalian Skeletal Muscle: An Electrophysiologigal Study

D. Conte-Camerino[1], V. Tortorella[2], E. Ferranini[3], and S. H. Bryant[4]

[1] Chair of Pharmacology and Pharmacognosy, Faculty of Pharmacy and [3]Neurological Clinic, Faculty of Medicine, University of Bari, Policlinico, Piazza G. Cesare, 70124 Bari, Italy
[2] Department of Medicinal Chemistry, Faculty of Pharmacy, University of Bari, Via Amendola 165, 70124 Bari, Italy
[4] Department Pharmacology and Cell Biophysics, College of Medicine, Bethesda AV, University of Cincinnati, Cincinnati, OH, USA

Abstract. Membrane electrical parameters of rat extensor digitorum longus muscles were analysed in vitro, with intracellular microelectrodes, after chronic treatment with clofibrate or after in vitro application of chlorophenoxyisobutyric acid, the in vivo metabolite of clofibrate. Clofibrate caused only a 38% decrease in the membrane chloride conductance while its metabolite induced a large decrease of chloride conductance and drastic changes in the excitability characteristics of the muscles sampled. The capability of clofibrate to induce two types of myotonia is discussed.

Key words: Clofibrate – Chlorophenoxyisobutyric acid – Skeletal muscle – Electrical parameters – Myotonia

Several authors by means of contractile and electromyographic (EMG) examinations have identified the myopathy caused by clofibrate in animals and man as a myotonic syndrome (Dromgoole et al. 1975; Kwiecinski 1978). Clofibrate (CL) in vivo is rapidly hydrolyzed to the free carboxylic acid, chlorophenoxyisobutyric acid (CPIB). In the present study electrophysiological investigations have been made in vivo and in vitro on the myotonic syndrome induced by CL and CPIB.

In the first series of experiments, Wistar male rats (250–300 g) were treated chronically (1–14 weeks) with CL (0.4 g/kg Atromidin, Icpharma) with daily subcutaneous injections. Rat extensor digitorum longus (EDL) muscles were studied in vitro at 30° C after 1–14 weeks of CL treatment. Fiber excitability, membrane potentials, membrane resistance and membrane conductances were observed using two intracellular microelectrodes, one for passing current and the

Abbreviations: EMG, Electromyography; CL, clofibrate; CPIB, chlorophenoxyisobutyric acid; EDL, extensor digitorum longus; G_{Cl}, chloride conductance

other for recording membrane potentials (Conte-Camerino et al. 1982). In a second series of experiments the effects of the in vitro application of sodium CPIB (0.5 mg/ml, Sigma) to EDL muscles from untreated rats were investigated using the electrical parameters mentioned above. During the treatment EMGs consistent with myotonia but variable in amplitude and frequency were observed.

The electrical parameters of the EDL (Table 1) during chronic treatment did not vary for the first 6 weeks of treatment; at this time the fibres were depolarized, the membrane resistance increased and the chloride conductance (G_{Cl}) decreased significantly. The excitability characteristics of these fibers were unchanged. In contrast intracellular recordings from the EDL treated in vitro with sodium CPIB (Table 1) showed prolonged latencies in the rheobase, multiple driven spikes and self-sustaining repetitive activity (Fig. 1) together with a drastic decrease in G_{Cl}. Different types of myotonia can be produced in animals by a variety of chemical agents. It is already known that in the myotonia induced by aromatic monocarboxylic acids there is a direct effect of the toxin on the chloride anion channel and the consequent abnormally low G_{Cl} is the basis for the repetitive activity and the after-discharge characteristic of this model of myotonia and typical of myotonia congenita (Bryant and Morales-Aguilera 1971; Adrian and Bryant 1974). In contrast a different mechanism seems be responsable for the myotonia induced by inhibitors of cholesterol synthesis such as 20,25-diazacholesterol. In fact, in this form of myotonia G_{Cl} seems not to be significantly changed (Furman and Barchi 1981) and appears to be secondary to an alteration in the lipid characteristics of the membrane.

These results suggest that CL is capable of inducing two different types of myotonic disorders. That due to sodium CPIB resembles that caused by monocarboxylic aromatic acids and it is similar to myotonia congenita. The myotonia due to chronic CL treatment resembles that caused by diazacholesterol.

Table 1. Mean membrane electrical parameters (± SEM) of rat extensor digitorum longus muscle after chronic treatment with clofibrate or after in vitro chlorophenoxyisobutyric acid application

Preparation	*n*	RP (mV)	Ith (nA)	Th (mV)	Lat (ms)	No. of spikes	n_1	G_{Cl} (μS/cm²)
Clofibrate (CL) chronic treatment								
Controls[a]	26/5	78 ± 2	93 ± 5	40 ± 2	3 ± 0.4	3 ± 0.1	34/6	3,827 ± 164
CL, 6–8 weeks	20/3	69 ± 3*	87 ± 3	33 ± 3	3 ± 0.6	2.5 ± 0.2	15/3	2,373 ± 254*
Chlorophenoxyisobutyric acid (CPIB) in vitro treatment								
Controls	13/3	75 ± 2	78 ± 6	27 ± 1	4 ± 0.2	4 ± 0.5	10/3	3,282 ± 738
CPIB treated	15/4	72 ± 4	38 ± 6*	26 ± 1	26 ± 7*	11 ± 1*	10/4	904 ± 229*

Values are as follows: Preparation; *n* and n_1 are the number of fibers from *n* of muscles examined; RP, resting potential; Ith, threshold current; Th, threshold depolarization; Lat, latency at rheobase; *n*, number of spikes elicited; G_{Cl}, chloride conductance

* Significantly different from mean of control group ($p < 0.01$ or less)

[a] Muscles from untreated rats

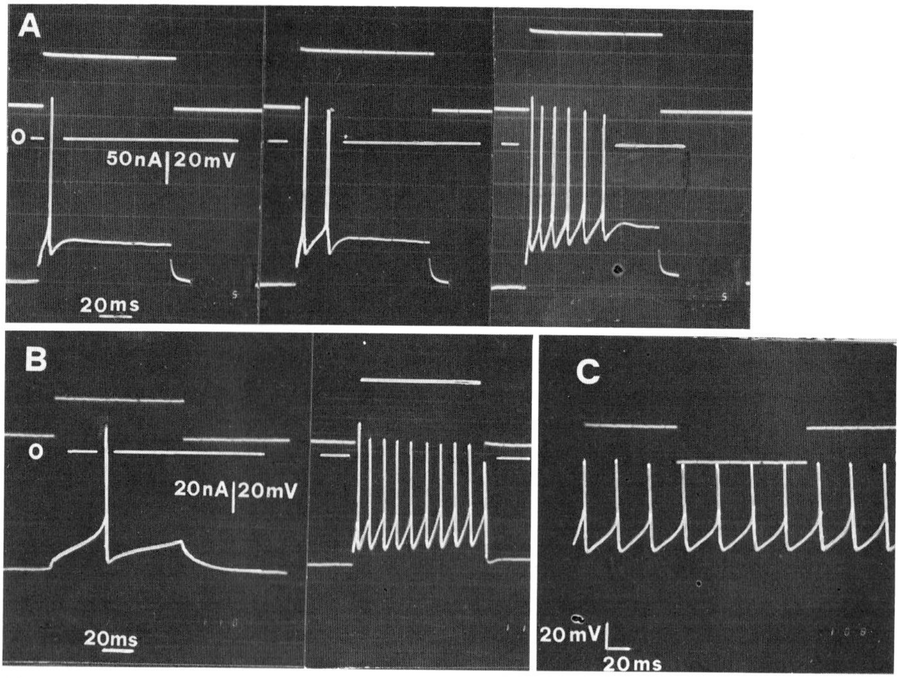

Fig. 1 A–C. Intracellular action potentials from EDL muscle fibers of the rat. **A** Control, **B** and **C** chlorophenoxyisobutyric acid. In C, spontaneous activity. The "*0*" line represents zero potential. *Upper trace,* depolarizing current; *lower trace,* membrane potential. In each fiber the membrane potential was artificially set to −80 mV before passing the depolarizing current. Temperature 30° C

Acknowledgments. We are grateful to Miss A. M. Cioce and to Mr. M. Persichella for expert assistance. This work was supported by grants CT 810014204 and 820212104 from Italian CNR.

References

Adrian RH, Bryant SH (1974) On the repetitive discharge in myotonic muscle fibres. J Physiol (Lond) 240: 500–515

Bryant SH, Morales-Aguilera A (1971) Chloride conductance in normal and mytotonic muscle fibres and the action of monocarboxylic aromatic acids. J Physiol (Lond) 219: 367–383

Conte-Camerino D, Bryant SH, Mitolo-Chieppa D (1982) Electrical properties of rat extensor digitorum longus muscle after chronic application of emetine to the motor nerve. Exp Neurol 77: 1–11

Dromgoole SH, Campion DS, Peter JB (1975) Myotonia induced by clofibrate and sodium chlorophenoxyisobutyrate. Biochem Med 14: 238–240

Furman RE, Barchi RL (1981) 20,25-Diazacholesterol myotonia an electrophysiological study. Ann Neurol 10: 251–260

Kwiecinski M (1978) Myotonia induced with clofibrate in rats. J Neurol 219: 107–116

Disease, Metabolism and Reproduction in the Toxic Response to Drugs and Other Chemicals
Arch. Toxicol., Suppl. 7, 485–487 (1984)

A Comparative Retrospective Analysis of Data from Short- and Long-Term Animal Toxicity Studies on 40 Pharmaceutical Compounds

S. R. Walker[1], E. Schuetz[2], D. Schuppan[2], and J. Gelzer[3]

[1] Centre for Medicines Research, Woodmansterne Road, Carshalton, Surrey SM5 4DS, Great Britain
[2] Bundesverband der Pharmazeutischen Industrie, Karlstrasse 21, 6000 Frankfurt am Main 1, Federal Republic of Germany
[3] INTERPHARMA, 4002 Basle, Switzerland

Abstract. A comparative retrospective survey of data from chronic toxicity studies has been carried out on 40 pharmaceutical compounds based on comprehensive information from 19 pharmaceutical companies. The results showed that no new salient toxicological effects were observed in tests of more than 6 months duration excluding carcinogenicity studies. Since no additional information was identified by dosing animals continuously for 12–18 months, the value of prolonging chronic toxicity studies in animals beyond 6 months should be carefully reassessed.

Key words: Short-term toxicity tests – Long-term toxicity tests – Pharmaceutical compounds – Rodent – Dog – Primate

Introduction

The last 20 years have witnessed an escalation in the number of toxicity studies carried out on new medicines together with a demand for more extensive pre-clinical safety assessment. These changes have been accompanied by a proliferation of guidelines detailing the requirements to be fulfilled before a drug can gain approval for long-term therapy in man. International and national guidelines for the evaluation of new drugs frequently describe a relationship between the minimum duration of animal toxicity studies and the length of time for which the drug can be administered to man. These data requirements vary substantially from one guideline to another and a rational basis for them is not apparent. A number of investigators over the past few years have declared that, apart from carcinogenicity experiments, there is questionable value in dosing animals continuously in chronic toxicity studies beyond 3 or 6 months, but their conclusions were either based on limited data, or they compared published toxicity investigations without common study criteria. In order to overcome these deficiences, a survey has been carried out to ascertain what additional toxicological information, if any, can be gained from animal studies lasting 12 or 18 months compared with those of 3 or 6 months duration.

Methodology

Nineteen pharmaceutical companies based in Germany, Switzerland and the United Kingdom were asked to participate in the survey. Detailed information was requested on those New Chemical Entities that they had studied since 1965 for which they had animal toxicity data from both short (1, 3, or 6 months) and long-term (12 or 18 months) studies which they considered were compatible with the objective of this study. Data was provided on a five page questionnaire that included details of the compound's therapeutic class, the animal species investigated, route of administration, elimination half-life, LD_{50}, dose levels utilised and the duration of the studies. Further details required, included: clinical signs relating to various body systems, laboratory findings (i.e., haematology, clinical chemistry and urinalysis) and salient pathological changes. The times and doses at which effects occurred were noted and in some instances the proportion of animals affected was recorded. Carcinogenicity studies were excluded from the survey.

Results

Toxicity findings were obtained from 62 case studies; each case study required data to be available from both short and long-term studies on the same compound investigated in the same species. These investigations included 50 pharmaceutical compounds from five major therapeutic drug classes: antiinfective, antiinflammatory, central nervous system, cardiovascular system and gastro-intestinal agents, the data having been obtained from the archives of 19 pharmaceutical companies. A significant number of the compounds had been marketed, but for some research had terminated because of toxicity in man or animal, commercial reasons or lack of therapeutic efficacy.

An evaluation of the 62 case studies resulted in rejection of eight because the study design was inappropriate for the analysis, i.e., certain parameters were not measured after both time periods or the number of animals included in the protocol was too small. A further six were subsequently rejected from the comparison as higher doses had been administered during the long-term study. Of the remaining 48 case studies on 40 compounds, in 18 there were tests of up to 18 months in rodents, and 22 and eight case studies included a maximum time span of 12 months in the dog and primate, respectively. Analysis of the data showed that no new salient toxicological features were observed after 1–3 months in 31 case studies and after 6 months for 17 case studies, although for the majority of the latter cases complete data at 3 months including pathological changes were not available for comparison. The salient effects seen included observations such as target organ weight changes, hepatic degeneration, renal tubular necrosis, myocardial fibrosis and necrosis, gastro-intestinal ulceration and blood dyscrasias.

Discussion

This study is the first comprehensive attempt to determine whether any additional information can be gained from toxicity studies of more than 6 months duration by using a survey technique, and obtaining data on investigational drugs direct from pharmaceutical companies in different countries. The companies were encouraged to provide details on as many compounds as possible with the proviso that the data from short and long-term studies should permit comparison of clinical effects, laboratory findings and pathological changes. The state of toxicological practice in the sixties has excluded a number of compounds from being submitted.

Data was provided from five major therapeutic groups; all compounds would have had to reach a late stage in their development to be included in this survey as many drugs under development do not proceed beyond the sub-acute toxicology stage, i.e., studies of 1 or 3 months duration. Few case studies had to be rejected on the basis of study design, although in six the dose for the short-term study was considered to be inappropriate as subsequently higher doses had been administered during the long-term study which made it impossible to include these in the final comparison.

Conclusions

The following conclusions are suggested by an analysis of the data from this preliminary study. First, in these series of chronic toxicity studies of varying duration no new salient toxicological effects were observed in studies beyond 3–6 months. Second, the dose is of fundamental importance in determining whether long-term toxicity studies may reveal different effects from shorter term investigations. Third, as a result of this survey the scientific basis for conventional long-term studies, beyond 6 months duration, excluding carcinogenicity tests, is questioned since organspecific effects, e.g., nephrotoxic or hepatotoxic effects might be investigated more rationally using specifically designed experimental protocols of shorter duration. Last, the implication of these findings is that current toxicological practice should be reassessed and this in turn could lead to a substantial reduction in the duration of experimental exposure and the number of animals required in toxicological evaluation.

Disease, Metabolism and Reproduction in the Toxic Response to Drugs and Other Chemicals
Arch. Toxicol., Suppl. 7, 488–493 (1984)

Cardiac Hypertrophy in the Dog and Rat Induced by Oxfenicine, an Agent Which Modifies Muscle Metabolism

P. Greaves, J. Martin, M. C. Michel, and P. Mompon

Centre de Recherche, Laboratories Pfizer, 37401 Amboise Cedex, France

Abstract. Oxfenicine (S-4-hydroxyphenyl glycine) has been shown to protect the rat and dog heart from experimentally induced myocardial ischaemia probably as a result of its ability to divert myocardial metabolism from fatty acid to carbohydrate utilization with a consequent reduction in oxygen consumption. When various dose levels of oxfenicine were administered to dogs for periods of up to 1 year and rats for periods of up to 2 years, dose-related increases in cardiac weight were observed. No increases in cardiac weight were observed in the rat after only 3 months of treatment but increases were observed in the dogs after a similar treatment period. Macroscopic, light, histochemical and electron microscopic examination of the myocardium revealed that the increase in heart weight was due to uniform myocardial fibre hypertrophy involving all cardiac chambers. Individual muscle fibres were increased in size but there was no clear disproportion of mitochondria and myofibrils. Although intracellular lipid was increased, vacuolated lysosomal structures were only occasionally observed. No histochemical differences in lysosomal enzyme activity were observed between the treated and the control rats. The structural changes were fully compatible with myocardial hypertrophy due to the decreased energy forming capacity of heart muscle resulting from inhibition of fatty acid oxidation by oxfenicine.

Key words: Cardiac hypertrophy – Oxfenicine – Ultrastructure – Histochemistry

Introduction

Oxfenicine (S-4-hydroxyphenyl glycine) has been shown to protect the rat and dog heart from experimentally induced myocardial ischaemia (Higgins et al. 1980; Burges et al. 1981) probably as a result of its ability to divert myocardial metabolism from fatty acid to carbohydrate utilization with consequent reduction in oxygen consumption. It has also been shown to reduce myocardial oxygen consumption in man (Atkinson et al. 1979). However when administered to dogs and rats for prolonged periods increases in heart weight were observed. The purpose of this study was to characterize the cardiac changes.

Material and Methods

The dogs used in this study were male and female Beagle dogs obtained from the Pfizer Sandwich (U.K.) breeding colony, aged 8–10 months at the start of each experiment. They were housed individually in stainless steel cages 80 × 55 × 75 cm, with free access to tap water. They were given 300 g (males) and 250 g (females) of pelleted animal feed 121 from Usine d'Alimentation Rationelle (U.A.R., Villemoisson-sur-Orge, France) once daily after treatment. Rats were of the Sprague-Dawley strain [Crl: COBS-CD(SD)BR] obtained as weanlings from Charles River, France. They were also housed separately in Makrolon shoe-box cages 43 × 30 × 18 cm and had free access to tap water and UAR powdered diet no. A04 was provided ad libitum. Moribund animals and all animals surviving to the scheduled dates of sacrifice were killed, the rats with carbon dioxide gas and the dogs with an overdose of intravenous sodium pentobarbitone. They were submitted to a detailed autopsy which included careful weighting of the heart, gently drained of blood. The organs were fixed in 10% formalin and standard histological sections were prepared.

At the end of the 2-year rat study, fragments of the anterior part of the left ventricular myocardium were taken for histochemical and electron microscopic study. Standard histochemical stains were performed on unfixed frozen tissue (Chayen et al. 1973) and included succinate dehydrogenase, glucose-6-phosphate dehydrogenase, adenosine triphosphatase (calcium activated), reduced nicotinamide dinucleotide phosphate dehydrogenase ($NADPH_2$, diaphorase), acid phosphatase, β-glucuronidase, leucylnaphthylamidase, P.A.S. and Oil red O. The electron microscopic techniques have been previously described (Greaves et al. 1982). The length of the studies and the dose regimens are recorded in Tables 1 and 2.

Results

The body weights, the absolute and relative heart weights of the dogs and rats in the various studies are listed in the tables. Although no increases in cardiac weight were observed in rats after 3 months of treatment with oxfenicine, definite increases were observed in cardiac weight of the dogs following a similar period of treatment with oxfenicine. Absolute heart weights in the dogs treated with 125, 250, or 750 mg/kg/day for 1 year were approximately 70% greater than those of the controls. After 1 year and 2 years of treatment rat heart weights were also greater than the respective controls although differences were less than in dogs.

Table 1. Body and heart weights of rats

	Period of test (3 months) Oral dose (mg/kg/day)			
	0	250	500	1,000
Male rats				
Number per group	15	15	15	15
Mean body weight (g)	475	459	459	438*
Mean absolute heart weight (g)	1.64	1.63	1.55	1.50*
Mean relative heart weight (%)	0.346	0.356	0.338	0.346
Female rats				
Number per group	15	15	15	15
Mean body weight (g)	274	277	262	260
Mean absolute heart weight (g)	1.16	1.09	1.05*	1.05*
Mean relative heart weight (%)	0.422	0.393	0.402	0.407
	Period of test (12 months) Oral dose (mg/kg/day)			
	0	100	300	900
Male rats				
Number per group	15	15	15	15
Mean body weight (g)	617	595	605	554**
Mean absolute heart weight (g)	1.89	1.92	2.07	2.22**
Mean relative heart weight (%)	0.309	0.332	0.343*	0.399***
Female rats				
Number per group	15	15	15	14
Mean body weight (g)	372	387	358	335
Mean absolute heart weight (g)	1.30	1.44*	1.29	1.38
Mean relative heart weight (%)	0.367	0.377	0.368	0.417**
	Period of test (24 months) Oral dose (mg/kg/day)			
	0	100	300	900
Male rats				
Number per group	63	36	40	35
Mean body weight (g)	655	672	669	600**
Mean absolute heart weight (g)	2.17	2.11	2.24	2.20
Mean relative heart weight (%)	0.331	0.318	0.339	0.371**
Female rats				
Number per group	61	25	30	33
Mean body weight (g)	430	459	409	392*
Mean absolute heart weight (g)	1.49	1.47	1.50	1.67***
Mean relative heart weight (%)	0.356	0.330	0.374	0.435***

Univariate analysis of variance separately for each sex. Groups compared to controls by Student's *t*-test

* Statistically significant at $p < 0.05$

** Statistically significant at $p < 0.01$

*** Statistically significant at $p < 0.001$

Table 2. Body and heart weights of dogs

	Period of test (3 months) Oral dose (mg/kg/day)			
	0	75	150	500
Male dogs				
Number per group	3	3	3	3
Mean body weight (g)	10,700	11,200	11,633	11,500
Mean absolute heart weight (g)	92.6	98.3	102.6	115.6
Mean relative heart weight (%)	0.86	0.88	0.88	1.00
Female dogs				
Number per group	3	3	3	3
Mean body weight (g)	10,300	10,600	10,333	10,533
Mean absolute heart weight (g)	87.3	87.3	94.3	103.3
Mean relative heart weight (%)	0.85	0.82	0.91	0.98
	Period of test (12 months) Oral dose (mg/kg/day)			
	0	125	250	750
Male dogs				
Number per group	4	4	4	4
Mean body weight (g)	11,600	11,300	10,900	10,800
Mean absolute heart weight (g)	102.0	113.3	125.5	175.5
Mean relative heart weight (%)	0.88	1.00	1.15	1.64***
Female dogs				
Number per group	4	4	4	4
Mean body weight (g)	10,500	10,500	11,000	10,200
Mean absolute heart weight (g)	87.0	99.8	110.5	150.7**
Mean relative heart weight (%)	0.83	0.95	1.02	1.48**

Univariate analysis of variance separately for each sex. Groups compared to controls by Student's *t*-test
** Statistically significant at $p < 0.01$
*** Statistically significant at $p < 0.001$

Macroscopic and light microscopic examination revealed that the increases in cardiac weight in both the rat and dog were due to symmetrical, increased thickening of the free walls and septum of all the cardiac chambers, with no evidence of cardiac dilatation. Myocardial fibres were enlarged although they were arranged in a normal manner. They generally showed no degenerative changes. Apart from very small foci of subendocardial fibrosis in the largest hearts of the dogs after 1 year of treatment, interstitial collagen or ground substance was not more marked in the treated animals. The coronary vasculature and heart valves were normal in both species at all dose levels.

Histochemical Findings

The only major finding in the rat after 2 years of treatment was the presence of diffuse fine lipid droplets in the myocardium of the rats treated with oxfenicine when compared with the control rats. All enzyme activities remained essentially similar in the controls and the treated rats.

Electron Microscopic Findings

A slight increase in intracellular lipid droplets was observed in the treated rats when compared with the controls and a few lipid-laden lysosomal structures were seen. However, there was no evidence of myofibrillar disarray or degeneration. The mitochondria and the sarcoplasmic reticulum appeared unaltered. There appeared to be no clear disproportion between the quantity of mitochondria relative to myofibrils.

Discussion

Prolonged administration of oxfenicine to dogs and rats produced cardiac hypertrophy. This effect was absent in mice treated according to comparable protocols (data not presented). The hypertrophy was more marked and occurred sooner in dogs than in rats.

The cardiac changes appeared morphologically dissimilar to those reported in most other forms of cardiac hypertrophy, for it was characterized by symmetrical involvement of all cardiac chambers including the atria, lipid accumulation and a general absence of myocardial fibre degeneration and disarray. Systemic hypertension and procedures such as aortic banding and administration of catecholamines tend to produce left ventricular hypertrophy in experimental animals (Laks et al. 1973). The increased cardiac weight observed in malnourished rats is usually accompanied by dilatation of the heart chambers and muscle fibre atrophy (Rossi and Zucoloto 1982). In man, hypertrophic cardiomyopathy is characterized by cardiac fibre disarray (Ferrans 1981), absent in this study. The most comparable morphological changes have been described following chronic administration of thyroxine to animals, which also produces biventricular hypertrophy in the absence of fibrosis or degenerative changes (Skelton and Sonnenblick 1974).

The increase in intracellular lipid observed in the rat heart after treatment with oxfenicine for 2 years is not a surprising finding in view of the fact that oxfenicine inhibits fatty acid utilization. Indeed, similar lipid droplet accumulation has been observed in the hearts of rats developing lipaemia following various dietary changes (Adams et al. 1981). Somewhat more surprising is the lack of marked changes in cytoplasmic organelles, particularly mitochondria and myofibrils, although detailed morphimetric analysis would be necessary to exclude minor changes. However the ultrastructural findings were fully consistent with the lack of histochemical alterations, particularly in mitochondrial and lysosomal enzyme activity. However the absence of major degenerative and enzymatic changes in this study support the concept that the hypertrophy induced by oxfenicine is a simple adaptive response to the decreased energy forming capacity of the heart muscle resulting from inhibition of fatty acid oxidation.

References

Adams MG, Barer R, Joseph S, Ominiabohs F (1981) Fat accumulation in the rat heart during fasting. J Pathol 135: 111–126

Atkinson L, Bergman G, Jackson N, Jewitt DE, Metcalfe JM (1979) Potential protective value of enhanced myocardial carbohydrate utilisation with reduced free fatty acid uptake after UK-25,842 in patients with coronary artery disease. Br J Pharmacol 66: 444

Burges RA, Gardiner DG, Higgins AJ (1981) Protection of the ischaemic dog heart by oxfenicine. Life Sci 29: 1847–1853

Chayen J, Bitensky L, Butcher R (1973) Practical histochemistry, part VI. Enzyme histochemistry. Wiley, London, pp 99–213

Ferrans VJ (1981) Overview of morphological reactions of the heart to toxic injury. In: Balaz T (ed) Cardiac toxicity, vol 3, chap 4. CRC Press, Boca Raton, pp 83–109

Greaves P, Martin J, Masson MT (1982) Spontaneous rat malignant tumors of fibrohistocytic origin: An ultrastructural study. Vet Pathol 19: 497–505

Higgins AJ, Morville M, Burges RA, Gardiner DG, Page MG, Blackburn KS (1980) Oxfenicine diverts rat muscle metabolism from fatty acid to carbohydrate oxidation and protects the ischaemic rat heart. Life Sci 27: 963–970

Laks MM, Morady F, Swan HJC (1973) Myocardial hypertrophy produced by chronic infusion of subhypertensive doses of norepinephrine in the dog. Chest 64: 75–78

Rossi MA, Zucoloto S (1982) Ultrastructural changes in nutritional cardiopathy of protein-calorie malnourished rats. Br J Exp Pathol 63: 242–253

Skelton CL, Sonnenblick EH (1974) Heterogeneity of contractile function in cardiac hypertrophy. Circ Res [Suppl 34–35] 2: 83–96

Disease, Metabolism and Reproduction in the Toxic Response to Drugs and Other Chemicals
Arch. Toxicol., Suppl. 7, 494–498 (1984)

An Epidemic of a "New" Haemorrhagic Disease in Infants Attributable to Talcum Powder Contaminated with Warfarin in Ho-Chi-Minh Ville (Vietnam)

G. Martin-Bouyer[1], N. B. Khanh[1], P. D. Linh[2], and J. Tourneau[3]

[1] INSERM, Unit 165, National Institute of Health and Medical Research, "Transmissible Diseases and Accidental Poisonings", 44, Chemin de Ronde, 78110 Le Vesinet, France
[2] Department of Health, Laboratory of Hygiene and Epidemiology, Ho-Chi-Minh Ville, Vietnam
[3] Toxicology Laboratory, Department of Police, Paris, France

Abstract. In August 1981, pediatric hospitals in Ho-Chi-Minh Ville (Saigon) began to report numerous cases of a haemorrhagic syndrome in infants. A collaborative study with a French epidemilogist began on September 24, 1981, with the aim of finding the cause of this "new" haemorrhagic disease. After having excluded the hypothesis of a viral or bacterial infection, a retrospective study, using questionnaires with 83 items, concerning products of hygiene and nutrition and living conditions, was undertaken. This epidemiological investigation showed this phenomenon was caused by an anticoagulant contained in talcum powder. Analysis of the talcum powders found warfarin; the concentrations ranged between 1.7% and 6.5%. This dramatic episode (741 cases with 177 deaths) ended when the contaminated talc was withdrawn from circulation. The hypothesis of accidental contamination or use of warfarin in lieu of a perfuming agent must be rejected. Accidental addition of a rat-killer seems highly improbable and the possibility of intentional and malevolent adulteration is now under study. An experimental study of hemostasis in two baboons was carried out, using dermal application of the contaminated talc powder. The intoxicated animal died on the 5th day with severe vitamin K deficiency. This accident together with the animal study, shows the transcutaneous uptake of the anticoagulant, which could be of considerable importance in toxicology and in pharmacokinetics.

Key words: Warfarin – Epidemiology – Toxicology – Vitamin K – Haemorrhage – Transcutaneous uptake

Beginning in August 1981, physicians at three pediatric hospitals in Ho-Chi-Minh Ville, Vietnam, reported numerous cases of haemorrhagic syndrome in infants. The clinical profile was characterized by sudden onset with miscellaneous haemorrhagic signs without capillary fragility. Prothrombin time and activated cephalin-koalin time were extremely high; the other coagulation tests were normal. Spinal taps yielded CSF contaminated with blood which could not be coagulated. Autopsy confirmed diffuse meningeal haemorrhage throughout the central nervous system, with the cerebral parenchyma remaining intact. Blood and CSF cultures wre negative; serology showed no evidence for viral infection.

This profile resembles that of severe vitamin K deficiency. However while therapy with intravenous vitamin K and blood transfusion yielded spectacular results in some patients, it was only moderately efficacious in others and the syndrome continued to prove fatal in half of all cases. Furthermore, after recovery some children showed relapse when they returned to the family environment.

All these findings led to a "new" disease profile and since no satisfactory explanation was found, a collaborative study began on September 24, 1981, with the aim of finding the cause.

Infectious aetiology could be eliminated on the basis of the initial observations and only a toxic aetiology was considered likely. The epidemiological study was thus aimed at identification of the toxic agent and the determination of its distribution among the population.

After a study and discussion of the files, four criteria were chosen to define the cases: (i) Infants more than 15 days of age; (ii) haemorrhagic syndrome characterized by ecchymoses, mucosal bleeding, and umbilical bleeding individually or together, but not by purpura or petechia; (iii) red and homogenous CSF from spinal tap; (iv) body temperature normal or below 38°.

Of 200 case-record charts for hospitalized children initially considered, 90 cases were retained (Fig. 1). The epidemic curve shows the beginning of the outbreak during the last week of July and the dramatic increase in the number of weekly cases which looks like an epidemic.

Distribution by age shows that half of the sick children were under 2 months of age (Fig. 2).

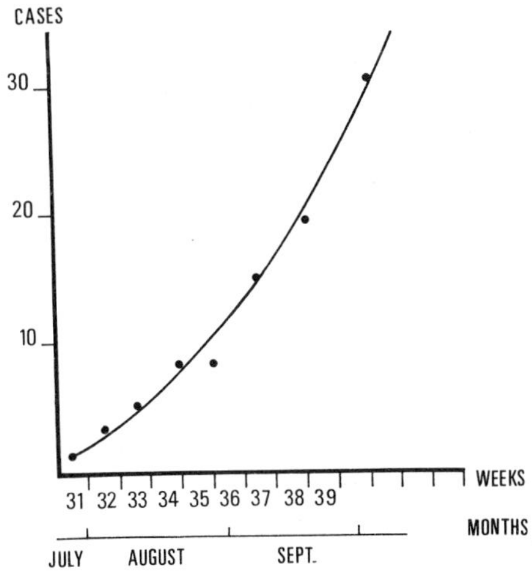

Fig. 1. Haemorrhagic syndrome in the infants. Ho-Chi-Minh Ville, 1981. First study. Epidemic curve

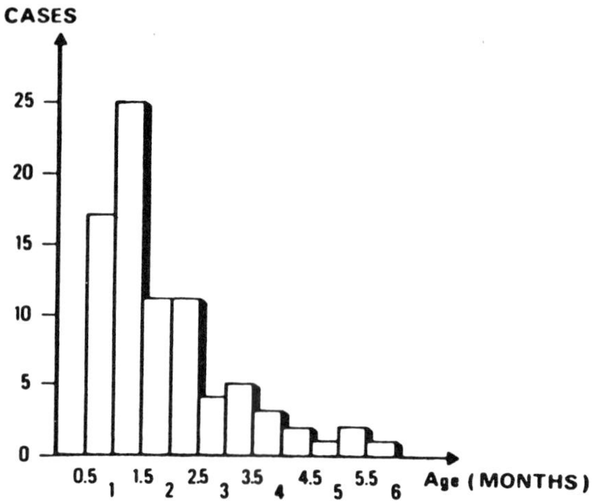

Fig. 2. Haemorrhagic syndrome in the infant. Ho-Chi-Minh Ville, 1981. Distribution of hospitalized patients by age-group

This first study having lead to confirm the existence of the epidemic, to define the age of the patients and to support the toxic aetiology, a retrospective survey was then undertaken in the stricken families.

This study, using questionnaires with 83 items, was made up of closed questions concerning possible factors ranging from insecticides to products for hygiene, nutrition, as well as living conditions. 100 families were chosen on the basis of the clinical signs of haemorrhagic syndrome in the infant or recent haemorrhagic incident.

The data were immediately analysed. The use of insecticides, rat poison, traditional or occidental medicines could be eliminated, as could factors related to the professional or domestic occupation of the parents. One factor appeared to be constant. The use of talcum for infant hygiene. The use of a talc contaminated with a coumarin-type anticoagulant was thus considered to be the most likely explanation.

The analytical results confirmed this hypothesis: Warfarin (α-phenyl-β-acetylethyl-4-hydroxy-coumarin) was found in talc with concentrations ranging from 1.7% to 6.5%. Identification of warfarin in the talcum powder was obtained by infra-red spectrum absorption.

The first seven samples of talcum powder analysed in Paris all contained warfarin. The concentrations were obtained by ultra-violet spectrum absorption using liquid chromatography.

Table 1 shows the different trademark powders found to contain warfarin.

A further study carried out using the same methods with the aim of covering the whole of the epidemic episode allowed identification of 741 cases by October 14 with a rise in the epidemic curve during September (360 new cases). The young age of the patients (55% were younger than 2 months) and the frequently fatal out come (177 deaths) were also confirmed (Fig. 3). The Ho-Chi-Minh city region was not the only area involved, and more than 200 cases were found in neighbouring provinces. This dramatic episode ended when the contaminated talc was withdrawn from circulation. At that time 799 cases were known.

Table 1. Trademark powders containing Warfarin

Can	Number labo	Colour	Perfume	Warfarin	
				Ultra-violet (%)	Liquid chromatography (%)
Fan bo talcum powder	1	White	0	3.4	3.45
White glass	2	Blue	+	1.7	2.3
White glass	3	Blue	+	2.5	2.5
Johnson's baby powder	4	Blue	+	2.5	2.66
Johnson's baby powder	5	Blue	+	2.2	2.28
Johnson's baby powder	6	Blue	+	2.5	2.7
Johnson's baby powder	7	Blue	+	1.75	1.92
Johnson's baby powder	8	White	0	0	0
Johnson's baby powder	9	Blue	+	2.5	3.0
Bong hong	10	White	0	0	0
Fan bo talcum powder	11	White	0	6.5	6.5

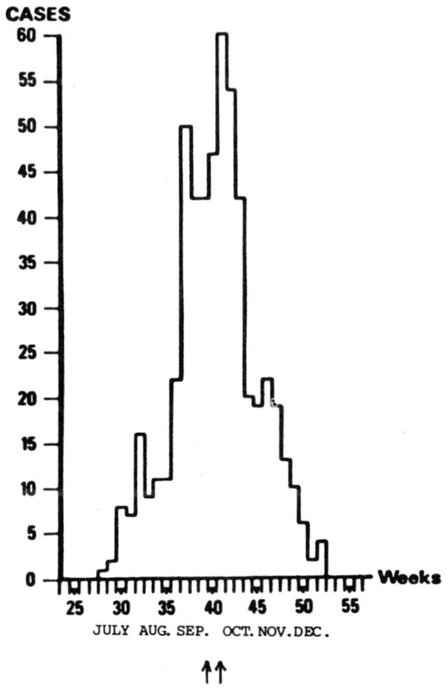

Fig. 3. Time distribution of toxic hemorrhagic syndromes. ↑, Time of epidemiological study

Animal Study

Two young female baboons were studied to discover how easily warfarin could cross the skin. Twice daily, the breech and lower part of the abdomen of the baboons were washed with soap and warm water, rinsed, and toweldried. Talc was applied to the buttock region and nappies (diapers) were put on, as for human infants. On each occasion one of the baboons received an application of 3 g of talc containing 3% warfarin. The other animal received uncontaminated talc under the same conditions. A femoral artery blood sample was taken from each animal before the first application of talc (day 0), on the 3rd day (day 3), and on the 5th day (day 5). For the first 4 days the animals were apparently well. On the 5th day the animal receiving warfarin talc appeared pale and listless; the nappy was spotted with blood. Malaena was noted and bleeding continued at the site of femoral puncture, despite compression. The animal became dyspnoeic, then comatose, and died. At necropsy there were two large subcutaneous haematomas on the skull and the peritoneal cavity was full of uncoagulated blood. There were no obvious visceral lesions.

Coagulation studies in the untreated animal were normal, but the baboon receiving warfarin talc had serious coagulation disturbances by day 3, confirmed as deficiencies of hepatic coagulation factors II, VII, and X.

This accident like the animal study shows the transcutaneous uptake of the anticoagulant warfarin, which could be of considerable importance in toxicology and in pharmacokinetics.

Disease, Metabolism and Reproduction in the Toxic Response to Drugs and Other Chemicals
Arch. Toxicol., Suppl. 7, 499 (1984)

Stress, Drugs, and Pregnancy: Experimental Studies on Embryo-Foetal Toxicity

B. Loscalzo, A. Agrusta, M. Agrusta, A. Crisci, L. Genovese, and M. Marino

Institute of Pharmacology and Toxicology, I Medical School, University of Naples, Naples Italy

Abstract. A research plan has been to evaluate the interference with the embryo-foetal toxicity of some drugs administered in pregnancy, simultaneously with stress factors.

To this aim two groups of pregnant albino rats were treated: the first group received oral hypoglycaemic drugs (glibenclamide + phenformin: GP, dose in mg/kg: 12.5 G and 125 P); the second group received an alcoholic extract of hashish (EH: 1 g of hashish in 100 ml of H_2O with ethanol 9.5%: 1 ml/100 g orally from the 5th to 18th day of pregnancy).

Both groups (total number, including controls: 169 females and 1,756 foetuses) were also exposed to stress by swimming in icy water (S.S.I.W.).

Each experimental group was evaluated according to embryo-foetal toxic parameters (litter size, pup mean weight and placental weight, resorptions, anomalies of bone nuclei by the alizarine technique). Some of these parameters (see Table 1) were significantly changed by S.S.I.W. and an increase of embryo-foetal-toxicity occurred.

The present study underlines the importance of concomitant factors in embryo-foetal damage induced by drugs administered during pregnancy.

Table 1

	A	B	C
Control	12.2 ± 0.98	1.71	5.21 ± 0.28
S.S.I.W.	11.3 ± 0.86	14.49	4.46 ± 0.34
GP	8.8 ± 0.74	7.54	3.46 ± 0.30
GP + S.S.I.W.	9.0 ± 0.70	45.10	2.65 ± 0.48
EH	7.9 ± 0.26	6.33	4.96 ± 0.24
EH + S.S.I.W.	7.0 ± 0.55	44.76	3.40 ± 0.30

A, Foetuses average per dam; B, resorptions % related to implantations; C, mean foetus weight in g

Key words: Embryo – Foetal toxicity – Hypoglycaemic drugs – Hashish – Stress

Acknowledgment. This work was supported in part by Grant from P.I. Min. 40%, 1981.

Disease, Metabolism and Reproduction in the Toxic Response to Drugs and Other Chemicals
Arch. Toxicol., Suppl. 7, 500–503 (1984)

Long-Lasting Hypothermic Effects of Vincristine in Rats

D. Rotiroti, F. Naccari, D. Ammendola, S. Gratteri,
N. De Gori, and G. Nisticò

Institute of Pharmacology, Faculty of Medicine, University of Messina
Piazza XX Settembre, 4, 98100 Messina, Italy

Abstract. The effects of vincristine given intravenously on deep and superficial body temperature were assessed in rats kept at ambient temperature within the thermoneutral range. Vincristine (0.5 and 1 mg/kg i. v.) produced a gradual but marked hypothermic response which was dose-dependent, reached its maximum after approximately 3 h and lasting approximately 48 h. Vincristine induced a decrease in deep body temperature which was accompanied by piloerection and a decrease in skin temperature. Pretreatment with phentolamine, an α-adrenoceptor blocking agent (0.5 mg/kg i.v. 15 min before) prevented the hypothermic effects induced by subsequent administration of vincristine (0.5 mg/kg i.v.).

These experiments showed that vincristine produced a marked hypothermic response in rats. However, the precise site of action remains to be established.

Key words: Vincristine – Vinca alkaloids – Body temperature – Neurotoxicity – Noradrenergic mechanisms

Vinblastine possesses several actions on adrenergic neurons including disruption of the microtubular system (Dählstrom 1971), blockade of axonal transport of enzymes (Wooten and Coyle 1973), reduction of impulse transmission followed by a 6-OH-dopamine-like degeneration of noradrenergic nerve endings (Hanbaurer et al. 1974) with depletion of noradrenaline levels in the heart and reduction of cardiac binding of labelled noradrenaline (Keen and Livingstone 1970; Cheney et al. 1973). There is evidence to suggest that these effects are not possessed by the vinblastine chemical analogue, vincristine (Cheney et al. 1973). On the other hand one of the limiting factors in the therapeutic use of vinca alkaloids as antineoplastic agents is their peripheral and central neurotoxicity (see Creasey 1979).

The aim of the present investigation was to assess the effects of vincristine, given intravenously, on body temperature in rats kept at ambient temperature within the thermoneutral range.

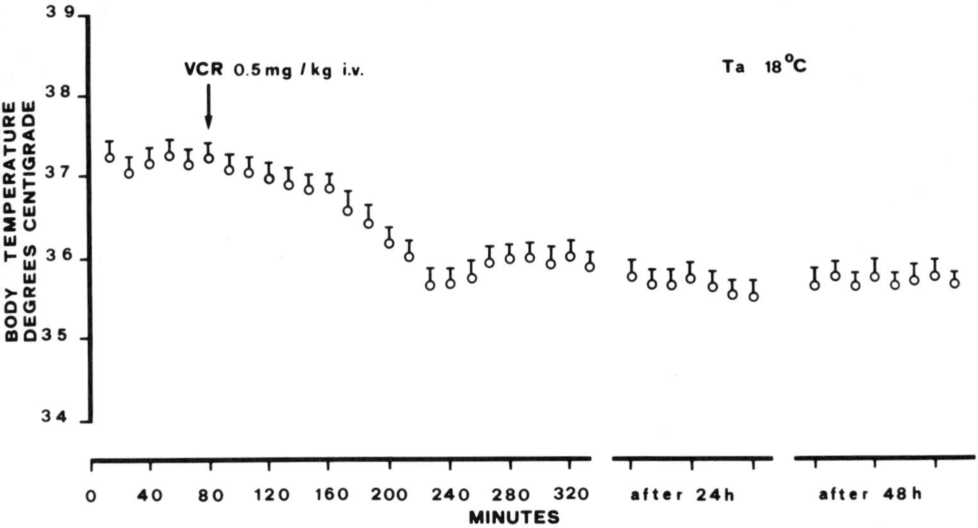

Fig. 1. Hypothermic effects of vincristine (0.5 mg/kg i.v.). Values are means ± SEM of six rats. Ta, Ambient temperature

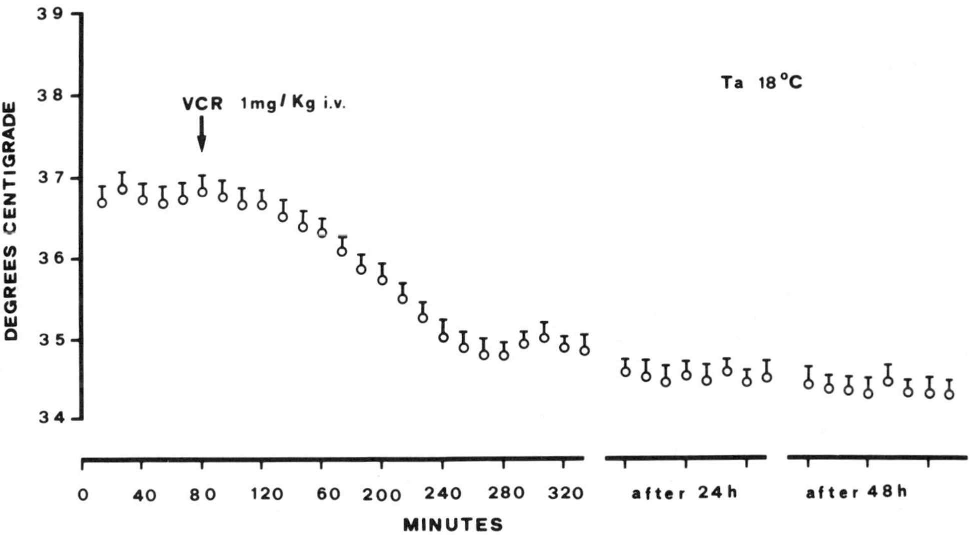

Fig. 2. Hypothermic effects of vincristine (1.0 mg/kg i.v.). Values are means ± SEM of eight rats. Ta, Ambient temperature

Male Wistar-Morini rats weighing 280–300 g were used. All operative procedures were carried out under general anaesthesia. A polyethylene tubing was inserted into a jugular vein and fixed to the skull with acrylic cement. Deep body temperature was recorded on a giant temperature recorder by means of a thermistor chronically implanted in the subcutaneous tissue of the cervical

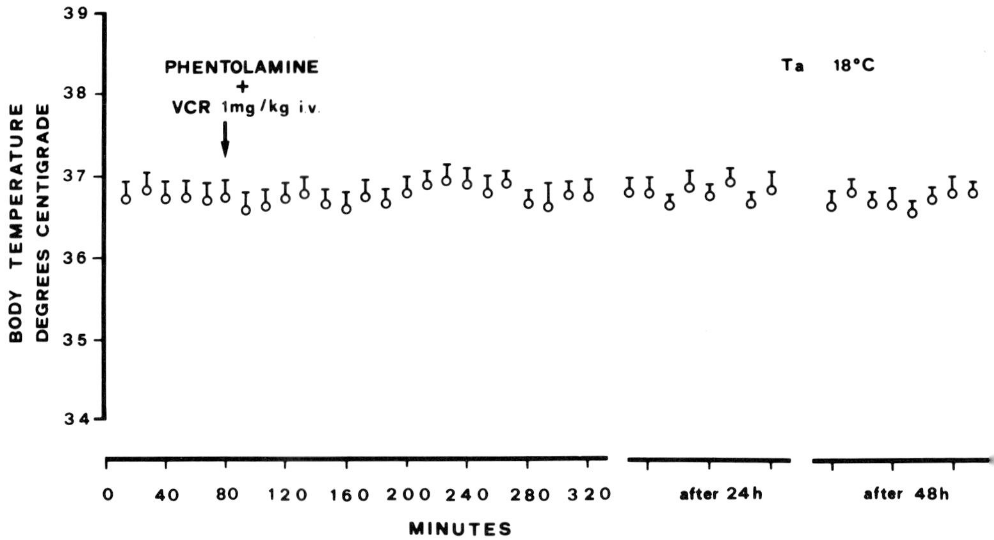

Fig. 3. Antagonism by phentolamine (0.5 mg/kg i.v. 15 min before) of the hypothermic effects induced by subsequent administration of vincristine (1 mg/kg). Values are means ± SEM of six experiments. Ta, Ambient temperature

region, whereas superficial body temperature was recorded from the tail skin.

Vincristine (0.5 and 1 mg/kg) given intravenously produced a gradual decrease in deep body temperature which was dose-dependent (Figs. 1 and 2) and reached its maximum after approximately 3 h and lasted approximately 48 h. However, a smaller dose (0.1 mg/kg i.v.) of vincristine was ineffective (n = 6). The hypothermic effect of vincristine was accompanied by piloerection, decrease in skin temperature and occasional sniffing and licking. Pretreatment with phentolamine (0.5 mg/kg i.v. 15 min before) prevented the hypothermic effects induced by subsequent administration of vincristine at 0.5 mg/kg or 1 mg/kg (Fig. 3).

In conclusion, the present experiments show that vincristine produces in rats marked hypothermic effects which very likely are due to noradrenaline release within the preoptic/anterior hypothalamic area; however, further studies are necessary before excluding the involvement of peripheral mechanisms.

References

Cheney DL, Hanin I, Massarelli R, Trabucchi M, Costa E (1973) Vinblastine and vincristine: A study of their action on tissue concentrations of epinephrine, norepinephreine and acetylcholine. Neuropharmacology 12 : 233–238

Creasey WA (1979) The vinca alkaloids. In: Hahn FE (ed) Antibiotics mechanism of action of antieukaryotic and antiviral compounds. Springer, Berlin Heidelberg New York, pp 414–438

Dählstrom A (1971) Axoplasmic transport (with particular respect to adrenergic neurons). Philos Trans R Soc Lond [Biol] 261 : 325–358

Hanbaurer I, Jacobowitz D, Kopin IJ (1974) Effects of vinblastine on noradrenergic axons. Br J Pharmacol 50 : 219–225

Keen P, Livingstone A (1970) Decline of tissue noradrenaline under the influence of a mitotic inhibitor. Nature 227 : 967–968

Wooten GF, Coyle JT (1973) Axonal transport of catecholamine synthesizing and metabolizing enzymes. J Neurochem 20 : 1361–1373

Disease, Metabolism and Reproduction in the Toxic Response to Drugs and Other Chemicals
Arch. Toxicol., Suppl. 7, 504–507 (1984)

Behavioural Changes in Rats After Prenatal Administration of Typical and Atypical Antidepressants

V. Cuomo[1], I. Cortese[1], R. Cagiano[1], G. Renna[1], and G. Racagni[2]

[1] Institute of Pharmacology, University of Bari, Piazza Giulio Cesare, 70124 Bari, Italy
[2] Institute of Pharmacology and Pharmacognosy, University of Milan,
Via A. del Sarto 21, 20129 Milan, Italy

Abstract. Prenatal administration of typical (desipramine, DMI) and atypical (viloxazine, VX and mianserin, MS) antidepressants, at dose levels which do not influence reproductive success or neonatal mortality, produces subtle behavioural changes in offspring of treated rats. Physical signs, such as pinna detachment (unfolding of external ear) and eye opening, were not modified by prenatal exposure to any of the antidepressants tested. However, at 23 days of age, DMI, MS and VX (only in males) pretreated rats showed higher levels of locomotor activity with respect to the control group. At 60 days of age, locomotor activity levels in DMI-exposed animals were still higher than in the saline-pretreated rats.

Key words: Prenatal administration – Desipramine – Viloxazine – Mianserin – Locomotion – Rat

Clinical studies indicate that neurological alterations have occurred in neonates of women treated during pregnancy with "typical antidepressants", such as tricyclic agent (Webster 1973; Musa and Smith 1979). These clinical reports have been paralleled by recent experimental findings showing that prenatal administration of tricyclic antidepressants (imipramine, amitriptyline) in rats can lead to profound neurobehavioural and neurochemical changes in offspring of exposed dams (Jason et al. 1981; Bigl et al. 1982). On the other hand, studies on the behavioural consequences of prenatal treatment with "atypical antidepressants" are lacking. Thus, the experiments reported here were performed in order to compare the effects induced by prenatal exposure to a typical antidepressant (desipramine) and to two atypical antidepressants (viloxazine and mianserin) on physical and behavioural development in rats.

On day 1 of gestation, the day on which sperm were present in vaginal smears, female rats (Sprague-Dawley) were randomly assigned to the control (saline) and the three antidepressant groups. From day 8 through to day 20 of gestation, the animals were weighed daily and received subcutaneous injections of one of the following: saline (1 ml/kg), DMI (1.25 mg/kg), VX (10 mg/kg) or MS (5 mg/kg). These dose levels, which influence some behavioural and biochemical parameters in the adult rat (Racagni et al. 1982), were chosen to produce the least possible maternal toxicity. The day of birth was designated postnatal day 0. On postnatal day 1 all litters were randomly reduced to a standard size of eight pups per litter (4 females and 4 males). Locomotor activity was measured with an apparatus (toggle-floor boxes) previously used for the study of locomotion in rats (Racagni et al. 1982).

The results show that prenatal antidepressant drug treatment did not influence the reproductive success or neonatal mortality. The number of pups produced per litter (mean ± SE) was as follows: saline (10.8 ± 0.75), DMI (11.3 ± 0.63), VX (11.0 ± 1.47), MS (12.0 ± 2.27). Moreover, the number of pups found dead on day 1 as a proportion of the total number born was as follows: saline (1/43), DMI (1/45), VX (0/44), MS (2/48). Figure 1 shows that the body weights of VX and MS exposed offspring were significantly higher than those of the control animals until postnatal day 18. However, from day 21 after birth no significant differences between the controls and the treated animals were found. Physical signs, such as pinna detachment (unfolding of external ear) and eye opening, were not influenced by prenatal treatment with all the antidepressants tested. The data are not shown. Concerning the effects of prenatal exposure to DMI, VX and MS on the locomotion of 23 day old rats, analysis of variance of activity crossings showed significant differences between treatments (F: 34.06; df: 3/56; $p < 0.01$), between sexes (F: 14.90; df: 1/56; $p < 0.01$) and between treatments × sexes (F: 3.62; df: 3/56; $p < 0.05$).

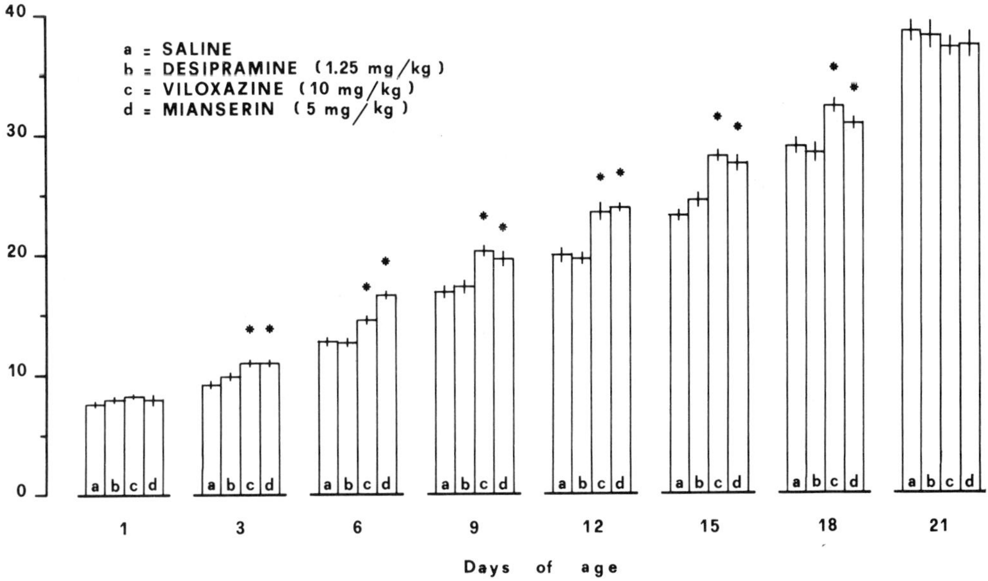

Fig. 1. Body weight of rats (males + females) prenatally treated with antidepressant agents. For pharmacological treatment, see the text. Antidepressants vs saline. * $p < 0.01$ (Student's *t*-test)

Table 1. Effect of prenatal antidepressant drug treatment on locomotor activity (15 min session) of 23 days old rats

Drugs (mg/kg)	Number of crossings (mean ± SE)	
	Males	Females
Saline	14.6 ± 1.41	12.4 ± 2.21
Desipramine (1.25)	24.0 ± 3.60*	23.0 ± 0.90*
Viloxazine (10)	21.3 ± 2.88*	12.9 ± 1.12
Mianserin (5)	25.1 ± 3.36*	23.1 ± 2.30*

Each group consisted of eight animals. For pharmacological treatment, see the text. Antidepressants vs saline: * $p < 0.001$ (test of least significant difference)

Table 2. Effect of prenatal antidepressant drug treatment on locomotor activity (15 min session) of 60 days old rats

Drugs (mg/kg)	Number of crossings (mean ± SE)	
	Males	Females
Saline	19.3 ± 1.53	20.5 ± 2.28
Desipramine (1.25)	28.8 ± 4.03*	31.1 ± 2.00**
Viloxazine (10)	21.4 ± 1.36	20.0 ± 1.40
Mianserin (5)	18.8 ± 2.72	23.5 ± 1.14

Each group consisted of eight animals. For pharmacological treatment, see the text. Desipramine vs saline: * $p < 0.01$, ** $p < 0.001$ (test of least significant difference)

Individual between treatments comparison indicated that locomotor activity levels of DMI and MS pretreated rats were significantly higher with respect to those of the control group; as regards the group pretreated with VX, only male rats exhibited a significant increased locomotion at 23 days of age (Table 1). At 60 days of age, analysis of variance of activity crossings showed the following differences: between treatments (F: 9.50; df: 3/56; $p < 0.01$), between sexes (F: 1.30; df: 1/56; n.s.) and between treatments × sexes (F: 0.69; df: 3/56; n.s.); individual between treatments comparison indicated that locomotor activity levels in DMI pretreated animals were still higher than in saline-pretreated ones, whereas VX and MS pretreated rats did not exhibit any significant difference with respect to the control group (Table 2).

The comparison of the present data with recent findings (Racagni et al. 1982; Cuomo et al. 1983a) shows that the locomotion of rats receiving prolonged treatment with DMI, VX and MS during adulthood was not modified with respect to the control animals. In this regard, it has been demonstrated that the behavioural and biochemical changes induced by chronic administration of other psychotropic drugs in adult rats completely differ from those produced by chronic treatment during neuronal maturation (Cuomo et al. 1983b). This study further suggests that the behavioural consequences of a prolonged treatment with some psychotropic agents are critically dependent upon the period of their administration. Furthermore, these findings indicate that DMI, VX and MS could be included in the class of chemical agents which cause behavioural changes in offspring of treated animals at subteratogenic doses.

References

Bigl V, Dalitz E, Kunert E, Biesold D, Leonard BE (1982) The effect of d-amphetamine and amitriptyline administered to pregnant rats on the locomotor activity and neurotransmitters of the offspring. Psychopharmacology 77: 371–375

Cuomo V, Cagiano R, Brunello N, Fumagalli R, Racagni G (1983a) Behavioural changes after acute and chronic administration of typical and atypical antidepressants in rats: Interactions with reserpine. Neurosci Lett 40: 315–319

Cuomo V, Cagiano R, Mocchetti I, Coen E, Cattabeni F, Racagni G (1983b) Biochemical and behavioural effects after early postnatal administration of neuroleptics in rats. In: Zbinden G, Cuomo V, Racagni G, Weiss B (eds) Application of behavioural pharmacology in toxicology. Raven, New York, pp 173–186

Jason KM, Cooper TB, Friedman E (1981) Prenatal exposure to imipramine alters early behavioral development and beta adrenergic receptors in rats. J Pharmacol Exp Ther 217: 461–466

Musa A, Smith C (1979) Neonatal effects of maternal chlorimipramine therapy. Arch Dis Child 54: 405–408

Racagni G, Mocchetti I, Renna G, Cuomo V (1982) In vivo studies on central noradrenergic synaptic mechanisms after acute and chronic antidepressant drug treatment: Biochemical and behavioral comparisons. J Pharmacol Exp Ther 223: 227–234

Webster P (1973) Withdrawal symptoms in neonates associated with maternal antidepressant therapy. Lancet 2: 318–319

Disease, Metabolism and Reproduction in the Toxic Response to Drugs and Other Chemicals
Arch. Toxicol., Suppl. 7, 508–509 (1984)

Side Effects of Drugs Stimulating Prolactin Secretion on the Behavior of Male Rats

F. Drago and U. Scapagnini

Institute of Pharmacology, University of Catania Medical School,
Viale A. Doria 6, 95125 Catania, Italy

Abstract. The behavioral effects of drugs stimulating PRL secretion have been studied in male rats. Acquisition of active avoidance behavior was facilitated by short- (SHPRL) and long-term hyperprolactinaemia (LHPRL) induced by pituitary homografts under the kidney capsule. Neuroleptics such as haloperidol and bromperidol, caused hyperprolactinaemia and suppressed the acquisition of active avoidance behavior. Sulpiride was not effective in this respect. SHPRL facilitated and LHPRL inhibited sexual behavior of male rats. Haloperidol, but not sulpiride suppressed the sexual capacity of these animals. Sulpiride and domperidone, but not haloperidol, increased the locomotor activity of male rats. These data suggest that differences in the behavioral effects of neuroleptics may depend on their capacity to compete with PRL at the central level.

Key words: Neuroleptics – Prolactin – Behavior

References

Bailey DJ, Herbert J (1982) Impaired copulatory behaviour of male rats with hyperprolactinaemia induced by domperidone or pituitary grafts. Neuroendocrinology 35: 186–192

Chen Y-F, Ramirez VD (1982) Prolactin stimulates dopamine release from male but not from female rat striatal tissue superfused in vitro. Endocrinology 111: 1740–1742

Cooper BR, Howard JL, Grant LD, Smith RD, Breese GR (1974) Alteration of avoidance and ingestive behaviour after destruction of central catecholamine pathways with 6-hydroxydopamine. Pharmacol Biochem Behav 2: 639–649

Doherty PC, Smith MS, Bartke A (1980) Hyperprolactinaemia and reproductive function in male rats. Effects of adrenalectomy and bromocriptine. Endocrinol Soc Meet Abst 704

Drago F, Bhous B (1981) Hyperprolactinaemia-induced excessive grooming in the rat: time course and element analysis. Behav Neurol Biol 33: 117–122

Drago F, Canonico PL, Bitetti R, Scapagnini U (1980) Systemic and intraventricular prolactin induces excessive grooming. Eur J Pharmacol 65: 547–458

Drago F, Pellegrini-Quarantotti B, Scapagnini U, Gessa GL (1981a) Short-term endogenous hyperprolactinaemia and sexual behavior of male rats. Physiol Behav 26: 277–279

Drago F, Ree JM van, Bohus B, Wied D de (1981b) Endogenous hyperprolactinaemia enhances amphetamine- and apomorphine-induced stereotypy. Eur J Pharmacol 72: 249–253
Drago F, Bohus B, Mattheij JAM (1982a) Endogenous hyperprolactinaemia and avoidance behaviors of the rat. Physiol Behav 28: 1–4
Drago F, Bohus B, Ree JM van, Scapagnini U, Wied D de (1982b) Behavioral responses of long-term hyperprolactinaemic rats. Eur J Pharmacol 79: 323–327
Fuxe K, Eneroth P, Gustafsson J-A, Löfström A, Skett P (1977) Dopamine in the nucleus accumbens: preferential increase of DA turnover by rat prolactin. Brain Res 122: 177–182
Fuxe K, Andersson K, Hökfelt T, Agnati LF (1978) Prolactin-monoamine interactions in the rat brain and their importance in regulation of LH and prolactin secretion. In: Robin C, Harter M (eds) Progress in prolactin physiology and pathology. Elsevier/North-Holland, Amsterdam, pp 95–109
Hruska RE, Pitman KT, Silbergeld EK, Ludmer LM (1982) Prolactin increases the density of striatal dopamine receptors in normal and hypophysectomized male rats. Life Sci 30: 547–553
Lichtensteiger W, Lienhart R (1975) Central action of α-MSH and prolactin: simultaneous responses of hypothalamic and mesencephalic dopamine systems. In: Endroczi E (ed) Cellular and molecular bases of neuroendocrine processes. Akadémiai Kiadò, Budapest, pp 211–221
Malmnas CD (1973) Monoaminergic influence on testosterone activated copulatory behavior in the castrated male rat. Acta Physiol Scand [Suppl] 39
Muller P, Seeman P (1975) Alterations in dopaminergic sensitivity in chronically pretreated rats. Soc Neurosci Abst 412
Muller P, Musch K, Wolf AS (1979) Prolactin variables of personality and sexual behavior. In: Zichella L, Pancheri P (eds) Psychoneuroendocrinology in reproduction. Elsevier-North-Holland, Amsterdam, pp 359–372
Neill JD (1980) Neuroendocrine regulation of prolactin secretion. In: Martini L, Ganong WF (eds) Frontiers in neuroendocrinology, vol 6. Raven, New York, pp 129–155
Paglietti E, Pellegrini-Quarantotti B, Mereu GP, Gessa GL (1978) Apomorphine and L-DOPA lower ejaculation threshold in the male rat. Physiol Behav 20: 559–562
Perkins NA, Westfall TC (1978) The effect of prolactin on dopamine release from rat striatum and medial basal hypothalamus. Neuroscience 3: 59–63
Ranje C, Ungerstedt U (1977) Lack of acquisition in dopamine denervated animals tested in an underwater Y-maze. Brain Res 134: 95–111
Svare B, Bartke A, Doherty P, Mason I, Michael SD, Smith MS (1979) Hyperprolactinemia suppresses copulatory behavior in male rats and mice. Biol Reprod 21: 529–535
Tagliamonte A, Fratta W, Del Fiacco M, Gessa GL (1974) Possible stimulatory role of brain dopamine in the copulatory behavior of male rats. Pharmacol Biochem Behav 2: 257–260
Wuttke W, Höhn KG, Honma K, Hilgendorf W, Lamberts R (1980) Interrelationship between prolactin and gonadotropins. In: MacLeod RM, Scapagnini U (eds) Central and peripheral regulation of prolactin function. Raven, New York, pp 221–236

Disease, Metabolism and Reproduction in the Toxic Response to Drugs and Other Chemicals
Arch. Toxicol., Suppl. 7, 510–514 (1984)

Possible Adverse Effects on the Cardiovascular System of an Antiarrhythmic Drug Mexiletine

F. Rossi, E. Ruggiero, M. A. Scafuro, M. Giasi, V. Mazzeo, G. Bile, E. Lamparelli, and E. Marmo

Institute of Pharmacology and Toxicology, Ist Faculty of Medicine and Surgery, University of Naples, Naples, Italy

Abstract. Mexiletine (MXT) is a drug endowed with a marked antiarrhythmic activity which may be included in 1B class of drugs employed in the therapy of arrythmias. In experimental cardiovascular research, MXT at very high doses induces a decrease in the arterial blood pressure and cardiac performance of dogs. MXT reduces the carotid baroreceptor responses, the fall in blood pressure following pharadic stimulation of the peripheral trunk of the vagus nerve and it also inhibits catecholamine uptake. All these effects may be related to the local anaesthetic activity which MXT possesses and which need careful consideration in the clinical use of the drug.

Key words: Adverse cardiovascular effects – Mexiletine

Introduction and Methods

Several studies were carried out in order to find antiarrhythmic drugs with a large therapeutic spectrum, a large manageable zone and with no toxic or unfavourable hemodynamic and cardiac effects. This ideal antiarrhythmic drug should be efficacious in every abnormal generation and conduction of impulses, such as increase of automaticity, reentrant arrhythmias and rhythms due to slow response by calcium-channels. It should have: minimum effect on normal excitation and conduction, and prolonged activity. It should be administrable by both the oral and intravenous route. It should not have significant interaction with other drugs (Marmo 1981).

Antiarrhythmic drugs can worsen cardiovascular performance and ventricular arrhythmias; for example, Pindolol induces an 18.5% increase in ventricular arrhythmias, quinidine sulphate 17%, aprindine 13.3%, mexiletine 10.9%, procainamide 7.5%, and propranolol 6.5% (Montgomery 1979).

Mexiletine (1-methyl-(2,6-xylyloxy)ethylamine · HCl) is an antiarrhythmic drug of the 1B class structurally analogous with lidocaine. It is used almost exclusively to treat ventricular arrhythmias. In therapeutic use mexiletine is given to adults as a single dose of 200 mg orally, or 250 mg intravenously (Marmo 1981).

Cardiovascular effects were observed at doses higher than those utilized in therapeutics. These experiments were carried out in order to evaluate probable negative effects of mexiletine on the cardiovascular system of anaesthetized dogs (α-chloralose 100 mg/kg given intravenously [i.v.]). Animals of both sexes were used weighing 6–10 kg. Arterial blood pressure, heart rate and respiration were recorded on a Hellige polygraph. In vitro studies were conducted on the isolated hearts of frogs (20–30 g) and albino rats (NOS strain, 220–280 g) perfused respectively by Goethlin and by Ringer-Locke solutions.

Results

In vitro mexiletine, administered in successive doses, induces a transitory and dose-dependent negative inotropic effect starting from concentrations of 5.5×10^{-7} M/l with isolated hearts of frogs and starting from concentrations of 5.5×10^{-8}–10^{-7} M/l with isolated hearts of rats (Fig. 1).

The perfusion of mexiletine for a period of 20 min through isolated hearts of rats induced a decrease of the inotropic effect starting from the concentration of 5.5×10^{-9} M/l. A decrease of coronary blood flow was induced at a concentration of 5.5×10^{-6} M/l. In vitro mexiletine starting from a concentration of 5.5×10^{-10} M/l produced a moderate and dose-proportional decrease of the positive inotropic effect induced by $CaCl_2$ (0.2–0.4 mg), by $BaCl_2$ (0.2–0.4 mg) and by isoprenaline (10^{-11} M/l). The coronary constriction by pitressin (0.01–0.1 IU) is not modified at concentrations between 5.5×10^{-11} and 5.5×10^{-9} M/l.

Mexiletine, given by the gastric route in single doses per kg corresponding to 50–100 mg to a bivagotomized dog, does not significantly modify the arterial blood pressure or the respiration, but it produces a moderate and transitory sinus bradycardia ($-11.8 \pm 2.1\%$ and $-21.6 \pm 2.9\%$, respectively, 2 h after mexiletine treatment).

Mexiletine, given by the intramuscular route at a dose of 10 mg/kg, does not significantly modify the arterial blood pressure, the respiration or the ECG, while at doses of 50–100 mg/kg, it caused 2 h after mexiletine treatment an hypotensive effect [-15 ± 1 and -36 ± 5 (mm Hg ± SE), respectively] associated with sinus bradycardia ($-18.6 \pm 3.8\%$ and $-36.9 \pm 6.2\%$, respectively). The respiration was not altered. At a dose of 250 mg/kg, it killed the animal.

Mexiletine, when given by the gastric route at a dose of 50 mg/kg, produced a moderate decrease in the hypertensive response induced by a 15 s occlusion of both common carotid arteries and it also induced a decrease of the hypotensive response due to faradic stimulation for 3–5 s of the peripheral end of the vagus nerve ($-82.5 \pm 6.1\%$ and $-61.5 \pm 4.5\%$, respectively, 2 h after mexiletine treatment).

The hypotensive response due to acetylcholine (0.1–1 µg/kg i.v.) is not significantly modified.

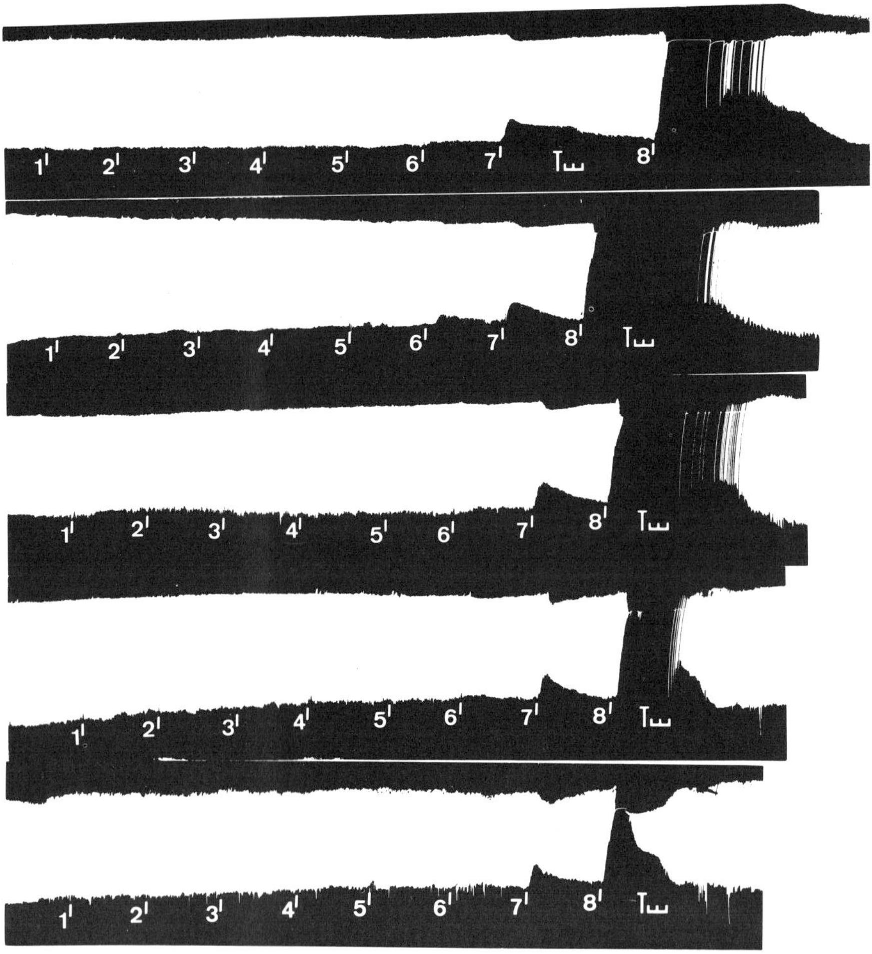

Fig. 1. Effect of mexiletine on isolated hearts of five rats. At positions *1–8* mexiletine was administered at concentrations of 5.5×10^{-13} (*1*), 5.5×10^{-12} (*2*), 5.5×10^{-11} (*3*), 5.5×10^{-10} (*4*), 5.5×10^{-9} (*5*), 5.5×10^{-8} (*6*), 5.5×10^{-7} (*7*), 5.5×10^{-6} (*8*), M/l. *T*: time of 60 s

Mexiletine, when given by the intravenous route to bivagotomized dogs at doses of 20–30 mg/kg, induced a moderate and transitory arterial hypotension; a dose of 50 mg/kg killed the animal.

Mexiletine, when given by the intravenous route at doses between 10–20 mg/kg, decreased the hypertensive response due to the occlusion of both common carotid arteries for × 15–30 s ($-13.3 \pm 2.1\%$ and $-41.6 \pm 2.8\%$, respectively), and it decreased the hypotensive response due to faradic stimulation for 3–5 s of the peripheral end of the vagus nerve ($-28.3 \pm 2.6\%$ and $-41.2 \pm 3.8\%$ respectively); at doses of 10–20 mg/kg it increased the hypertensive response induced by e-norepinephrine (1 µg/kg i.v. in 5 s) ($+16 \pm 3\%$ and $+31 \pm 4.2\%$, respectively) associated with sinus bradycardia.

Table 1. Effects induced by infiltration with mexiletine into both the carotid sinus walls in dogs

No. animals used	Treatment	% Reduction ± SE of the hypertension induced by occlusion of carotid arteries for 30 sec 5 min after infiltration	Maximal variation (mm Hg ± SE) of arterial pressure by infiltration of NaCl 0.9% solution or mexiletine solution
4	NaCl 0.9% (0.2 ml solution)	0	0
4	Mexiletine (0.001% solution)	0	0
4	Mexiletine (0.01% solution)	− 14 ± 1	+ 14 ± 2
4	Mexiletine (0.1% solution)	− 18 ± 3	+ 19 ± 2
4	Mexiletine (1% solution)	− 20 ± 2	+ 23 ± 3

Table 2. Effects of mexiletine injected into the common carotid artery

No. animals used	Treatment mg/kg into the common carotid artery (each injection in 5 sec)	% Reduction ± SE of the hypertension induced by occlusion of both common carotid arteries for 30 s 5 min after mexiletine injection into the common carotid artery		Maximal variation (mm Hg ± SE) of arterial pressure 5 min after mexiletine injection into the common carotid artery	
		with sinus denervation	without sinus denervation	with sinus denervation	without sinus denervation
4	Mexiletine 0.01	− 10 ± 2.4	− 13 ± 1.3	0	0
4	Mexiletine 0.1	− 24 ± 6.1	− 33 ± 4.1	0	0
4	Mexiletine 1	− 32 ± 4.7	− 44 ± 5.6	− 10 ± 1	− 11 ± 1
4	Mexiletine 10	− 46 ± 7.1	− 58 ± 6.8	− 16 ± 2	− 17 ± 3

The hypotensive response induced by acetylcholine (0.1–1 μg/kg i.v.) is not significantly modified.

Infiltration of both walls of the carotid sinus of bivagotomized dogs was carried out with 0.2 ml per sinus of mexiletine at concentrations of 0.001–1%. At the concentrations of 0.1–1%, a transitory increase of the arterial blood pressure associated was produced with a decrease of the hypertension induced by carotid endosinusal hypotension (Table 1).

Mexiletine when administered into the common carotid artery, with or without sinus denervation, of bivagotomized dogs, prepared according to Heymans et al. (1931), starting from a dose of 0.01 mg/kg reduced the hypertensive response due to an occlusion of the contralateral common carotid sinus (Table 2).

Starting from doses of 1–10 mg/kg, it induced a slow and progressive arterial hypotension.

Discussion

In conclusion mexiletine at doses higher than those necessary for antiarrhythmic activity (0.8–4.16 mg/kg) exhibits hypotensive, bradycardial and negative inotropic effects. The hypotension is dependent on an intact peripheral and central nervous effect. The bradycardia and the reduction of cardiac contractility are related to the peripheral effects of mexiletine independent of interference with β-adrenergic receptors.

High dosages of mexiletine reduce the baroreceptor response of the carotid sinus by both direct and central nervous effects. It also affects acetylcholine release, as seen in the reduction of the response to peripheral vagus stimulation which was not associated with the hypotensive response induced by acetylcholine.

The increase in norepinephrine induced hypertension showed that mexiletine inhibited catecholamine uptake. These last effects are due to its local anaesthetic activity (Marmo 1981).

Acknowledgment. This research was supported by grants from CNR and MPI.

References

Heymans C, Bouckaert JJ, Dautrebande A (1931) Sinus carotidien et réflexes respiratoires. III. Sensibilité des sinus carotidiens aux substances chemiques. Action stimulante respiratoire réflexe du sufure de sodium, du cyanure de potassium, de la nicotine et de la lobéline. Arch Int Pharmacodyn Ther 40: 54–91

Marmo E (1981) Farmacologia delle aritmie cardiache. Minerva, Torino

Montgomery BJ (1979) Antiarrhythmic agents may cause sudden dealth drug testing urged. JAMA 241: 1771–1793

Novel and New Techniques in Toxicology

Disease, Metabolism and Reproduction in the Toxic Response to Drugs and Other Chemicals
Arch. Toxicol., Suppl. 7, 517–520 (1984)

A Single Step Method for the Separation of Rat Liver Cytosolic Glutathione S-Transferase Isozymes

B. Botti-Cacciari[1], M. T. Moslen[2], E. S. Reynolds[2] †, and V. Vannini[1]

[1] Istituto di Patologia Generale, Universitá di Modena, 41100 Modena, Italy
[2] Chemical Pathology Laboratory, UTMB, Galveston, TX, USA

Abstract. A simple, single step chromatographic method was developed to separate the liver cytosolic glutathione S-transferase (GSH-S-t) isozymes from each other and from the bulk of the cytosolic protein.

Five peaks of GSH-S-t activity, tested with 1-chloro-2,4-dinitrobenzene (CDNB) as a substrate, were eluted. By comparison of the activities with CDNB and the other substrate 3,4-dichloronitrobenzene (DCNB) the five peaks could be identified as GSH-S-t isozymes C, B, A, and AA, being GSH-S-t isozyme C eluted in two different peaks.

The method was used to detect a decrease of specific GSH-S-t isozymes in the cytosol of rats intoxicated with carbon tetrachloride, as compared with control rats.

Key words: Carbon tetrachloride – Glutathione S-transferase isozymes

It was recently found that liver cytosolic glutathione S-transferase (GSH-S-t) activities were rapidly decreased in rats given carbon tetrachloride (CCl_4), 1,2-dibromoethane (Botti and Moslen 1982) or 1,1-dichloroethylene (Moslen and Reynolds 1981). Each toxin decreased GSH-S-t activities with two or three of the following substrates: 1-chloro-2,4-dinitrobenzene (CDNB), 3,4-dichloronitrobenzene (DCNB), 1,2-epoxy-3-(p-nitro-phenoxy)propane and ethacrynic acid. This apparent substrate specificity could be due to deactivation of specific cytosolic GSH-S-t isozymes. It was decided, therefore, to verify this possibility in the case of CCl_4 treatment.

Chemicals. DNCB and CDNB were obtained from Aldrich Chemical Co., and were recrystallized from ethanol-water twice before use. GSH was obtained from Sigma Chemical Co. CCl_4 was from Fisher Scientifc Co.

Abbreviations: CCl_4, Carbon tetrachloride; CDNB, 1-chloro-2,4-dinitrobenzene; DCNB, 3,4-dichloronitrobenzene; GSH, reduced glutathione; GSH-S-t, Glutathione S-transferase

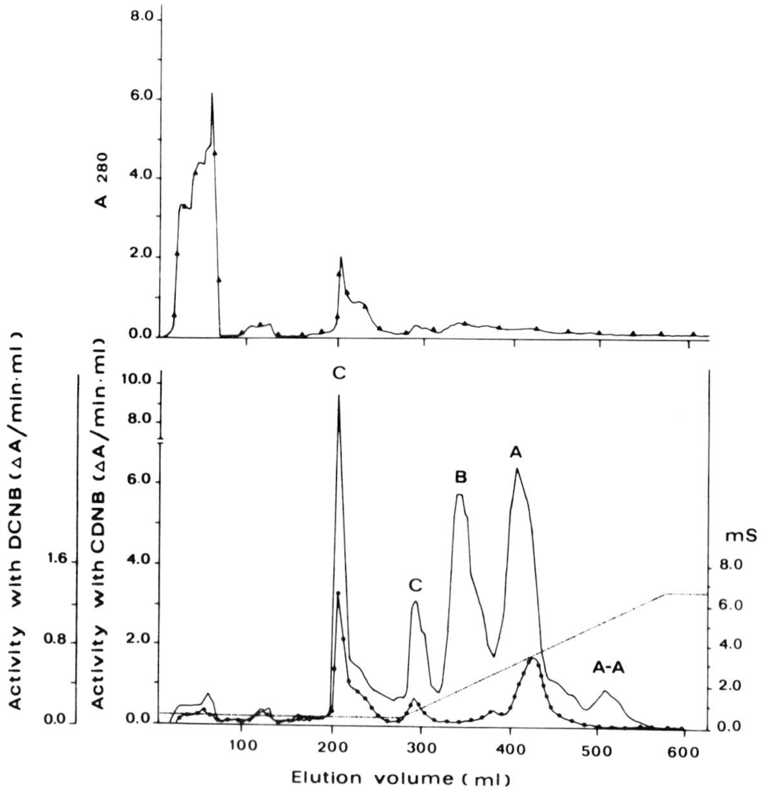

Fig. 1. Elution pattern from CM-Sephadex C-50 column of liver cytosolic protein and glutathione S-transferase isozymes from control rats. (———) activity with 1-chloro-2,4-dinitrobenzene (CDNB); (●) activity with 3,4-dichloronitrobenzene (DCNB); (▲) absorbance at 280 nm; (------) conductivity in milliSiemens (mS)

Treatment of Animals. Male Sprague-Dawley (Charles River Laboratories, Calco, Italy) rats, acclimatized in a 12 h light/dark cycle animal room for at least one week, were used. Rats weighing 200–250 g and fasted from the previous evening were given CCl_4 by gavage in the dose of 4.0 mmol/kg in mineral oil 2 h before sacrifice, in a total volume of 2.5 ml/kg; control rats received only mineral oil.

Separation of GSH-S-t Isozymes. A single step chromatographic method was developed to separate liver GSH-S-t isozymes from each other and from the bulk of the cytosolic protein.

Liver cytosol was prepared as previously described (Botti and Moslen 1982) with the exception that the homogenate was in 5 mM sodium-phosphate buffer, pH 6.7 containing 0.25 M sucrose. Cytosol from three control rats was dialyzed (4° C, 15 h) against two changes, each of 4 l of 5 mM sodium phosphate buffer pH 6.7 containing 1.4 mM mercaptoethanol (initial buffer). The dialyzed cytosolic protein (400 mg) was applied to a CM-Sephadex C-50 (Pharmacia) column (2.6 × 17 cm) which was equilibrated with the initial buffer. After the

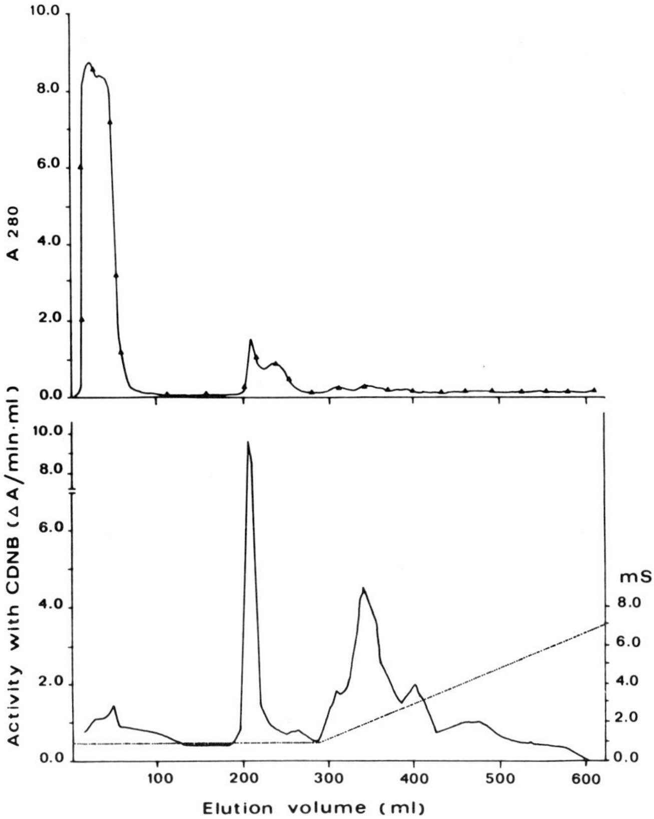

Fig. 2. Elution pattern from CM-Sephadex C-50 column of liver cytosolic protein and glutathione S-transferase isozymes from CCl_4 treated rats. (———) activity with 1-chloro-2,4-dinitrobenzene (CDNB); (▲) absorbance at 280 nm; (------) conductivity in milliSiemens (mS)

bulk of the cytosolic protein had been washed out by eluting with 100 ml of the initial buffer (18 ml/h, 4° C), the GSH-S-t isozymes, which were retained by the ion exchanger, were then eluted by the application of approximatively 120 ml of 5 mM sodium-phosphate buffer pH 7.4 containing 1.4 mM mercaptoethanol followed by the application of a continuous 0–80 mM NaCl gradient in 10 mM sodium-phosphate buffer pH 7.4 containing 1.4 mM mercaptoethanol. The fraction volume was 3.3 ml. Five peaks of GSH-S-t activity, measured by following the conjugation of GSH with the substrate CDNB (according to the method of Habig 1974), were eluted at the following elution volumes: peak 1, 200–285 ml; peak 2, 285–320 ml; peak 3, 320–385 ml; peak 4, 385–480 ml; peak 5, 480–555 ml. Only the material eluted in peak 1, 2 and 4 was also able to catalyse the conjugation of GSH with DCNB, while the material eluted in the peak 3 and 5 was unable to catalyse the conjugation of GSH with this substrate. By the comparison of the enzymatic activities with CDNB and DCNB and on the basis of the ratio of the activities with the two substrates reported for purified GSH-S-t isozymes (Jakoby 1978), the five peaks could therefore be identified as

GSH-S-t isozyme C, B, A and AA respectively. GSH-S-t isozyme C is the first eluted at the lowest ionic strength and, in this system, is eluted in two different peaks; GSH-S-t isozyme AA is the last one eluted at the highest ionic strength (Fig. 1). Recovery of enzymatic activity, measured with CDNB, was greater than 90%.

When the same amount of liver cytosolic protein from CCl_4 treated rats was applied to the column, dramatic changes were seen in the elution pattern (Fig. 2). Particularly, compared with the control on the basis of the total units of enzymatic activity with CDNB eluted in the peaks at corresponding elution volumes, GSH-S-t isozyme A was reduced to 30% of the control value and the second eluted peak of GSH-S-t C was practically undetectable, while the first eluted peak of GSH-S-t C was unaffected. GSH-S-t isozyme B was reduced to 73% of the control value and AA was 85%. Recovery of enzymatic activity, measured with CDNB, was 90%.

It is therefore suggested that the CCl_4 treatment deactivates specific GSH-S-t isozymes. It is possible that the effects observed are due to "sacrificial" covalent linkages between selective GSH-S-t isozymes and CCl_4 or its reactive metabolites.

Acknowledgments. The authors would like to thank Dr. Yogesh C. Awasthi for helpful advice and Dr. Ronald P. Pelley for constructive criticism.

This work was supported in part by a grant from the Italian C.N.R. to Dr. Vanio Vannini and by grants AM 27135 and ES 02102 from N.I.H.

References

Botti B, Moslen MT, Trieff NM, Reynolds ES (1982) Transient decrease of liver cytosolic glutathione S-transferase activities in rats given 1,2-dibromoethane or CCl_4. Chem Biol Interact 42 : 259–270

Habig WH, Pabst MJ, Jakoby WB (1974) Glutathione S-transferases: the first enzymatic step in mercapturic acid formation. J Biol Chem 249 : 7130–7139

Jakoby WB (1978) The glutathione S-transferases: a group of multifunctional detoxification proteins. Adv Enzymol 46 : 383–414

Moslen MT, Reynolds ES (1981) Early loss of hepatic glutathione S-transferase activities in 1,1-dichloroethylene poisoned rats. The Toxicologist 1 : 68

Disease, Metabolism and Reproduction in the Toxic Response to Drugs and Other Chemicals
Arch. Toxicol., Suppl. 7, 521 (1984)

In Vitro Mouse Fertilization as an Experimental Model for the Monitoring of Adverse Effects on Gametes and Gamete Fusion

B. P. Schmid and R. R. Racine

Sandoz Ltd., Preclinical Research, Toxicology, 4002 Basle, Switzerland

Abstract. In vitro fertilization of mice gametes is frequently used to assess different factors that disturb human in vitro fertilization, as almost identical conditions prevail for both species. The mouse in vitro fertilization technique was considered to be a suitable model to evaluate chemically induced effects on male and female gametes. Optimal results were obtained with gametes of the C57B1/6J and $B_6C_3F_1$ mouse inbred strains cultured in Toyoda's modified medium. The spermatozoa were preincubated for 90 min prior to being added to the oocytes; the sperm concentration was 1×10^6/ml medium. This system's response to the heavy metal cadmium chloride ($CdCl_2$), present in the environment worldwide, was investigated. In vivo tests of this chemical's effects on the reproductive systems have resulted in controversial findings.

0.4, 0.8, and 1.6 μM of $CdCl_2$ were added, together with the spermatozoa, to the medium. Spermatozoa, oocytes and $CdCl_2$ were then incubated for 6 h, after which the oocytes were washed several times and cultured for another 18 h, up to the 2-cell stage. 0.4 and 0.8 μM of $CdCl_2$ had no effects on sperm motility, whereas 1.6 μM affected sperm motility slightly. Nevertheless, cleaveage rates were unaffected in all groups, thus indicating that $CdCl_2$ had no direct effect on the processes of gamete fusion, such as sperm-ovum binding, penetration of the oocyte by the spermatozoon, syngamy fusion of the male and female pronuclei, and cleavage.

Key words: In vitro Fertilization – Mouse – Cadmium

Disease, Metabolism and Reproduction in the Toxic Response to Drugs and Other Chemicals
Arch. Toxicol., Suppl. 7, 522 (1984)

Repeat Dermal Models for Systemic Toxicity: A Comparison of the Rabbit, Rat and Guinea Pig

R. J. Staab[1] and W. J. Tierney[2]

[1] Essochem Europe, Inc., Machelen, Belgium
[2] Biodynamics, Inc., East Millstone, NJ, USA

Abstract. The rabbit repeated dermal toxicity study has been a standard model for skin irritation for years. Reasons for the adoption of this model for systemic toxicity has not been clear. This report presents a complete comparative investigation of three species to determine the utility of each as a model for predicting systemic toxicity by the dermal route. Aqueous mercuric chloride (1% and 7%) was applied, at a dosage of 2 ml/kg body weights to the clipped, unabraded dorsal surface of 10/sex/group/species 5 days per week for 4 weeks. Physical and dermal assessments were performed twice in pretest and weekly thereafter. Hematology, clinical chemistry and urinalysis were performed at termination. Blood, urine and kidney tissue were collected and analyzed for mercury content. Selected tissues were examined microscopically following organ weight analysis. Rats were the most resistant to mortality due to mercuric chloride, whereas mortality in rabbits was demonstrated to be dose related. Dose related incidences in atonia and desquamation were evident in all three species, as was the effect on body weight, protein and occult blood in the urine, BUN elevations, kidney weights, and renal and skin histopathology.

The major observations can be summarised as follows:

Topical application of mercuric chloride at a dose level of 7% (w/v) as conducted in this study causes severe kidney changes, nephritis and mineralization, leading to death in rabbits. The same treatment level in rats cause some kidney tubular damage leading to tubular epithelial regeneration; deaths did not occur. One of ten male and one of ten female guinea pigs receiving the higher dosage level died, but the cause of death was not obvious by microscopic examination of tissue sections. The test compound, mercuric chloride also produced varying degrees of cutaneous lesions when applied topically at the higher level. Changes consisted of ulcerative dermatitis, eschar, acanthosis, and hyperkeratosis. They are most severe in rabbits, somewhat less in rats, and least in guinea pigs. This study verifies the sensitivity of the rabbit model.

Key words: Dermal toxicity – Skin irritation – Systemic toxicity

Disease, Metabolism and Reproduction in the Toxic Response to Drugs and Other Chemicals
Arch. Toxicol., Suppl. 7, 523 (1984)

A New Cation-Exchange and Thin Layer Chromatography Technique for the Identification of Pethidine in Urine

M. Henneberg and E. Kwasek

Medical Postgraduate Education Centre, Warsaw, Poland

Abstract. Pethidine is placed second after self-preparations from poppy-heads, as a drug of abuse in Poland.

To detect pethidine use and to discriminate between it, natural opiates and heroin use, an indicatory rapid test on cation-exchange rods together with thin layer chromatography (TLC) methods for testing urine were developed by the authors.

A proficiency survey of the tests, i.e., their sensitivity, specifity and validity was performed. It was found that: The tests are sufficiently specific for differentiation of pethidine from morphine and heroin. The sensitivity of the indicatory test is 10^{-6} g/ml urine and the TLC confirmation test was 10^{-6} g/ml, too. Validity (i.e., incidence of positive urine samples in the precise time interval between drug administration and urine collection) was workable during 88 h for the indicatory test and greater than 96 h in most cases for the TLC test.

It is believed that this ion-exchange–TLC analytical system offers a rapid, reliable screening and confirmation procedure in testing urine specimens for the presence or absence of pethidine, on a large scale. It is also useful for distinguishing pethidine abuse cases from the other opiate addictions.

Key words: Cation-exchange – Pethidine – Thin layer chromatography – Urine

Author Index

Subject Index

Toxicology in the Use, Misuse and Abuse of Food, Drugs and Chemicals

Proceedings of the European Society of Toxicology Meeting Held in Tel Aviv, March 21–24, 1982

Editors: **P. L. Chambers, S. Gitter, C. M. Chambers**
1983. 125 figures. X, 403 pages.
(Archives of Toxicology, Supplement 6)
ISBN 3-540-12392-X

Contents: Effects of Foreign Substances on Blood. – Drugs of Abuse – With Special Reference to Marijuana and Phencyclidine. – Toxic Agents in Food. – Xenobiotics. – Novel and New Techniques in Toxicology. – Miscellaneous Toxic Effects. – Author Index. – Subject Index.

This publication deals in detail with three particular areas of toxicology. The first of these considers the effects of foreign substances on the formed elements of the blood. The second area covers the toxic effects of drugs of abuse, and in particular an updating of the methodology for the detection of drugs of abuse. The third major section deals with toxic agents which are found in food, especially those which occur naturally. Further papers deal with the toxicity of xenobiotics and new and novel developments in the methodology of toxicology. Free Communications in interesting and unusual toxic affects due to drugs are included, as are some new techniques now of use in forensic toxicology.

Springer-Verlag
Berlin
Heidelberg
New York
Tokyo

Archives of Toxicology, Supplement 7

The major part of this publication concerns four topics. The first of these is the present understanding of how disease processes may influence or change the expected toxic response to drugs. Much toxicological testing disregards the diseased state in its models, although the drugs are designed for use in these conditions. The section dealing with the second topic presents new ideas in the approach to an assessment of the toxic effects drugs and other chemicals may have on the male reproductive system and testicular function. Somewhat akin to the first topic, the third involves the metabolism of drugs and chemicals and the consequent changes in the toxicological response. This section discusses fundamental concepts involved in the part active metabolites play in toxicological studies and how species differences in metabolism can be used to advantage in interpreting the toxic response. The toxicity of nonsteroidal antirheumatic drugs is the fourth major topic. Molecular, biochemical and clinical aspects of the production of the toxic response are dealt with and lead to suggestions for further areas of study.

A review of cardiotoxicology is the first item in the book, emphasizing the importance of this field. Short papers are presented on the toxicity of heavy metals, xenobiotic toxicology and miscellaneous toxic effects. There is also a brief section on new techniques in toxicology.

ISBN 3-540-12452-7
ISBN 0-387-12452-7